现代高级
中国针灸治疗学

Advanced Modern
Chinese Acupuncture Therapy

—A Practical Handbook for Intermediate and Advanced Study

Ganglin Yin

Zhenghua Liu

NEW WORLD PRESS

First Edition 2000

Edited by Li Shujuan

Cover Design by Tang Shaowen

ISBN 7-80005-558-2/R • 046

Published by
New World Press
24 Baiwanzhuang Road, Beijing 100037, China

Distributed by
China International Book Trading Corporation
35 Chegongzhuang Xilu, Beijing 100044, China
P.O. Box 399, Beijing, China

Printed in the People's Republic of China

现代高级
中国针灸治疗学
Advanced Modern
Chinese Acupuncture Therapy
—A Practical Handbook for Intermediate and Advanced Study

Editor-in-Chief:	**主编：**
Ganglin Yin	尹钢林
Zhenghua Liu	刘正华
Associate Editor-in-Chief:	**副主编：**
Walton Che	车卫东
Zhiguang Hu	胡志光
Ming Zeng	曾明
Assitant Editors:	**协编：**
Linda Li	李力丹
Jian Peng	彭坚
Xin He	何馨
Jianxin Liu	刘建新
Alice Huang	黄凤仙
Jinyuan Tang	唐金元
Kit Wang	黄杰
Dan Schalm	*Dan Schalm*
Masanobu Kikukawa	*Masanobu Kikukawa*
Terry Sigurdson	*Terry Sigurdson*
Shelly Sawada	*Shelly Sawada*
Eileen Sowerby	*Eileen Sowerby*
English Counsellors:	**英语审校：**
Eileen Sowerby	*Eileen Sowerby*
Dan Schalm	*Dan Schalm*
Shelly Sawada	*Shelly Sawada*
Stephen Miller	*Stephen Miller*
Kit Wang	黄杰
Electronic Typesetting by:	**电子排版：**
Yuhong Li	李宇宏
Dan Schalm	*Dan Schalm*

ACKNOWLEDGEMENTS

The authors of the book would like to express their thanks to:

Prof. Dashun Chen, principal of Hunan University of Traditional Chinese Medicine, Ph. D., adviser of graduate students.

Prof. Renxian Li, former principal of Guangzhou University of Traditional Chinese Medicine, . Ph. D., adviser of graduate students.

Prof. Jiashan Yang, Ph. D., adviser of graduate students, in Beijing University of Traditional Chinese Medicine.

Prof. Jie Yan, Ph. D., adviser of graduate students, in Hunan University of Traditional Chinese Medicine.

Mr. Huang Lixin, president of American College of Traditional Chinese Medicine, San Francisco, USA, for his support and consideration.

Prof. Wally Mui, principal of International College of Traditional Chinese Medicine of Victoria, Canada, for his support and suggestions.

Dr. Tosiko Oshio, principal of Oshio College of Acupuncture & Herbology, Victoria, BC, Canada, for her support.

Prof. Henry Lu, principal of the International College of Traditional Chinese Medicine of Vancouver, for his advice and support.

Ms. Shujuan Li, director of English Department of New World Press, for her guidance in designing and editing.

Mr. Weimin Hu, Ph. D., of the Health Ministry of British Columbia, for his support.

Mr. Rong Zhen and his wife Ze Chen, and Mr. Jianghua Lu and his wife Zhiyi Yang for their help in designing the illustrations.

Dr. Berte Marr, Dr. Willo Walker, Dr.Graham Robertson, Dr. Louis Fasjbind, Dr.Byron Fauth, Dr. Tammy Henry, Dr. Jacque O'Connor, Dr. Warren Brander, Dr. Colt Oswald, Ms. Maggie Yip, Mr. Moses Cooper, Miss Chris Smitheram, for their help and suggestions.

Mr. Zhang and Mr. Huang for their support.

PREFACE

Each passing year, Chinese acupuncture and moxibustion (Zhenjiu) attracts the attention of more and more people from countries all over the world. Modern research also is clearly proving that acupuncture is a credible form of health care. As a result the demand for knowledge in this field has dramatically increased, not only from students and practitioners of Chinese medicine and acupuncture, but from the Western medical community as well. The numbers of students and practitioners of Chinese Zhenjiu has dramatically increased too.

We decided to publish this book, "Advanced Modern Chinese Acupuncture Therapy", to meet the demand for an advanced textbook and an advanced clinical handbook of Chinese Zhenjiu for students and practitioners of Chinese Zhenjiu. It is meant as a comprehensive text and/or handbook for students and practitioners of Zhenjiu, and a reference for those within the field of Western medicine who may be interested to learn about Chinese medicine.

The book has two parts. Part One introduces a basic knowledge of Zhenjiu, including Jingluo (meridians and collaterals), standard locations, properties, actions, point indications and Zhenjiu methods, specific points and clinical applications, treatment principles and selection of points. It also comprehensively details the arts of Zhenjiu and its techniques. Part Two discusses in detail 105 common clinical diseases and morbid conditions which respond well to the application of Zhenjiu. Each disease is described in Western medical terms and differentiated in accordance with the Chinese theory of syndromes. Treatment is divided into standard treatment and experiential treatment, in which many simple and effective methods are described. Indexes of acupoints in Chinese Pinyin, symptoms and diseases known to Western medical science, and diseases known to Traditional Chinese Medicine (TCM) in both Pinyin and characters are provided.

As Professors of Acupuncture and experienced acupuncture practitioners both in China and overseas (Canada, the United States, Russia and Singapore), we have had many years of experience combining theory with practice and teaching Zhenjiu in English. Our book in English includes information on basic theoretical knowledge of Zhenjiu and regular principles and methods of Zhenjiu in the treatment of diseases (which are always seen in the main current textbooks of Zhenjiu in English). It also contains other important information on Zhenjiu, including actions of points, combination of points, Zhenjiu manipulations and invaluable clinical experience, which is seldom given in texts and reference manuals in English.

We believe that a good Zhenjiu doctor must not only know the basic theory and techniques of his/her discipline. It is also imperative that the doctor has an advanced knowledge of Zhenjiu and experiential knowledge must be part of the picture. Zhenjiu is based on the common theory and common clinical techniques of Chinese medicine as well as advanced theoretical knowledge and clinical experiences of practitioners. Having a good knowledge of the former can make one a Zhenjiu doctor, but having a good knowledge of the latter, based on the former, can make one an outstanding doctor.

We are also dedicated to the process of combining Zhenjiu with Western medicine. Blending acupuncture and moxibustion with Western medicine is very important in improving the results of Zhenjiu treatment, summarizing treatment experiences, and widening its application to the prevention and treatment of disease. The diseases in Part Two are named and introduced briefly according to Western medical practice and translated into the terms of Chinese medicine. As now more and more students and practitioners of Chinese medicine in Western countries have a knowledge of Western medicine, the book is designed so that they can take advantage of that knowledge. Also almost every practitioner of Chinese medicine has to have some knowledge of Western medicine and the book is designed so that he or she might learn the necessary knowledge of Western medicine.

This unique book should meet an increasing demand for knowledge of TCM, and shows specifically how Zhenjiu can be used effectively to treat diseases in a modern acupuncture clinic.

Ganglin Yin, Zhenghua Liu

August 1, 1999

USING GUIDE

1. Symbols:

In this book, symbols are used to represent certain words in order to make reading more convenient. They are as the follows:

⊥ = perpendicular acupuncture;

↘ = oblique acupuncture;

↳ = subcutaneous or horizontal acupuncture;

ʃ = moxibustion;

~ = disease or diseases.

2. Special Marks in This Book:

In order to save the space and to be easy to read, there are four special marks, which follow the acupoints, used for explaining manipulation in treatment. They are:

- "+" means puncturing the point with reinforcing manipulation;

- "-" means puncturing the point with reducing manipulation;

- "/" means puncturing the point with uniform reinforcing and reducing manipulation;

- "^" means applying moxibustion on the point.

For examples:
Point Prescription & Manipulation:
Primary points:
- Tianshu ST-25 - (This is explained by that acupuncture with reducing manipulation should be applied on Tianshu ST-25.)
- Zusanli ST-36 + ^ (This is explained by that acupuncture with reinforcing manipulation and moxibustion — usually the moxibustion for warming the needle is suggested, should be applied on Zusanli ST-36.)
- Yinlingquan SP-9 / (This is explained by that acupuncture with uniform reinforcing and reducing manipulation should be applied on Yinlingquan SP-9.)

Secondary points:
- Hegu LI-4 [-] and Dazhui DU-14 [-] are added for high fever. (This is explained that acupuncture with reducing manipulation should be applied on Hegu LI-4 and Dazhui DU-14 if there is high fever.)

3. Abbreviation of Some Terms:

TCM — Traditional Chinese Medicine
Ot. — Otopoint, i.e., ear acupuncture point
Zhenjiu — Acupuncture or acupuncture and moxibustion
LU — Lung Meridian or Its Point
LI — Large Intestine Meridian or Its Point
ST — Stomach Meridian or Its Point
SP — Spleen Meridian or Its Point
HT — Heart Meridian or Its Point
SI — Small Intestine Meridian or Its Point
BL — Bladder Meridian or Its Point
KI — Kidney Meridian or Its Point
PC — Pericardium Meridian or Its Point
SJ — Sanjiao Meridian or Its Point
GB — Gallbladder Meridian or Its Point
LR — Liver Meridian or Its Point
DU — Du Meridian or Its Point
RN — Ren Meridian or Its Point

CONTENTS

PART ONE
BASIC KNOWLEDGE

CHAPTER ONE
THE MERIDIANS &
COLLATERALS

CHAPTER TWO
THE ACUPOINTS OF THE FOURTEEN ERIDIANS & EXTRAORDINARY POINTS

CHAPTER THREE
ZHENJIU MANIPULATIONS

CHAPTER FOUR
EAR ACUPUNCTURE, SCALP ACUPUNCTURE, & WRIST-ANKLE ACUPUNCTURE

CHAPTER FIVE
TREATMENT PRINCIPLES

CHAPTER SIX
SELECTION OF POINTS

PART TWO
TREATMENT OF
COMMON DISEASES

CHAPTER ONE
INTERNAL DISEASES

CHAPTER THREE
GYNECOLOGICAL
DISEASES

CHAPTER FOUR
CHILDREN'S DISEASES

CHAPTER FIVE
DISEASES OF EYE, EAR,
NOSE & THROAT

CHAPTER SIX
SKIN DISEASES

INDEXES

PART ONE

BASIC KNOWLEDGE

CHAPTER ONE
THE MERIDIANS & COLLATERALS

The meridians and collaterals (named Jing and Luo in Chinese, and collectively termed Jingluo) are pathways in which the qi and blood circulate. They pertain to the zang-fu organs interiorly and extend over the body exteriorly, forming a network and linking the tissues and organs into an organic whole. The meridians, which constitute the main trunks of the Jingluo system, run longitudinally and interiorly; while the collaterals, which represent branches of the meridians, run transversely and superficially from the meridians.

The theory of meridians and collaterals deals with the courses, physiological functions, pathological changes of the meridians and collaterals of the human body, and their relationship to the zang-fu (viscera) organs. It is one of the important components of Traditional Chinese Medicine (TCM). Just like the other basic TCM theories, such as that of the zang-fu organs, of qi and blood, etc., the theory of meridians and collaterals is of great significance in guiding diagnosis and treatment, especially in acupuncture and moxibustion (Zhenjiu).

I. NOMENCLATURE & COMPOSITION OF THE MERIDIANS & COLLATERALS

The meridians comprise twelve regular meridians, the eight extra meridians, and those subordinate to the twelve regular meridians, i.e. the twelve divergent meridians, twelve muscle regions, and the twelve cutaneous regions. The collaterals include fifteen collaterals, superficial collaterals, and minute collaterals. (See Tab. I-1)

1. The Twelve Regular Meridians

The twelve regular meridians include the three yin and three yang meridians of the hand (the Lung Meridian of Hand-Taiyin, the Pericardium Meridian of Hand-Jueyin, the Heart Meridian of Hand-Shaoyin, the Large Intestine Meridian of Hand-Yangming, the Sanjiao Meridian of Hand-Shaoyang and Small Intestine Meridian of Hand-Taiyang), and the three yin and three yang meridians of the foot (the Spleen Meridian of Foot-Taiyin, the Liver Meridian of Foot-Jueyin, the Kidney Meridian of Foot-Shaoyin, the Stomach

Meridian of Foot-Yangming, the Gallbladder Meridian of Foot-Shaoyang and the Bladder Meridian of Foot-Taiyang). They are called regular meridians, and they are the major trunks in the Jingluo system.

Their nomenclature is based on three factors:
    a. Zang or fu
    b. Hand or foot
    c. Yin or yang

The twelve regular meridians pertain to the twelve zang-fu organs respectively, each of them is named after the organ which it pertains to. The meridians are distributed on the upper limbs are named *hand meridians*, and those on the lower limbs, *foot meridians*. Both the upper limbs and lower limbs are divided into six regions, which are supplied respectively by the three yin (Taiyin, Shaoyin and Jueyin) and three yang (Yangming, Taiyang and Shaoyang) meridians. There exists an exterior-interior relationship between the three yin and three yang meridians:
    Taiyin—Yangming
    Jueyin—Shaoyang
    Shaoyin—Taiyang

In accordance with the fact that the zang organs pertain to yin, the fu organs to yang, and the medial aspect is attributed to yin, the lateral aspect, to yang, the meridians that pertain to the zang organs are yin meridians, which are mainly distributed on the medial aspect of the limbs. Those distributed on the medial aspect of the upper limbs are the three yin meridians of hand, while those distributed on the medial aspect of the lower limbs are the three yin meridians of foot. The meridians that pertain to the fu organs are yang meridians, which mainly travel along the lateral aspect of the limbs. Those travelling along the lateral aspect of the upper limbs are the three yang meridians of the hand; while those travelling along the lateral aspect of the lower limbs are the three yang meridians of the foot.

2. The Eight Extra Meridians & the Fourteen Meridians

The eight extra meridians are the Du, Ren, Chong, Dai, Yangqiao, Yinqiao, Yangwei and Yinwei Meridians. They are different from the twelve regular meridians because none of them pertain to or connect with the zang or fu organs, and they are not exteriorly-interiorly related.

- Du means governing. Running along the midline of the back, the Du Meridian (Governor Vessel) governs all the yang meridians.

- Ren means fostering and responsibility. Going along the midline of the abdomen, the Ren Meridian (Conception Vessel) is responsible for all the yin meridians.

- Chong means a vital pass. As it regulates the flow of qi and blood in the twelve regular meridians, the Chong Meridian is called "the sea of the twelve regular meridians".

- Dai means a girdle. The Dai Meridian goes around the waist, binding up all the meridians.

- Qiao means the heel. The one starting below the external malleolus is the Yangqiao Meridian, while the one starting below the internal malleolus is the Yinqiao Meridian.

- Wei means connection and network. The Yangwei Meridian connects and networks with the exterior yang of the whole body, while the Yinwei Meridian connects and networks with the interior yin of the whole body.

The twelve regular meridians and the Du and Ren Meridians are called *"the fourteen meridians."*

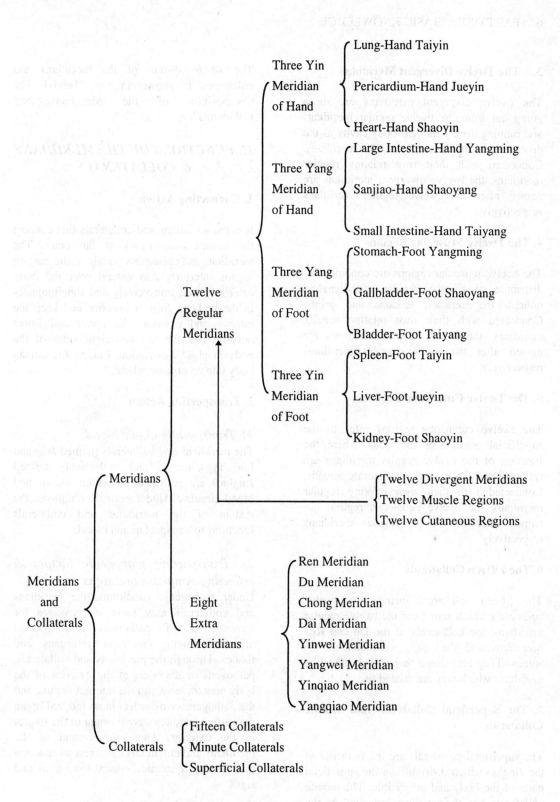

Tab. I-1 The Composition of the Meridians and Collaterals

The structure diagram contains the following:

Meridians and Collaterals
- Meridians
  - Twelve Regular Meridians
    - Three Yin Meridian of Hand
      - Lung-Hand Taiyin
      - Pericardium-Hand Jueyin
      - Heart-Hand Shaoyin
    - Three Yang Meridian of Hand
      - Large Intestine-Hand Yangming
      - Sanjiao-Hand Shaoyang
      - Small Intestine-Hand Taiyang
    - Three Yang Meridian of Foot
      - Stomach-Foot Yangming
      - Gallbladder-Foot Shaoyang
      - Bladder-Foot Taiyang
    - Three Yin Meridian of Foot
      - Spleen-Foot Taiyin
      - Liver-Foot Jueyin
      - Kidney-Foot Shaoyin
    - Twelve Divergent Meridians
    - Twelve Muscle Regions
    - Twelve Cutaneous Regions
  - Eight Extra Meridians
    - Ren Meridian
    - Du Meridian
    - Chong Meridian
    - Dai Meridian
    - Yinwei Meridian
    - Yangwei Meridian
    - Yinqiao Meridian
    - Yangqiao Meridian
- Collaterals
  - Fifteen Collaterals
  - Minute Collaterals
  - Superficial Collaterals

3.   The Twelve Divergent Meridians

The twelve divergent meridians are those going out from the twelve regular meridians and running deeply into the body cavity as the divergent part of the twelve regular meridians. Connected with their own relating regular meridians, the twelve divergent meridians are named after the twelve regular meridians respectively.

4. The Twelve Muscular Regions

The twelve muscular regions are conduits that distribute qi of the regular meridians to nourish the muscles, tendons and joints. Connected with their own relating regular meridians, the twelve muscular regions are named after the twelve regular meridians respectively.

5. The Twelve Cutaneous Regions

The twelve cutaneous regions refer to the superficial portion of the body where the function of the twelve regular meridians are reflected and the qi of the collaterals spreads. Connected with their own relating regular meridians, the twelve cutaneous regions are named after the twelve regular meridians respectively.

6. The Fifteen Collaterals

The fifteen collaterals include the twelve collaterals which start from the twelve regular meridians, the collaterals of the Du and Ren Meridians and the major collateral of the spleen. They are named respectively after the meridians which they are related to.

7. The Superficial Collaterals and Minute Collaterals

The superficial collaterals are the branches of the Jingluo which distribute on the superficial parts of the body and are visible. The minute collaterals are the smallest branches of the Jingluo.

The whole system of the meridians and collaterals is shown in the "Tab.I-1 The Composition of the Meridians and Collaterals".

II. FUNCTIONS OF THE MERIDIANS & COLLATERALS

1. Connecting Action

It is the meridians and collaterals that connect the tissues and organs of the body. The meridians and collaterals pertain to the zang-fu organs interiorly and extend over the body exteriorly, run transversely and longitudinally in the body to form a network and keep the interior and exterior, the upper and lower portions and the left and right sides of the body in close association, linking the human body into an organic whole.

2. Transporting Action

1). Transporting qi and blood
The meridians and collaterals (named Jing and Luo in Chinese, and collectively termed Jingluo) are pathways in which the qi and blood circulate. Under normal conditions, the system of the meridians and collaterals functions to transport qi and blood.

2). Transporting pathogenic factors & reflecting symptoms and signs
Under pathogenic conditions, the meridians and collaterals may serve as passages for transmission of pathogens and morbid affection among the zang-fu organs and tissues. Through the meridians and collaterals, pathogens or disorders at the exterior of the body may traverse into the internal organs, and the pathogens or disorders in an internal organ may affect another internal organ or the tissues in the exterior. Thus, the system of the meridians and collaterals can exert its function of reflecting systemic or local symptoms and signs.

3). Transporting treatment effect

In treatment, the effects of acupuncture and moxibustion or medicine are mainly transported to the diseased zang-fu organs or tissues through the system of the meridians and collaterals.

3. Regulating Action

The meridians and collaterals are passages for the circulation of qi and blood. They transport qi and blood to adjust yin and yang, and maintain a relative equilibrium of normal life.

4. Defending Action

The Ying Qi (nutrient qi) flows inside the meridians and Wei Qi (defensive qi) runs outside the meridians. Through the system of the meridians and collaterals, the nutrient qi and defensive qi are distributed all over the body to defend the body. Thus, the system of the meridians and collaterals exerts its function of combating pathogens.

III. THE TWELVE REGULAR MERIDIANS

1. The Lung Meridian of Hand-Taiyin (LU)

1). The running course

It originates in the middle-jiao, runs downwards to connect with the large intestine (1). Turning back to run along the cardiac orifice (2), it passes through the diaphragm (3), and enters its pertaining organ—the lung (4). From the portion connecting the trachea with the larynx, it comes out transversely (5), passes downwards along the radial side of the medial aspect of the upper arm (6), and runs through the cubital fossa (7). Then, it goes continuously downwards along the radial side of the medial aspect of the forearm (8), and enters the site where the radial pulse is felt (9). Passing through LU-11 Yuji (10), it goes along the border of the thenar (11), and enters at the radial side of the tip of the thumb (12).

A branch proximal to the wrist starts from LU-7 Lieque, and runs to the radial side of the tip of the index finger to connect with the Large Intestine Meridian of Hand-Yangming (13).

The line made by its acupoints distributed on the body surface: It originates from LU-1 Zhongfu at the latero-superior aspect of the chest, runs along the radial border of the medial aspect of the upper limb and goes downwards to the site where the radial artery beats. Then, it passes along the margin of the thenar and ends at the tip of the radial side of the thumb at LU-11 Shaoshang. (See Fig. I-1)

2). The inner organs concerned

The lung, large intestine and throat.

3). Indications

a. Disorders of the respiratory system: Common cold, cough, asthma, hemoptysis, rhinitis, epistaxis, sore throat.

b. Disorders in the regions along the course of the meridian: Pain in the chest, shoulder and back, and the anterior border of the medial aspect of the upper limbs, feverish sensation in the palms.

c. Other disorders: Frequent urination with small amounts of urine.

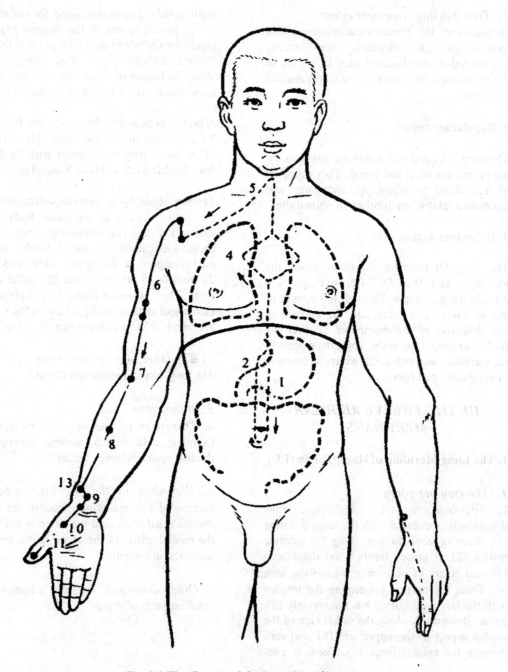

Fig. I-1 The Course of the Lung Meridian

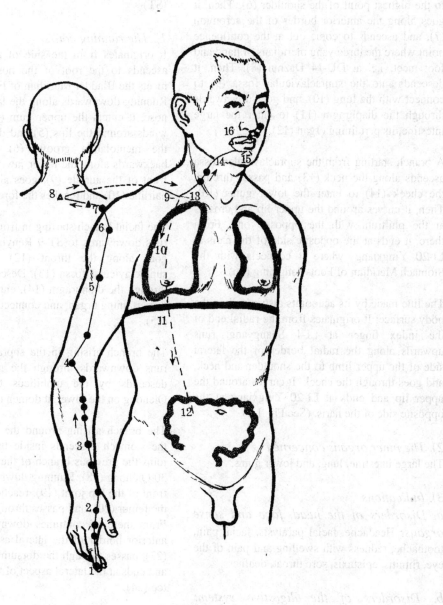

Fig.I-2 The Course of Large Intestine Meridian

2. The Large Intestine Meridian of Hand-Yangming (LI)

1). The running course

It starts from the tip of the index finger at LI-1 Shangyang (1). Running upwards along the radial side of the index finger, and passing through the 1st metacarpal space, it dips into the depression between the tendon of m. extensor pollicis longus and brevis (2), and goes along the radial border of the lateral aspect of the forearm (3) to reach the lateral side of the elbow (4). It goes upwards along the latero-anterior border (5) to the highest point of the shoulder (6). Then, it goes along the anterior border of the acromion (7), and ascends to come out at the confluence point where the three yang meridians of hand and foot meet, i.e. at DU-14 Dazhui (8). Then, it descends into the supraclavicular fossa (9) to connect with the lung (10), and goes downwards through the diaphragm (11) to enter the large intestine, its pertaining organ (12).

A branch starting from the supraclavicular fossa ascends along the neck (13) and passes through the cheek (14) to enter the lower gums (15). Then, it curves around the upper lip and crosses at the philtrum with the opposite one. From there, it ends at the opposite side of the naris at LI-20 Yingxiang, where it connects with the Stomach Meridian of Foot-Yangming (16).

The line made by its acupoints distributed on the body surface: It originates from the radial end of the index finger at LI-1 Shangyang, runs upwards along the radial border of the lateral side of the upper limb to the shoulder and neck, and goes through the cheek. It curves around the upper lip and ends at LI-20 Yingxiang at the opposite side of the naris. (See Fig. I-2)

2). The inner organs concerned
The large intestine, lung, and lower gums.

3). Indications
a. Disorders of the head, face and sense organs: Headache, facial paralysis, facial pain, toothache, redness with swelling and pain of the eye, rhinitis, epistaxis, sore throat, deafness.

b. Disorders of the digestive system: Diarrhea, constipation, abdominal distention and/or pain.

c. Disorders in the regions along the course of the meridian: Pain and swelling in the neck, shoulder pain, pain in the elbow, arm and hand.

d. Other disorders: Common cold, fever, cough, skin diseases.

3. The Stomach Meridian of Foot-Yangming (ST)

1). The running course
It originates from the side of the ala nasi and ascends to the root of the nose (1), where it meets the Bladder Meridian of Foot-Taiyang (2). Running downwards along the lateral side of the nose, it enters the upper gum (4). Emerging, it winds around the lips (5) and descends to meet the mentolabila groove (6). Then, running backwards along the lower jaw (7), it ascends in front of the auricle (9), goes along the anterior hairline (10) and reaches the forehead (11).

The facial branch starting in front of ST-5 Dayin runs downwards to ST-9 Renyin. From there, it goes along the throat (12) and enters the supraclavicular fossa (13). Descending, it passes through the diaphragm (14), enters the stomach, its pertaining organ, and connects with the spleen (15).

The branch arising in the supraclavicular fossa runs downwards through the nipple (16), and descends by the umbilicus to enter ST-30 Qichong on the lower abdomen (17).

The branch arising around the lower orifice of the stomach descends inside the abdomen and joins the previous branch of the meridian at ST-30 Qichong (18). Running downwards, it goes in front of the hip joint (19), reaches ST-32 Futu at the femur (20), and passes through the knee (21). From there, it continues downwards along the anterior border of the lateral aspect of the tibia (22), passes through the dorsum of the foot (23), and ends at the lateral aspect of the tip of the 2nd toe (24).

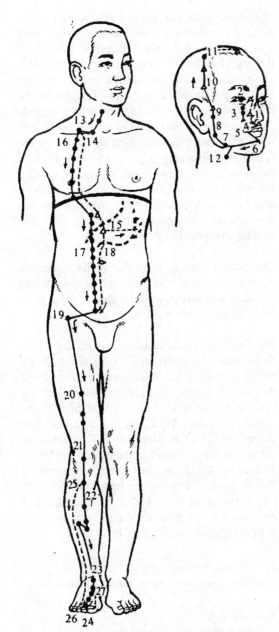

Fig.I-3 The Course of the Stomach Meridian

connects with the Spleen Meridian of Foot-Taiyin.

The line made by its acupoints distributed on the body surface: It starts from ST-1 Chengqi below the eye, and runs around the cheek and in front of the auricle. Then, it ascends to ST-8 Touwei at the corner of the forehead. Its branch comes out from the angle of the mandible, runs downwards to the neck , and descends along the line 4 cun lateral to the midline of the chest and 2 cun lateral to the midline of the abdomen. Then it goes downwards along the lateral anterior border of the lower limb, passes through the dorsum of the foot and ends at ST-45 Lidui at the lateral side of the tip of the corner of the nail of the 2nd toe. (See Fig. I-3)

2). The organs concerned
The stomach, spleen and throat.

3). Indications
a. *Disorders of the digestive system:* Stomachache, vomiting, diarrhea, abdominal distention, borborygmus.

b. *Disorders of the head, face and sense organs:* Headache, toothache, facial paralysis, sore throat, epistaxis.

c. *Disorders in the regions along the course of the meridian:* Pain, paralysis and atrophy of the lower limbs, chest pain.

d. *Other disorders:* Hypertension, mastitis, mental disorders, edema, febrile diseases.

4. The Spleen Meridian of Foot-Taiyin (SP)

1). The running course

It originates from SP-1 Yinbai at the tip of the great toe (1). Then, it runs along the dorsoventral boundary at the medial aspect of the great toe and passes behind the first metatarsal

The tibial branch comes out 3 cun below the knee (25), and enters the lateral side of the tip of the middle toe (26).

The branch arising in the dorsum of the foot starts at ST-42 Chongyang (27) and terminates at the medial side of the tip of the big toe, where it

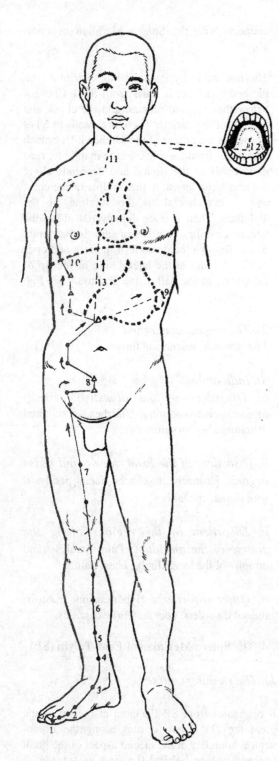

Fig. I-4 the Course of the Spleen Meridian

phalangeal joint (2). From there, it ascends in front of the medial malleolus (3), and runs upwards along the medial aspect of the calf of the leg (4). Then, it runs behind the tibia (5), crosses and runs in front of the Liver Meridian of Foot-Jueyin at the area 8 cun proximal to the medial alleolus (6). Running upwards, it ascends along anterior medial border of the knee and thigh (7), enters the abdomen (8) and then the spleen, its pertaining organ, and connects with the stomach (9). From there, it ascends, passing through the diaphragm (10) and running alongside the esophagus (11). When it reaches the root of the tongue, it spreads over the sublingual region (12).

The branch starting from the stomach ascends through the diaphragm (13), and disappears into the heart to connect with the Heart Meridian of Hand Shaoyin (14).

The line made by its acupoints distributed on the body surface: Starts from SP-1 Yinbai at the tip of the medial border of the great toe, runs along the medial border of the first phalanx and the first metatarsal bone, and passes in front of the medial malleolus. Ascending, it crosses and runs in front of the Liver Meridian of Foot-Jueyin at the area 8 cun proximal to the medial malleolus. Ascending again, it runs along the anterior medial border of the lower limb and along the line 4 cun lateral to the abdominal midline and 6 cun lateral to the midline of the chest, and ends at SP-21 Dabao below the axillus. (See Fig. I-4)

2). The inner organs concerned
The spleen, stomach, heart, throat, and tongue.

3). Indications
a. Disorders of the digestive system: Stomachache, vomiting, diarrhea, abdominal distention, borborygmus, dysentery, indigestion, jaundice.

b. Disorders of the reproductive & urinary systems: Irregular menstruation, uterine bleeding, seminal emission, dysuria, enuresis.

c. Disorders in the regions along the course of the meridian: Paralysis and pain of the lower limbs.

d. Other disorders: Edema, skin diseases, insomnia.

5. The Heart Meridian of Hand-Shaoyin (HT)

1). The running course

It originates from the heart. Emerging, it spreads over the "heart system" (i.e., the tissues

connecting the heart with the other zang-fu organs) (1). It passes through the diaphragm to connect with the small intestine (2).

The ascending portion of the meridian from the "heart system" (3) runs alongside the esophagus (4) to connect with the "eye system" (i.e., the tissues connecting the eyes with the brain) (5).

The straight portion of the meridian from the "heart system" goes upward to the lung (6). Then it turns downward and emerges from the axilla (HT-1 Jiquan).   From there it goes along the

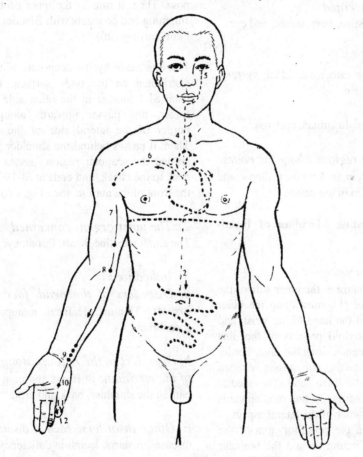

Fig. I-5 The Course of the Heart Meridian

posterior border of the medial aspect of the upper arm behind the Lung Meridian of Hand-Taiyin and the Pericardium Meridian of Hand-Jueyin (7) down to the cubital fossa (8). From

there it descends along the posterior border of the medial aspect of the forearm to the pisiform region proximal to the palm (9) and enters the palm (10). Then, it follows the medial aspect of the little finger to its tip (HT-9 Shaochong) (11) and links with the Small Intestine Meridian of Hand-Taiyang.

The line made by the acupoints of the meridian distributed on the body surface: It originates from the axilla at HT-1 Jiquan, passes along the ulnar border of the palmar surface of the arm, and enters the area between the 4th and 5th metacarpal bones of the palm. Then, it ends at HT-9 Shaochong at the radial side of the little finger. (See Fig. I-5)

2). The organs concerned
The heart, small intestine, lung, throat, and eye.

3). Indications
a. Disorders of the cardiovascular system: Palpitation, cardiac pain.

b. Mental disorders: Insomnia, epilepsy.

c. Disorders in the regions along the course of the meridian: Pain in the chest, elbow and arm, feverish sensation in the palms.

6. The Small Intestine Meridian of Hand-Taiyang (SI)

1). The running course
It starts from SI-1 Shaoze at the ulnar side of the tip of the little finger (1), runs along the ulnar side of the dorsum of the hand to the wrist, and passes through the styloid process of the ulna (2). From there, it ascends along the ulnar border of the lateral side of the forearm, passes between the olecranon of the ulna and the medial epicondyle of the humerus (3), and runs upwards along the posterior border of the lateral aspect of the upper arm (4) to the posterior area of the shoulder joint (5). Circling around the scapular region (6), it meets DU-14 Dazhui (7). Then, it runs downwards into the supraclavicular fossa (8) to connect with the heart (9). From there, it

goes downwards along the esophagus (10), passes through the diaphragm (11), reaches the stomach (12), and finally enters the small intestine, its pertaining organ (13).

The branch arising in the supraclavicular fossa (14) runs along the neck (15), and ascends to the cheek (16). Then, it reaches the outer canthus (17). From there it turns to end at SI-19 Tinggong in front of the ear (18).

The branch arising in the cheek (19) ascends to the infraorbital region, and to the side of the nose. Then, it runs to the inner canthus at BL-1 Jingming and connects with Bladder Meridian of Foot-Taiyang (20).

The line made by the acupoints of the meridian distributed on the body surface: It originates from SI-1 Shaoze at the ulnar side of the little finger, and passes upwards along the ulnar border of the lateral side of the upper limb. Then, it passes behind the shoulder joint, circles around the scapular region, passes through the neck to the cheek, and ends at SI-19 Tinggong in the front of the auricle. (See Fig. I-6)

2). The inner organs concerned
The small intestine, heart, throat, eye, and ear.

3). Indications
a. Disorders of the head, face and sense organs: Tinnitus, deafness, mumps, toothache, sore throat.

b. Disorders in the regions along the course of the meridian: Stiffness and pain of the neck, pain in the shoulder, back and arm.

c. Other disorders: Mental disorders, febrile diseases, malaria, lactation deficiency.

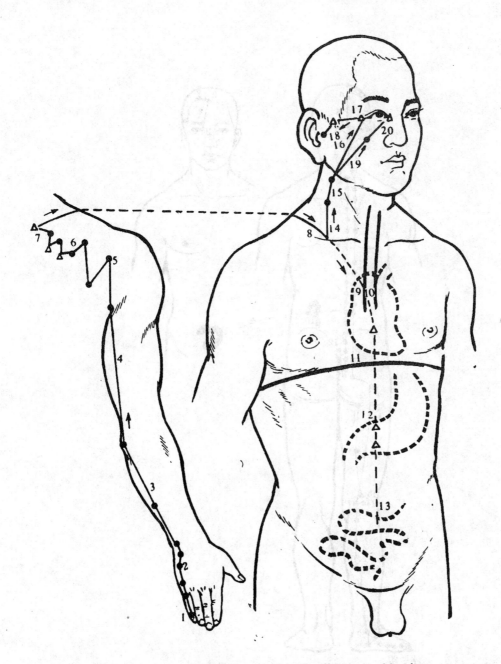

Fig. I-6 The Course of the Small Intestine Meridian

7. The Bladder Meridian of Foot-Taiyang (BL)

1). The running course
It starts from BL-1 Jingming at the inner canthus

(1). Ascending to the forehead (2), it meets DU-20 Baihui at the vertex (3).

The branch arising at the vertex runs to the temple (4).

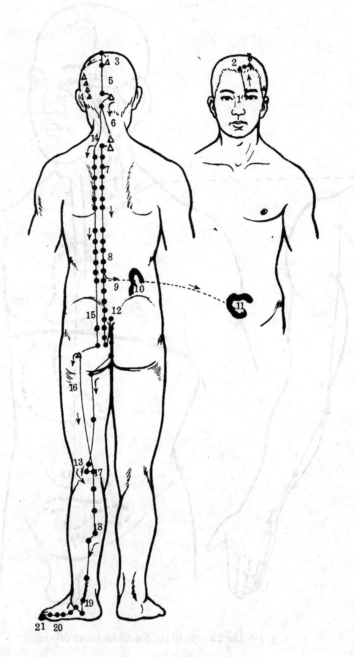

Fig. I-7 The Course of The Bladder Meridian

Another straight branch arising at the vertex enters and communicates with the brain (5). Then, it emerges and bifurcates to descend to the posterior aspect of the neck (6). Running downwards along the medial side of the scapula and parallel to the vertebral column (7), it reaches the lumbar region (8), and enters the body cavity via the paravertebral muscle (9) to connect with the kidney (10). Then, it enters the urinary bladder, its pertaining organ.

The branch arising in the lumbar region runs downwards through the gluteal region (12), and ends at the center of the popliteal fossa (13).

The branch arising in the nape passes downwards along the medial border of the scapula (14). Passing through the gluteal region (15) downwards along the postero-lateral aspect of the thigh (16), it meets the branch from the lumbar region at the center of the popliteal fossa (17). From there, it runs downwards through the gastrocnemius (18) to the posterior aspect of the external malleolus (19). Then, it runs along the tuberosity of the 5th metatarsal bone (20) to reach BL-67 Zhiyin at the lateral border of the tip of the small toe, where it connects with the Kidney Meridian of Foot-Shaoyin (21).

The line made by the acupoints of the meridian distributed on the body surface: It starts at BL-1 Jingming at the inner canthus, ascends through the medial end of the eyebrow to the side of the midline of the head, then descends through the back of neck. From there, it divides into two to go respectively downwards along the two lines, which are 1.5 cun and 3 cun lateral to the vertebral column to the gluteal region, and along the posterior aspect of the thigh. These two lines join each other in the popliteal fossa. From there, it goes downwards along the posterior aspect of the lower leg to the posterior aspect of the external malleolus, and passes through the lateral side of the dorsum of the foot. Then, it ends at BL-67 Zhiyin at the lateral border of the tip of the little toe. (See Fig. I-7)

2). The inner organs concerned
The urinary bladder, kidney and brain.

3). Indications
a. Disorders in the regions along the course of the meridian: Headache, eye disorders, nasal disorders, pain of the nape and back, paralysis and pain of the lower limbs.

b. Disorders of the zang-fu organs: The Back-Shu Points are indicated for disorders of the relevant zang-fu organs.

c. Other disorders: Mental illness, malaria.

8. The Kidney Meridian of Foot-Shaoyin (KI)

1). The running course
It starts from the plantar area of the small toe, runs obliquely to KI-1 Yongquan at the sole of the plantar foot (1). Emerging from the lower area of the tuberosity of the navicular bone (2) and running behind the medial malleolus (3), it enters the heel (4). Then, it ascends along the medial side of the calf of the leg (5) to the medial side of the popliteal fossa (6), and goes further upwards along the posterior medial border of the thigh (7) towards the vertebral column (DU-1 Changqiang), where it enters the kidney, its pertaining organ (8), and connects with the urinary bladder (9).

The trunk starting from the kidney (10) ascends and passes through the liver and the diaphragm (11), and enters the lung (12). Then, it further ascends along the throat (13), and terminates at the root of the tongue (14).

The branch starting from the lung comes out from the lung to connect with the heart. Then, it distributes in the chest to connect with the Pericardium Meridian of Hand-Jueyin (15).

The line made by the acupoints of the meridian distributed on the body surface: It starts from the sole at KI-1 Yongquan, runs behind the medial malleolus, and ascends along the posterior border of the medial side of the lower limb to reach the lower abdomen. Then, it further ascends along the line 0.5 cun lateral to the midline of the abdomen and 2 cun lateral to the midline of the chest, and ends at the point KI-27 Shaofu below the clavicle. (See Fig. I-8)

2). The organs concerned
The kidney, urinary bladder, liver, lung, heart, vertebral column, throat, and the root of the tongue.

3). Indications

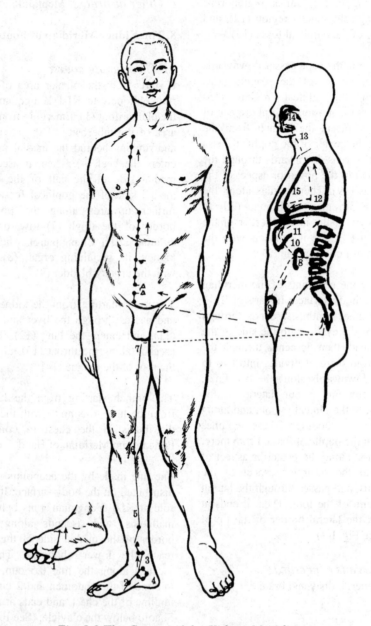

Fig. I-8 The Course of the Kidney Meridian

a. Disorders of the urinary and reproductive systems: Enuresis, retention of urine, seminal emission, impotence, irregular menstruation.

b. Disorders of the five sense organs: Tinnitus, deafness, toothache, sore throat.

c. Disorders of the respiratory system: Asthma, hemoptysis.

d. Disorders in the regions along the course of the meridian: Pain in the lower back and the posterior border of the medial aspect of the lower limbs.

e. Emergency conditions: Wind stroke, sun stroke.

9. The Pericardium Meridian of Hand-Jueyin (PC)

1). The running course
It originates from the chest. Emerging, it enters its pertaining organ, the pericardium (1). Then, it descends through the diaphragm (2) to the abdomen, and connects successively with the upper-, middle- and lower-jiao in order from the chest to the abdomen.

The branch arising in the chest runs inside the chest (4), emerges at the lateral aspect of the chest, and descends to the point 3 cun below the axilla at PC-1 Tianchi (5). Then, it ascends to the axilla (6). From there, it runs downwards along the medial aspect of the upper arm and between the meridians of Hand-Taiyin and Hand-Shaoyin (7) to the cubital fossa (8). Then it further descends between the tendons of m.palmaris longus and m. flexor carpi radialis of the forearm (9) to the palm (10). From there, it runs along the middle finger to its tip at PC-9 Zhongchong (11).

The branch arising in the palm originates from PC-8 Laogong, and runs along the ring finger to its tip at SJ-1 Guangchong, where it connects with the Sanjiao Meridian of Hand-Shaoyang (12).

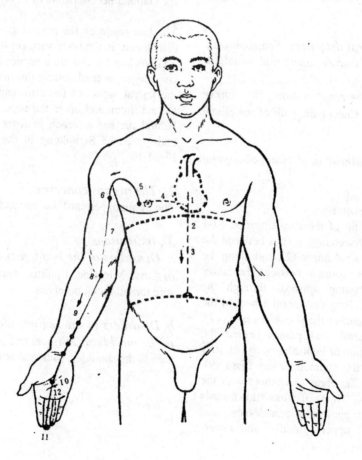

Fig. I-9 The Course of the Pericardium Meridian

The line made by the acupoints of the meridian distributed on the body surface: It starts from PC-1 Tianchi at the point lateral to the nipple, and ascends to the axilla. Then, it runs downwards between the tendons of the m. palmaris longus and m. flxor carpi radialis at the medial aspect of the arm to the palm. Finally, it ends at PC-9 Zhongchong at the tip of the middle finger. (See Fig. I-9)

2). The organs concerned
The pericardium and Sanjiao.

3). Indications
a.   Disorders of the cardiovascular system: Tachycardia, arrhythmia, bradycardia, angina pectoris.

b. Mental & neural disorders: Schizophrenia, hysteria, epilepsy, neurosis, intercostal neuralgia.

c. Disorders in the regions along the course of the meridian: Chest pain, pain of the elbow and arm.

10. The Sanjiao Meridian of Hand-Shaoyang (SJ)

1). The running course
It starts from the tip of the ring finger at SJ-1 Guangchong (1). Ascending, it runs between the 4th and 5th metacarpal bones (2), and along the dorsal aspect of the forearm between the radius and ulna (4). Passing upwards through the olecranon (5) and along the lateral aspect of the upper arm (6), it reaches the shoulder region (7), where it runs across and passes behind the Gallbladder Meridian of Foot-Shaoyang (8), runs forward to enter the supraclavicular fossa (9), and distributes in the chest to connect with the pericardium (10). Then, it runs downwards through the diaphragm to the abdomen, and connects with the upper-, middle- and lower-jiao, its pertaining organ, from the chest to the abdomen (11).

The branch arising in the chest runs upwards (12) and emerges from the supraclavicular fossa (13). From there, it ascends to the nape (14), running upwards behind the ear and above the ear (15), and going to the corner of the forehead (16). Then, it turns downwards to the cheek and reaches the infraorbital region (17).

The branch arising in the ear runs from the retroauricular region and enters the ear. Then, it emerges in front of the ear, crosses the previous branch at the cheek (18), and reaches the outer canthus below SJ-23 Sizhukong to connect with the Gallbladder Meridian of Foot-Shaoyang (19).

The line made by the acupoints of the meridian distributed on the body surface: It starts from SJ-1 Guanchong at the ulnar aspect of the tip of the ring finger, ascends along the middle portion of the lateral aspect of the arm, and passes behind the acromion and up to the nape. Then, it winds behind the ear to reach in front of the ear and ends at SJ-23 Sizhukong in the eyebrow. (See Fig. I-10)

2). The organs concerned
The Sanjiao, pericardium, ear and eye.

3). Indications
a. Disorders of the head, face and five sense organs: Migraine, tinnitus, deafness, eye pain, sore throat, facial paralysis.

b. Disorders in the regions along the course of the meridian: Stiffness and pain of the neck, pain in the shoulder, back and arm.

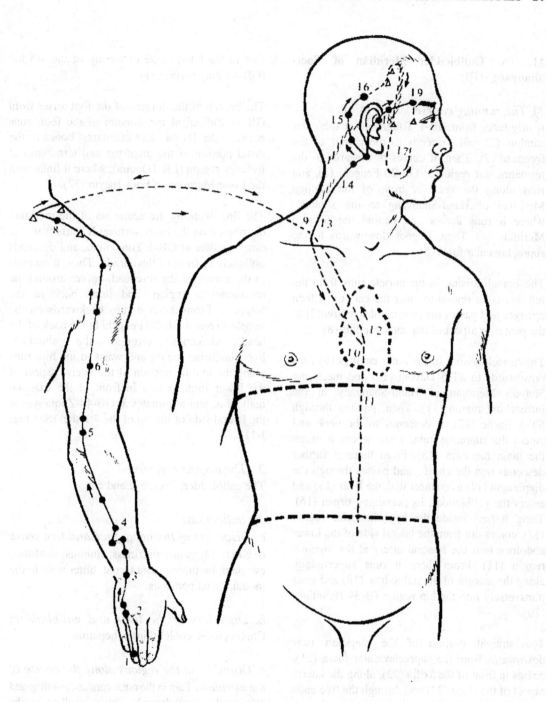

Fig. I-10 The Course of the Sanjiao Meridian

11. The Gallbladder Meridian of Foot-Shaoyang (GB)

1). The running course

It originates from GB-1 Tongziliao at the outer canthus (1) and descends to the corner of the forehead (2). Then, it curves downwards to the retroauricular region at GB-20 Fengchi (3), and runs along the neck in front of the Sanjiao Meridian of Hand-Shaoyang to the shoulder where it runs across and behind the Sanjiao Meridian (4). Then, it goes downwards to the supraclavicular fossa (5).

The branch arising in the auricle runs from the retroauricular region to enter the ear (6). It then emerges and passes the precuricular region (7) to the posterior aspect of the outer canthus (8).

The branch arising in the outer canthus (9) runs downwards to ST-5 Daying (10) and meets the Sanjiao Meridian of Hand-Shaoyang in the infraorbital region (11). Then, passing through ST-6 Jiache (12), it descends to the neck and enters the supraclavicular fossa where it meets the main meridian (13). From there it further descends into the chest and passes through the diaphragm (14) to connect with the liver (15) and enters the gallbladder, its pertaining organ (16). Then, it runs inside the hypochondriac region (17), comes out from the lateral side of the lower abdomen near the femoral artery at the inguinal region (18). From there it runs superficially along the margin of the pubic hair (19) and goes transversely into the hip region (B-34 Huantiao) (20).

The straight portion of the meridian runs downwards from the supraclavicular fossa (21), passes in front of the axilla (22), along the lateral aspect of the chest (23) and through the free ends of the floating ribs (24) to the hip region where it meets the previous branch (25). Then, it descends along the lateral aspect of the thigh (26) to the lateral side of the knee (27). Going further downward along the anterior aspect of the fibula (28) to its lower end (GB-39 Xuanzhong) (29), it reaches the anterior aspect of the external malleolus (30). It then follows the dorsum of the

foot to the lateral side of the tip of the 4th toe (GB-44 Zuqiaoyin) (31).

The branch of the dorsum of the foot arises from GB-41 Zulinqi at the dorsum of the foot, runs between the 1st and 2nd metatarsal bones to the distal portion of the great toe and terminates at its hairy region (LR-1Dadun), where it links with the Liver Meridian of Foot-Jueyin (32).

The line made by the acupoints of the meridian distributed on the body surface: It starts from the outer canthus at GB-1 Tongziliao, and descends obliquely in front of the auricle. Then, it ascends to the corner of the forehead, curves around the retroauricular region, and turns back to the forehead. From there, it runs backwards on the temple to reach GB-20 Fengchi at the back of the head, descends through the shoulder, hypochondriac region and waist to the hip, runs along the middle portion of the lateral aspect of the lower limb, passes in front of the external malleolus, and terminates at GB-44 Zuqiaoyin at the lateral side of the tip of the 4th toe. (See Fig. I-11)

2). The organs concerned

The gallbladder, liver, eye and ear.

3). Indications

a. Disorders of the head, face and five sense organs: Migraine, dizziness, tinnitus, deafness, eye pain, toothache, sore throat, bitter taste in the mouth, facial paralysis.

b. Disorders of the liver and gallbladder: Cholecystitis, cholelithiasis, hepatitis.

c. Disorders in the regions along the course of the meridian: Pain in the outer canthus, swelling and pain in the supraclavicular fossa, swelling in the axilla, pain in the chest, hypochondriac region and lateral side of the lower limb, feverish sensation at the lateral side of the foot.

d. Other disorders: Febrile diseases, epilepsy.

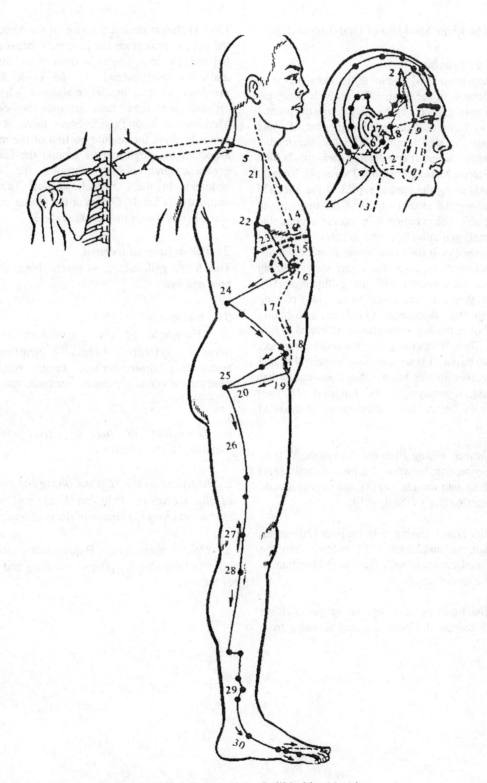

Fig. I-11 The Course of the Gallbladder Meridian

12. The Liver Meridian of Foot-Jueyin (LR)

1). The running course
It starts from LR-1 Dadun at the hairy region of the dorsum of the big toe (1), ascends along the dorsum of the foot (2), passes through the point 1 cun in front of the medial malleolus (3), and reaches the area 8 cun proximal to the medial malleolus, where it crosses and then runs behind the Spleen Meridian of Foot-Taiyin (4). Then, it ascends along the medial aspect of the knee (5) and along the medial aspect of the thigh (6) to the pubic hairy region (7), curves around the external genitalia (8), and reaches the lower abdomen (9). It then runs upwards and encircles the stomach to enter the liver, its pertaining organ, and connects with the gallbladder (10). From there, it continues to ascend, passing through the diaphragm (11) and distributing itself over the hypochondrium and costal region (12). Then, it ascends along the posterior aspect of the throat (13) to the nasopharynx (14) and connects with the brain (15). Running further upward, it emerges at the forehead (16) and meets the Du Meridian at the vertex of the head (17).

The branch arising from the "eye system" (i.e., the connection between the eyeball and brain) descends into the cheek (18) and curves around the inner surface of the lips (19).

Another branch arising from the liver (20) passes through the diaphragm (21), ascends into the lung, and connects with the Lung Meridian of Hand-Taiyin (22).

The line made by the acupoints of the meridian distributed on the body surface: It starts from LR-1 Dadun at the hairy region of the dorsum of the big toe, runs along the interspace between the big and 2nd toes, passes in front of the internal malleolus, and ascends to the point 8 cun proximal to the medial malleolus where it crosses and then runs behind the Spleen Meridian of Foot-Taiyin. From there, it runs upwards along the middle portion of the medial aspect of the thigh, curves around the external genitalia, and ascends through the lower abdomen to the hypochondrium. Then, it terminates at LR-14 Qimen at the 6th intercostal space below the nipple. (See Fig. I-12)

2). The organs concerned
The liver, gallbladder, stomach, lung, throat, nose and eye.

3). Indications
a. Disorders of the reproductive and urinary systems: Irregular menstruation, amenorrhea, dysmenorrhea, uterine bleeding, seminal emission, impotence, enuresis, retention of urine, hernia.

b. Disorders of the digestive system: Vomiting, hiccup, diarrhea.

c. Disorders in the regions along the course of the meridian: Pain, numbness and motor impairment long the course of the meridian.

d. Other disorders: Hypertension, stroke, infantile convulsion, epilepsy, swelling and pain of the eye.

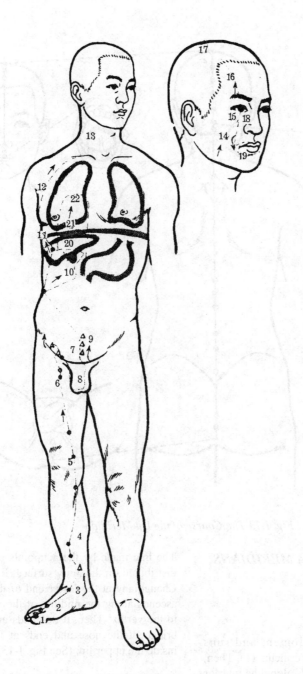

Fig. I-12 The Course of the Liver Meridian

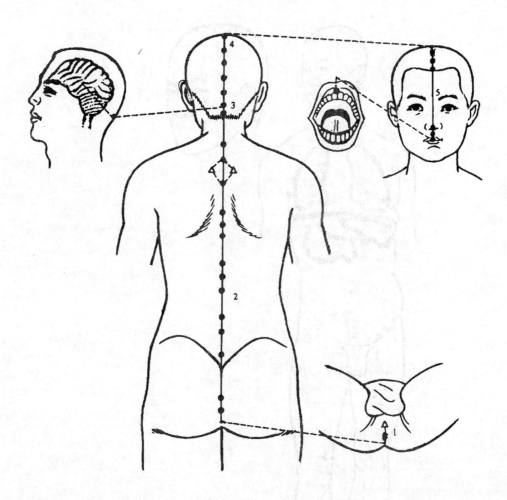

Fig. I-13 The Course of the Du Meridian

IV. THE EIGHT EXTRA MERIDIANS

1. The Du Meridian (DU)

1). The running course
It starts in the lower abdomen, and runs downwards to emerge at the perineum (1). Then, it turns backwards and ascends along the interior of the spine column (2) to DU-16 Fengfu at the nape, where it enters the brain (3). Then, it further ascends to the vertex (4) and turns to

descend along the forehead to the bridge of the nose (5).

The line made by the acupoints of the meridian distributed on the body surface: It starts at DU-1 Changqiang at the lower end of the coccyx, and ascends along the midline of the waist and back to the vertex. Then, it descends anteriorly to the bridge of the nose and ends at DU-28 Yinjiao inside the upper lip. (See Fig. I-13)

2). The organs concerned
The uterus, brain and spinal column.

3). Indications

a. Disorders of the reproductive & urinary systems: Sterility in women, impotence, difficulty in urination, enuresis.

b. Disorders in the regions along the course of the meridian: Stiffness of the back, opisthotonos.

c. Mental disorders: Epilepsy, poor development of intelligence.

d. Other disorders: Fever, haemorrhoids.

2. The Ren Meridian (RN)

1). The running course

It starts from the inside of the lower abdomen, and descends to emerge at the perineum (1). It ascends through the pubic hairy region (2) and along the interior of the abdomen, passing through RN-4 Guanyuan and the other points along the front midline (3) to the throat (4). Ascending further, it curves around the lips (5), passes through the face (6) and enters ST-1 Chengqi at the infraorbital region (7).

The line made by the acupoints of the meridian distributed on the body surface: It starts at RN-1 Huiyin between the front and back lower orifices, and runs upwards along the midline of the abdomen and chest and through the neck and throat. Then, it ends at RN-24 Chengjiang at the center below the chin. (See Fig. I-14)

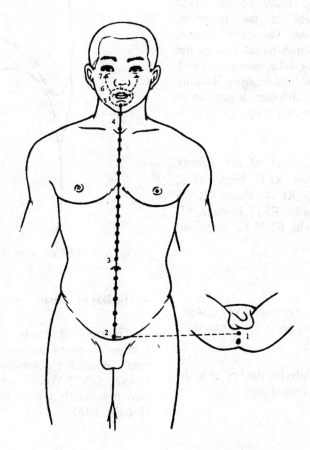

Fig. I-14 The Course of the Ren Meridian

2). The organs concerned
The uterus, throat, lip and eye.

3). Indications

a. Disorders of the reproductive & urinary systems: Sterility in women, impotence, difficulty in urination, enuresis, masses in the lower abdomen in women.

b. Digestive disorders: Abdominal pain and/or distention, vomiting, diarrhea.

3. The Chong Meridian

1). The running course
It originates from the inside of the lower abdomen and emerges at the perineum. Ascending, it runs inside the spinal column, where its superficial branch passes through the region of ST-30 Qichong and communicates with the Kidney Meridian of Foot-Shaoyin. Running along both sides of the abdomen, it goes up to the throat and curves around the lips. (See Fig. I-15)

2). The coalescent points of the Chong Meridian: RN-1 Huiyin, KI-11 Hegu, KI-12 Dahe, RN-13 Xixue, KI-14 Simen, KI-15 Zhongzhu, KI-16 Huangshu, KI-17 Shangqu, KI-18 Shiguan, KI-19 Yindu, KI-20 Futonggu and KI-21 Youmen.

3). Indications

a. Disorders of the reproductive system: Irregular menstruation, amenorrhea, dysmenorrhea, infertility.

b. Other disorders: Adverse flow of qi in the abdomen and chest, abdominal pain.

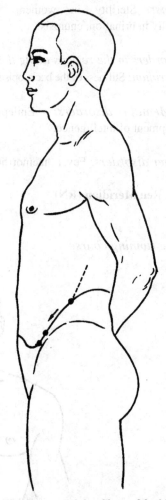

Fig. I-15 The Course of the Chong Meridian

4. The Dai Meridian

1). The running course
It originates below the hypochondriac region and runs obliquely downwards though GB-26 Daimai, GB-27 Wuchu, and GB-28 Weidao. It runs transversely around the waist like a belt. (See Fig. I-16)

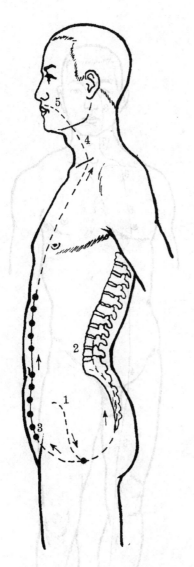

Fig. I-16 The Course of the Dai Meridian

2). The coalescent points of the Dai Meridian: GB-26 Daimai, GB-27 Wuchu and GB-28 Weidao.

3). Indications
a. Disorders in women: Leukorrhea.

b. Disorders in the waist: Pain or/and weakness in the lower back.

5. The Yangqiao Meridian

1). The running course
It starts from the lateral side of the heel (BL-62 Shenmai and BL-61 Pushen). It runs upwards along the external malleolus and passes the posterior border of the fibula. It then goes along the lateral side of the thigh and posterior side of the hypochondrium to the posterior axillary fold. From there, it winds over to the shoulder and ascends along the neck to the corner of the mouth. Then it enters the inner canthus (BL-1 Jingming) to communicate with the Yinqiao Meridian. Running further upward along the Bladder Meridian of Foot-Taiyang to the forehead, it meets the Gallbladder Meridian of Foot-Shaoyang at GB-20 Fengchi. (See Fig. I-17).

2). The coalescent points of the Yangqiao Meridian: BL-62 Shenmai, BL-61 Pushen, BL-59 Fuyang, GB-29 Juliao, SJ-10 Naoshu, LI-15 Jianyu, LI-16 Jugu, ST-4 Dicang, SI-3 Juliao, ST-1 Chengqi, BL-1 Jingming and GB-20 Fengchi.

3). Indications: Eye pain starting from the inner canthus, insomnia.

6. The Yinqiao Meridian

1). The running course
It starts from the posterior aspect of the navicular bone (KI-6 Zhaohai). Ascending to the upper portion of the medial malleolus, it runs straight upwards along the posterior border of the medial aspect of the thigh to the external genitalia. Then it goes upward along the chest to the supraclavicular fossa and runs further upwards lateral to the "Adam's apple" in front of ST-9 Renyin and then along the zygoma. From there, it reaches the inner canthus (BL-1 Jingming) and communicates with the Yangqiao Meridian. (See Fig. I-18)

2). The coalescent points of the Yinqiao Meridian: KI-6 Zhaohai, KI-8 Jiaoxin and BL-1 Jingming.

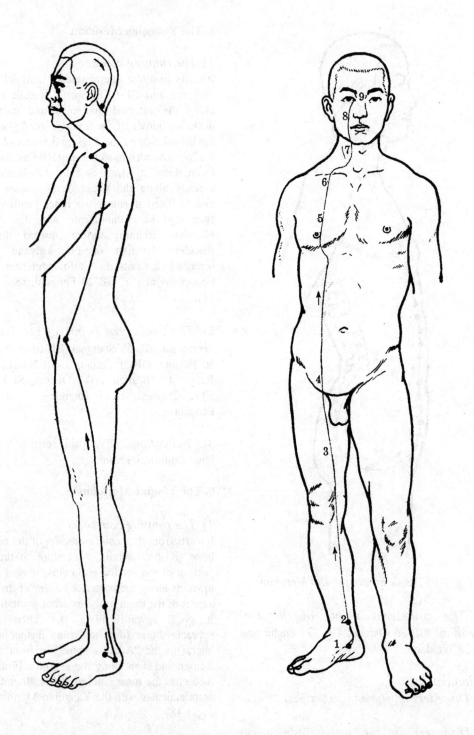

Fig. I-17 The Course of the Yangqiao Meridian   *Fig. I-18 The Course of the Yinqiao Meridian*

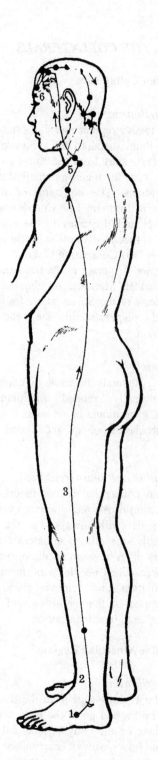

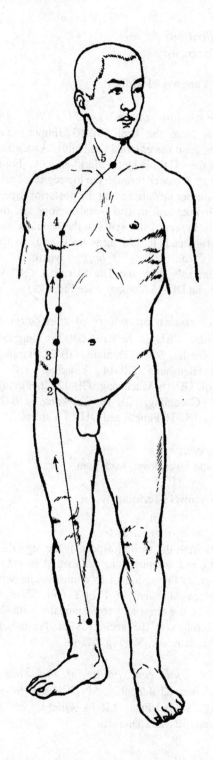

Fig. I-19 The Course of the Yangwei Meridian   *Fig. I-20 The Course of the Yinwei Meridian*

3). Indications
Somnolence, dysuria.

7. The Yangwei Meridian

1). The running course
It starts from the heel (BL-63 Jinmen) and emerges from the external malleolus. Ascending along the Gallbladder Meridian of Foot-Shaoyang, it passes through the hip region. Then, it runs further upwards along the posterior aspect of the hypochondriac and costal regions and the posterior aspect of the axilla to the shoulder and to the forehead. It then turns backwards to the back of the neck, where it communicates with the Du Meridian (DU-16 Fengfu and DU-15 Yamen). (See Fig.I-19)

2). The coalescent points of the Yangwei Meridian: BL-63 Jinmen, GB-35 Yangjiao, SI-10 Naoshu, SJ-15 Tianliao, GB-21 Jianjing, GB-13 Benshen, GB-14 Yangbai, GB-15 Toulinqi, GB-16 Muchuang, GB-17 Zhengying, GB-18 Chengling, GB-19 Naokong, GB-20 Fengchi, DU-16 Fengfu and DU-15 Yamen.

3). Indications
Chills and fever, lower back pain.

8. The Yinwei Meridian

1). The running course
It starts from the medial aspect of the leg (KI-9 Zhubin), and ascends along the medial aspect of the thigh to the abdomen to communicate with the Spleen Meridian of Foot-Taiyin. Then, it runs along the chest and communicates with the Ren Meridian at the neck (RN-22 Tiantu and RN-23 Lianquan). (See Fig. I-20)

2). The coalescent points of the Yinwei Meridian: KI-9 Zhubin, SP-13 Fushe, SP-15 Daheng, SP-16 Fuai, LR-14 Qimen, RN-22 Tiantu and RN-23 Lianquan.

3). Indications
Cardiac pain, melancholia.

V. THE COLLATERALS

1. The Fifteen Collaterals

1). The distribution
Each of the twelve regular meridians has a Luo-Connecting Point distal to the elbow or knee. Their collaterals start from the Luo-Connecting Points and run to their externally-internally related meridians. The collateral of the Ren Meridian starts from its Luo-Connecting Point RN-15 Jiuwei and disperses in the abdominal region. The collateral of the Du Meridian starts from its Luo-Connecting Point DU-1 Changqiang and disperses in the head and joints with the Bladder Meridian on the back. The major collateral of the Spleen starts from SP-21 Dabao and disperses in the chest and hypochondrium.

2). Functions
The fifteen collaterals function to connect the externally-internally related meridians and transport the local qi and blood so as to promote the free circulation of qi and blood of the meridians.

3). Indications and their treatment
If the fifteen collaterals do not function well, blood stagnation of the meridians or even in the internal organs will always be the result. Therapeutically, the fifteen collaterals may be stimulated by plum blossom needle or pricked to bleed by three edged needle to promote qi and blood circulation and remove blood stasis, treating diseases of the meridians and zang-fu organs with/due to blood stagnation.

2. The Twelve Muscular Regions

1). The distribution
The muscular regions start from the distal ends of the extremities and go to the head and trunk. They distribute on the body surface and knot at the joints and bones without entering the zang-fu organs. The three yang muscular regions of foot originate from the toes, ascend along the lateral aspect of the lower limbs and knot at the face. The three yin muscular regions of foot originate

from the toes, ascend along the medial aspect of the lower limbs and knot at the external genitalia. The three yang muscular regions of hand originate from the fingers, ascend along the lateral aspect of the upper limbs and knot at the head. The three yin muscular regions of hand originate from the fingers, ascend along the medial aspect of the upper extremities and knot at the chest. On their courses, the muscular regions also knot at the joints and areas full of muscles, i.e. the ankle, popliteal fossa, knee, thigh, hip, wrist, elbow, armpit, shoulder and neck, etc. The muscular region of Foot-Jueyin (liver) not only knots at the external genitalia but also connects all the tendons.

2). Functions
The main function of the twelve muscular regions is to connect all the bones and joints of the body to maintain the normal motion of the body.

3). Indications and their treatment
Abnormal qi and blood circulation of the muscular regions may cause muscular problems, such as pain, contracture, stiffness, spasm and muscular atrophy. These problems are usually treated by stimulating the tender points in the local area.

3. The Twelve Cutaneous Regions

1). The distribution
The cutaneous regions are twelve distinct areas on the body surface within the domains of the twelve regular meridians.

2). Functions
The twelve cutaneous regions function to protect the organism.

3). Indications and their treatment
Since the cutaneous regions are the most superficial part of the body, they bear the protective function of the body. When this function is not good, the external pathogen may penetrate the skin to invade the collaterals and gain access to meridians and zang-fu organs. Conversely, symptoms and signs of internal diseases can also be projected onto the skin through the cutaneous regions and meridians. Therapeutically, the cutaneous regions can be stimulated by plum blossom needle or intradermal needle to treat diseases of the meridians and zang-fu organs.

VI.   CYCLICAL FlOW OF QI IN THE TWELVE MERIDIANS

The twelve regular meridians link one another in a fixed order. A cyclical flow of qi is maintained by the connection of the meridians of the hand and foot, yin and yang, exterior and interior. (See Tab. I-2)

Tab.I-2 The Flow of Qi in the Twelve Meridians

(——→pertaining and communicative   ←- - - ——exterior and interior relations)

Zang Organs (Yin Meridians) (Interior)	Fu Organs (Yang Meridians) (Exterior)
→ Lung (1)	(2) Large Intestine
Spleen (4)	(3) Stomach
Heart (5)	(6) Small Intestine
Kidney (8)	(7) Bladder
Pericardium (9)	(10) Sanjiao
Liver (12)	(11) Gallbladder

CHAPTER TWO
THE ACUPOINTS OF THE FOURTEEN MERIDIANS & EXTRAORDINARY POINTS

Acupoints are the specific sites through which the qi of the zang-fu organs and meridians is transported to the body surface. "Acupoint" in Chinese is two characters, meaning respectively "transportation" and "hole". In the medical literature of the past dynasties, acupoints, the sites where acupuncture treatment is applied, have other terms such as "qi point" and "aperture". Acupoints are not only the pathways for the circulation of qi and blood, but also the sites of response to diseases. In acupuncture and moxibustion treatment, proper techniques are applied on the acupoints to regulate the functional activities of the body, strengthen body resistance so as to prevent and treat diseases. TCM practitioners of past ages have left plentiful recordings describing the locations, actions and indications of acupoints, and manipulations of needles and moxibustion on acupoints, formulating a systematical theory.

I. CLASSIFICATION & NOMENCLATURE OF ACUPOINTS

There are numerous acupoints distributed over the human body. A great deal of work has been accomplished by TCM specialists in the past to generalize and systematize acupoints, which have been classified either by "meridians" or by "body parts". Generally speaking, acupoints fall into the following three categories in terms of their evolution.

1. Acupoints of the Fourteen Meridians

Also known as "regular point", acupoints of the fourteen meridians are distributed along the twelve regular meridians, the Du and the Ren Meridians, totally amounting to 361. According to ancient medical records, the acupoints of this category are the crystallization of rich clinical experience of TCM practitioners in the past. All the points in this category can be used to treat disorders of the related meridians, collaterals and zang-fu organs. They are the most commonly used points and form the main part of all acupoints. Those of the twelve regular meridians are distributed symmetrically in pairs on the left and right sides of the body, while those of the Du and the Ren Meridians are singly ones, aligning on the posterior and anterior midlines respectively.

2.   Extraordinary Points

They are named "extra points" in short. They are experiential points with specific names and definite locations, but are not attributed to the fourteen meridians. They are effective in the treatment of certain diseases. Although scattered over the body, they are still related to the meridian system. Moreover, a lot of them are just located on the meridians. A survey of the ancient acupuncture literature has revealed that some regular points were developed from the extraordinary points. Therefore, extraordinary points are said to be the preceding counterparts of regular points. Clinically, they are supplement to regular points and, in treatment of some syndromes or diseases, are more effective than regular points. Generally speaking, points in "new acupuncture therapy", such as scalp puncture, ear puncture, face puncture, wrist-ankle puncture, foot puncture, etc., can also be put into this category if they have specific names and definite locations, but are not listed into the regular point system.

3.   Ashi Points

They are also called "reflecting points", "unfixed points" or "tender points". They do not have specific names or definite locations. Clinically, they are mainly used for pain syndromes.

Additionally, some points are named "specific points". But they are not something apart from the above three categories. Actually, specific points are those points of the fourteen meridians (a few of them do not belong to the fourteen meridians) that have special properties and are grouped under special names.

II.   NOMENCLATURE OF ACUPOINTS

1.   Nomenclature Based on Analogy

Most of the acupoints are nominated by way of analogy. The flow of qi and blood is similized by that of water; the prominence and depression of the tendons and bones are compared to mountains and valleys; the characteristic local shape of the body is signified by certain animals or utensils; and the acupoint functions are analogized by architectural structures, astronomical or meteorological phenomena.

1). Names bearing analogy to water flow, mountains and valleys
For example, HT-3 Shaohai means "young sea" in Chinese; BL-57 Chengshan means "sustaining mountain" in Chinese; and LI-4 Hegu means "connected valleys" in Chinese.

2). Names bearing analogy to animals, plants or utensils
For example, ST-35 Dubi means "calf nose" in Chinese; BL-2 Cuanzhu means "assembled bamboo" in Chinese; and LI-17 Tianding means "heavenly cooking vessel" in Chinese.

3). Names bearing analogy to architectural structure
For example, HT-7 Shenmen means "spiritual gate" in Chinese, and SI-19 Tinggong means "hearing palace" in Chinese.

4). Names bearing analogy to astronomical and meteorological phenomena
For example, GB-24 Riyue means "sun and moon" in Chinese; and LU-2 Yunmen means "cloud door" in Chinese.

2.   Nomenclature Based on Therapeutic Properties

A lot of points are named according to their therapeutic properties. For example, BL-1 Jingming means "brightening eyes" in Chinese; and BL-23 Shenshu means "kidney point" in Chinese.

Most of extraordinary points are named in this way.

III.   THE BASIS AND METHODS FOR THE LOCATION OF POINTS

The Methods for Point Location

There are three methods for locating points: 1). Surface anatomical landmarks; 2). Bone proportional measurement and; 3). Finger measurement. They should be used in combination, but the first one is the fundamental and the other two the supplemental ones.

1. Surface Anatomical Landmarks

This is a method to determine the location of points on the body surface based on anatomical landmarks that are divided into fixed and movable categories.

The fixed landmarks include the prominence and depressions formed by the joints and muscles, the configuration of the five sense organs, hairline, fingernails and toenails, nipples and umbilicus. For example, GB-34 Yanglingquan is in the depression anterior and inferior to the head of the fibula; LI-14 Binao is at the end of the insertion of the deltoid muscle; BL-2 Cuanzhu is at the medial end of the eyebrow; EX-HN-3 Yintang is midway between the eyebrows; And RN-17 Danzhong is at the midpoint between the two nipples.

The movable landmarks refer to the clefts, depressions, wrinkles or prominence appearing on the joints, muscles, tendons and skin during motion. For example, SI-19 Tinggong is between the tragus and mandibular joint, where a depression is formed when the mouth is slightly open; LI-11 Quchi is in the depression at the lateral end of the cubital crease when the elbow is flexed.

The major anatomical landmarks on the human body surface are listed as follows:

On the head:

1)   The midpoint of the anterior hairline.
2)   The midpoint of the posterior hairline.
3)   The corner of the forehead (at the corner of the anterior hairline).
4)   The mastoid process.

On the face:

1)   EX-HN-3 Yintang (at the midpoint between the eyebrow).
2)   The pupil, or the center of the eye (at the midpoint of the line between the inner and outer canthi).

On the neck:

1)   The laryngeal protuberance.

On the chest:

1)   The suprasternal fossa (in the depression above the suprasternal notch).
2)   The midpoint of the sternoxiphoid symphysis (at the conjunction of the sternum and xiphoid process).
3)   The nipple (the center of the nipple).

On the abdomen:

1)   The umbilicus (RN-8 Shenque, the center of the umbilicus).
2)   The upper border of the pubic symphysis at the crossing point of the upper border of the pubic symphysis and the anterior midline.
3)   The anterior superior iliac spine.

On the lateral side of the chest and abdomen:

1)   The apex of the axilla (the highest point of the axillary fossa).
2)   The free end of the 11th rib.

On the back, low back and sacrum:

1)   The spinous process of the 7th cervical vertebra.
2)   The spinous process from the 1st to the 12th thoracic vertebra and from the 1st to the 5th lumbar vertebra, the median sacral crest and the coccyx.
3)   The medial and the scapular spine (on the medial border of the scapula).
4)   The acromial angle.
5)   The posterior superior iliac spine.

On the upper limbs:

1)   Anterior axillary fold (the anterior end of the axillary crease).
2)   The posterior axillary fold (the posterior end of the axillary crease).

3) The cubital crease.
4) The tip of the elbow (olecranon).
5) The dorsal and ventral creases of the wrist (the styloid crease between the distal ends of the styloid processes of the ulna and radius).

On the lower limbs:

1) The greater trochanter of the femur.
2) The medial epicondyle of the femur.
3) The medial epicondyle of the tibia.
4) The inferior gluteal crease (the border between the buttocks and thigh).
5) ST-35 Dubi (in the center of the depression lateral to the patella ligament).
6) The popliteal crease.
7) The tip of the medial malleolus.
8) The tip of the lateral malleolus.

2. Bone Proportional Measurement

In this method, the joints are taken as the main landmarks to measure the length and width of various portions of the human body. The proportional measurements of various portions of the human body defined in Ling Shu (*Miraculous Pivot*), are taken as the basis for the location of points in combination with the modified methods introduced by acupuncturists through the ages. **The length between two joints is divided into several equal portions, each portion as one cun**. Cun was used as a length unit in China, 1 cun=3.3 cm. It should be pointed out that in location of acupuncture points, cun is taken as the length unit only based on the proportional measurement and finger measurement. As this reason, the length of one cun on different individuals can be actually different in length.

The descriptions of the portions of the human body in TCM are not always the same as those in modern anatomy. For example, the palmar (flexor) side of the upper limbs is named the "medial side", while the dorsal (extensor) side is known as the "lateral side". The side of the lower limbs facing the sagittal plane of the body is called the "medial side", while the side opposite to the lateral side is called as "lateral side" or the "posterior side".

The main bone-proportional measurements are listed in the following tables and figures.

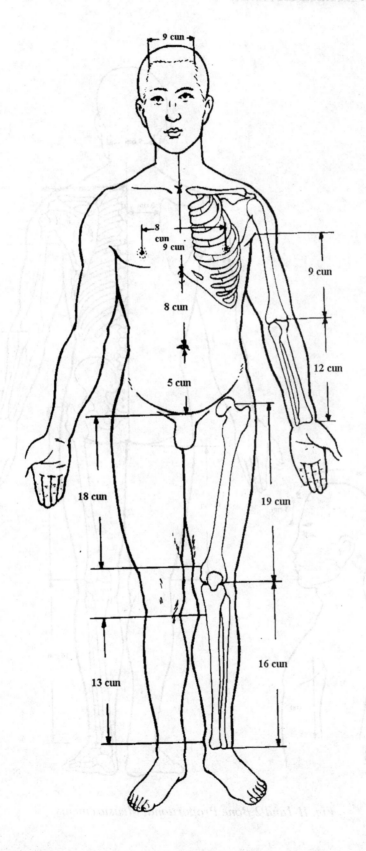

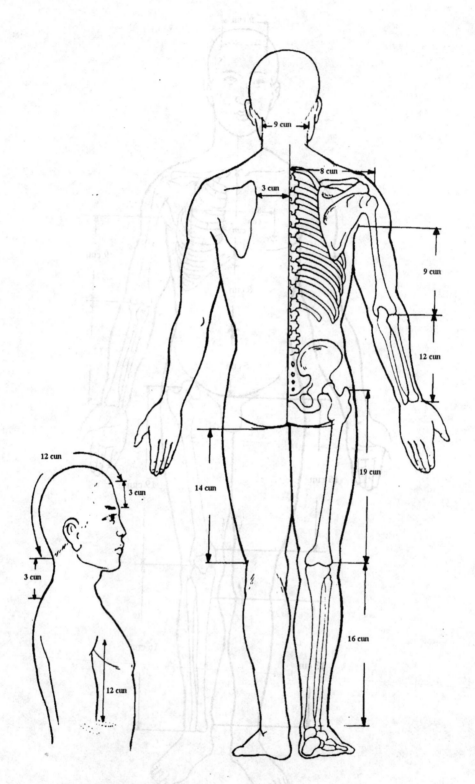

Fig. II-1and 2 Bone Proportional Measurements

Tab. II-1: Bone Proportional Measurements

Distance	Proportional measurement	Method	Remarks
From the midpoint of the anterior hairline to the midpoint of the posterior hairline.	12 cun	Longitudinal measurement	Used for measuring the longitudinal distance when locating the points on the head.
From EX-HN-3 Yintang to the midpoint of the anterior hairline.	3 cun	Longitudinal measurement	Used for measuring the longitudinal distance when locating the points on the anterior or posterior hairline and the head.
From the point below the spinous process of the 7th cervical vertebra DU-14 Dazhui to the midpoint of the posterior hairline.	3 cun	Longitudinal measurement	Used for measuring the longitudinal distance when locating the points on the anterior or posterior hairline and the head.
From EX-HN-3 Yintang to the midpoint of the posterior hairline and then to the point below the spinous process of the 7th cervical vertebra. (DU-14 Dazhui)	18 cun	Longitudinal measurement	Used for measuring the longitudinal distance when locating the points on the anterior or posterior hairline and the head.
Between the corners of the forehead. (ST-8 Touwei)	9 cun	Transverse measurement	Used for measuring the transverse distance when locating the points on the anterior part of the head.
Between the mastoid processes.	9 cun	Transverse measurement	Used for measuring the transverse distance when locating the points on the posterior part of the head.
From the suprasternal fossa (RN-22 Tiantu) to the midpoint of the sternoxiphoid symphysis.	9 cun	Longitudinal measurement	Used for measuring the longitudinal distance when locating the points of the Ren Meridian on the chest.
From the midpoint of the sternoxiphoid symphysis to the center of the umbilicus.	8 cun	Longitudinal measurement	Used for measuring the longitudinal distance when locating the points on the upper abdomen.
From the center of the umbilicus to the upper border of the pubic symphysis. (RN-2 Qugu)	5 cun	Longitudinal measurement	Used for measuring the longitudinal distance of the points on the lower abdomen.

Tab. II-1: Bone Proportional Measurements

Distance	Proportional measurement	Method	Remarks
Between the two nipples.	8 cun	Transverse measurement	Used for measuring the transverse distance when locating the points on the chest and abdomen.
From the apex of the axilla to the free end of the 11th rib. (LR-13 Zhangmen)	12 cun	Longitudinal measurement	Used for measuring the longitudinal distance when locating the points on the hypochondrium.
From the medial border of the scapula to the posterior midline.	3 cun	Transverse measurement	Used for measuring the transverse distance when locating the points on the back.
From the acromial angle to the posterior midline.	8 cun	Transverse measurement	Used for measuring the transverse distance when locating the points on the shoulder and back.
From the anterior and posterior axillary folds to the cubital crease.	9 cun	Longitudinal measurement	Used for measuring the longitudinal distance when locating the points on the arm.
From the cubital crease to the dorsal crease of the wrist.	12 cun	Longitudinal measurement	Used for measuring the longitudinal distance when locating the points on the forearm.
From the upper border of the pubic symphysis to the upper border of the medial epicondyle of the femur.	18 cun	Longitudinal measurement	Used for measuring the longitudinal distance when locating the points on the three yin meridians of the foot which are on the medial side of the lower limbs .
From the lower border of the medial epicondyle of the tibia to the tip of the medial malleolus.	13 cun	Longitudinal measurement	Used for measuring the longitudinal distance when locating the points on the three yin meridians of the foot which are on the medial side of the lower limbs.
From the greater trochanter to the popliteal crease.	19 cun	Longitudinal measurement	Used for measuring the longitudinal distance when locating the points on the side of the lower limbs. (The distance from the gluteal groove to the popliteal crease is equivalent to 14 cun.)

Tab. II-1: Bone Proportional Measurements

Distance	Proportional measurement	Method	Remarks
From the popliteal crease to the tip of the lateral malleolus.	16 cun	Longitudinal measurement	Used for measuring the longitudinal distance when locating the points on the three yang meridians of the foot which are on the lateral-posterior side of the lower limbs.

3. Finger Measurement

This is a method to locate acupoints by measuring distance with either the length or width of the patient's finger(s).

a. Middle finger measurement: When the middle finger is flexed, the distance between the radial ends of the two interphalangeal creases of the patient's middle finger is taken as 1 cun.

b. Thumb measurement: The width of the interphalangeal joint of the patient's thumb is taken as 1 cun.

c. Four-finger measurement: When the four fingers (index, middle, ring and little fingers) are extended and held close together, their width on the level of the proximal interphalangeal crease of the middle finger is taken as 3 cun.

The finger measurement is usually used in combination with some simple movable landmarks based on the bone proportional measurement.

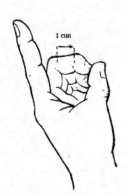 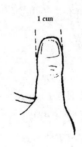 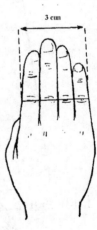

Fig. II-3 Proportional "Cun" Measurements (3)

IV. LOCATION, ACTION & INDICATIONS OF THE POINTS OF THE 14 MERIDIANS

In the following tables, symbols are used to represent certain words in order to make reading more convenient. They are as the follows:

↓ = perpendicular acupuncture;

↘ = oblique acupuncture;

↪ = subcutaneous or horizontal acupuncture;

ᵭ = Moxibustion.

1. The Points of the Lung Meridian of Hand-Taiyin (LU)

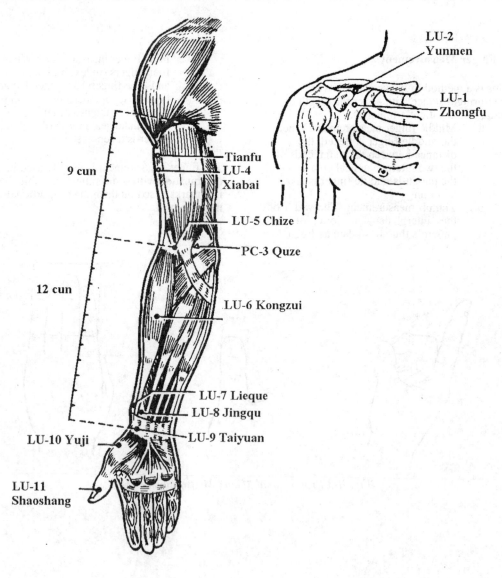

Fig. II-4 Points of the Lung Meridian (1)

Tab. II-2 Points of the Lung Hand-Taiyin Meridian (LU)

Point, Property, Method & Remarks	Location & Action	Categories of Disease & Indications
LU-1 Zhongfu ⌖ *0.5-0.8 cun towards lateral aspect of chest.* ᵟ *is applicable.*	In the superior lateral part of the anterior thoracic wall, 1 cun below LU-2 Yunmen, in the 1st intercostal space, 6 cun lateral to the anterior midline. 1. Regulates lung qi and stops cough. 2. Descends lung qi. 3. Disperses fullness from chest and stops pain.	1. Head and sense organs: Nasal obstruction, rhinorrhea, sinusitis, sore throat. 2. Respiratory: Cough, asthma, shortness of breath, feeling of fullness and pain in chest, hemoptysis. 3. Digestive: Vomiting, anorexia, abdominal distention, edema of limbs. 4. Other: Shoulder pain, goiter, abdominal pain that is referring to the lumbar area.
LU-2 Yunmen ⌖ *0.5-0.8 cun towards lateral aspect of chest.* ᵟ *is applicable.*	In the superior lateral part of the anterior thoracic wall, superior to the coracoid process of the scapula, in the depression of the infraclavicular fossa, 6 cun lateral to the anterior midline. 1. Disperses fullness from chest. 2. Descends lung qi and stops cough.	1. The meridian course: Shoulder pain, pain in supraclavicular fossa, hypochondriac pain referring to back, cold limbs. 2. Respiratory: Cough, asthma, pain and fullness in chest, sensation of heat and oppression in chest. 3. Other: Heat sensation in limbs caused by cold, sudden pain in cardiac region and abdomen, irregular pulse, goiter.
LU-3 Tianfu ⌖ *0.5-0.8 cun.* ᵟ *is applicable.*	On the medial side of the upper arm and on the radial border of the biceps muscle, 3 cun below the anterior end of the axillary fold. 1. Dispels pathogens from lung. 2. Clears heat from lung and cools blood.	1. The meridian course: Pain and numbness of shoulder and arm. 2. Head and sense organs: Epistaxis, vertigo. 3. Respiratory: Cough, asthma. 4. Mental: Trance, amnesia, grief. 5. Other: General edema, heavy sensation of body.

Tab. II-2 Points of the Lung Hand-Taiyin Meridian (LU)

Point, Property, Method & Remarks	Location & Action	Categories of Disease & Indications
LU-4 Xiabai ⊥ *0.5-0.8 cun.* *δ is applicable.*	On the medial side of the upper arm and on the radial border of the biceps muscle, 4 cun below the anterior end of the axillary fold, or 5 cun above the cubital crease. 1. Disperses lung qi. 2. Regulates qi and relieves chest stuffiness.	1. The meridian course: Pain in medial aspect of upper arm and shoulder, tinea. 2. Respiratory: Cough, asthma, shortness of breath. 3. Digestive: Stomachache, nausea.
LU-5 Chize *He-Sea Point* ⊥ *0.3-0.5 cun, or prick to cause bleeding.* *δ is applicable.*	In the cubital crease, in the depression on the radial side of the tendon of the biceps muscle. 1. Clears heat from lung and nourishes lung yin. 2. Descends lung qi. 3. Expels phlegm from lung. 4. Benefits bladder.	1. The meridian course: Spasmodic pain of elbow and arm, pain in medial aspect of shoulder, sudden swelling of four limbs, inability to extend arm, paralysis of upper arms. 2. Head and sense organs: Sore throat, aphasia. 3. Digestive: Acute vomiting and diarrhea, dryness of tongue, spitting blood. 4. Respiratory: Cough, asthma, hemoptysis, afternoon fever, feeling of fullness in chest and hypochondrium. 5. Urinary: Enuresis, incontinence of urine. 6. Mental: Sadness, infantile convulsions, epilepsy. 7. Other: General pain, stiffness and pain in back and lumbar region, swelling and pain of knee, mastitis, erysipelas, fever.
LU-6 Kongzui *Xi-Cleft Point* ⊥ *0.5-1 cun.* *δ is applicable.*	On the radial side of the palmar surface of the forearm, and on the line connecting LU-5 Chize, and LU-9 Taiyuan, 7 cun above the cubital crease. 1. Regulates lung qi and descends lung qi. 2. Clears heat from lung and stops bleeding.	1. The meridian course: Shoulder pain, pain of elbow and arm, hemiplegia. 2. Head and sense organs: Sore throat, aphasia. 3. Respiratory: Hemoptysis, cough, asthma, febrile diseases without sweating. 4. Other: Hemorrhoids.

Tab. II-2 Points of the Lung Hand-Taiyin Meridian (LU)

Point, Property, Method & Remarks	Location & Action	Categories of Disease & Indications
LU-7 Lieque *Luo-Connecting Point; One of Eight Confluent Points communicating with RN* ↘ *0.5-0.8 cun.* *ᵟ is applicable.*	On the radial side of the forearm, proximal to the styloid process of the radius, 1.5 cun above the crease of the wrist, between the brachioradial muscle and the tendon of the long abductor muscle of the thumb. 1. Descends and disperses lung qi. 2. Circulates defensive qi and releases exterior. 3. Benefits bladder and opens water passages. 4. Opens nose.	1. The meridian course: Pain of arm and shoulder, numbness of fingers, hemiparalysis. 2. Head and sense organs: Headache, migraine, deviation of eye and mouth, facial spasm, trigeminal neuralgia, sore throat, toothache. 3. Respiratory: Cough, asthma, common cold. 4. Digestive: Abdominal pain, diarrhea, dysentery, hemoptysis, dysphasia. 5. Cardiovascular: Chest pain, hypertension. 6. Urinary: Hematuria, penile pain, hotness of urine, difficulty and pain in micturition, dysuria. 7. Genital: Nocturnal emission, retention of dead fetus. 8. Other: Lumbago, sudden swelling of limbs, mastitis.
LU-8 Jingqu *Jing-River Point.* ⊥ *or* ↘ *0.3-0.5 cun.* *ᵟ is contraindicated.*	On the radial side of the palmar surface of the forearm, 1 cun above the crease of the wrist, in the depression between the styloid process of the radius and radial artery. 1. Stops cough and relieves asthma.	1. The meridian course: Pain in medial aspect of shoulder, forearm and wrist, neuralgia and paralysis of radial nerve. 2. Head and sense organs: Sore throat. 3. Respiratory: Cough, asthma, fullness and pain in chest. 4. Digestive: Epigastric pain, vomiting. 5. Other: Malaria, phrenospasm, esophagospasm.

Tab. II-2 Points of the Lung Hand-Taiyin Meridian (LU)

Point, Property, Method & Remarks	Location & Action	Categories of Disease & Indications
LU-9 Taiyuan *Shu-Stream Point;* *Yuan-Source Point;* *One of Eight Influential Points dominating pulse and vessels.* ⊥ *0.2-0.3 cun.* ᶺ *is applicable.*	At the radial end of the crease of the wrist, lateral to the point where the pulsation of the radial artery is palpable. 1. Regulates lung qi and stops cough. 2. Tonifies lung and promotes blood circulation. 3. Clears heat from lung and liver and resolves phlegm.	1. The meridian course: Pain in arm and elbow, hemiparalysis, injury of wrist and soft tissue. 2. Head and sense organs: Cataract, dryness of throat, inflammation of throat. 3. Respiratory: Cough, asthma, hemoptysis, pain in chest and back. 4. Digestive: Abdominal distention, belching, vomiting with bleeding. 5. Other: Amenorrhea, dysmenorrhea, deafness and mutism, intercostal neuralgia.
LU-10 Yuji *Ying-Spring Point* ⊥ *0.2-0.3 cun.* ᶺ *is applicable.*	In the depression proximal to the 1st metacarpophalangeal joint, on the radial side of the midpoint of the 1st metacarpal bone, and on the junction of the red and white skin. 1. Clears heat from lung and heart. 2. Benefits throat.	1. The meridian course: Shoulder pain, spasmodic pain of elbow, numbness of fingers. 2. Head and sense organs: Headache, dry throat, sore throat, aphasia. 3. Respiratory: Cough, asthma, hemoptysis, pain in chest and back, common cold, fever. 4. Mental: Susceptibility to sorrow and fright, mental confusion. 5. Digestive: Abdominal pain, vomiting. 6. Other: Mastitis, arrhythmia.
LU-11 Shaoshang *Jing-Well Point* ⊥ *0.1 cun, or prick to cause bleeding.* ᶺ *is applicable.*	On the radial side of the distal segment of the thumb, 0.1 cun from the corner of the fingernail. 1. Expels wind and clears heat. 2. Disperses and descends lung qi. 3. Benefits throat. 4. Opens orifices and promotes resuscitation.	1. The meridian course: Numbness and spasmodic pain of fingers. 2. Head and sense organs: Sore throat, epistaxis, mumps, toothache, tinnitus. 3. Respiratory: Cough, asthma. 4. Mental: Coma, loss of consciousness, trismus, epilepsy, mania, infantile convulsion. 5. Other: Heatstroke, febrile diseases, apoplexy.

2. The Points of the Large Intestine Meridian of Hand-Yangming (LI)

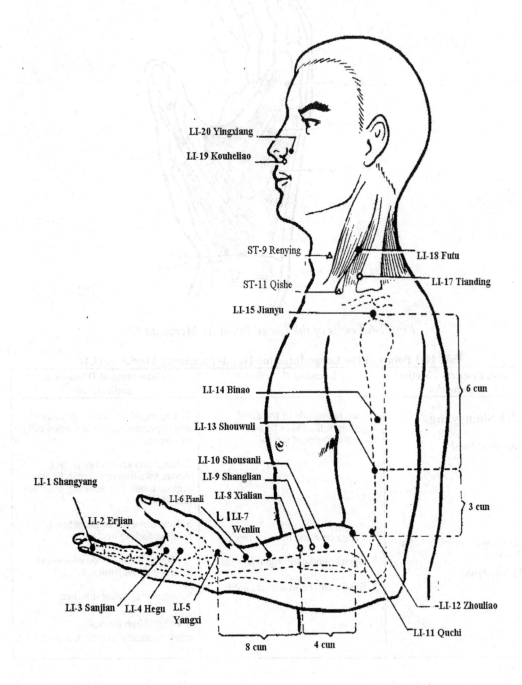

LI-20 Yingxiang
LI-19 Kouheliao

ST-9 Renying
ST-11 Qishe
LI-15 Jianyu

LI-18 Futu
LI-17 Tianding

LI-14 Binao
LI-13 Shouwuli

6 cun

LI-1 Shangyang
LI-2 Erjian

LI-10 Shousanli
LI-9 Shanglian
LI-8 Xialian
LI-6 Pianli
LI-7 Wenliu

3 cun

LI-3 Sanjian   LI-4 Hegu   LI-5 Yangxi

LI-12 Zhouliao
LI-11 Quchi

8 cun   4 cun

Fig. II-5 Points of the Large Intestine Meridian (1)

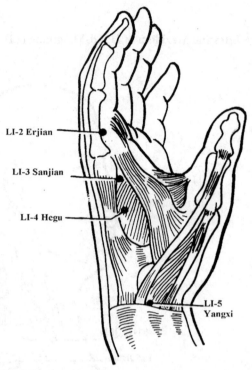

LI-2 Erjian

LI-3 Sanjian

LI-4 Hegu

LI-5
Yangxi

Fig. II-6 Points of the Large Intestine Meridian (2)

Tab. II-3 Points of the Large Intestine Hand-Yangming Meridian (LI)

Point, Property , Method & Remarks	Location & Action	Categories of Diseases & Indications
LI-1 Shangyang *Jing-Well Point* *± 0.1 cun, or prick to cause bleeding.* *Ƌ is applicable.*	On the radial side of the distal segment of the index finger, 0.1 cun from the corner of the nail. 1. Clears heat and benefits throat. 2. Opens mind and brightens eyes. 3. Expels wind and scatters cold.	1. The meridian course: Shoulder and supraclavicular pain, numbness of fingers. 2. Head and sense organs: Sore throat, swelling of submandibular region, toothache, tinnitus, deafness and glaucoma. 3. Respiratory: Cough, asthma, fullness feeling in chest. 4. Mental: Loss of consciousness, infantile convulsion. 5. Digestive: Acute diarrhea. 6. Other: High fever, cerebrovascular accident, sunstroke.

Tab. II-3 Points of the Large Intestine Hand-Yangming Meridian (LI)

Point, Property, Method & Remarks	Location & Action	Categories of Diseases & Indications
LI-2 Erjian *Ying-Spring Point* ⊥ *0.3 cun.* *ϑ is applicable.*	In the depression on the radial side, distal to the 2nd metacarpophalangeal joint when a loose fist is made. 1. Clears heat and relieves swelling.	1. The meridian course: Pain of arm and shoulder, numbness and pain of finger. 2. Head and sense organs: Headache, sore throat, swelling of submandibular region, epistaxis, vertigo, toothache, facial paralysis. 3. Digestive: Intestinal disorders, stool with blood. 4. Mental: Timidity. 5. Other : Lumbar pain, somnolence, fever, dry mouth.
LI-3 Sanjian *Shu-Stream Point* ⊥ *0.3-05 cun, or* ↘ *towards LI-4 Hegu.* *ϑ is applicable.*	In the depression of the radial side, proximal to the 2nd metacarpophalangeal joint when a loose fist is made. 1. Dispels external wind. 2. Clears heat and Benefits throat. 3. Relieves abdominal fullness and diarrhea.	1. The meridian course: Pain of arm and shoulder, redness and swelling of fingers. 2. Head and sense organs: Pain in eyes, toothache, sore throat, running nose and epistaxis, dry mouth. 3. Respiratory: Cough, asthma, fullness of chest. 4. Digestive: Abdominal fullness, borborygmus, diarrhea, dysentery, constipation.

Tab. II-3 Points of the Large Intestine Hand-Yangming Meridian (LI)

Point, Property , Method & Remarks	Location & Action	Categories of Diseases & Indications
LI-4 Hegu *Yuan-Source Point* ⊥ *0.3 cun.* ᵷ *is applicable.* ⊥ *& ᵷ are contraindicated in pregnancy.*	On the dorsum of the hand, between the 1st and 2nd metacarpal bones, and on the radial side of the midpoint of the 2nd metacarpal bone. 1. Dispels wind and releases exterior. 2. Promotes dispersing function of lung. 3. Removes obstruction from meridian. 4. Tonifies qi and stabilizes exterior. 5. Harmonizes ascending and descending activities of qi.	1. The meridian course: Pain of shoulder, arm, elbow and wrist, numbness of fingers, hemiplegia, arthralgia syndrome, flaccidity syndrome, frozen shoulder. 2. Head and sense organs: Headache, dizziness, redness, swelling and pain in the eye, night blindness, epistaxis, sinusitis, toothache, trismus, mumps, swelling of face, furuncles on the face, deviated eye and mouth, deafness, tinnitus, sore throat, loss of voice. 3. Respiratory: Common cold, fever cough, asthma. 4. Digestive : Stomachache, vomiting, diarrhea, dysentery, constipation. 5. Gynecopathies: Amenorrhea, dysmenorrhea, delayed labor, retention of placenta, lochiostasis, insufficient lactation, mastitis. 6. Cardiovascular: Cardiac pain, acrotism. 7. Mental: Apoplexy, infantile convulsion, tetanus, coma, depression, mania, epilepsy, spasm, opisthotonos. 8. Other: Malaria, edema, diabetes, retention of urine, scabies.
LI-5 Yangxi *Jing-River Point* ⊥ *0.3-0.5 cun.* ᵷ *is applicable.*	At the radial end of the crease of the wrist, in the depression between the tendons of the short extensor and long extensor muscles of the thumb when the thumb is tilted upwards . 1. Expels wind and releases exterior. 2. Clears heat and benefits throat. 3. Stops pain.	1. The meridian course: Pain of shoulder and arm, hemiplegia, pain and weakness of wrist and elbow, stiffness of fingers. 2. Head and sense organs: Headache, tinnitus, deafness, stiffness of tongue, frequent involunary protrusion of tongue, sore throat, toothache, redness and pain in eyes, cataract. 3. Digestive: Diarrhea, indigestion. 4. Mental: Epilepsy, convulsion, ravings, over-susceptibility to laughter. 5. Other: Fever, malaria.

Tab. II-3 Points of the Large Intestine Hand-Yangming Meridian (LI)

Point, Property , Method & Remarks	Location & Action	Categories of Diseases & Indications
LI-6 Pianli *Luo-Connecting Point* ⊥ *0.3 cun, or* ⊾ *0.3-0.5 cun.* ᵹ *is applicable.*	With the elbow slightly flexed, on the radial side of the dorsal surface of the forearm and on the line connecting LI -5 Yangxi and LI-11 Quchi, 3 cun above the crease of the wrist. 1. Opens water passages. 2. Improves visual and hearing acuity.	1. The meridian course: Pain of shoulder, arm, elbow and wrist. 2. Head and sense organs: Headache, epistaxis, redness of eyes, blurring of vision, deafness, tinnitus, deviation of mouth and eye, toothache, sore throat, dry throat, cheek swelling. 3. Urogenital: Dysuria, edema. 4. Other: Malaria.
LI-7 Wenliu *Xi-Cleft Point* ⊥ *0.5-0.8 cun.* ᵹ *is applicable.*	With the elbow flexed, on the radial side of the dorsal surface of the forearm and on the line connecting LI-5 Yangxi, and LI-11 Quchi, 5 cun above the crease of the wrist. 1. Clears heat and relieves swelling and pain. 2. Calms mind.	1. The meridian course: Pain and motor impairment of shoulder and arm, stiffness and pain of neck. 2. Head and sense organs: Headache, dizziness, dry lips, salivation, toothache, redness, pain and swelling of eyes. 3. Digestive: Abdominal pain or distention, borborygmus. 4. Mental: Ravings, mania, epilepsy. 5. Respiratory: Pulmonary tuberculosis, asthma. 6. Other: Mastitis, furuncles.
LI-8 Xialian ⊥ *0.5-0.8 cun.* ᵹ *is applicable.*	On the radial side of the dorsal surface of the forearm and on the line connecting LI-5 Yangxi and LI-11 Quchi, 4 cun below the cubital crease. 1. Regulates qi and benefits bowel movement.	1. The meridian course: Pain of arm and shoulder, hemiplegia. 2. Head and sense organs: Headache, dizziness, pain of eyes, dry lips, salivation. 3. Digestive: Abdominal pain, or distention, masses due to disorders of qi, distending pain in the abdomen and hypochondrium, indigestion, diarrhea. 4. Mental: Ravings, mania. 5. Other: Mastitis.

Tab. II-3 Points of the Large Intestine Hand-Yangming Meridian (LI)

Point, Property , Method & Remarks	Location & Action	Categories of Diseases & Indications
LI-9 Shanglian ⊥ *0.5-0.8 cun.* ठ *is applicable.*	On the radial side of the dorsal surface of the forearm and on the line connecting LI-5 Yangxi and LI-11 Quchi, 3 cun below the cubital crease. 1. Regulates qi and benefits bowel movement.	1. The meridian course: Hemiplegia, numbness of hand and foot, soreness and pain of arm, hand and shoulder. 2. Head and sense organs: Headache. 3. Digestive: Abdominal pain, borborygmus, diarrhea, pain around umbilicus. 4. Respiratory: Chest pain, asthma, cough.
LI-10 Shousanli ⊥ *0.5-0.8 cun.* ठ *is applicable.*	On the radial side of the dorsal surface of the forearm and on the line connecting LI-5 Yangxi and LI-11 Quchi, 2 cun below the cubital crease. 1. Removes obstruction from meridian. 2. Regulates qi and benefits bowel movement. 3. Tonifies qi. 4. Clears heat and brightens eyes.	1. The meridian course: Pain of arm and shoulder, numbness of arm, hemiplegia. 2. Head and sense organs: Toothache, loss of voice, swelling of cheek, eye disorders, pain in the tongue, facial paralysis. 3. Digestive: Abdominal distention, vomiting, diarrhea, stomach pain, distention of stomach. 4. Other: Scrofula, discomfort of arm due to improper needling, common cold, lower back pain.

Tab. II-3 Points of the Large Intestine Hand-Yangming Meridian (LI)

Point, Property , Method & Remarks	Location & Action	Categories of Diseases & Indications
LI-11 Quchi *He-Sea Point* ⊥ *0.8-1.5 cun.* *ß is applicable.*	With the elbow flexed, at the lateral end of the cubital crease, at the midpoint of the line connecting LU-5 Chize and the external humeral epicondyle. 1. Expels wind and arrests itching. 2. Clears heat and cools blood. 3. Resolves dampness. 4. Regulates nutritive qi and blood. 5. Benefits sinews and joints.	1. The meridian course: Hemiplegia, thin and weak arm, stiffness or flaccidity of elbow and arm, pain around shoulder, pain and limited movement of elbow, redness and swelling of arm. 2. Head and sense organs: Headache, dizziness, tinnitus, deafness, pain of anterior side of ear, redness and pain of eyes, blurred vision, toothache, swelling of neck, sore throat. 3. Mental: Manic depression and insanity, timidity. 4. Digestive: Abdominal pain, vomiting, diarrhea, dysentery, constipation, appendicitis. 5. Respiratory: Fullness in chest, cough, asthma. 6. Other: Scrofula, goiter, eczema, urticaria, scabies, erysipelas, furuncle, dry skin, hypertension, febrile diseases, prolonged fever, malaria, common cold, diabetes, back pain, lumbago, edema.
LI-12 Zhouliao ⊥ *0.5-0.8 cun.* *ß is applicable.*	With the elbow flexed, on the lateral side of the upper arm, 1 cun above LI-11 Quchi, on the border of the humerus. 1. Removes obstruction from meridians and collaterals.	1. The meridian course: Pain and motor impairment of elbow and arm, stiffness, numbness and pain of elbow, paralysis of upper limb.
LI-13 Shouwuli ⊥ *0.5-0.8 cun.* *ß is applicable.*	On the lateral side of the upper arm and on the line connecting LI-11 Quchi and LI-15 Jianyu, 3 cun above LI-11 Quchi. 1. Relieves cough and stops bleeding. 2. Transforms phlegm and relieves swelling.	1. The meridian course: Stiffness, pain and motor impairment of elbow and arm, swelling of arm. 2. Respiratory: Cough, hemoptysis. 3. Digestive : Distention and pain in epigastric region, jaundice. 4. Other: Malaria, scrofula, timidity, somnolence.

Tab. II-3 Points of the Large Intestine Hand-Yangming Meridian (LI)

Point, Property , Method & Remarks	Location & Action	Categories of Diseases & Indications
LI-14 Binao *Crossing Point of the Collateral of LI* ⊥ *0.5-0.8 cun, or* ↘ *upwards 1-1.5 cun.* ᵟ *is applicable.*	On the lateral side of the arm, at the insertion of the deltoid muscle and on the line connecting LI-11 Quchi and LI-15 Jianyu, 7 cun above LI-11 Quchi. 1. Removes obstruction from meridian. 2. Brightens the eyes. 3. Resolves phlegm and disperses masses.	1. The meridian course: Stiffness and pain of neck, paralysis of arm. 2. Head and sense organs: Headache, swelling, pain and redness of eyes, excessive lacrimation. 3. Other: Chills and fever, scrofula.
LI-15 Jianyu *Crossing Point of LI & Yangqiao M.* ⊥ *0.5-1 cun.* ᵟ *is applicable.*	On the shoulder, superior to the deltoid muscle, in the depression anterior and inferior to the acromion when the arm is abducted or raised to the level of the shoulder. 1. Benefits sinews, promotes qi circulation to stop pain. 2. Expels wind and clears heat.	1. The meridian course: Hemiplegia, stiffness of hand and arm, atrophy and weak arm, soreness and pain of tendon and bone, pain and swelling of arm and shoulder, motor impairment of arm and hand. 2. Other: Urticaria, scrofula, goiter.
LI- 16 Jugu *Crossing Point of LI & Yangqiao M.* ⊥ *0.5 cun.* ᵟ *is applicable.*	On the shoulder, in the depression between the acromial extremity of the clavicle and scapular spine. 1. Removes obstructions from meridian and benefits joints. 2. Tranquilizes convulsion and subdues rebellious qi.	1. The meridian course: Pain of shoulder and back, pain and motor impairment of upper limbs, hemiparalysis. 2. Mental: Convulsion. 3. Other: Scrofula, goiter, urticaria, hemoptysis.
LI-17 Tianding ⊥ *0.3-0.5 cun.* ᵟ *is applicable.*	On the lateral side of the neck, at the posterior border of the sternocleidomastoid muscle beside the laryngeal protuberance, at the mid point of the line connecting LI-18 Futu and ST-12 Quepen. 1. Clears heat and relieves swelling. 2. Regulates and transforms phlegm.	1. Head and sense organs: Sore throat, sudden loose of voice, throat mass, wheezing due to retention of phlegm in throat. 2. Other : Scrofula, goiter.

Tab. II-3 Points of the Large Intestine Hand-Yangming Meridian (LI)

Point, Property , Method & Remarks	Location & Action	Categories of Diseases & Indications
LI-18 Futu ⊥ *0.5-0.8 cun.* ⊘ *is applicable.*	On the lateral side of the neck, beside laryngeal protuberance, between the anterior and posterior borders of the sternocleidomastoid muscle. 1. Benefits throat. 2. Relieve cough and asthma. 3. Resolves phlegm and disperses masses.	1. Head and sense organs: Sore throat, sudden loss of voice, mass in throat, bleeding from the root of the tongue. 2. Respiratory: Asthma, cough, wheezing due to retention of phlegm in throat. 3. Other: Scrofula, goiter, hiccup.
LI-19 Kouheliao ⊥ *0.2-0.4 cun.*	On the upper lip, directly below the lateral border of the nostril, on the level of DU-26 Shuigou. 1. Clears lung and benefits nose.	1. Head and sense organs: Soreness of the nose, nasal polyps, nasal obstruction, deviation of mouth. 2. Mental: Syncope, trismus.
LI-20 Yingxiang ↘ *towards root of nose 0.3-0.5 cun.*	In the nasolabial groove, beside the midpoint of the lateral border of the nasal ala. 1. Dispels external wind and clears heat. 2. Removes obstruction from nasal orifice.	1. Head and sense organs: Nasal obstruction, epistaxis, rhinitis, deviation of mouth and eyes, itching and swelling of face, nasal polyps, headache. 2. Other: Biliary ascariasis.

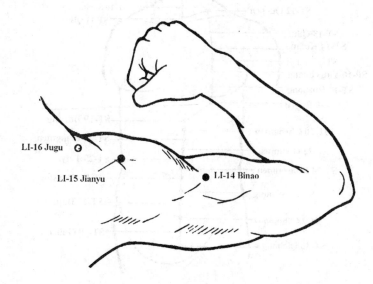

Fig. II-7 Points of the Large Intestine Meridian (3)

3. The Points of the Stomach Meridian of Foot-Yangming (ST)

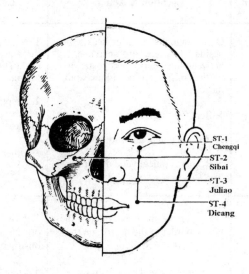

Fig. II-8 Points of the Stomach Meridian (1)

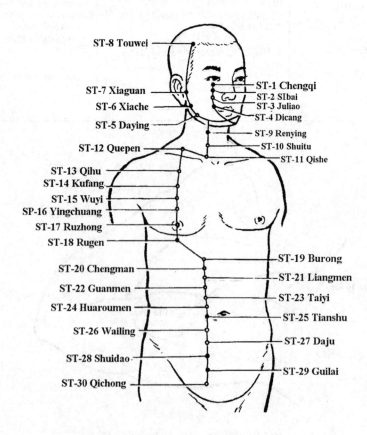

Fig. II-9 Points of the Stomach Meridian (2)

Tab. II-4 Points of the Stomach Meridian of Foot-Yangming (ST)

Point, Property , Method & Remarks	Location & Action	Categories of Diseases & Indications
ST-1 Chengqi *Crossing Point of Yangjiao M., RN & ST* ⊥ *0.5-1 cun along infraorbital ridge without lifting, thrusting or rotating manipulation.*	On the face, directly below the pupil, between the eyeball and the infraorbital ridge. 1. Expels wind and clears heat. 2. Brightens eyes and stops excessive lacrimation.	1. Head and sense organs: Eye lid tremors and spasms, conjunctival congestion with swelling and pain, epiphora induced by wind, nyctalopia, myopia, glaucoma, facial hemiparalysis, tinnitus, deafness. 2. Other: Hiccup, acute lumbar sprain, diabetes insipidus.
ST-2 Sibai ⊥ *0.2-0.3 cun.*	On the face, directly below the pupil, in the depression of the infraorbital foramen. 1. Expels wind and brightens eyes. 2. Comforts sinews and activates collaterals.	1. Head and sense organs: Eye lid tremors and spasms, conjunctival congestion with swelling and pain, epiphora induced by wind, nyctalopia, facial paralysis, vertigo, headache and facial pain, trigeminal neuralgia. 2. Other: Biliary ascariasis.
ST-3 Juliao *Crossing Point of Yangqiao M. & ST* ⊥ *0.3-0.4 cun.* *ᵐ is applicable.*	On the face, directly below the pupil, on the level of the lower border of the nasal ala, beside the nasolabial groove. 1. Expels wind and brightens eyes. 2. Comforts sinews and activates collaterals.	1. Head and sense organs: Facial pain, facial paralysis, eye lid tremors, clustered nebula, redness and pain in eye, conjunctival congestion and pain in lower orbit, blocked nose, epistaxis, toothache, swelling of lip and cheek, swelling of jaw. 2. Other: Beriberi, knee swelling.
ST-4 Dicang *Crossing Point of Yangqiao M., LI & ST* ⬊ *0.-5-1.5 cun.* *ᵐ is applicable.*	On the face, directly below the pupil, beside the mouth angle. 1. Expels wind, removes obstruction from meridian. 2. Benefits tendons and muscles.	1. Head and sense organs: Flaccid muscle with difficulty in closing mouth, eye lid tremors, deviation of mouth, toothache and cheek swelling, excessive salivation.

Tab. II-4 Points of the Stomach Meridian of Foot-Yangming (ST)

Point, Property , Method & Remarks	Location & Action	Categories of Diseases & Indications
ST-5 Daying ⊥ 0.3-0.4 cun. ᵭ is applicable. *Avoid puncturing the artery.*	Anterior to the mandibular angle, on the anterior border of the masseter muscle, where the pulsation of the facial artery is palpable. 1. Dispels wind and stops pain. 2. Activates collaterals and relieves swelling.	1. Head and sense organs: Trismus, deviation of mouth, cheek swelling, facial swelling, lip tremors, poor mobility of the tongue with difficulty in speaking and chewing. 2. Other: Fever with chills, cervical pain, apoplexy.
ST-6 Jiache ⊥ 0.3-0.4 cun, or ↪ towards ST-4 Dicang. ᵭ is applicable.	On the cheek, one finger breadth (middle finger) anterior and superior to the mandibular angle, in the depression where the masseter muscle is prominent. 1. Expels wind and clears heat. 2. Removes obstruction from meridian.	1. Head and sense organs: Toothache, facial paralysis, apoplexy, lockjaw, aphonia, difficulty in chewing, parotitis.
ST-7 Xiaguan *Crossing Point of GB & ST* ⊥ 0.3-0.5 cun. ᵭ is applicable.	On the face, anterior to the ear, in the depression between the zygomatic arch and mandibular notch. 1. Removes obstruction from meridian and relieves swelling & pain. 2. Benefits ear.	1. Head and sense organs: Facial pain, toothache, gingival swelling and pain, trismus with difficulty in opening and closing mouth, facial paralysis, deafness, tinnitus, ear pain, suppurative otitis media, vertigo.
ST-8 Touwei *Crossing Point of GB & Yangwei M.* ↪ 0.5-1 cun.	On the lateral side of the head, 0.5 cun above the anterior hairline at the corner of the forehead, and 4.5 cun lateral to the midline of the head. 1. Expels wind and clears heat. 2. Relieves pain and brightens eyes.	1. Head and sense organs: Headache, migraine, vertigo, eye pain, excessive lacrimation induced by wind, eyelid tremors.

Tab. II-4 Points of the Stomach Meridian of Foot-Yangming (ST)

Point, Property , Method & Remarks	Location & Action	Categories of Diseases & Indications
ST-9 Renying ⊥ 0.3-0.4 cun. *Avoid puncturing the common carotid artery.*	On the neck, beside the laryngeal protuberance, and on the anterior border of the sternocleidomastoid muscle where the pulsation of the common carotid artery is palpable. 1. Soothes chest oppression and relieves asthma. 2. Removes masses. 3. Benefits throat.	1. Head and sense organs: Headache, vertigo, sore throat. 2. Respiratory: Fullness sensation in chest, asthma. 3. Digestive: Cholera, vomiting, difficulty in swallowing.
ST-10 Shuitu ⊥ 0.3-0.5 cun. ᵟ is applicable.	On the neck and on the anterior border of sternocleidomastoid muscle, at the midpoint of the line connecting ST-9 Renying and ST-11 Qishe. 1. Descends lung qi. 2. Regulates qi and transforms phlegm.	1. Respiratory: Cough with dyspnea, shortness of breath with inability to fall sleep, sore throat. 2. Other: Scrofula, goiter, hiccup, swelling of shoulder.
ST-11 Qishe ⊥ 0.3-0.5 cun. ᵟ is applicable.	On the neck and on the upper border of the medial end of the clavicle, between the sternal and clavicular heads of sternocleidomastoid muscle. 1. Relieves swelling and benefits throat. 2. Subdues rebellious qi and relieves asthma.	1. Respiratory: Cough with dyspnea, asthma, choking sensation in chest, sore throat. 2. Other: Swollen shoulder, stiffness and pain of neck and nape.
ST-12 Quepen ⊥ 0.3-0.5 cun. ᵟ is applicable. *Deep ⊥ is prohibited.*	At the center of the supraclavicular fossa, 4 cun lateral to the anterior midline. 1. Subdues rebellious qi. 2. Relieves cough and asthma.	1. Respiratory: Cough, shortness of breath, hemoptysis, sore throat, choking sensation in chest, feverish sensation in chest.

Tab. II-4 Points of the Stomach Meridian of Foot-Yangming (ST)

Point, Property , Method & Remarks	Location & Action	Categories of Diseases & Indications
ST-13 Qihu ⊻ 0.3-0.5 cun. ᵟ is applicable.	On the chest, below the midpoint of the lower border of the clavicle, 4 cun lateral to the anterior midline. 1. Promotes descending and dispersing function of lung. 2. Relieves chest oppression and stops pain.	1. Respiratory: Cough, dyspnea, fullness sensation in chest and hypochondrium, sore throat. 2. Digestive: Hiccup, dysphasia, hematemesis.
ST-14 Kufang ⊻ 0.3-0.5 cun. ᵟ is applicable.	On the chest, in the 1st intercostal space, 4 cun lateral to the anterior midline. 1. Soothes chest oppression and dispels pus. 2. Relieves cough and asthma.	1. Respiratory: Cough, dyspnea, hemoptysis with pus, fullness sensation in chest and hypochondrium.
ST-15 Wuyi ⊻ 0.3-0.5 cun. ᵟ is applicable.	On the chest, in the 2nd intercostal space, 4 cun lateral to the anterior midline. 1. Transforms phlegm and stops cough. 2. Dredges water passages.	1. Respiratory: Cough, asthma, hemoptysis with pus, fullness sensation in chest and hypochondrium. 2. Other: Pruritis of whole body, rough and painful skin, acute mastitis.
ST-16 Yingchuang ⊻ 0.3-0.5 cun. ᵟ is applicable.	On the chest, in the 3rd intercostal space, 4 cun lateral to the anterior midline. 1. Clears heat and relieves edema. 2. Relieves cough and asthma.	1. Respiratory: Cough, asthma, distention and pain in chest and hypochondrium, shortness of breath. 2. Digestive: Diarrhea, borborygmus. 3. Other: Mastitis, swollen lips.
ST-17 Ruzhong *Puncture and ᵟ are contraindicated.*	On the chest, in the 4th intercostal space, at the center of the nipple, 4 cun lateral to the anterior midline.	This point serves as a reference only, it has no therapeutic value.

Tab. II-4 Points of the Stomach Meridian of Foot-Yangming (ST)

Point, Property , Method & Remarks	Location & Action	Categories of Diseases & Indications
ST-18 Rugen ⩤ *0.3-0.5 cun.* *ᵹ is applicable.*	On the chest, directly below the nipple, on the lower border of the breast, in the 5th intercostal space, 4 cun lateral to the anterior midline. 1. Regulates stomach qi. 2. Regulates breast and lactation. 3. Disperses stagnation.	1. Respiratory: Cough, feeling of oppression in chest, swelling pain in chest. 2. Digestive: Dysphasia, regurgitation with vomiting, acute abdominal distention, difficulty in breathing with sensation of qi ascending to heart and chest. 3. Other: Mastitis, shortness of lactation.
ST-19 Burong ⩒ *0.5-0.8 cun.* *ᵹ is applicable.*	On the upper abdomen, 6 cun above the center of the umbilicus and 2 cun lateral to the anterior midline. 1. Regulates stomach to stop vomiting. 2. Descends rebellious qi to relieve asthma.	1. Respiratory: Cough, hemoptysis, asthma. 2. Digestive: Epigastralgia, vomiting, abdominal distention, borborygmus, hematemesis, dry mouth, poor appetite, indigestion with food retention in children. 3. Cardiovascular: Precordial pain, chest pain radiating to back, pain in hypochondrium. 4. Other: Hernia, nyctalopia.
ST-20 Chengman ⩒ *0.5-1 cun.* *ᵹ is applicable.*	On the upper abdomen, 5 cun above the center of the umbilicus and 2 cun lateral to the anterior midline. 1. Regulates qi and stomach. 2. Subdues rebellious qi and stops vomiting.	1. Respiratory: Asthma, tense pain in chest and hypochondrium. 2. Digestive: Stomachache, vomiting, hematemesis, abdominal distention, borborygmus, dysentery, poor appetite, indigestion, loose stool. 3. Other: Phlegm retention, general body swelling, convulsion.
ST-21 Liangmen ⩒ *0.5-1 cun.* *ᵹ is applicable.*	On the upper abdomen, 4 cun above the center of the umbilicus and 2 cun lateral to the anterior midline. 1. Regulates stomach and subdues rebellious qi. 2. Stops vomiting. 3. Removes food stagnation and relieves pain.	1. Digestive: Stomachache, vomiting, poor appetite, loose stool, fullness in hypochondrium and abdomen. 2. Other: Rectal prolapse, abdominal mass in women.

Tab. II-4 Points of the Stomach Meridian of Foot-Yangming (ST)

Point, Property , Method & Remarks	Location & Action	Categories of Diseases & Indications
ST-22 Guanmen ⊥ 0.5-1 cun. ᗡ is applicable.	On the upper abdomen, 3 cun above the center of the umbilicus and 2 cun lateral to the anterior midline. 1. Strengthens spleen and stomach. 2. Promotes urination to relieve edema.	1. Digestive: Abdominal pain or distention, borborygmus and diarrhea, poor appetite. 2. Urinary: Enuresis, ascites, general body swelling.
ST-23 Taiyi ⊥ 0.5-1 cun. ᗡ is applicable.	On the upper abdomen, 2 cun above the center of the umbilicus and 2 cun lateral to the anterior midline. 1. Clears heart and calms mind. 2. Regulates stomach and transforms phlegm.	1. Digestive: Stomachache, dysphagia. 2. Mental: Manic-depressive psychosis, involuntary movements of the tongue, vexation. 3. Other: Hernia, beriberi, enuresis.
ST-24 Huaroumen ⊥ 0.5-1 cun. ᗡ is applicable.	On the upper abdomen, 1 cun above the center of the umbilicus and 2 cun lateral to the anterior midline. 1. Transforms phlegm and calms mind. 2. Regulates stomach and stops vomiting.	1. Digestive: Stomachache, vomiting, hematemesis, rectal prolapse. 2. Mental: Manic-depressive psychosis, epilepsy, involuntary movements of the tongue, poor mobility of the tongue.

Tab. II-4 Points of the Stomach Meridian of Foot-Yangming (ST)

Point, Property , Method & Remarks	Location & Action	Categories of Diseases & Indications
ST-25 Tianshu *Front Mu Point of Large Intestine* ⊥ *0.7-1.2 cun.* Ꝼ *is applicable.*	On the middle abdomen, 2 cun lateral to the center of the umbilicus. 1. Promotes function of intestines. 2. Clears heat and removes dampness. 3. Regulates qi. 4. Relieves food retention.	1. Digestive: Diarrhea, dysentery, constipation, abdominal distention, borborygmus, acute appendicitis, stomachache, vomiting, jaundice. 2. Gynecopathies: Irregular menstruation, continuous menstruation, mass in abdomen, metrorrhagia and metrostaxis, dysmenorrhea, amenorrhea, leukorrhea, postpartum colic, sterility. 3. Urinary: Difficult urination, edema, stranguria with turbid urine. 4. Mental: Convulsion, ravings, trance. 5. Other: Tympanites, umbilical hernia, pain around navel, sensation of gas moving, malaria, lumbago, vertigo, chronic wasting syndromes.
ST-26 Wailing ⊥ *0.7-1.2 cun.* Ꝼ *is applicable.*	On the lower abdomen, 1 cun below the center of the umbilicus and 2 cun lateral to the anterior midline. 1. Promotes qi flow to stop pain. 2. Regulates menstruation.	1. Acute appendicitis, hernia, dysmenorrhea.
ST-27 Daju ⊥ *0.7-1.2 cun.* Ꝼ *is applicable.*	On the lower abdomen, 2 cun below the center of the umbilicus and 2 cun lateral to the anterior midline. 1. Promotes qi flow to relieve distention. 2. Regulates intestines to remove water.	1. Urogenital: Distention in lower abdomen, difficult urination, spontaneous seminal emission, impotence, premature ejaculation. 2. Mental: Palpitation due to fright with difficulty in falling sleep. 3. Other: Hemiplegia.
ST-28 Shuidao ⊥ *0.7-1.2 cun.* Ꝼ *is applicable.*	On the lower abdomen, 3 cun below the center of the umbilicus and 2 cun lateral to the anterior midline. 1. Promotes urination. 2. Opens water passages. 3. Regulates menstruation and helps improve women's fertility.	1. Urogenital: Difficult urination, dysmenorrhea, lower abdominal pain radiating to external genitals. 2. Other: Constipation, hernia, rigidity and pain in spine and around waist.

Tab. II-4 Points of the Stomach Meridian of Foot-Yangming (ST)

Point, Property , Method & Remarks	Location & Action	Categories of Diseases & Indications
ST-29 Guilai ⊥ *0.7-1.2 cun.* *ʓ is applicable.*	On the lower abdomen, 4 cun below the center of the umbilicus, and 2 cun lateral to the anterior midline. 1. Soothes liver and promotes qi flow. 2. Relieves stagnation of blood. 3. Regulates menstruation and arrests leukorrhagia.	1. Reproductive: Amenorrhea, leukorrhea, sterility, retraction of testis into abdomen, pain in penis.
ST-30 Qichong ⊥ *0.5-1 cun.* *ʓ is applicable.*	Slightly above the inguinal groove, 5 cun below the center of the umbilicus and 2 cun lateral to the anterior midline. 1. Soothes liver and reinforces kidney. 2. Regulates Chong Meridian and menstruation. 3. Nourishes essence and helps improve women's fertility.	1. Reproductive: Pain and swelling of vulva, irregular menstruation, sterility, difficult labor, retention of placenta; impotence, penile pain, testicular pain. 2. Other: Sensation of gas moving in abdomen or chest, lumbago, rectal prolapse.
ST-31 Biguan ⊥ *1-1.5 cun.* *ʓ is applicable.*	On the anterior side of the thigh, on the line connecting the anterio-superior iliac spine and the superolateral corner of the patella, at the level of the perineum when the thigh is flexed, in the depression lateral to the sartorius muscle. 1.Removes obstruction from meridian and collaterals.	1. The meridian course: Pain in the waist and lower limbs, muscular contracture, flaccidity of thigh muscles, numbness in lower limbs, coldness in knees, lower abdominal pain radiating to leg.
ST-32 Futu ⊥ *1-1.5 cun.* *ʓ is applicable.*	On the anterior side of the thigh, on the line connecting the anterio-superior iliac spine and the supero-lateral corner of the patella, 6 cun above this corner. 1. Removes obstruction from meridian and collaterals. 2. Dispels cold and removes dampness.	1. The meridian course: Pain in waist and hip, coldness and pain in legs and knees with numbness. 2. Other: Diabetes, periumbilical colic due to invasion of cold, beriberi, abdominal pain, edema.

Tab. II-4 Points of the Stomach Meridian of Foot-Yangming (ST)

Point, Property , Method & Remarks	Location & Action	Categories of Diseases & Indications
ST-33 Yinshi ↓ *1-1.5 cun.* 𝄃 *is applicable.*	On the anterior side of the thigh and on the line connecting anteriosuperior iliac spine and the superolateral corner of the patella, 3 cun above this corner. 1. Warms meridians and dispels cold.	1. The meridian course: Numbness and pain in leg and knee with difficulty in bending and stretching, paralysis, lumbago, beriberi, edema of lower limbs. 2. Digestive: Abdominal distention, abdominal pain, edema.
ST-34 Liangqiu *Xi-Cleft Point* ↓ *0.5-1 cun.* 𝄃 *is applicable.*	With the knee flexed, on the anterior side of the thigh and on the line connecting the anterio-superior iliac spine and the supero-lateral corner of the patella, 2 cun above this corner. 1. Subdues rebellious stomach qi. 2. Removes obstruction from the meridian.	1. The meridian course: Paralysis, swollen knee, swelling and pain in the waist and knee, cold limbs with difficulty in flexing and extending, mastitis. 2. Digestive: Stomachache.
ST-35 Dubi ↓ *0.5-1 cun.* 𝄃 *is applicable.*	With the knee flexed, on the knee, in the depression lateral to the patella and its ligament. 1. Invigorates meridians and collaterals. 2. Relieves swelling and stops pain.	1. Pain in the knee with difficulty in kneeling, flaccidity of lower limbs.

Tab. II-4 Points of the Stomach Meridian of Foot-Yangming (ST)

Point, Property , Method & Remarks	Location & Action	Categories of Diseases & Indications
ST-36 Zusanli *He-Sea Point* ± *0.5-1.2 cun.* ᵟ *is applicable.*	On the antero-lateral side of the leg, 3 cun below ST-35 Dubi, one finger breadth (middle finger) from the anterior crest of the tibia. 1. Benefits stomach and spleen. 2. Tonifies qi and blood and strengthens body resistance. 3. Regulates nutritive and defensive qi. 4. Regulates intestines and stomach, transforms phlegm and resolves dampness. 5. Raises yang.	1. The meridian course: Paralysis, flaccidity, swelling and pain in the foot and knee. 2. Head and sense organs: Blurred vision, dryness in nose, stuffy nose, deafness, tinnitus, facial paralysis, sore throat. 3. Digestive: Stomachache, poor appetite, fullness of abdomen, vomiting, hiccup, borborygmus, diarrhea, abdominal pain, dysentery, children's indigestion with food retention, constipation. 4. Cardiovascular: Palpitation, feeling of oppression in chest and shortness of breath, sudden precordial pain. 5. Respiratory: Cough, asthma, excessive expectoration, pulmonary tuberculosis. 6. Urinary: Enuresis, difficult urination, edema. 7. Reproductive: Postpartum vertigo, abdominal pain after childbirth, leukorrhea, morning sickness. 8. Mental: Manic-depressive psychosis, inappropriate wild or maniacal laughter, hysteria, apoplexy. 9. Skin: Furuncle, urticaria. 10. Other: Insufficient vitality qi, severe emaciation, weakness caused by seven emotional impairments, pain and swelling of lower abdomen.

Tab. II-4 Points of the Stomach Meridian of Foot-Yangming (ST)

Point, Property , Method & Remarks	Location & Action	Categories of Diseases & Indications
ST-37 Shangjuxu *Lower He-Sea Point of Large Intestine* ⊥ *0.5-1 cun.* 𝛿 *is applicable.*	On the anterolateral side of the leg, 6 cun below ST-35 Dubi, one finger breadth (middle finger) from the anterior crest of the tibia. 1. Regulates function of stomach and intestines. 2. Eliminates damp heat. 3. Dispels retention of food. 4. Calms asthma.	1. The meridian course: Paralysis, flaccidity with pain and numbness, pain in waist and knees with difficulty in bending and stretching, general edema of lower limbs. 2. Digestive: Acute appendicitis, abdominal colic, abdominal distention and borborygmus, dysentery, stomachache, constipation, diarrhea, poor appetite. 3. Other: Insufficient vitality qi, emaciation with weakness, beriberi, retention of urine, sensation of gas flowing from abdomen to chest, fullness in chest and hypochondrium.
ST-38 Tiaokou ⊥ *0.5-1 cun.* 𝛿 *is applicable.*	On the superolateral side of the leg, 8 cun below ST-35 Dubi, one finger breadth (middle finger) from the anterior crest of the tibia. 1. Removes dampness and warms meridians. 2. Relieves rigidity of muscles and activates collaterals.	1. The meridian course: Pain of shoulder and arm, painful numbness of thigh and knee, spasm, flaccidity of feet, cold feet, heat sensation and pain in sole. 2. Digestive: Stomachache, abdominal pain, dysentery. 3. Other: Beriberi, pain in enterocele, sore throat.
ST-39 Xiajuxu *Lower He-Sea Point of Small Intestine* ⊥ *0.5-1 cun.* 𝛿 *is applicable.*	On the anterolateral side of the leg, 9 cun below ST-35 Dubi, one finger breadth (middle finger) from the anterior crest of the tibia. 1. Regulates function of stomach and intestines. 2. Eliminates damp-heat. 3. Eliminates wind-damp. 4. Stops pain.	1. The meridian course: Paralysis, flaccidity of lower limbs with difficulty in walking, plantar fasciitis or pain in the toes, edema of lower limbs. 2. Digestive: Diarrhea, stool with pus and blood, dysentery, stomachache, poor appetite, emaciation. 3. Head and sense organs: Dry lips, salivation, inflammation of throat. 4. Mental: Epilepsy, sudden terror, ravings. 5. Other: Pain in lower abdomen, pain in waist and spine radiating to lower abdomen, pain in chest and hypochondrium, breast pain.

Tab. II-4 Points of the Stomach Meridian of Foot-Yangming (ST)

Point, Property , Method & Remarks	Location & Action	Categories of Diseases & Indications
ST-40 Fenglong *Luo-Connecting Point* ⊥ *0.5-1 cun.* ᵭ *is applicable.*	On the anterolateral side of the leg, 8 cun above the tip of the external malleolus, lateral to ST-38 Tiaokou, and two finger breadths (middle finger) from the anterior crest of the tibia. 1. Resolves phlegm. 2. Eliminates dampness. 3. Calms asthma. 4. Clears heat. 5. Calms and clears mind. 6. Relieves chest oppression.	1. The meridian course: Flaccidity of lower limbs, swelling and pain or flaccidity of legs, difficulty in plantar or solar flexion. 2. Digestive: Colic in abdomen, diarrhea, dysentery, constipation. 3. Head and sense organs: Headache, vertigo, sore throat, aphonia. 4. Respiratory: Cough, asthma, excessive expectoration. 5. Cardiovascular: Cardiac pain, pain in chest and hypochondrium. 6. Urinary: Retention of urine, edema of limbs, heavy sensation in limbs, edema of face. 7. Gynecopathies: Amenorrhea, metrorrhagia. 8. Mental: Madness, epilepsy, susceptibility to inappropriate laughter, dysphoria, apoplexy, insomnia. 9. Other: Beriberi.
ST-41 Jiexi *Jing-Well Point* ⊥ *0.5-0.7 cun.* ᵭ *is applicable.*	In the central depression of the crease between the dorsum of the foot and leg, between the tendons of the long extensor muscle of the great toe and the long extensor muscle of the toes. 1. Clears heat from stomach and intestines and subdues rebellious qi. 2. Tranquilizes convulsion and calms mind.	1. The meridian course: Flaccidity in lower limbs with swelling, pain and heavy sensation. 2. Head and sense organs: Edema of head and face, flushed face, eye pain, nebula, headache, vertigo, pain in supra-orbital bone. 3. Digestive: Abdominal distention, constipation, stomachache. 4. Mental: Epilepsy, convulsion, delirium. 5. Other: Malaria, muscle spasm, febrile diseases with difficulty in sweating, palpitation.

Tab. II-4 Points of the Stomach Meridian of Foot-Yangming (ST)

Point, Property , Method & Remarks	Location & Action	Categories of Diseases & Indications
ST-42 Chongyang *Yuan-Source Point* ⊥ *0.3-0.5 cun.* δ *is applicable.* *Avoid puncturing the artery.*	On the dome of the dorsum of the foot, between the tendons of the long extensor muscle of the great toe and the long extensor muscle of the toes, where the pulsation of the dorsal artery of the foot is palpable. 1. Tonifies stomach and spleen. 2. Calms mind. 3. Removes obstruction from meridian.	1. The meridian course: Flaccidity of feet with weakness, red and swollen instep, paralysis. 2. Head and sense organs: Headache, pain in forehead, edema of face, facial hemiparalysis. 3. Digestive: Stomachache, abdominal distention, poor appetite. 4. Mental: Manic psychosis, susceptibility to fright, convulsion. 5. Other: Malaria, fever with anhidrosis.
ST-43 Xiangu *Shu-Stream Point* ⊥ *0.3-0.5 cun.* δ *is applicable.*	On the instep of the foot, in the depression distal to the junction of the 2nd and 3rd metatarsal bones. 1. Regulates stomach and intestines. 2. Strengthens spleen to remove water.	1. Digestive: Epigastric pain, borborygmus, abdominal distention and pain, ascites, over-susceptibility to eructations. 2. Head and sense organs: Edema of face, conjunctival congestion with pain, weakness of upper eyelid. 3. Other: Swelling and pain of instep, febrile diseases without sweating, malaria, hysteria, night sweating, hypochondriac pain, hiccup, hernia.
ST-44 Neiting *Ying-Spring Point* ⊥ *0.3-0.5 cun.* δ *is applicable.*	On the instep of the foot, at the junction of the red and white skin proximal to the margin of the web between the 2nd and 3rd toes. 1. Clears heat from stomach and intestines. 2. Regulates spleen and stomach and promotes digestion.	1. The meridian course: Pain in tibia with difficulty in bending the leg. 2. Head and sense organs: Toothache, swollen gums, deviation of mouth, trismus, epistaxis, inflammation of throat, edema of face, deafness. 3. Digestive: Stomachache, abdominal pain, diarrhea, constipation, dysentery, acute appendicitis. 4. Other: Urticaria, hysteria, enterocele, bloody urine, fever with chills, malaria with poor appetite.

Tab. II-4 Points of the Stomach Meridian of Foot-Yangming (ST)

Point, Property , Method & Remarks	Location & Action	Categories of Diseases & Indications
ST-45 Lidui *Jing-Well Point* ↳ *0.1 cun, or prick to cause bleeding.* δ *is applicable.*	On the lateral side of the distal segment of the 2nd toe, 0.1 cun from the corner of the toenail. 1. Clears heat and dampness. 2. Regulates stomach and calms mind. 3. Relieves food retention.	1. The meridian course: Swelling and pain in front of knee, cold in dorsum of foot, pain in breast. 2. Head and sense organs: Edema of face, toothache,　deviation of mouth, edema of lips, edema of neck, epistaxis, nasal obstruction, running nose. 3. Digestive: Abdominal fullness, jaundice, polyphagia. 4. Mental: Madness, susceptibility to palpitation, corpse-like syncope with lockjaw. 5. Other: Febrile diseases without sweating, edema, malaria with chills, dark urine.

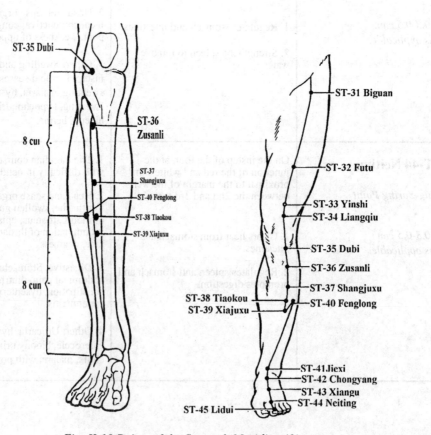

Fig. II-10 Points of the Stomach Meridian (3)

4. The Points of the Spleen Meridian of Foot-Taiyin (SP)

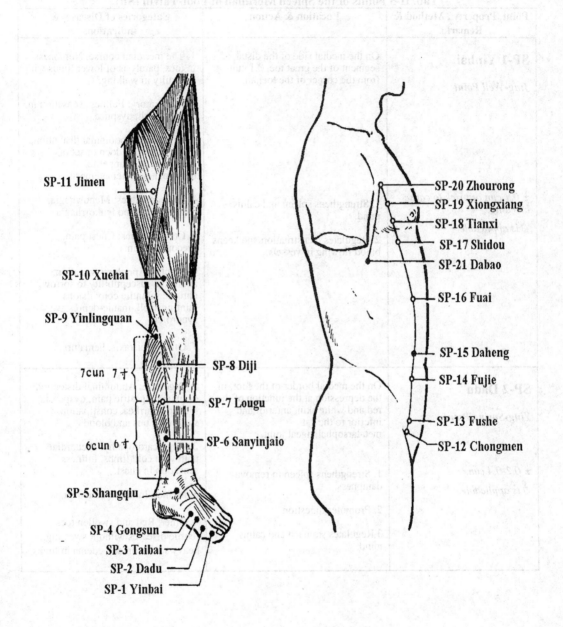

Fig. II-11 Points of the Spleen Meridian (1)

Tab. II-5 Points of the Spleen Meridian of Foot-Taiyin (SP)

Point, Property , Method & Remarks	Location & Action	Categories of Diseases & Indications
SP-1 Yinbai *Jing-Well Point* *⊥ 0.1 cun or prick to cause bleeding.* *◊ is applicable.*	On the medial side of the distal segment of the great toe, 0.1 cun from the corner of the toenail. 1. Strengthens spleen and calms mind. 2. Regulates menstruation and keeps blood flowing in vessels.	1. The meridian course: Numbness in toes, paralysis of lower limbs with difficulty in walking. 2. Respiratory: Fullness sensation in chest, cough, dyspnea. 3. Digestive: Abdominal distention, diarrhea with sudden onset of vomiting, poor appetite, hematochezia, hematemesis. 4. Gynecopathies: Menorrhagia, metrorrhagia and leukorrhagia. 5. Cardiopathies: Chest pain, precordial pain. 6. Mental: Apoplexy, vexation, abnormal susceptibility to sorrow, chronic infantile convulsions, fainting spell, manic-depressive syndrome. 7. Other: Epistaxis, hematuria.
SP-2 Dadu *Ying-Spring Point* *⊥ 0.2-0.4 cun.* *◊ is applicable.*	On the medial border of the foot, in the depression at the junction of the red and white skin, anterior and inferior to the 1st metatarsophalangeal joint. 1. Strengthens spleen to remove dampness. 2. Promotes digestion. 3 Regulates stomach and calms mind.	1. Digestive: Abdominal distention or pain, epigastric pain, dyspepsia, hiccup, diarrhea, constipation, stool with pus and blood. 2. Angiocardiopathy: Precordial pain with cold limbs, fullness sensation in chest. 3. Mental: Infantile convulsions. 4. Other: Red and swollen toes, febrile diseases without sweating, heavy sensation and edema in limbs.

Tab. II-5 Points of the Spleen Meridian of Foot-Taiyin (SP)

Point, Property , Method & Remarks	Location & Action	Categories of Diseases & Indications
SP-3 Taibai *Shu-Stream and Yuan-Source Point* ⊥ *0.3-0.5 cun.* ᵇ *is applicable.*	On the medial border of the foot, in the depression at the junction of the red and white skin, posterior and inferior to the 1st metatarsophalangeal joint. 1. Strengthens spleen to resolve dampness. 2. Regulates qi and stomach, strengthens spine.	1. The meridian course: Soreness of thigh and knee, heavy sensation of body, flaccidity syndrome. 2. Digestive: Stomachache, abdominal distention or pain, borborygmus, vomiting, diarrhea, dysentery, constipation, anorexia, eructation, dyspepsia. 3. Angiocardiopathy: Precordial pain with slow pulse, sensation of fullness and pain in the chest and hypochondrium. 4. Other: Beriberi, feverish sensation accompanied with restlessness.
SP-4 Gongsun *Luo-Connecting Point;* *Yuan-Source Point;* *One of Eight Confluent Points, linking to Chong M.* ⊥ *0.5-0.8 cun.* ᵇ *is applicable.*	On the medial border of the foot, anterior and inferior to the proximal end of the 1st metatarsal bone. 1. Tonifies stomach and spleen. 2. Regulates Chong Meridian and stops bleeding. 3. Dispels abdominal fullness. 4. Regulates menstruation.	1. Digestive: Stomachache, vomiting, diarrhea, dyspepsia, borborygmus, abdominal distention or pain, dysentery, hematochezia, excessive drinking of alcohol. 2. Gynecopathies: Irregular menstruation, metrorrhagia and metrostaxis, leukorrhagia. 3. Mental: Mania, epilepsy, excessive vexation, insomnia. 4. Other: Edema of face and head, general edema, drowsiness, jaundice, beriberi, malarial, hot sensation in the soles.

Tab. II-5 Points of the Spleen Meridian of Foot-Taiyin (SP)

Point, Property , Method & Remarks	Location & Action	Categories of Diseases & Indications
SP-5 Shangqiu *Jing-River Point* ⊥ *0.2-0.4 cun.* ᪲ *is applicable.*	In the depression anterior and inferior to the medial malleolus, at the midpoint of the line connecting the tuberosity of the navicular bone and the tip of the medial malleolus. 1. Strengthens spleen and stomach. 2. Resolves dampness. 3. Subdues rebellious qi of lung.	1. The meridian course: Pain of medial side of thigh, red and swollen medial malleolus, foot weakness. 2. Respiratory: Cough, dyspnea. 3. Digestive: Abdominal distention, borborygmus, diarrhea, constipation, dyspepsia, jaundice, stomachache. 4. Gynecopathy: Sterility. 5. Mental: Manic-depressive syndrome, susceptibility to laugh, infantile convulsion, melancholia. 6. Other: Hemorrhoids, poor mobility of tongue.
SP-6 Sanyinjiao *Crossing Point of SP, LR & KI* ⊥ *0.5-1 cun.* ᪲ *is applicable.*	On the medial side of the leg, 3 cun above the tip of the medial malleolus, posterior to the medial border of the tibia. 1. Strengthens spleen and resolves dampness. 2. Promotes liver function and soothes liver qi. 3. Tonifies kidney and nourishes blood and yin. 4. Promotes urination. 5. Regulates menstruation. 6. Moves blood and eliminates stasis. 7. Stops pain and calms mind.	1. The meridian course: Hemiplegia due to apoplexy, poliomyelitis, pain in medial side of thigh. 2. Head and sense organs: Inflammation of throat, poor mobility of the tongue, epistaxis. 3. Respiratory: Cough, pulmonary tuberculosis. 4. Digestive: Vomiting, hiccup, fullness and pain in chest and abdomen, epigastralgia, indigestion, anorexia, borborygmus, abdominal pain, diarrhea, dysentery, jaundice, edema, heavy sensation in body. 5. Urinary: Uroschesia, enuresis, stranguria, gonorrhea. 6. Reproductive: Seminal emissions, impotence, premature ejaculation, pain in penis, hernia, irregular menstruation, dysmenorrhea, amenorrhea, leukorrhea with reddish discharge, prolapse of uterus, lochiostasis or lochiorrhea, sterility, mass in abdomen, retention of placenta, metrorrhagia and metrostaxis.

Tab. II-5 Points of the Spleen Meridian of Foot-Taiyin (SP)

Point, Property , Method & Remarks	Location & Action	Categories of Diseases & Indications
SP-7 Lougu ⊥ *0.5-1 cun.* ᵭ *is applicable.*	On the medial side of the leg and on the line connecting the tip of the medial malleolus and SP-9 Yinlingquan, 6 cun from the tip of the medial malleolus, posterior to the medial border of the tibia. 1. Strengthens spleen and relieves edema. 2. Promotes urination and removes dampness.	1. The meridian course: Arthralgia, beriberi, coldness and numbness of knees and legs, painful and swollen ankle. 2. Digestive: Abdominal distention, borborygmus, dyspepsia, emaciation. 3. Urogenital: Dysuria, seminal emission.
SP-8 Diji *Xi-Cleft Point* ⊥ *0.5-1 cun.* ᵭ *is applicable.*	On the medial side of the leg and on the line connecting the tip of the medial malleolus and SP-9 Yinlingquan, 3 cun below SP-9 Yinlingquan. 1. Strengthens spleen and removes dampness. 2. Regulates menstruation. 3. Regulates qi and blood and stops pain.	1. The meridian course: Pain in medial side of thigh. 2. Digestive: Abdominal distention, borborygmus, vomiting, diarrhea, anorexia. 3. Reproductive: Pain in penis, seminal emission, irregular menstruation, dysmenorrhea, prolapse of uterus. 4. Urinary: Dysuria, incontinence of urine, edema. 5. Mental: Insomnia, neurasthenia.
SP-9 Yinlingquan *He-Sea Point* ⊥ *0.5-1 cun.* ᵭ *is applicable.*	On the medial side of the leg, in the depression posterior and inferior to the medial condyle of the tibia. 1. Strengthens spleen and removes dampness. 2. Reinforces kidney and consolidates essence. 3. Benefits lower-jiao and promotes urination.	1. The meridian course: Hemiplegia, painful and swollen legs and knees. 2. Digestive: Abdominal distention or pain, anorexia, vomiting, diarrhea, jaundice. 3. Reproductive: Seminal emission, pain in penis, leukorrhea, prolapse of uterus. 4. Urinary: Dysuria, edema, incontinence of urine, stranguria. 5. Other: Emaciation, headache.

Tab. II-5 Points of the Spleen Meridian of Foot-Taiyin (SP)

Point, Property , Method & Remarks	Location & Action	Categories of Diseases & Indications
SP-10 Xuehai ⊥ *0.5-1.2 cun* ᵹ *is applicable.*	With the knee flexed, on the medial side of the thigh, 2 cun above the superior medial corner of the patella, on the prominence of the medial head of the quadriceps muscle of the thigh. 1. Strengthens spleens and removes dampness. 2. Regulates menstruation. 3. Cools blood. 4. Removes blood stasis. 5. Tonifies blood.	1. Digestive: Abdominal distention. 2. Gynecopathies: Irregular menstruation, dysmenorrhea, amenorrhea, metrorrhagia and metrostaxis, leukorrhea, pruritis vulvae, swelling and pain of vulva, lochiostasis. 3. Urinary: Stranguria. 4. Skin: Eczema, urticaria, pruritis, erysipelas, any sores on the medial thigh. 5. Other: Anemia.
SP-11 Jimen ⊥ *0.5-1 cun* ᵹ *is applicable.*	On the medial side of the thigh and on the line connecting SP-10 Xuehai and SP-12 Chongmen, 6 cun above SP-10 Xuehai. 1. Strengthens spleen and removes dampness. 2. Clears heat and promotes urination.	1. Urinary: Dysuria, enuresis, stranguria. 2. Skin and surgical: Swelling and pain in groin, soreness of the thighs, scrotal eczema.
SP-12 Chongmen ***Crossing Point of SP & LR*** ⊥ *0.5-1 cun.* ᵹ *is applicable.* ***Avoid puncturing the artery.***	At the lateral end of the inguinal groove, 3.5 cun lateral to the midpoint of the upper border of the symphysis pubis and lateral to the pulsation of the external iliac artery. 1. Strengthens spleen and removes dampness. 2. Promotes qi flow and relieves hemorrhoids.	1. Digestive: Abdominal distention or pain. 2. Gynecopathies: Edema during pregnancy, leukorrhea, postpartum hemorrhage. 3. Urinary: Dysuria. 4. Other: Hemorrhoids, hernia, abdominal mass.
SP-13 Fushe ⊥ *0.5-1 cun.* ᵹ *is applicable.*	On the lower abdomen, 4 cun below the center of the umbilicus, 0.7 cun above SP-12 Chongmen, and 4 cun lateral to the anterior midline. 1. Strengthens spleen and relieves abdominal fullness. 2. Regulates stomach.	1. Digestive: Vomiting and diarrhea due to cholera, constipation. 2. Other: Pain in theabdomen due to a mass, fullness and pain in lower abdomen.

Tab. II-5 Points of the Spleen Meridian of Foot-Taiyin (SP)

Point, Property , Method & Remarks	Location & Action	Categories of Diseases & Indications
SP-14 Fujie ⊥ *0.5-1 cun.* ∂ *is applicable.*	On the lower abdomen, 1.3 cun below SP-15 Daheng, and 4 cun lateral to the anterior midline. 1. Warms spleen and arrests diarrhea. 2. Relieves pain and stops cough.	1. Digestive: Diarrhea, dysentery, pain around the navel. 2. Other: Hernia.
SP-15 Daheng ⊥ *0.5-1 cun.* ∂ *is applicable.*	On the middle abdomen, 4 cun lateral to the center of the umbilicus. 1. Strengthens spleen & limbs. 2. Regulates qi & stops pain. 3. Promotes function of large intestine.	1. Digestive: Diarrhea, dysentery, constipation, abdominal pain, ascariasis, gastroptosis. 2. Other: Coldness and spasm of limbs, hyperhidrosis.
SP-16 Fu'ai ⊥ *0.5-1 cun.* ∂ *is applicable.*	On the upper abdomen, 3 cun above the center of the umbilicus, and 4 cun lateral to the anterior midline. 1. Strengthens spleen and improves digestion. 2. Improves function of large intestine.	1. Digestive: Stomachache, pain around navel, dysentery, dyspepsia.
SP-17 Shidou ⊾ *0.3-0.5 cun.* ∂ *is applicable.*	On the lateral side of the chest and in the 5th intercostal space, 6 cun lateral to the anterior midline. 1. Promotes digestion. 2. Regulates stomach and subdues rebellious qi.	1. Respiratory: Fullness in chest and hypochondrium, edema, dyspnea. 2. Digestive: Abdominal distention, borborygmus, abdominal pain, frequent vomiting.
SP-18 Tianxi ⊾ *0.3-0.5 cun.* ∂ *is applicable.*	On the lateral side of the chest and in the 4th intercostal space, 6 cun lateral to the anterior midline. 1. Soothes chest oppression and promotes lactation. 2. Stops cough and relieves edema.	1. Respiratory: Cough, dyspnea, excessive expectoration. 2. Breast: Acute mastitis, poor lactation.

Tab. II-5 Points of the Spleen Meridian of Foot-Taiyin (SP)

Point, Property , Method & Remarks	Location & Action	Categories of Diseases & Indications
SP-19 Xiongxiang ⩗ 0.3-0.5 cun. ᵷ is applicable.	On the lateral side of the chest and in the 3rd intercostal space, 6 cun lateral to the anterior midline. 1. Promotes qi flow and relieves chest oppression. 2. Soothes liver and alleviates pain.	1. Respiratory: Difficulty in lying and turning the body due to chest pain, cough. 2. Breast: Acute mastitis, poor lactation.
SP-20 Zhourong ⩗ 0.3-0.5 cun. ᵷ is applicable.	On the lateral side of the chest and in the 2nd intercostal space, 6 cun lateral to the anterior midline. 1. Promotes qi flow and relieves chest oppression. 2. Descends lung qi to stop cough.	1. Respiratory: Cough, dyspnea, pain in chest and hypochondrium. 2. Other: Poor appetite.
SP-21 Dabao *Luo-Connecting Point* ⩗ 0.3-0.5 cun. ᵷ is applicable.	On the lateral side of the chest and on the middle axillary line, in the 6th intercostal space. 1. Promotes blood circulation and removes blood stasis. 2. Promotes qi flow and relieves chest oppression.	1. Respiratory: Dyspnea, oppressive feeling in the chest, pain in the chest and hypochondrium. 2. Other: General pain, myasthenia of limbs.

5. The Points of the Heart Meridian of Hand-Shaoyin (HT)

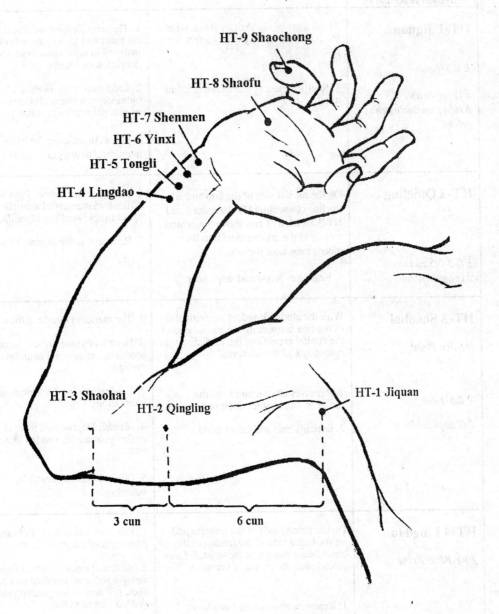

Fig. II-12 Points of the Heart Meridian (1)

Tab. II-6   Points of the Heart Meridian of Hand-Shaoyin (HT)

Point, Property, Method & Remarks	Location & Action	Categories of Diseases & Indications
HT-1 Jiquan ⊥ 0.5-1 cun. ᵟ is applicable. **Avoid puncturing the artery.**	At the apex of the axillary fossa, where the pulsation of the axillary artery is palpable. 1. Soothes chest oppression and calms mind.	1. The meridian course: Paralysis, coldness and pain in the elbow, inability to raise arms, pain and distention of fingers. 2. Cardiovascular: Feeling of oppression in chest, shortness of breath, palpitation, cardiac pain. 3. Other: Insufficient lactation, intercostal neuralgia, axillary odor.
HT-2 Qingling ⊥ 0.3-0.5 cun. ᵟ is applicable.	On the medial side of the arm and on the line connecting HT-1 Jiquan and HT-3 Shaohai, 3 cun above the cubital crease, in the groove medial to the biceps muscle of the arm. 1. Regulates blood and stops pain.	1. The meridian course: Pain and difficult movement of shoulder and upper limbs, swelling of axilla. 2. Head and sense organs: Headache.
HT-3 Shaohai *He-Sea Point* ⊥ 0.5-1 cun. ᵟ is applicable.	With the elbow flexed, at the midpoint of the line connecting the medial end of the cubital crease and the medial epicondyle of the humerus. 1. Removes obstruction from the meridian and soothes chest oppression. 2. Benefits heat and calms mind.	1. The meridian course: Elbow pain. 2. Head and sense organs: Headache, toothache, trigeminal neuralgia, vertigo. 3. Cardiovascular: Cardiac pain, palpitation. 4. Mental: Depression, mania, epilepsy, amnesia, sudden loss of voice. 5. Other: Furuncle, scrofula, vomiting.
HT-4 Lingdao *Jing-River Point* ⊥ 0.3-0.5 cun. ᵟ is applicable.	On the palmar side of the forearm and on the radial side of the tendon of the ulnar flexor muscle of the wrist, 1.5 cun proximal to the crease of the wrist. 1. Removes obstruction from heart meridian. 2. Relieves chest oppression and promotes qi circulation.	1. The meridian course: Pain and numbness of elbow and arm. 2. Head and sense organs: Dizziness, vertigo, redness, swelling and pain in eyes, stiffness of tongue, aphasia, sudden loss of voice. 3. Cardiovascular: Cardiac pain, palpitation. 4. Mental: Hysteria, convulsion, schizophrenia. 5. Digestive: Stomachache, nausea.

Tab. II-6   Points of the Heart Meridian of Hand-Shaoyin (HT)

Point, Property , Method & Remarks	Location & Action	Categories of Diseases & Indications
HT-5 Tongli *Luo-Connecting Point* ⊥ *0.3-0.5 cun.* ᵰ *is applicable.*	On the palmar side of the forearm and on the radial side of the tendon of the ulnar flexor muscle of the wrist, 1 cun proximal to the crease of the wrist. 1. Tonifies heart yin and calms the mind. 2. Benefits bladder.	1. The meridian course: Pain of posterior aspect of shoulder, upper arm and elbow, wrist pain, spasm of finger. 2. Head and sense organs: Headache, vertigo, pain and redness of eyes, sore throat, flushing of face, tonsillitis, hypomobility of tongue, sublingual swelling, sore tongue. 3. Cardiovascular: Cardiac pain, palpitation, shortness of breath, irritability. 4. Mental: Mania, depression, epilepsy, hysteria, sudden loss of voice, amnesia, insomnia. 5. Respiratory: Cough, asthma. 6. Gynecopathies: Irregular menstruation, dysmenorrhea, menorrhagia. 7. Urinary: Incontinence of urine, hematuria.
HT-6 Yinxi *Xi-Cleft Point* ⊥ *0.3-0.5 cun.* ᵰ *is applicable.*	On the palmar side of the forearm and on the radial side of the tendon of the ulnar flexor muscle of the wrist, 0.5 cun proximal to the crease of the wrist. 1. Nourishes heart yin, clears heat and calms mind. 2. Stops sweating.	1. The meridian course: Pain and numbness of posterior-medial aspect of shoulder, arm and elbow, spasmodic pain of little finger. 2. Head and sense organs: Headache, vertigo, tonsillitis, acute glossolysis, sudden loss of voice. 3. Cardiovascular: Cardiac pain, palpitation, shortness of breath, feverish sensation in chest. 4. Mental: Irritability, timidity, tremor, depression, epilepsy. 5. Digestive: Epigastric pain, cholera, vomiting, diarrhea, hematemesis. 6. Urogenital: Incontinence of urine, hematuria, irregular menstruation, dysmenorrhea, metrorrhagia. 7. Other: Hectic fever due to yin deficiency, night sweating, feeling cold.

Tab. II-6 Points of the Heart Meridian of Hand-Shaoyin (HT)

Point, Property , Method & Remarks	Location & Action	Categories of Diseases & Indications
HT-7 Shenmen *Shu-Stream Point; Yuan-Source Point* ⊥ *0.3-0.5 cun.* 𝄐 *is applicable.*	On the wrist, at the ulnar end of the crease of the wrist, in the depression on the radial side of the tendon of the ulnar flexor muscle of the wrist. 1. Nourishes heart blood and calms mind. 2. Opens heart orifice.	1. The meridian course: Paralysis, spasm and numbness of elbow, arm, wrist and fingers. 2. Head and sense organs: Headache, vertigo, icteric sclera, flushed face, sore tongue, swelling of tongue. 3. Cardiovascular: Cardiac pain, palpitation, timidity. 4. Mental: Dementia, crying due to sadness and mania with laughter, depression, epilepsy, sudden loss of voice, insomnia, amnesia, hysteria. 5. Digestive: Stomachache, dry mouth, anorexia, hematemesis, stools with blood and pus, jaundice. 6. Urogenital: Enuresis, hematuria, pain in vagina, irregular menstruation, metrorrhagia. 7. Respiratory: Asthma, cough, hemoptysis. 8. Other: Malaria, emaciation with weakness, fever and aversion to cold.
HT-8 Shaofu *Yin-Spring Point* ⊥ *0.3-0.5 cun.* 𝄐 *is applicable.*	In the palm, between the 4th and 5th metacarpal bones, at the part of the palm touching the tip of the little finger when a fist is made. 1. Clears heart fire, heart deficiency heat and heart phlegm-fire. 2. Calms mind.	1. The meridian course: Spasmodic pain of elbow and arm, feverish sensation in palm, spasm of little finger. 2. Head and sense organs: Pain and dryness of throat, globus hystericus, epistaxis, dryness of nose. 3. Cardiovascular: Cardiac pain, palpitation, fullness in chest, shortness of breath. 4. Mental: Susceptibility to laugh and fear, hysteria. 5. Reproductive: Pruritis vulvae, prolapse of uterus, menorrhagia. 6. Other: Enuresis, dysuria, acute appendicitis, malaria.

Tab. II-6   Points of the Heart Meridian of Hand-Shaoyin (HT)

Point, Property, Method & Remarks	Location & Action	Categories of Diseases & Indications
HT-9 Shaochong *Jing-Well Point* $\perp$ *0.1 cun or prick to cause bleeding.* ∂ *is applicable.*	On the radial side of the distal segment of the little finger, 0.1 cun from the corner of the nail. 1. Clears heat and dispels wind. 2. Opens heart orifice and restores consciousness.	1. The meridian course: Pain in posterior border of medial aspect of arm, feverish sensation in palm, spasm and numbness of hand and finger. 2. Head and sense organs: Icteric sclera, stiffness of tongue, tonsillitis. 3. Cardiovascular: Cardiac pain, palpitation. 4. Mental: Coma, infantile convulsion. 5. Digestive: Hematemesis, stools with blood and pus, jaundice. 6. Other: High fever, apoplexy, sunstroke, shock.

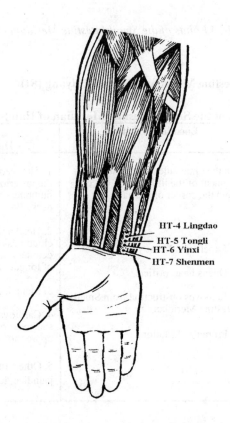

Fig. II-13 Points of the Heart Meridian (2)

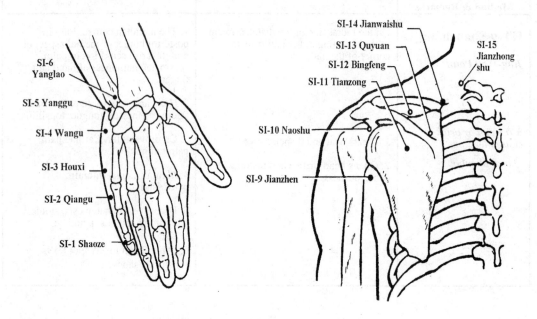

Fig. II-14 Points of the Small Intestine Meridian (1)

6. The Points of the Small Intestine Meridian of Hand-Taiyang (SI)

Tab. II-7 Points of the Small Intestine Meridian of Hand-Taiyang (SI)

Point, Property, Method & Remarks	Location & Action	Categories of Diseases & Indications
SI-1 Shaoze *Jing-Well Point* ⊥ *0.1 cun, or prick to cause bleeding.* 𝄞 *is applicable.*	On the ulnar side of the distal segment of the little finger, 0.1 cun from the corner of the nail. 1. Expels wind-heat. 2. Opens heart orifice. 3. Removes obstruction from Small Intestine Meridian. 4. Promotes lactation.	1. The meridian course: Pain in theposterior aspect of shoulder and arm, numbness of the 5th finger, stiffness of neck. 2. Head and sense organs: Sore throat, cloudiness of cornea, pterygium, deafness, tinnitus, epistaxis, immobility of tongue, aphasia, excessive salivation. 3. Mental: Apoplexy, coma, depression. 4. Cardiovascular: Cardiac pain, shortness of breath, feeling of oppression in chest. 5. Other: Insufficient lactation, mastitis, jaundice, febrile diseases, cough.

Tab. II-7 Points of the Small Intestine Meridian of Hand-Taiyang (SI)

Point, Property, Method & Remarks	Location & Action	Categories of Diseases & Indications
SI-2 Qiangu *Ying-Spring Point* ⊥ *0.3-0.5 cun.* 𝄽 *is applicable.*	At the junction of the red and white skin along the ulnar border of the hand, at the ulnar end of the crease distal to the 5th metacarpophalangeal joint when a loose fist is made. 1. Soothes liver and clears heart. 2. Improves visual and hearing acuity.	1. The meridian course: Pain of forearm, spasm of elbow, numbness, redness, swelling and difficulty in moving fingers, feverish sensation in palm. 2. Head and sense organs: Tinnitus, deafness, pain in eyes, cloudiness of cornea, nasal obstruction, epistaxis, sore throat, mumps. 3. Mental: Depression, mania, epilepsy. 4. Respiratory: Cough, hemoptysis. 5. Other: Insufficient lactation, anhidrosis in febrile diseases, malaria.
SI-3 Houxi *Shu-Stream Point; One of Eight Confluent Points, connecting with DU* ⊥ *0.5-0.7 cun.* 𝄽 *is applicable.*	At the junction of the red and white skin along the ulnar border of the hand, at the ulnar end of the distal palmar crease, proximal to the 5th metacarpophalangeal joint when a loose fist is made. 1. Eliminates interior wind from Du Meridian and benefits sinews. 2. Clears heat and eliminates dampness and resolves jaundice.	1. The meridian course: Stiffness, pain and difficulty in moving neck, pain of shoulder and arm, hemiplegia, torticollis, lower back pain. 2. Head and sense organs: Headache, deafness, redness of eye, cloudiness of cornea, epistaxis. 3. Mental: Depression, mania, epilepsy, insomnia, hysteria. 4. Urinary: Dysuria with reddish urine. 5. Other: Night sweating, jaundice, febrile diseases, malaria, scabies, warts.
SI-4 Wangu *Yuan-Primary Point* ⊥ *0.3-0.5 cun.* 𝄽 *is applicable.*	On the ulnar border of the hand, in the depression between the proximal end of the 5th metacarpal bone and hamate bone, and at the junction of the red and white skin. 1. Removes obstruction from Hand-Taiyang Meridian. 2. Eliminates damp-heat. 3. Benefits gallbladder.	1. The meridian course: Rigidity of neck, limited movement of elbow and arm, pain of arm and finger, weakness of wrist, hemiplegia, lower back pain. 2. Head and sense organs: Excessive lacrimation induced by wind, cloudiness of cornea, tinnitus, deafness, nasal obstruction, epistaxis, swelling of submandibular region. 3. Mental: Infantile convulsion. 4. Other: Febrile diseases with anhidrosis, cholecystitis, pleurisy.

Tab. II-7 Points of the Small Intestine Meridian of Hand-Taiyang (SI)

Point, Property, Method & Remarks	Location & Action	Categories of Diseases & Indications
SI-5 Yanggu *Jing-River Point* ⊥ *0.3-0.5 cun.* ᵟ *is applicable.*	On the ulnar border of the wrist, in the depression between the styloid process of the ulna and triangular bone. 1. Clears heart and calms mind. 2. Removes obstruction from Small Intestine Meridian. 3. Benefits visual and hearing acuity.	1. The meridian course: Swelling of the neck and submandibular region, pain of the posterior aspect of arm and wrist, hemiplegia. 2. Head and sense organs: Redness, pain and swelling of eyes, vertigo, tinnitus, deafness, toothache, aphthous ulcer. 3. Mental: Depression, incoherent speech, convulsion. 4. Other: Febrile diseases with anhidrosis, hemorrhoids, scabies, hypochondriac pain.
SI-6 Yanglao *Xi-Cleft Point* ⊥ *0.3-0.5 cun.* ᵟ *is applicable.*	On the ulnar side of the posterior surface of the forearm, in the depression proximal to and on the radial side of the head of the ulna. 1. Benefits sinews and brightens eyes. 2. Removes obstruction from Small Intestine Meridian.	1. The meridian course: Torticollis. 2. Head and sense organs: Blurring of vision, redness, pain and swelling of eye. 3. Other: Acute lumbar sprain.
SI-7 Zhizheng *Luo-Connecting Point* ⊥ *0.5-0.8 cun.* ᵟ *is applicable.*	On the ulnar side of the posterior surface of the forearm and on the line connecting SI-5 Yanggu and SI-8 Xiaohai, 5 cun proximal to the dorsal crease of the wrist. 1. Removes obstruction from Small Intestine Meridian. 2. Calms mind. 3. Clears heat and releases exterior.	1. The meridian course: Neck rigidity, spasmodic pain in elbow and fingers, numbness of fingers, swelling of submandibular region. 2. Head and sense organs: Headache, hordeolum. 3. Mental: Depressive psychosis, timidity, abnormal susceptibility to laugh, and amnesia. 4. Other: Scabies, diabetes, febrile diseases.

Tab. II-7 Points of the Small Intestine Meridian of Hand-Taiyang (SI)

Point, Property, Method & Remarks	Location & Action	Categories of Diseases & Indications
SI-8 Xiaohai *He-Sea Point* ⊥ *0.3-0.5 cun.* ᕰ *is applicable.*	On the medial side of the elbow, in the depression between the olecranon of the ulna and the medial epicondyle of the humerus. 1. Resolves damp-heat. 2. Removes obstruction from Small Intestine Meridian. 3. Soothes liver and calms mind.	1. The meridian course: Pain in shoulder and back, spasmodic pain in elbow, pain in posterior-lateral aspect of arm. 2. Head and sense organs: Headache, dizziness, vertigo, deafness, tinnitus, hordeolum. 3. Mental: Depressive psychosis, epilepsy. 4. Other: Scrofula, ulceration of skin, lower abdominal pain, irritability.
SI-9 Jianzhen ⊥ *0.5-1 cun.* ᕰ *is applicable.*	Posterior and inferior to the shoulder joint, 1 cun above the posterior end of the axillary fold with the arm adducted. 1. Transforms phlegm and relieves swelling. 2. Clears heat and improves hearing acuity. 3. Soothes the meridian to stop pain.	1. The meridian course: Pain, numbness and motor impairment of hand and arm, pain in scapular region. 2. Head and sense organs: Tinnitus, deafness, toothache. 3. Other: Scrofula.
SI-10 Naoshu ***Crossing Point of SI, Yangwei & Yangqiao M.*** ⊥ *0.5-1 cun.* ᕰ *is applicable.*	On the shoulder, above the posterior end of the axillary fold, in the depression below the lower border of the spine of the scapula. 1. Transforms phlegm and relieves swelling. 2. Comforts sinews and activates collaterals.	1. The meridian course: Swelling of shoulder, pain and weakness of arm and shoulder, scrofula in neck.
SI-11 Tianzong ⊥ *0.5-1 cun.* ᕰ *is applicable.*	On the scapula, in the depression at the center of the subscapular fossa, and at the level of the 4th thoracic vertebra. 1. Descends rebellious lung qi. 2. Relieves rigidity of muscles and activates collaterals.	1. The meridian course: Pain in scapular region and inability to raise arms, numbness and soreness of upper limbs along the meridian course. 2. Other: Mastitis.

Tab. II-7 Points of the Small Intestine Meridian of Hand-Taiyang (SI)

Point, Property, Method & Remarks	Location & Action	Categories of Diseases & Indications
SI-12 Bingfeng *Crossing Point of LI, SI, SJ & GB* ⊥ *0.5-0.7 cun.* ᶜ *is applicable.*	On the scapula, at the center of the suprascapular fossa, directly above SI-11 Tianzong, in the depression produced when the arm is raised. 1. Relieves rigidity of muscles and activates collaterals.	1. The meridian course: Pain in scapular region, soreness and numbness of upper limbs on the meridian course, stiffness and motor impairment of neck.
SI-13 Quyuan ⊥ *0.3-0.5 cun.* ᶜ *is applicable.*	On the scapula, at the medial end of the suprascapular fossa, at the midpoint of the line connecting SI-10 Naoshu and the spinous process of the 2nd thoracic vertebra. 1. Relieves rigidity of muscles and activates collaterals.	1. The meridian course: Spasmodic pain in shoulder and scapular region.
SI-14 Jianwaishu ⊥ *0.3 -0.7 cun.* ᶜ *is applicable.*	On the back, below the spinous process of the 1st thoracic vertebra, 3 cun lateral to posterior midline. *1.* Relieves rigidity of muscles and activates collaterals.	1. The meridian course: Stiffness of neck, soreness and pain in shoulder and back.
SI-15 Jianzhongshu ⬂ *0.3-0.6 cun.* ᶜ *is applicable.*	On the back, below the spinous process of the 7th cervical vertebra, 2 cun lateral to posterior midline. 1. Disperses lung and relieves exterior.	1. The meridian course: Pain in shoulder and back, torticollis. 2. Head and sense organs: Blurring of vision. 3. Respiratory: Cough, asthma, fever and chills.
SI-16 Tianchuang ⊥ *0.3-0.7 cun.* ᶜ *is applicable.*	On the lateral side of the neck, posterior to the sternocleidomastoid muscle and LI-18 Futu, at the level of the laryngeal protuberance. 1. Improves hearing acuity and benefits orifices in head. 2. Extinguishes wind and calms mind.	1. The meridian course: Pain and stiffness of neck, soreness and numbness of arm and hand. 2. Head and sense organs: Sore throat, deafness, tinnitus, sudden loss of voice, deviation of eye and/or mouth.

Tab. II-7 Points of the Small Intestine Meridian of Hand-Taiyang (SI)

Point, Property, Method & Remarks	Location & Action	Categories of Diseases & Indications
SI-17 Tianrong ⊥ 0.3-0.7 cun. ᚹ is applicable.	On the lateral side of the neck, posterior to the mandibular angle, in the depression on the anterior border of the sternocleidomastoid muscle. 1. Resolves damp-heat. 2. Eliminates fire-poison to benefit throat and ear. 3. Removes obstruction from Small Intestine Meridian.	1. The meridian course: Muscular sprain of neck, furuncle on neck. 2. Head and sense organs: Tinnitus, deafness, sore throat, globus hystericus. 3. Respiratory: Asthma, fever and aversion to cold. 4. Other: Scrofula.
SI-18 Quanliao **Crossing Point of SJ & SI** ⊥ 0.5-0.8 cun.	On the face, directly below the outer canthus, in the depression below the zygomatic bone. 1. Expels wind and relieves pain.	1. Head and sense organs: Deviation of eye and/or mouth, twitching of eyelids, flushed face, toothache, swelling of cheek, trigeminal neuralgia.
SI-19 Tinggong **Crossing Point of SJ, GB & SI** ⊥ 0.5-1 cun. ᚹ is applicable.	On the face, anterior to the tragus and posterior to the mandibular condyloid process, in the depression produced when the mouth is open. 1. Benefits ear and relieves swelling.	1. Head and sense organs: Tinnitus, deafness, tympanites, earache, toothache. 2. Other: Lower back pain.

7. The Points of the Bladder Meridian of Foot-Taiyang (BL)

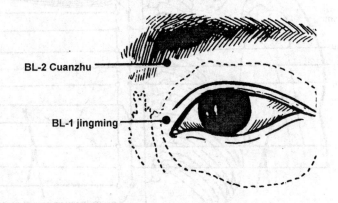

Fig. II-15 Points of the Bladder Meridian (1)

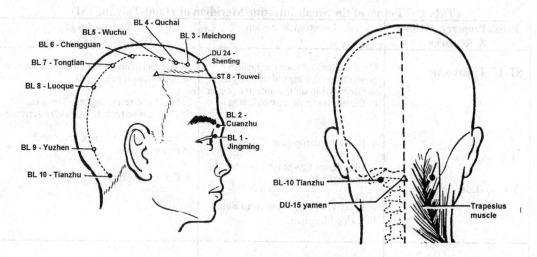

Fig. II-16 Points of the Bladder Meridian (2)

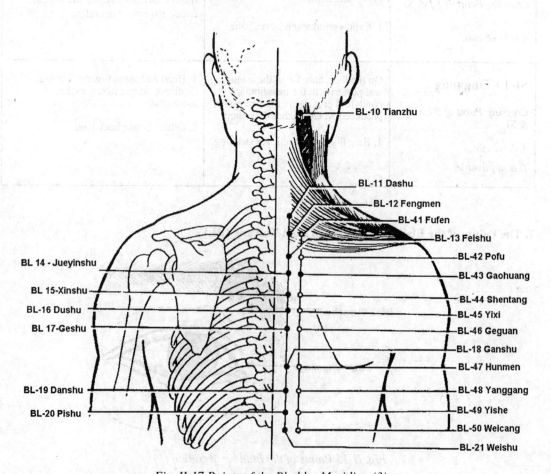

Fig. II-17 Points of the Bladder Meridian (3)

Tab. II-8   Points of the Bladder Meridian of Foot-Taiyang (BL)

Point, Property , Method & Remarks	Location & Action	Categories of Diseases & Indications
BL-1 Jingming *Crossing Point of SI, BL, ST, Yinqiao & Yangqiao M.* ⊥ *0.3-0.7 cun along infraorbital ridge.* *Twisting or manipulating needle with large amplitude is prohibited.* ʃ *is prohibited.*	On the face, in the depression slightly above the inner canthus. 1. Expels wind and clears heat. 2. Improves visual acuity and removes nebula.	1. Ophthalmopathy: Conjunctival congestion, epiphora, itching and pain around inner canthus, pterygium, nebula, blurred vision, myopia, night blindness, color blindness, eye disorders in children due to malnutrition. 2. Other: Aversion to cold, headache, lumbago, dizziness.
BL-2 Cuanzhu ↳ *0.3-0.5 cun.*	On the face, in the depression at the medial end of the eyebrow, at the supraorbital notch. 1. Expels wind, clears heat and brightens eyes. 2. Soothes liver, removes obstruction from Bladder Meridian and stops pain.	1. Head and sense organs: Headache, pain in supra-orbital bone, facial paralysis, flushed face, swollen cheeks, epistaxis, dizziness, conjunctivitis, blurred vision, conjunctival congestion, epiphora, itching and pain of eyes, myopia, night blindness, twitching eyelids. 2. Mental: Coma, manic-depressive psychosis, epilepsy, convulsion.
BL-3 Meichong ↳ *0.3-0.5 cun.*	On the head, directly above BL-2 Cuanzhu, 0.5 cun above the anterior hairline, on the line connecting DU-24 Shenting and BL-4 Qucha. 1. Dispels wind and clears heat. 2. Tranquilizes convulsion and calms mind.	1. Head and sense organs: Conjunctival congestion, blurred vision, stuffy nose, headache, vertigo. 2. Other: Epilepsy.
BL-4 Qucha ↳ *0.3-0.5 cun.* ʃ *is applicable.*	On the head, 0.5 cun directly above the midpoint of the anterior hairline and 1.5 cun lateral to the midline, at the junction of the medial third and middle third of the line connecting DU-24 Shenting and ST-8 Touwei. 1. Relieves asthma and descends rebellious qi. 2. Brightens eyes and calms mind.	1. Head and sense organs: Headache, blurred vision, dizziness, ophthalmalgia, stuffy nose, epistaxis.

Tab. II-8   Points of the Bladder Meridian of Foot-Taiyang (BL)

Point, Property , Method & Remarks	Location & Action	Categories of Diseases & Indications
BL-5 Wuchu ↳ *0.3-0.5 cun.* *δ is applicable.*	On the head, 1 cun directly above the midpoint of the anterior hairline and 1.5 cun lateral to the midline. 1. Dispels wind and clears heat. 2. Tranquilizes convulsion and brightens eyes.	1. Head and sense organs: Headache, dizziness. 2. Mental: Infantile convulsion, epilepsy.
BL-6 Chengguang ↳ *0.3-0.5 cun.*	On the head, 2.5 cun directly above the midpoint of the anterior hairline and 1.5 cun lateral to the midline. 1. Dispels wind and clears heat. 2. Brightens eyes and descends rebellious qi.	1. Head and sense organs: Headache, dizziness, stuffy nose, running nose. 2. Other: Febrile disease without sweating, vomiting, dysphoria.
BL-7 Tongtian ↳ *0.3-0.5 cun.* *δ is applicable.*	On the head, 4 cun directly above the midpoint of the anterior hairline and 1.5 cun lateral to the midline. 1. Dispels wind and clears heat. 2. Promotes dispersing function of lung and benefits nose.	1. Head and sense organs: Headache, heaviness in head, dizziness, vertigo, deviation of mouth and face, stuffy nose with watery discharge, epistaxis, pyogenic infection of nose, stuffy nose. 2. Other: Goiter, neck pain which causes difficulty in turning head, torticollis.
BL-8 Luoque ↳ *0.3-0.5 cun.* *δ is applicable.*	On the head, 5.5 cun directly above the midpoint of the anterior hairline and 1.5 cun lateral to the midline. 1. Extinguishes wind and soothes liver. 2. Clears heat and calms mind.	1. Head and sense organs: Dizziness, vertigo, tinnitus, stuffy nose, deviation of mouth and face, blurred vision. 2. Other: Goiter, manic-depressive psychosis, epilepsy, swelling in neck.

Tab. II-8   Points of the Bladder Meridian of Foot-Taiyang (BL)

Point, Property , Method & Remarks	Location & Action	Categories of Diseases & Indications
BL-9 Yuzhen ↳ *0.3-0.5 cun.* ⊘ *is applicable.*	On the occiput, 2.5 cun directly above the midpoint of the posterior hairline and 1.3 cun lateral to the midline, in the depression at the level of the upper border of the external occipital protuberance. 1. Dispels wind and clears heat. 2. Brightens eyes and descends rebellious qi.	1. Head and sense organs: Headache, myopia, opthalmalgia, stuffy nose. 2. Other: Aversion to cold and wind, vomiting.
BL-10 Tianzhu ⊥ *0.5-0.8 cun.* ⊘ *is applicable.*	On the nape, in the depression of the lateral border of the trapezius muscle and 1.3 cun lateral to the midpoint of the posterior hairline. 1. Expels wind and cold. 2. Clears brain and brightens eyes. 3. Removes obstruction and invigorates lower back.	1. Head and sense organs: Headache, vertigo, stuffy nose, anosmia, sore throat, conjunctival congestion. 2. Other: Torticollis, stiffness of nape and neck, pain in shoulder and back.
BL-11 Dazhu *Influential Point of Bone; Crossing Point of SI & BL* ↘ *0.5-0.7 cun.* ⊘ *is applicable.*	On the back, below the spinous process of the 1st thoracic vertebra, 1.5 cun lateral to the posterior midline. 1. Nourishes blood, soothes sinews, strengthens bones. 2. Expels wind and releases exterior.	1. The meridian course: Scapular pain, pain and stiffness in neck, pain in back and waist, pain in knees with inability to flex. 2. Head and sense organs: Splitting sensation of headache, dizziness, inflammation of throat. 3. Respiratory: Cough, asthma, exogenous febrile disease without sweating, oppressive feeling in chest. 4. Mental: Epilepsy, stroke.
BL-12 Fengmen *Crossing Point of BL & DU* ↘ *0.5-0.7 cun.* ⊘ *is applicable.*	On the back, below the spinous process of the 2nd thoracic vertebra, 1.5 cun lateral to the posterior midline. 1. Expels exterior wind and releases exterior. 2. Promotes lung's dispersing function and regulates nutritive and defensive qi.	1. Respiratory: Cough due to attack by pathogenic cold, asthma, stuffy nose, excessive discharge from nose, fever, headache. 2. Mental: Epilepsy, wind stroke, unconsciousness, convulsion. 3. Other: Arthralgia, carbuncle, cellulitis, urticaria, dizziness, neck stiffness and various febrile diseases.

Tab. II-8   Points of the Bladder Meridian of Foot-Taiyang (BL)

Point, Property , Method & Remarks	Location & Action	Categories of Diseases & Indications
BL-13 Feishu *Back-Shu Point of Lung* ⤵ *0.5-0.7 cun.* ᶿ *is applicable.*	On the back, below the spinous process of the 3rd thoracic vertebra, 1.5 cun lateral to the posterior midline. 1. Promotes lung's dispersing function and regulates nutritive and defensive qi. 2. Regulates & tonifies lung qi. 3. Clears heat from lung.	1. Respiratory: Cough, fullness in chest, abundant expectoration, asthma, pulmonary tuberculosis, high fever, night sweating, hematemesis and inflammation of throat. 2. Digestive: Stomachache, vomiting, diarrhea, hiccup, loss of appetite, dysentery, infantile malnutrition. 3. Metal: Manic-depression, epilepsy, convulsion. 4. Other: General pruritis, urticaria, deafness, diabetes, jaundice, goiter, pain in back and loin.
BL-14 Jueyinshu *Back-Shu Point of Pericardium* ⤵ *0.5-0.7 cun.* ᶿ *is applicable.*	On the back, below the spinous process of the 4th thoracic vertebra, 1.5 cun lateral to the posterior midline. 1. Relieves chest stuffiness and pain. 2. Regulates heart and calms mind.	1. Cardiovascular: Cardiac pain, palpitation, chest pain radiating to the back, fullness and oppressive feeling in chest. 2. Respiratory: Cough, asthma. 3. Digestive: Stomachache, vomiting. 4. Other: Toothache, costalgia.
BL-15 Xinshu *Back-Shu Point of Heart* ⤵ *0.5-0.7 cun.* ᶿ *is applicable.*	On the back, below the spinous process of the 5th thoracic vertebra, 1.5 cun lateral to the posterior midline. 1. Relieves chest stuffiness and pain. 2. Invigorates blood and nourishes heart. 3. Clears heat and calms mind.	1. Cardiovascular: Cardiac pain, palpitation, chest pain radiating to back, chest fullness and oppressive feeling. 2. Respiratory: Cough, asthma, hemoptysis. 3. Digestive: Vomiting, poor appetite. 4. Mental: Manic-depressive psychosis, epilepsy, schizophrenia, palpitation due to fright, insomnia, amnesia. 5. Other: Stroke, hemiplegia, nocturnal emission, white or cloudy urine, jaundice, pain in shoulder and back.

Tab. II-8   Points of the Bladder Meridian of Foot-Taiyang (BL)

Point, Property , Method & Remarks	Location & Action	Categories of Diseases & Indications
BL-16 Dushu ↘ *0.5-0.7 cun.* *δ is applicable.*	On the back, below the spinous process of the 6th thoracic vertebra, 1.5 cun lateral to the posterior midline. 1. Relieves chest stuffiness and pain. 2. Regulates heart and invigorates blood.	1. Cardiovascular: Pricordial pain, palpitations. 2. Digestive: Epigastric and abdominal pain, distention of abdomen, borborygmus, hiccup. 3. Other: Fever and aversion to cold.
BL-17 Geshu *Influential Point of Blood* ↘ *0.5-0.7 cun.* *δ is applicable.*	On the back, below the spinous process of the 7th thoracic vertebra, 1.5 cun lateral to the posterior midline. 1. Activates blood and stops bleeding. 2. Nourishes blood and regulates qi. 3. Soothes chest oppression and descends rebellious qi.	1. Digestive: Distending pain over epigastrium, hiccup, vomiting, hematemesis, hematochezia, loss of appetite, distention of abdomen, solid mass in abdomen, jaundice, dysphagia. 2. Respiratory: Asthma, cough, hemoptysis, inflammation of throat, high fever, spontaneous sweating, night sweating. 3. Cardiovascular: Pricordial pain, sensation of fullness in chest. 4. Other: Anemia, urticaria, pruritis, metrorrhagia, pantalgia, febrile disease without sweating, lassitude, hypochondriac pain.
BL-18 Ganshu *Back-Shu Point of Liver* ↘ *0.5-0.7 cun.* *δ is applicable.*	On the back, below the spinous process of the 9th thoracic vertebra, 1.5 cun lateral to the posterior midline. 1. Benefits liver and gallbladder. 2. Calms mind and brightens eyes.	1. The meridian course: Hypochondriac pain. 2. Head and sense organs: Headache, dizziness, conjunctival congestion, blurred vision, night blindness, optic atrophy, nebula, pterygium and epiphora. 3. Digestive: Dysfunction of liver, jaundice, epigastralgia, anorexia, abdominal pain, diarrhea. 4. Mental: Epilepsy, mania. 5. Other: Wind stroke, insufficient lactation, flaccidity syndrome, pain along spinal column.

Tab. II-8   Points of the Bladder Meridian of Foot-Taiyang (BL)

Point, Property , Method & Remarks	Location & Action	Categories of Diseases & Indications
BL-19 Danshu *Back-Shu Point of Gallbladder* ⟍ *0.5-0.7 cun.* ᵹ *is applicable.*	On the back, below the spinous process of the 10th thoracic vertebra, 1.5 cun lateral to the posterior midline. 1. Clears damp-heat in liver and gallbladder. 2. Benefits gallbladder to stop pain.	1. The meridian course: Hypochondriac pain, subaxillary swelling. 2. Head and sense organs: Headache, sore throat. 3. Digestive: Jaundice, bitter taste, dry tongue, vomiting, poor appetite, distention and pain in stomach and abdomen.
BL-20 Pishu *Back-Shu Point of Spleen* ⟍ *0.5-0.7 cun.* ᵹ *is applicable.*	On the back, below the spinous process of the 11th thoracic vertebra, 1.5 cun lateral to the posterior midline. 1. Strengthens spleen and eliminates damp. 2. Reinforces stomach to nourish blood. 3. Raises yang qi to stop diarrhea.	1. Digestive: Stomachache, distention and pain in abdomen, vomiting, diarrhea, dysentery, jaundice, dysphagia, tympanites, lassitude, drowsiness, polyphagia with emaciated body or loss of appetite, chronic infantile convulsions due to dysfunction of spleen. 2. Respiratory: Cough, abundant expectoration. 3. Other: Stiffness of back and loin. distention and fullness in chest and hypochondrium, abdominal masses.
BL-21 Weishu *Back-Shu Point of Stomach* ⟍ *0.5-0.8 cun.* ᵹ *is applicable.*	On the back, below the spinous process of the 12th thoracic vertebra, 1.5 cun lateral to the posterior midline. 1. Reinforces stomach and spleen. 2. Regulates middle-jiao and descends stomach qi.	1. Digestive: Cold feeling in stomach, vomiting of watery fluid, pain in epigastrium, regurgitation, vomiting, poor appetite, dysphagia, polyphagia with emaciated body, vomiting of milk in children, abdominal pain, borborygmus, diarrhea, dysentery, indigestion, infantile malnutrition, convulsion due to dysfunction of spleen, prolapse of rectum. 2. Respiratory: Cough, pulmonary tuberculosis. 3. Other: Pain in chest and hypochondrium, spinal pain, flaccidity syndrome, amenorrhea, edema, tympanites, abdominal masses.

Tab. II-8   Points of the Bladder Meridian of Foot-Taiyang (BL)

Point, Property , Method & Remarks	Location & Action	Categories of Diseases & Indications
BL-22 Sanjiaoshu *Back-Shu Point of Sanjiao* ⊥ *0.5-1 cun.* *δ is applicable.*	On the lower back, below the spinous process of the 1st lumbar vertebra, 1.5 cun lateral to the posterior midline. 1. Benefits Sanjiao and regulates water passages. 2. Strengthens spleen to resolve dampness.	1. Digestive: Abdominal distention, borborygmus, indigestion, vomiting, abdominal pain, diarrhea, dysentery, infantile malnutrition. 2. Urinary: Dysuria, edema. 3. Other: Muscular spasm of shoulder and back, stiffness and pain of spine, headache, dizziness, fever without sweating, jaundice, abdominal mass in women.
BL-23 Shenshu *Back-Shu Point of Kidney* ⊥ *1-1.2 cun.* *δ is applicable.*	On the lower back, below the spinous process of the 2nd lumbar vertebra, 1.5 cun lateral to the posterior midline. 1. Tonifies kidney yin and strengthens kidney yang. 2. Resolves dampness and benefits reception of qi.	1. Head and sense organs: Vertigo, dizziness, deafness, tinnitus, blurred vision, night blindness, aphonia. 2. Urogenital: Enuresis, frequent micturition, dysuria, dribbling urination, hematuria, edema, impotence, seminal emission, painful and swollen testis, leukorrhagia, irregular menstruation, dysmenorrhea. 3. Respiratory: Cough with shortness of breath, asthma which is exacerbated with movement. 4. Digestive: Stomachache, abdominal dissension, borborygmus, diarrhea, indigestion. 5. Other: Epilepsy, soreness and pain in lower back and knees, cold sensation in back, diabetes, pain in lower abdomen, fullness and distention of hypochondrium.
BL-24 Qihaishu ⊥ *0.8-1.2 cun.* *δ is applicable.*	On the lower back, below the spinous process of the 3rd lumbar vertebra, 1.5 cun lateral to the posterior midline. 1. Reinforces qi and tonifies kidney. 2. Regulates menstruation and stops pain.	1. Urogenital: Irregular menstruation, dysmenorrhea, metrorrhagia and metrostaxis, leukorrhea, seminal emission, impotence, premature ejaculation, cloudy urine, stranguria, dysuria, incontinence of urine. 2. Anal: Hemorrhoid and hematochezia. 3. Other: Pain along spinal column, flaccidity and numbness of lower limbs.

Tab. II-8   **Points of the Bladder Meridian of Foot-Taiyang (BL)**

Point, Property , Method & Remarks	Location & Action	Categories of Diseases & Indications
BL-25 Dachangshu *Back-Shu Point of Large Intestine* ⊥ *0.8-1.2 cun.* δ *is applicable.*	On the lower back, below the spinous process of the 4th lumbar vertebra, 1.5 cun lateral to the posterior midline. 1. Descends qi of stomach and large intestine and promotes bowel movement. 2. Regulates qi to stop pain.	1. Digestive: Abdominal pain, severe pain around umbilicus, abdominal distention, borborygmus, diarrhea, indigestion, constipation, dysentery, periappendicular abscess, polyphagia with emaciated body, prolapse of rectum. 2. Urogenital: Enuresis, difficulty in micturition, menorrhagia. 3. Other: Pain in loins and knees, spinal rigidity with difficulty in lying flat.
BL-26 Guanyuanshu ⊥ *0.8-1.2 cun.* δ *is applicable.*	On the lower back, below the spinous process of the 5th lumbar vertebra, 1.5 cun lateral to posterior midline. 1. Tonifies primary qi. 2. Promotes bowel movement and urination.	1. Digestive: Abdominal distention, diarrhea. 2. Urogenital: Dysuria, enuresis, frequent micturition, menorrhagia, irregular menstruation, abdominal mass. 3. Other: Lumbago, cold and overstrain, diabetes.
BL-27 Xiaochangshu *Back-Shu Point of Small Intestine* ⊥ *0.8-1.2 cun.* δ *is applicable.*	On the sacrum, at the level of the 1st posterior sacral foramen, 1.5 cun lateral to the median sacral crest. 1. Promotes bowel movement and urination. 2. Resolves dampness.	1. Digestive: Diarrhea, dysentery, stool with purulent and bloody discharge, hemorrhoids, constipation, anorexia. 2. Urogenital: Seminal emission, leukorrhea, enuresis, hematuria, dysuria with dark urine, stranguria. 3. Other: Numbness and pain in waist and legs, hernia, diabetes.
BL-28 Pangguanshu *Back-Shu Point of Bladder* ⊥ *0.8-1.2 cun.* δ *is applicable.*	On the sacrum, at the level of the 2nd posterior sacral foramen, 1.5 cun lateral to the median sacral crest. 1. Removes damp-heat. 2. Removes obstruction from meridians and activates collaterals.	1. Digestive: Abdominal pain, flatulence and fullness of abdomen, constipation, dyspepsia. 2. Urogenital: Seminal emission, abdominal mass in women, swelling, pain and sores in pudendal area, dampness and pruritis vulvae, dysuria with dark urine, enuresis, dysuria, stranguria. 3. Other: Rigidity and pain of spine, coldness and weakness of the knees and feet with spasms.

Tab. II-8   Points of the Bladder Meridian of Foot-Taiyang (BL)

Point, Property , Method & Remarks	Location & Action	Categories of Diseases & Indications
BL-29 Zhonglushu ⊥ *0.8-1.2 cun.* *ð is applicable.*	On the sacrum, at the level of the 3rd posterior sacral foramen, 1.5 cun lateral to the median sacral crest. 1. Descends large intestine qi to promote bowel movement. 2. Reinforces kidney to strengthen waist.	1. Digestive: Abdominal distension, diarrhea. 2. Other: Stiffness and pain along spinal column with difficulty in lying flat, hernia.
BL-30 Baihuanshu ⊥ *0.8-1.2 cun.* *ð is applicable.*	On the sacrum, at the level of the 4th posterior sacral foramen, 1.5 cun lateral to the median sacral crest. 1. Reinforces kidney and consolidates essence. 2. Regulates menstruation and leukorrhea.	1. Urogenital: Leukorrhea, irregular menstruation, metrorrhagia and metrostaxis, seminal emission, cloudy urine, dysuria, dark urine. 2. Other: Pain in lower back and legs, flaccidity and numbness in lower limbs, hernia.
BL-31 Shangliao ⊥ *0.8-1.2 cun.* *ð is applicable.*	On the sacrum, at the midpoint between the posterosuperior iliac spine and the posterior midline, in the 1st posterior sacral foramen. 1. Regulates menstruation to improve reproductive function. 2. Tonifies qi to restore it from collapse.	1. Urogenital: Irregular menstruation, hysteroptosis, leukorrhagia with reddish and whitish discharge, vulval pruritis, dysmenorrhea, sterility, seminal emissions, impotence, dysuria, stranguria with turbid urine. 2. Other: Lumbosacral rigidity and pain, flaccidity and pain of knees and legs.
BL-32 Ciliao ⊥ *0.8-1.2 cun.* *ð is applicable.*	On the sacrum, medial and inferior to the posterosuperior iliac spine, at the 2nd posterior sacral foramen. 1. Clears damp-heat. 2. Regulates qi and menstruation.	1. Urogenital: Irregular menstruation, leukorrhagia with reddish and whitish discharge, dysmenorrhea, pudendal pain, impotence, dysuria with dark urine, stranguria with turbid urine. 2. Other: Pain along spinal column with inability to twist spine, lumbar numbness radiating down to feet.

Tab. II-8   Points of the Bladder Meridian of Foot-Taiyang (BL)

Point, Property , Method & Remarks	Location & Action	Categories of Diseases & Indications
BL-33 Zhongliao ⊥ *0.8-1.2 cun.* ᶿ *is applicable.*	On the sacrum, medial and inferior to BL-32Ciliao, at the 3rd posterior sacral foramen. 1. Promotes bowel movement and urination. 2. Regulates menstruation and arrests leukorrhagia.	1. Digestive: Abdominal pain, constipation, dysentery, diarrhea. 2. Urogenital: Irregular menstruation, leukorrhagia with reddish and whitish discharge, sterility, dysuria, stranguria with turbid urine. 3. Other: Lumbosacral pain.
BL-34 Xialiao ⊥ *0.8-1.2 cun.* ᶿ *is applicable.*	On the sacrum, medial and inferior to BL-33 Zhongliao, at the 4th posterior sacral foramen. 1. Clears damp-heat. 2. Promotes bowel movement and urination.	1. Digestive: Borborygmus, diarrhea, constipation, hematochezia, acute pain in lower abdomen. 2. Urogenital: Dysuria, leukorrhagia, dysmenorrhea. 3. Other: Lumbago with difficulty in turning the trunk.
BL-35 Huiyang ⊥ *0.5-1 cun.* ᶿ *is applicable.*	On the sacrum, 0.5 cun lateral to the tip of the coccyx. 1. Reinforces kidney and arrests leukorrhagia. 2. Promotes bowel movement and urination.	1. Digestive: Abdominal pain and coldness, dysentery, hematochezia, hemorrhoids. 2. Urogenital: Leukorrhagia with reddish and whitish discharge, lower back pain during menstruation, sweating, moisture and pruritis in vulval area; impotence. 3. Other: Lumbago.
BL-36 Chengfu ⊥ *1-1.5 cun.* ᶿ *is applicable.*	On the posterior side of the thigh, at the midpoint of the inferior gluteal crease. 1. Promotes bowel movement and cures hemorrhoids. 2. Relieves rigidity of muscles and activates collaterals.	1. The meridian course: Pain in lumbosacral region, pain along spinal column, coldness and pain in the lower back, swelling and pain in the perineum. 2. Urinary: Dysuria. 3. Anal: Hemorrhoids, difficult bowel movement.

Tab. II-8 Points of the Bladder Meridian of Foot-Taiyang (BL)

Point, Property , Method & Remarks	Location & Action	Categories of Diseases & Indications
BL-37 Yinmen ⊥ *1-2 cun.* ᵦ *is applicable.*	On the posterior side of the thigh and on the line connecting BL-36 Chengfu and BL-40 Weizhong, 6 cun below BL-36 Chengfu. 1. Dredges meridians and collaterals.	1. Rigidity and pain of spinal column with difficulty in lying on back, pain in leg and in lateral side of thigh.
BL-38 Fuxi ⊥ *0.5-1 cun.* ᵦ *is applicable.*	At the lateral end of the popliteal crease, 1 cun above BL-39 Weiyang, medial to the tendon of the biceps muscle of the thigh. 1. Clears heat. 2. Relieves rigidity of muscles and activates collaterals.	1. Numbness of gluteal area and thigh, muscular stiffness of upper arm.
BL-39 Weiyang *Lower He-Sea Point of SJ* ⊥ *0.5-1 cun.* ᵦ *is applicable.*	At the lateral end of the popliteal crease, medial to the tendon of the biceps femoris muscle. 1. Promotes urination to remove dampness. 2. Regulates qi activities.	1. The meridian course: Rigidity and pain in loins and spine, pain and muscular contracture of legs and feet, flaccidity and numbness of limbs. 2. Urinary: Dysuria, retention of urine, enuresis, stranguria, distending pain in lower abdomen. 3. Other: Epilepsy, febrile diseases, hemorrhoids, constipation.

Tab. II-8   Points of the Bladder Meridian of Foot-Taiyang (BL)

Point, Property , Method & Remarks	Location & Action	Categories of Diseases & Indications
BL-40 Weizhong *He-Sea Point* ⊥ *0.5-1 cun or prick to cause bleeding.* ∂ *is applicable.*	At the midpoint of the popliteal crease, between the tendons of the biceps muscle of the thigh and the semitendinosus muscle. 1. Promotes blood circulation and removes blood stasis to relieve swelling and pain. 2. Clears heat and mind.	1. The meridian course: Pain in loins and back, heaviness and pain in lumbosacral region, flaccidity and numbness due to wind and dampness, paralysis of lower limbs, muscular contracture of upper arms, knee pain with limited movement. 2. Digestive: Cholera morbus, epigastric pain, vomiting, diarrhea. 3. Mental: Wind stroke, coma, epilepsy, convulsion. 4. Dermatoses: Lumbodorsal cellulitis, erysipelas, eczema, breast abscess, vulval pruritis, leprosy. 5. Other: Febrile disease without sweating, summer-heat disease, malaria, epistaxis, sore throat, spontaneous sweating, night sweating.
BL-41 Fufen ***Crossing Point of SI & BL*** ↘ *0.3-0.5 cun.* ∂ *is applicable.*	On the back, below the spinous process of the 2nd thoracic vertebra, 3 cun lateral to the posterior midline. 1. Dispels wind and cold. 2. Comforts sinews and activates collaterals.	1. Muscular spasm of shoulder and back, rigidity and pain of neck with difficulty in turning head, numbness of upper arm.
BL-42 Pohu ↘ *0.5 cun.* ∂ *is applicable.*	On the back, below the spinous process of the 3rd thoracic vertebra, 3 cun lateral to the posterior midline. 1. Promotes dispersing function of lung and descends lung qi. 2. Comforts sinews and activates collaterals.	1. Respiratory: Cough, asthma, impairment of lung due to overstrain, pulmonary tuberculosis, hectic fever due to yin deficiency. 2. Digestive: Cholera, vomiting. 3. Other: Neck rigidity causing difficulty in turning the head, pain in waist and back, brachialgia, choking sensation in chest.

Tab. II-8   Points of the Bladder Meridian of Foot-Taiyang (BL)

Point, Property , Method & Remarks	Location & Action	Categories of Diseases & Indications
BL-43 Gaohuang ↘ 0.3-0.5 cun. ᵟ is applicable.	On the back, below the spinous process of the 4th thoracic vertebra, 3 cun lateral to the posterior midline. 1. Tonifies yin and clears heat from heart. 2. Relieves cough and asthma.	1. Respiratory: Hemoptysis, hectic fever, night sweating, cough, dyspnea. 2. Digestive: Deficiency syndrome of spleen and stomach, indigestion, dysphagia, vomiting, consumptive syndrome. 3. Reproductive: Nocturnal emissions. 4. Mental: Amnesia, sleeplessness, vertigo, dizziness. 5. Other: Pain in shoulder and back, carbuncle, cellulitis, breast abscess, weakness of limbs.
BL-44 Shentang ↘ 0.5 cun. ᵟ is applicable.	On the back, below the spinous process of the 5th thoracic vertebra, 3 cun lateral to the posterior midline. 1. Soothes chest oppression and regulates qi. 2. Calms mind and relieves asthma.	1. Cardiovascular: Severe palpitation, cardialgia, fullness and oppressive sensation in chest, shortness of breath. 2. Respiratory: Cough with dyspnea, fever, aversion to cold. 3. Mental: Vexation, insomnia. 4. Other: Pain in shoulder and back, rigidity of spinal column which causes difficulty in lying on back.
BL-45 Yixi ↘ 0.5 cun. ᵟ is applicable.	On the back, below the spinous process of the 6th thoracic vertebra, 3 cun lateral to the posterior midline. 1. Regulates qi to stop pain. 2. Clears heat and promotes dispersing function of lung.	1. Respiratory: Cough with dyspnea, chest pain. 2. Other: Febrile disease without sweating, malaria, insomnia, restlessness, dizziness, ophthalmalgia, epistaxis.
BL-46 Geguan ↘ 0.5 cun. ᵟ is applicable.	On the back, below the spinous process of the 7th thoracic vertebra, 3 cun lateral to the posterior midline. 1. Soothes chest oppression, subdues rebellious qi, and regulates stomach.	1. Digestive: Loss of appetite, vomiting, hiccup, eructations, ptyalism. 2. Other: Pain along spinal column, strongly colored yellow urine, feeling of choking and oppression in chest, various blood diseases.

Tab. II-8   Points of the Bladder Meridian of Foot-Taiyang (BL)

Point, Property , Method & Remarks	Location & Action	Categories of Diseases & Indications
BL-47 Hunmen ⊾ 0.5 cun. ᵭ is applicable.	On the back, below the spinous process of the 9th thoracic vertebra, 3 cun lateral to the posterior midline. 1. Soothes liver and reinforces spleen. 2. Regulates stomach to subdue rebellious qi.	1. Digestive: Loss of appetite, borborygmus, diarrhea. 2. Head and sense organs: Headache, dizziness. 3. Other: Distending pain in chest and hypochondrium, pain in back and loins, epigastric pain radiating to back, muscular contracture with arthralgia, reddish urine.
BL-48 Yanggang ⊾ 0.5 cun. ᵭ is applicable.	On the back, below spinous process of the 10th thoracic vertebra, 3 cun lateral to the posterior midline. 1. Soothes liver and benefits gallbladder. 2. Strengthens spleen and transforms dampness.	1. Digestive: Abdominal pain, borborygmus, diarrhea, abdominal fullness and distention, loss of appetite. 2. Other: Distension and pain over chest and hypochondrium, jaundice, fever, diabetes.
BL-49 Yishe ⊾ 0.5 cun. ᵭ is applicable.	On the back, below the spinous process of the 11th thoracic vertebra, 3 cun lateral to the posterior midline. 1. Strengthens spleen and transforms dampness. 2. Regulates stomach and benefits gallbladder.	1. Digestive: Abdominal distention and fullness, borborygmus, diarrhea, vomiting, loss of appetite. 2. Other: Diabetes, fever with jaundice, urine with reddish and strong yellowish color, spinal pain, aversion to cold and wind.
BL-50 Weicang ⊾ 0.5 cun. ᵭ is applicable.	On the back, below the spinous process of the 12th thoracic vertebra, 3 cun lateral to the posterior midline. 1. Strengthens spleen and regulates stomach. 2. Promotes digestion and resolves food retention.	1. Digestive: Abdominal pain, stomachache, infantile dyspepsia, constipation. 2. Other: Edema, pain along spinal column.

Tab. II-8   Points of the Bladder Meridian of Foot-Taiyang (BL)

Point, Property , Method & Remarks	Location & Action	Categories of Diseases & Indications
BL-51 Huangmen ⊥ *0.5-1 cun.* ᵦ *is applicable.*	On the lower back, below the spinous process of the 1st lumbar vertebra, 3 cun lateral to the posterior midline. 1. Regulates qi and relieves depression. 2. Clears heat and relieves swelling.	1. Digestive: Abdominal pain, stomachache, abdominal mass, constipation. 2. Other: Postpartum disorders.
BL-52 Zhishi ⊥ *0.7-1 cun.* ᵦ *is applicable.*	On the low back, below the spinous process of the 2nd lumbar vertebra, 3 cun lateral to the posterior midline. 1. Tonifies kidney and consolidates essence. 2. Clears damp-heat.	1. Urogenital: Seminal emission, impotence, swelling and pain in pudendal area, stranguria, edema. 2. Digestive: Dyspepsia, abdominal distension, vomiting. 3. Mental: Insomnia, amnesia, dreaminess. 4. Other: Backache, rigidity and pain of spinal column which causes difficulty in lying flat, acute pain in hypochondrium.
BL-53 Baohuang ⊥ *0.8-1.2 cun.* ᵦ *is applicable.*	On the buttock and at the level of the 2nd posterior sacral foramen, 3 cun lateral to the median sacral crest. 1. Clears heat and removes dampness. 2. Promotes bowel movement and urination.	1. Urogenital: Dysuria, stranguria, distension of lower abdomen, uroschesis, swelling of the vulva. 2. Digestive: Borborygmus, abdominal distension, constipation. 3. Other: Pain along spinal column.
BL-54 Zhibian ⊥ *1-1.5 cun.* ᵦ *is applicable.*	On the buttock and at the level of the 4th posterior sacral foramen, 3 cun lateral to the median sacral crest. 1. Clears heat and removes dampness. 2. Relives swelling and cures hemorrhoids.	1. The meridian course: Lumbosacral pain which causes difficulty in lying flat, heavy sensation in lumbosacral region with limited movement, flaccidity and numbness of lower limbs. 2. Two Lower Orifices: Dysuria, reddish urine, pudendal pain, dyschezia, hemorrhoids.

Tab. II-8   Points of the Bladder Meridian of Foot-Taiyang (BL)

Point, Property , Method & Remarks	Location & Action	Categories of Diseases & Indications
BL-55 Heyang ↧ 0.7-1 cun. ᵹ is applicable.	On the posterior side of the leg and on the line connecting BL-40 Weizhong and BL-57 Chengshan, 2 cun below BL-40Weizhong. 1. Dispels cold and regulates qi. 2. Regulates menstruation and arrests metrorrhagia and metrostaxis.	1. The meridian course: Back pain, pain and numbness of lower limbs, heaviness, swelling and pain of knees and calves. 2. Reproductive: Metrorrhagia and metrostaxis, leukorrhea, pudendal pain, testicular inflammation, impotence. 3. Mental: Epilepsy, muscular spasm, convulsion. 4. Other: Hernia, pain in upper and lower abdomen.
BL-56 Chengjin ↧ 1-1.5 cun. ᵹ is applicable.	On the posterior side of the leg and on the line connecting BL-40 Weizhong and BL-57 Chengshan, at the center of the gastrocnemius muscle belly, 5 cun below BL-40 Weizhong. 1. Regulates middle-jiao. 2. Clears heat from intestines.	1. The meridian course: Spasm and pain in back, soreness, heaviness, pain or numbness of knees and calves, cramp in cholera morbus, pain and contracture of feet with edema of the dorsum. 2. Head and sense organs: Dizziness, headache, epistaxis. 3. Digestive: Vomiting, diarrhea, constipation, hemorrhoids.
BL-57 Chengshan ↧ 1-1.5 cun. ᵹ is applicable.	On the posterior midline of the leg, between BL-40 Weizhong and BL-60 Kunlun, in the pointed depression formed below the gastrocnemius muscle belly when the leg is stretched or the heel is lifted. 1. Promotes qi circulation to stop pain. 2. Relieves hemorrhoids and rigidity of muscles.	1. The meridian course: Spasm and pain in legs, back pain, pain in heel, contracture of foot which causes pain in lower abdomen, beriberi. 2. Head and sense organs: Epistaxis, running nose, sore throat. 3. Digestive Tract: Hemorrhoids, constipation, vomiting, diarrhea. 4. Mental: Epilepsy, infantile convulsion. 5. Other: Hernia.

Tab. II-8   Points of the Bladder Meridian of Foot-Taiyang (BL)

Point, Property , Method & Remarks	Location & Action	Categories of Diseases & Indications
BL-58 Feiyang ⊥ *1-1.5 cun.* ᵷ *is applicable.*	On the posterior side of the leg, 7 cun directly above BL-60 Kunlun BL 60 and 1 cun lateral and inferior to BL-57 Chengshan. 1. Dispels wind and clears heat. 2. Calms mind and relieves hemorrhoids.	1. The meridian course: Pain in back and loins, lassitude and weakness of legs, contracture of muscles and tendons which causes difficulty in flexing, leprosy. 2. Head and sense organs: Headache, dizziness, stuffy nose, epistaxis. 3. Mental: Epilepsy. 4. Other: Hemorrhoids, fever without sweating.
BL-59 Fuyang ⊥ *1-1.5 cun.* ᵷ *is applicable.*	On the posterior side of the leg, posterior to the lateral malleolus, 3 cun directly above BL-60 Kunlun. 1. Dispels wind and transforms dampness. 2. Dredges meridians and activates collaterals.	1. The meridian course: Shoulder pain, torticollis, lumbago, flaccidity and numbness of lower limbs, hemiplegia, beriberi, calf spasm. 2. Head and sense organs: Headache, heavy sensation in head, vertigo. 3. Mental: Epilepsy, convulsion.
BL-60 Kunlun *Jing-River point* ⊥ *0.5 cun.* ᵷ *is applicable.*	Posterior to the lateral malleolus, in the depression between the tip of the external malleolus and Achilles tendon. 1. Clears heat and relieves malaria. 2. Tranquilizes convulsion and relieves epilepsy.	1. The meridian course: Neck rigidity, cramping of shoulder and back, lumbosacral pain, pain in heel, swelling of feet causing inability to stand. 2. Head and sense organs: Headache, dizziness, unbearable pain in eyes, epistaxis. 3. Gynecopathies: Dystocia, retained placenta, swelling and pain in vulva. 4. Mental: Epilepsy, clonic convulsion, epilepsy. 5. Digestive: Abdominal pain, diarrhea. 6. Other: Malaria, epigastric pain radiating to back, fullness sensation in chest with sudden acute attack of asthma.

Tab. II-8   Points of the Bladder Meridian of Foot-Taiyang (BL)

Point, Property , Method & Remarks	Location & Action	Categories of Diseases & Indications
BL-61 Pucan ⊥ 0.2-0.3 cun. δ is applicable.	On the lateral side of the foot, posterior and inferior to the external malleolus, directly below BL 60 Kunlun, lateral to the calcaneum, at the junction of the red and white skin. 1. Regulates middle-jiao. 2. Tranquilizes convulsion and relieves rigidity of muscles.	1. The meridian course: Heel pain, lumbago, cramps due to cholera morbus, beriberi, pain in knees, flaccidity and weakness of lower limbs. 2. Mental: Manic-depressive psychosis, epilepsy, corpse-like syncope. 3. Other: Vomiting, regurgitation, stranguria with turbid urine.
BL-62 Shenmai *One of Eight Confluent Points, connecting with Yangqiao M.* ⊥ 0.2-0.3 cun. δ is applicable.	On the lateral side of the foot, in the depression directly below the external malleolus. 1. Tranquilizes convulsion and relieves epilepsy. 2. Calms mind.	1. The meridian course: Cold-pain in lower back and coccyx, pain in waist and legs, foot and calf pain, swelling of external ankle, paralysis of lower limbs. 2. Head and sense organs: Headache, dizziness, tinnitus, conjunctival congestion, epistaxis, distortion of face. 3. Mental: Manic-depressive psychosis, daily epileptic attacks, aphasia due to apoplexy, opisthotonos. 4. Other: Aversion to cold.
BL-63 Jinmen *Xi-Cleft Point* ⊥ 0.3-0.5 cun. δ is applicable.	On the lateral side of the foot, directly below the anterior border of the external malleolus, on the lower border of the cuboid bone. 1. Calms mind and tranquilizes epilepsy. 2. Dredges meridians and collaterals.	1. The meridian course: Lumbago, flaccidity or numbness of lower limbs, soreness and pain in knees and calves, cramping due to cholera morbus, swelling and pain in external ankle. 2. Head and sense organs: Headache, tinnitus, deafness. 3. Mental: Epilepsy, coma, corpse-like syncope, infantile convulsion. 4. Other: Acute hernia, pain in lower abdomen.

Tab. II-8 Points of the Bladder Meridian of Foot-Taiyang (BL)

Point, Property , Method & Remarks	Location & Action	Categories of Diseases & Indications
BL-64 Jinggu ***Yuan-Source Point*** *⊥ 0.3-0.5 cun.* *♁ is applicable.*	On the lateral side of the foot, below the tuberosity of the 5th metatarsal bone, at the junction of the red and white skin. 1. Tranquilizes convulsion and relieves epilepsy. 2. Brightens eyes and relieves rigidity of muscles.	1. The meridian course: Neck rigidity, acute pain in waist which causes difficulty in lying flat, pain in lower back and legs, knee pain with contracture of feet. 2. Head and sense organs: Headache, dizziness, erosion in inner canthus, nebula, epistaxis. 3. Mental: Manic-depressive psychosis, epilepsy, infantile convulsion. 4. Digestive: Diarrhea, fullness sensation in abdomen, loss of appetite. 5. Cardiovascular: Precordial pain, palpitation. 6. Other: Malaria, alternating fever and chills.
BL-65 Shugu ***Shu-Stream Point*** *⊥ 0.3 cun.* *♁ is applicable.*	On the lateral side of the foot, posterior to the 5th metatarsophalangeal joint, at the junction of the red and white skin. 1. Calms mind, clears heat and relieves edema.	1. The meridian course: Neck rigidity causing difficulty in turning head, acute pain of upper and lower back with difficulty in lying flat, pain in legs and loins, pain in back of lower limbs. 2. Head and sense organs: Headache, dizziness, erosion in inner canthus, hyperdacryosis, deafness. 3. Digestive: Diarrhea, dysentery. 4. Gynecopathies: Metrorrhagia and metrostaxis. 5. External: Hemorrhoids, carbuncle, cellulitis and carbuncle on back, furuncle. 6. Mental: Manic-depressive psychosis. 7. Other: Fever, aversion to cold.

Tab. II-8   Points of the Bladder Meridian of Foot-Taiyang (BL)

Point, Property , Method & Remarks	Location & Action	Categories of Diseases & Indications
BL-66 Zutonggu *Ying-Spring Point* ⊥ *0.2-0.3 cun.* ᵟ *is applicable.*	On the lateral side of the foot, anterior to the 5th metatarsophalangeal joint, at the junction of the red and white skin. 1. Calms mind. 2. Clears heat and stops malaria.	1. The meridian course: Heaviness and pain in head, neck rigidity, vertigo, stuffy nose. 2. Head and sense organs: Dizziness and epistaxis. 3. Respiratory: Cough with fullness sensation in chest. 4. Gynecopathies: Metrorrhagia and metrostaxis. 5. Mental: Manic-depressive psychosis, hyper-susceptibility to fright.
BL-67 Zhiyin *Jing-Well Point* ⟍ *0.1 cun.* ᵟ *is applicable.*	On the lateral side of the distal segment of the little toe, 0.1 cun from the corner of the toenail. 1. Removes obstruction from nose and benefits eyes. 2. Relieves rigidity of muscles and corrects malposition of fetus.	1. The meridian course: Swollen knees and feet, hot sensation in sole. 2. Head and sense organs: Headache, rigidity and pain in neck, ophthalmalgia, stuffy nose, epistaxis. 3. Urogenital: Dysuria, seminal emission, abnormal fetal position, dystocia, retained placenta. 4. Other: Hernia, generalized pruritis, non-sweating syndrome, dysphoria, convulsion.

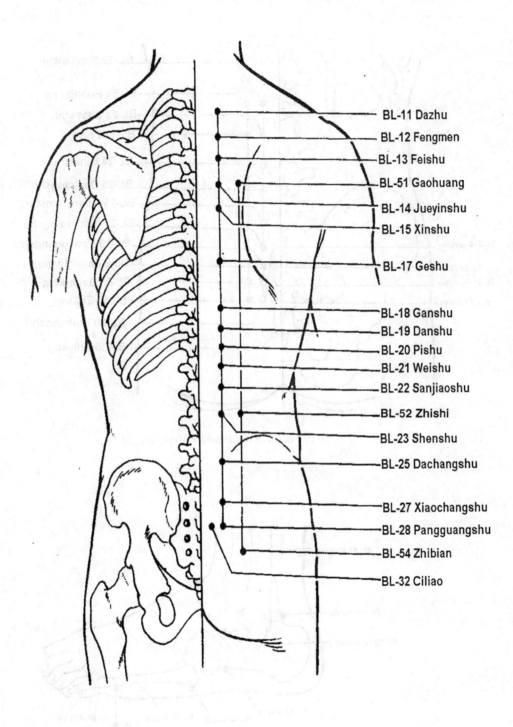

BL-11 Dazhu
BL-12 Fengmen
BL-13 Feishu
BL-51 Gaohuang
BL-14 Jueyinshu
BL-15 Xinshu
BL-17 Geshu
BL-18 Ganshu
BL-19 Danshu
BL-20 Pishu
BL-21 Weishu
BL-22 Sanjiaoshu
BL-52 Zhishi
BL-23 Shenshu
BL-25 Dachangshu
BL-27 Xiaochangshu
BL-28 Pangguangshu
BL-54 Zhibian
BL-32 Ciliao

Fig II-18 Points of the Bladder Meridian (4)

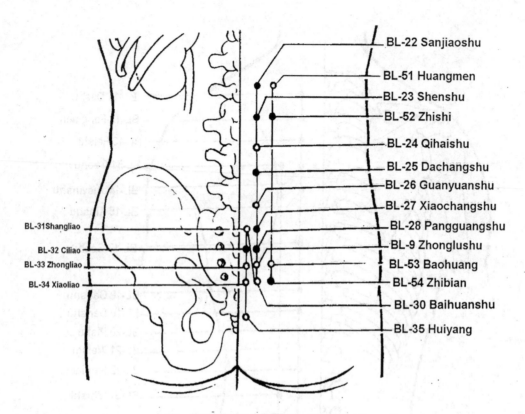

Fig. II-19 Points of the Bladder Meridian (5)

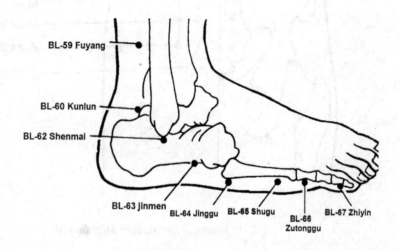

Fig. II-20 Points of the Bladder Meridian (6)

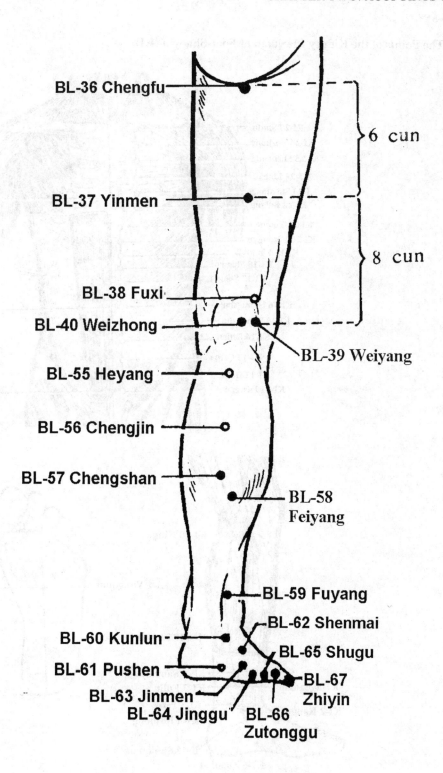

Fig. II-21 Points of the Bladder Meridian (7)

8. The Points of the Kidney Meridian of Foot-Shaoyin (KI)

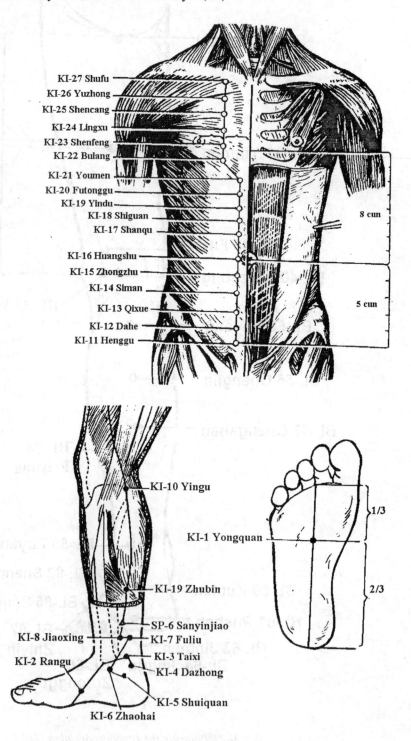

KI-27 Shufu
KI-26 Yuzhong
KI-25 Shencang
KI-24 Lingxu
KI-23 Shenfeng
KI-22 Bulang
KI-21 Youmen
KI-20 Futonggu
KI-19 Yindu
KI-18 Shiguan
KI-17 Shanqu
KI-16 Huangshu
KI-15 Zhongzhu
KI-14 Siman
KI-13 Qixue
KI-12 Dahe
KI-11 Henggu

8 cun

5 cun

KI-10 Yingu

KI-1 Yongquan

1/3

2/3

KI-19 Zhubin

SP-6 Sanyinjiao
KI-8 Jiaoxing
KI-7 Fuliu
KI-2 Rangu
KI-3 Taixi
KI-4 Dazhong
KI-5 Shuiquan
KI-6 Zhaohai

Fig.I-20 Points of the Kidney Meridian (1)

Tab. II-9 Points of the Kidney Meridian of Foot-Shaoyin (KI)

Point, Property, Method & Remarks	Location & Action	Categories of Diseases & Indications
KI-1 Yongquan *Jing-Well Point* ↓ *0.3-0.5 cun.* Ⴘ *is applicable.*	On the sole, in the depression appearing on the anterior part of the sole when the foot is in plantar flexion, approximately at the junction of the anterior third and posterior two-thirds of the line connecting the base of the 2nd and 3rd toes and the heel. 1. Tonifies kidney and promotes urination. 2. Pacifies liver and extinguishes wind.	1. The meridian course: Cold and pain in feet and knees, hot sensation on the center of the sole. 2. Head and sense organs: Vertex pain, dizziness, vertigo, dull complexion, blurring of vision, inflammation of throat, stiffness of root of tongue, aphonia, epistaxis. 3. Respiratory: Cough, shortness of breath, hemoptysis. 4. Digestive: Nausea, vomiting, epigastralgia, diarrhea, dyschesia, gastrointestinal neurosis. 5. Urogenital: Retention of urine, edema, sterility, impotence. 6. Cardiovascular: Vexation, precordial pain. 7. Mental: Coma, convulsion, epilepsy, apoplexy, hyper-susceptibility to fright, amnesia and anger. 8. Other: Hernia, fever, jaundice, hypertension.

Tab. II-9 Points of the Kidney Meridian of Foot-Shaoyin (KI)

Point, Property, Method & Remarks	Location & Action	Categories of Diseases & Indications
KI-2 Rangu *Ying-Spring Point* ⊥ *0.3-0.5 cun.* ᵟ *is applicable.*	On the medial border of the foot, below the tuberosity of the navicular bone, and at the junction of the red and white skin. 1. Tonifies kidney and arrests diarrhea. 2. Promotes urination to clear heat from heart.	1. The meridian course: Pain and numbness of legs, swelling on dorsum of foot, sprain, beriberi. 2. Head and sense organs: Painful throat, stiffness of tongue, aphonia. 3. Respiratory: Hemoptysis, shortness of breath. 4. Digestive: Diarrhea, dysentery, anorexia. 5. Urogenital: Irregular menstruation, prolapse of uterus, pruritis vulvae, impotence, spontaneous emission, cloudy urine, dysuria, retention of urine. 6. Cardiovascular: Precordial pain, spontaneous perspiration, night sweating. 7. Mental: Infantile convulsion, tetanus, hypersensitivity to fright, manic depressive psychosis, tetanus. 8. Other: Diabetes, jaundice, fullness and pain in lower abdomen.

Tab. II-9 Points of the Kidney Meridian of Foot-Shaoyin (KI)

Point, Property, Method & Remarks	Location & Action	Categories of Diseases & Indications
KI-3 Taixi *Shu-Stream Point* *Yuan-Source Point* ± *0.3-0.5 cun.* ᶿ *is applicable.*	On the medial side of the foot, posterior to the medial malleolus, in the depression between the tip of the medial malleolus and Achilles tendon. 1. Tonifies kidney to assist its function of receiving qi. 2. Strengthens spleen to nourish lung.	1. The meridian course: Arthralgia, pain and cold sensation of lower limbs, limited movement of legs, painful and swollen heel and medial malleolus. 2. Head and sense organs: Headache, dizziness, painful and swollen throat, toothache, tinnitus, deafness, epistaxis. 3. Respiratory: Cough, dyspnea, hemoptysis, chest pain, fullness in chest and hypochondrium, sticky phlegm. 4. Digestive: Cholera morbus, diarrhea, constipation. 5. Urogenital: Irregular menstruation, mass in abdomen, spontaneous emission, impotence, whitish and cloudy urine, frequent micturition, dark urine. 6. Cardiovascular: Palpitation, precordial pain. 7. Mental: Insomnia, amnesia, vexation, irritability, over-susceptibility to fright. 8. Other: Diabetes, acute mastitis, hernia due to cold.
KI-4 Dazhong *Luo-Connecting Point* ± *0.3-0.5 cun.* ᶿ *is applicable.*	On the medial side of the foot, posterior and inferior to the medial malleolus, in the depression on the medial side of and anterior to the attachment of the Achilles tendon. 1. Tonifies kidney and stops asthma. 2. Promotes bowel movement and urination.	1. The meridian course: Pain of heel. 2. Head and sense organs: Pharyngodynia, bleeding tongue. 3. Respiratory: Cough, dyspnea, fullness sensation of chest. 4. Digestive: Dysphasia, constipation, abdominal fullness, vomiting, sensation of heat in mouth, dry tongue. 5. Urogenital: Dysuria, retention of urine, stranguria, irregular menstruation. 6. Mental: Dementia, timidity, over-susceptibility to anger, insomnia, amnesia, dreaminess, hysteria.

Tab. II-9 Points of the Kidney Meridian of Foot-Shaoyin (KI)

Point, Property, Method & Remarks	Location & Action	Categories of Diseases & Indications
KI-5 Shuiquan *Xi-Cleft Point* ⊥ *0.3-0.5 cun.* ᵟ *is applicable.*	On medial side of the foot, posterior and inferior to the medial malleolus, 1 cun directly below KI-3 Taixi, in the depression at the medial side of the tuberosity of the calcacneum. 1. Tonifies kidney and clears heat. 2. Activates blood and dredges meridians.	1. Gynecopathies: Irregular menstruation, dysmenorrhea, amenorrhea, prolapse of uterus, metrorrhagia and metrostaxis. 2. Urinary: Dysuria, stranguria. 3. Other: Blurred vision, myopia, abdominal pain,.
KI-6 Zhaohai *One of Eight Confluent Points, connecting with Yinqiao M.* ⊥ *0.3-0.5 cun.* ᵟ *is applicable.*	On the medial side of the foot, in the depression below the tip of the medial malleolus. 1. Regulates yin and calms mind. 2. Regulates and benefits functions of the external genitalia and anus.	1. Head and sense organs: Heaviness of head, blurring of vision, dry and · painful throat, tetanus, conjunctival congestion, dull complexion. 2. Respiratory: Cough, asthma, abundant expectoration, hemoptysis. 3. Digestive: Anorexia, constipation, gastrointestinal neurosis. 4. Gynecopathies: Irregular menstruation, leukorrhea with reddish discharge, prolapse of uterus, pruritis vulvae, dystocia, lochiostasis, postpartum abdominal pain. 5. Urinary: Frequent micturition, dark urine, stranguria. 6. Mental: Night epilepsy, terror, insomnia, depressive syndrome, over susceptibility to sorrow. 7. Other: Hernia, flaccid feet.

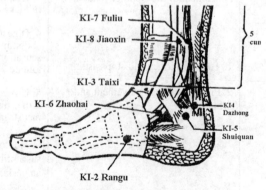

Fig. II-21 Points of the Kidney Meridian (2)

Tab. II-9 Points of the Kidney Meridian of Foot-Shaoyin (KI)

Point, Property , Method & Remarks	Location & Action	Categories of Diseases & Indications
KI-7 Fuliu *Jing-River Point* ⊥ *0.5-0.7 cun.* ᵟ *is applicable.*	On the medial side of the leg, 2 cun directly above KI-3 Taixi, anterior to the Achilles tendon. 1. Tonifies kidney and nourishes yin. 2. Regulates water passage.	1. The meridian course: Weakness of feet, limited movement of waist. 2. Head and sense organs: Dry mouth, pain inside nose. 3. Digestive: Diarrhea, borborygmus, abdominal pain or distention, constipation, dysentery with pus and blood, hemorrhoids. 4. Urogenital: Retention of urine, stranguria, spontaneous emission, metrorrhagia and metrostaxis.. 5. Mental: Manic-depressive syndrome, susceptibility to anger. 6. Other: Stiffness and pain along spinal column, edema, swollen limbs, weak and thready pulse, fever, lassitude, profuse sweating, night sweating, diabetes.
KI-8 Jiaoxin *Xi-Cleft Point of Yinqiao M.* ⊥ *0.5-0.7 cun.* ᵟ *is applicable.*	On the medial side of the leg, 2 cun above KI-3 Taixi and 0.5 cun anterior to KI-7 Fuliu, posterior to the medial border of the tibia. 1. Tonifies kidney and regulates menstruation. 2. Regulates and benefits functions of the external genitalia and anus.	1. The meridian course: Numbness and pain along medial side of legs. 2. Urogenital: Irregular menstruation, metrorrhagia and metrostaxis, amenorrhea, prolapse of uterus. pruritis vulvae, painful and swollen testicles, stranguria, retention of urine. 3. Digestive: Diarrhea, constipation, dysentery.
KI-9 Zhubin *Xi-Cleft Point of Yinwei M.* ⊥ *0.5-0.7 cun.* ᵟ *is applicable.*	On the medial side of the leg and on the line connecting KI-3 Taixi and KI-10 Yingu, 5 cun above KI-3 Taixi, medial and inferior to the gastrocnemius muscle belly. 1. Tonifies kidney, calms heart. 2. Promotes qi flow to stop pain.	1. The meridian course: Numbness and pain along medial side of legs. 2. Mental: Manic-depressive syndrome, epilepsy, water brash. 3. Other: Swollen and painful tongue, hernia, infantile umbilical hernia.

Tab. II-9 Points of the Kidney Meridian of Foot-Shaoyin (KI)

Point, Property , Method & Remarks	Location & Action	Categories of Diseases & Indications
KI-10 Yingu *He-Sea Point* ± *0.8 -1 cun.* ẟ *is applicable.*	On the medial side of the popliteal fossa, between the tendons of the semitendinous and semimembranosus muscles when the knee is flexed. 1. Tonifies kidney and reinforces yang. 2. Regulates function of external genitalia.	1. The meridian course: Pain in medial aspect of thigh, pain in knees joint. 2. Digestive: Abdominal distention, epigastralgia. 3. Urogenital: Irregular menstruation, menorrhagia and metrostaxis, leukorrhea, pudendal pain, impotence, eczema of scrotum, dysuria. 4. Other: Hernia, involuntary repeated protrusion of tongue with salivation, manic-depressive syndrome.
KI-11 Henggu *Crossing Point of KI and Chong M.* ± *0.5 -1 cun.* ẟ *is applicable.*	On the lower abdomen, 5 cun below the center of the umbilicus and 0.5 cun lateral to the anterior midline. 1. Tonifies kidney and reinforces yang. 2. Clears heat and promotes urination.	1. Urogenital: Pain in pudendum, amenorrhea, spontaneous emission, impotence, enuresis, stranguria, retention of urine, pain in lower abdomen. 2. Other: Hernia, lumbago, red, swollen and painful eyes.
KI-12 Dahe *Crossing Point of KI and Chong M.* ± *0.5 -1 cun.* ẟ *is applicable.*	On the lower abdomen, 4 cun below the center of the umbilicus and 0.5 cun lateral to the anterior midline. 1. Tonifies kidney and consolidates essence. 2. Regulates menstruation and improves reproductive ability.	1. Digestive: Diarrhea, dysentery, pain in lower abdomen. 2. Urogenital: Pain in pudendum, prolapse of uterus, irregular menstruation, dysmenorrhea, spontaneous emission, leukorrhea, pain in penis, enuresis, retention of urine, stranguria. 3. Other: Red, swollen and painful eyes.
KI-13 Qixue *Crossing Point of KI and Chong M.* ± *0.5 -1 cun.* ẟ *is applicable.*	On the lower abdomen, 3 cun below the center of the umbilicus and 0.5 cun lateral to the anterior midline. 1. Reinforces Chong and Ren Meridians. 2. Regulates functions of external genitalia and anus.	1. Digestive: Diarrhea, dysentery, intestinal colic. 2. Urogenital: Irregular menstruation, leukorrhea, impotence, sterility, retention of urine, stranguria. 3. Other: Pain along spinal column, gastrointestinal neurosis, red, painful and swollen eyes.

Tab. II-9 Points of the Kidney Meridian of Foot-Shaoyin (KI)

Point, Property , Method & Remarks	Location & Action	Categories of Diseases & Indications
KI-14 Siman *Crossing Point of KI and Chong M.* ⊥ *0.5 -1 cun.* *ᵬ is applicable.*	On the lower abdomen, 2 cun below the center of the umbilicus and 0.5 cun lateral to the anterior midline. 1. Regulates qi and relieves hernia. 2. Regulates menstruation and improves reproductive ability.	1. Urogenital: Irregular menstruation, metrorrhagia and metrostaxis, leukorrhea, sterility, lochiorrhea, spontaneous emission, gonorrhea, enuresis, dysuria. 2. Digestive: Constipation, diarrhea, dysentery, gastrointestinal neurosis. 3. Other: Pain below the umbilicus, red, painful and swollen eyes.
KI-15 Zhongzhu *Crossing Point of KI and Chong M.* ⊥ *0.5 -1 cun.* *ᵬ is applicable.*	On the lower abdomen, 1 cun below the center of the umbilicus and 0.5 cun lateral to the anterior midline. 1. Regulates menstruation. 2. Regulates large intestine function.	1. Urogenital: Irregular menstruation, stranguria. 2. Digestive: Constipation, diarrhea, dysentery. 3. Other: Cold sensation, pain in waist and abdomen, pain below the umbilicus, red, painful and swollen eyes.
KI-16 Huangshu *Crossing Point of KI and Chong M.* ⊥ *0.5 -1 cun.* *ᵬ is applicable.*	On the middle of the abdomen, 0.5 cun lateral to the center of the umbilicus. 1. Regulates qi and stops pain. 2. Moistens dryness to promote bowel movement.	1. Digestive: Vomiting, abdominal distension, pain around umbilicus, sensation of heat in lower abdomen, dysentery, diarrhea, constipation. 2. Gynecopathies: Irregular menstruation. 3. Other: Pain along spinal column, hernia, painful and red eyes.
KI-17 Shangqu *Crossing Point of KI and Chong M.* ⊥ *0.5 -1 cun.* *ᵬ is applicable.*	On the upper abdomen, 2 cun above the center of the umbilicus, and 0.5 cun lateral to the anterior midline. 1. Strengthens spleen and harmonizes stomach. 2. Eliminates food stagnation to stop pain.	1. Digestive: Diarrhea, dysentery, abdominal pain, poor appetite. 2. Other: Red and painful eyes.

Tab. II-9 Points of the Kidney Meridian of Foot-Shaoyin (KI)

Point, Property , Method & Remarks	Location & Action	Categories of Diseases & Indications
KI-18 Shiguan *Crossing Point of KI and Chong M.* ⊥ *0.5 -1 cun.* ∂ *is applicable.*	On the upper abdomen, 3 cun above the center of the umbilicus and 0.5 cun lateral to the anterior midline. 1. Resolves masses and fullness. 2. Tonifies kidney and improves reproductive ability.	1. Digestive: Vomiting, hiccup, stomachache, fullness and stiffness in epigastrium, constipation, 2. Gynecopathies: Abdominal pain after childbirth, sterility, irregular menstruation, dysmenorrhea.
KI-19 Yindu *Crossing Point of KI and Chong M.* ⊥ *0.5 -1 cun.* ∂ *is applicable.* *To avoid injuring liver, deep puncture is prohibited.*	On the upper abdomen, 4 cun above the center of the umbilicus and 0.5 cun lateral to the anterior midline. 1. Soothes chest oppression and subdues rebellious qi. 2. Regulates qi and harmonizes stomach.	1. Digestive: Abdominal distension, borborygmus, stomachache, constipation, fullness of upper abdomen, jaundice. 2. Gynecopathies: Sterility. 3. Respiratory: Asthma, dyspnea. 3. Other: Malaria, pain in chest and hypochondrium, red and painful eyes.
KI-20 Futonggu *Crossing Point of KI and Chong M.* ⊥ *0.5 -1 cun.* ∂ *is applicable.* *To avoid injuring liver, deep puncture is prohibited.*	On the upper abdomen, 5 cun above the center of the umbilicus and 0.5 cun lateral to the anterior midline. 1. Strengthens spleen and harmonizes stomach. 2. Soothes chest oppression and calms mind.	1. Respiratory: Cough, asthma. 2. Digestive: Abdominal pain or distention. 3. Cardiovascular: Precordial pain, palpitation, pain in chest and hypochondrium. 4. Mental: Epilepsy, palpitation due to fright.
KI-21 Youmen *Crossing Point of KI and Chong M.* ⊥ *0.3-0.7 cun.* ∂ *is applicable.* *To avoid injuring liver, deep puncture is prohibited.*	On the upper abdomen, 6 cun above the center of the umbilicus and 0.5 cun lateral to the anterior midline. 1. Strengthens spleen and harmonizes stomach. 2. Subdues rebellious qi and stops vomiting.	1. Digestive: Stomachache, abdominal distention, vomiting, diarrhea, dysentery. 2. Gynecopathies: Galactostasis, acute mastitis. 3. Other: Pain in chest which involves the waist and back, red and painful eyes.

Tab. II-9 Points of the Kidney Meridian of Foot-Shaoyin (KI)

Point, Property , Method & Remarks	Location & Action	Categories of Diseases & Indications
KI-22 Bulang *↘ 0.3-0.5 cun.* *ẞ is applicable.* ***To avoid injuring heart & lung, deep puncture is prohibited.***	On the chest, in the 5th intercostal space, 2 cun lateral to the anterior midline. 1. Soothes chest oppression and subdues rebellious qi. 2. Relieves cough and asthma.	1. Respiratory: Fullness and pain in chest and hypochondrium, cough, asthma, nasal obstruction. 2. Digestive: Vomiting, poor appetite. 3. Other: Acute mastitis.
KI-23 Shenfeng *↘ 0.3-0.5 cun.* *ẞ is applicable.* ***To avoid injuring heart & lung, deep puncture is prohibited.***	On the chest, in the 4th intercostal space, 2 cun lateral to the anterior midline. 1. Soothes chest oppression and stops cough. 2. Subdues rebellious qi and harmonizes stomach.	1. Respiratory: Cough, dyspnea, restlessness due to fullness in chest. 2. Digestive: Vomiting, poor appetite. 3. Other: Acute mastitis.
KI-24 Lingxu *↘ 0.3-0.5 cun.* *ẞ is applicable.* ***To avoid injuring heart & lung, deep puncture is prohibited.***	On the chest, in the 3rd intercostal space, 2 cun lateral to the anterior midline. 1. Soothes liver and chest oppression. 2. Subdues rebellious lung qi.	1. Respiratory: Cough, dyspnea, abundant expectoration. 2. Digestive: Vomiting, poor appetite. 3. Other: Acute mastitis, fullness and pain in chest and hypochondrium.
KI-25 Shencang *↘ 0.3-0.5 cun.* *ẞ is applicable.* ***To avoid injuring lung, deep puncture is prohibited.***	On the chest, in the 2nd intercostal space, 2 cun lateral to the anterior midline. 1. Soothes chest oppression and regulates qi. 2. Stops cough and transforms phlegm.	1. Respiratory: Cough, asthma, profuse sputum, oppression and feeling of fullness in chest and hypochondrium. 2. Digestive: Vomiting, poor appetite. 3. Other: Acute mastitis.
KI-26 Yuzhong *↘ 0.3-0.5 cun.* *ẞ is applicable.* ***To avoid injuring lung, deep puncture is prohibited.***	On the chest, in the 1st intercostal space, 2 cun lateral to the anterior midline. 1. Stops cough and asthma. 2. Harmonizes stomach and subdues rebellious qi.	1. Respiratory: Cough, dyspnea, abundant expectoration, fullness and pain in chest and hypochondrium. 2. Digestive: Vomiting, poor appetite. 3. Other: Acute mastitis.

Tab. II-9 Points of the Kidney Meridian of Foot-Shaoyin (KI)

Point, Property , Method & Remarks	Location & Action	Categories of Diseases & Indications
KI-27 Shufu ⊻ *0.3-0.5 cun.* *δ is applicable.*	On the chest, below the lower border of the clavicle, 2 cun lateral to the midline. 1. Stops cough and asthma. 2. Harmonizes stomach and subdues rebellious qi.	1. Respiratory: Cough, dyspnea, pain in chest, restlessness due to fullness sensation in chest. 2. Digestive: Abdominal distension, vomiting, poor appetite.

9. The Points of the Pericardium Meridian of Hand-Jueyin (PC)

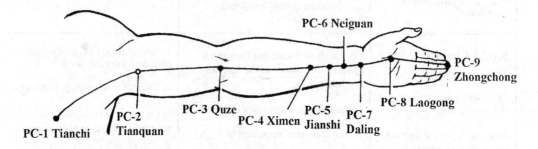

Fig. II-22 Points On The Pericardium Meridian (1)

Tab. II-10 Points of the Pericardium Meridian of Hand-Jueyin (PC)

Point, Property, Method & Remarks	Location & Action	Categories of Diseases & Indications
PC-1 Tianchi *Crossing Point of PC & GB* ⊻ *0.2-0.4 cun.* *δ is applicable.* **Deep puncture is prohibited.**	On the chest, in the 4th intercostal space, 1 cun lateral to the nipple and 5 cun lateral to the anterior midline. 1. Soothes chest oppression, regulates qi and stops pain.	1. Cardiovascular: Cardiac pain, feeling of pain and oppression in chest, fullness in chest. 2. Respiratory: Cough, asthma, excessive phlegm, wheezing sound in throat. 3. Other: Scrofula in axilla, mastitis, pain in hypochondrium.

Tab. II-10 Points of the Pericardium Meridian of Hand-Jueyin (PC)

Point, Property, Method & Remarks	Location & Action	Categories of Diseases & Indications
PC-2 Tianquan ⟂ *0.5-0.7 cun.* *ᵹ is applicable.*	On the medial side of the arm, 2 cun below the anterior end of the axillary fold, between the long and short heads of the biceps muscle of the arm. 1. Soothes chest oppression and regulates qi. 2. Stops cough.	1. The meridian course: Pain in chest and medial aspect of upper limbs. 2. Cardiovascular: Cardiac pain, palpitation, fullness in chest and hypochondrium. 3. Respiratory: Cough, pain in chest. 4. Other: Hiccup, failure of lower limbs when walking, blurring of vision.
PC-3 Quze *He-Sea Point* ⟂ *0.5-0.7 cun or prick to cause bleeding.* *ᵹ is applicable.*	At the midpoint of the cubital crease, on the ulnar side of the tendon of the biceps muscle of the arm. 1. Clears heart and stops pain. 2. Harmonizes stomach and subdues rebellious qi.	1. The meridian course: Pain in arm and elbow, tremor in upper limbs. 2. Cardiovascular: Cardiac pain, palpitation. 3. Respiratory: Cough. 4. Digestive: Stomachache, vomiting, hematemesis, cholera, diarrhea. 5. Other: Heatstroke, febrile disease, dry mouth.
PC-4 Ximen *Xi-Cleft Point* ⟂ *0.5-1 cun.* *ᵹ is applicable.*	On the palmar side of the forearm and on the line connecting PC-3 Quze and PC-7 Daling, 5 cun above the crease of the wrist. 1. Clears heart and relieves cough. 2. Cools blood and arrests bleeding.	1. The meridian course: Hemiplegia, numbness and pain of arm and shoulder. 2. Cardiovascular: Cardiac pain, palpitation, irritability, chest pain. 3. Respiratory: Hemoptysis. 4. Digestive: Hematemesis. 5. Mental: Epilepsy, timidity, hysteria. 6. Other: Uterine bleeding, furuncle, mastitis.

Tab. II-10 Points of the Pericardium Meridian of Hand-Jueyin (PC)

Point, Property, Method & Remarks	Location & Action	Categories of Diseases & Indications
PC-5 Jianshi *Jing-River Point* ⊥ *0.5-1 cun.* *ᵭ is applicable.*	On the palmar side of the forearm and on the line connecting PC-3 Quze and PC-7 Daling, 3 cun above the crease of the wrist, between the tendons of the palmaris longus muscle and radial flexor muscle of the wrist. 1. Soothes chest oppression and relieves depressed qi. 2. Calms heart and subdues rebellious qi.	1. The meridian course: Swelling of axilla, pain of arm, spasm of elbow, feverish sensation in palm. 2. Cardiovascular: Cardiac pain, palpitation, slow and irregular pulse. 3. Digestive: Stomachache, vomiting, cholera, diarrhea. 4. Head and sense organs: Sore throat. 5. Mental: Epilepsy, mania, depression, apoplexy, infantile convulsion, aphasia, hysteria. 6. Other: Metrorrhagia and metrostaxis, scabies, malaria.
PC-6 Neiguan *Luo-Connecting Point; One of Eight Confluent Points, joining Yinwei M.* ⊥ *0.5-0.8 cun.* *ᵭ is applicable.*	On the palmar side of the forearm and on the line connecting PC-3 Quze and PC-7 Daling, 2 cun above the crease of the wrist, between the tendons of the palmaris longus muscle and radial flexor muscle of the wrist. 1. Calms mind and stops pain. 2. Soothes liver and regulates middle-jiao.	1. The meridian course: Spasmodic pain of arm, elbow and wrist, hemiplegia. 2. Cardiovascular: Cardiac pain, palpitation, pain in chest and hypochondrium. 3. Respiratory: Cough, asthma, fullness sensation in chest, shortness of breath. 4. Head and sense organs: Migraine, vertigo. 5. Digestive: Stomachache with distention, vomiting, hiccups, gastric and abdominal distention, diarrhea. 6. Genital: Irregular menstruation, vomiting due to pregnancy, postpartum vertigo, nocturnal emission. 7. Mental: Insomnia, amnesia, depression, mania, epilepsy, melancholia, apoplexy. 8. Other: Heatstroke, malaria, anhidrosis.

Tab. II-10 Points of the Pericardium Meridian of Hand-Jueyin (PC)

Point, Property, Method & Remarks	Location & Action	Categories of Diseases & Indications
PC-7 Daling *Shu-Stream Point* ⊥ *0.3-0.5 cun.* ᵟ *is applicable.*	At the midpoint of the crease of the wrist, between the tendons of the palmaris longus muscle and radial flexor muscle of the wrist. 1. Calms heart and mind. 2. Soothes chest oppression and regulates stomach.	1. The meridian course: Spasmodic pain of arm, elbow and wrist, feverish sensation in palms. 2. Cardiovascular: Cardiac pain, palpitation, fullness sensation in chest, shortness of breath. 3. Digestive: Stomachache, vomiting, appendicitis, cholera, hematemesis, halitosis. 4. Head and sense organs: Headache, sore throat, pain, swelling and redness of eyes, stiffness of tongue. 5. Mental: Timidity, depression, mania, epilepsy, capriciousness, over-susceptibility to fright and anger. 6. Other: Eczema, urticaria, scabies, sores, anhidrosis
PC-8 Laogong *Ying-Spring Point* ⊥ *0.3-0.5 cun.* ᵟ *is applicable.*	At the center of the palm, between the 2nd and 3rd metacarpal bones, but close to the latter, and in the part touching the tip of the middle finger when a fist is made. 1. Clears heat and calms heart. 2. Relieves swelling and arrests itching.	1. The meridian course: Anhidrosis in palm, numbness of fingers, feverish sensation in palms. 2. Cardiovascular: Pain in chest and hypochondrium, cardiac pain. 3. Digestive: Epigastric pain, vomiting, poor appetite, blood in stool. 4. Head and sense organs: Headache, trigeminal neuralgia, halitosis, epistaxis, swelling of throat, aphasia. 5. Mental: Coma, infantile epilepsy, hysteria. 6. Other: Lower abdominal mass, hematuria, fever, wind stroke, heatstroke.

Tab. II-10 Points of the Pericardium Meridian of Hand-Jueyin (PC)

Point, Property, Method & Remarks	Location & Action	Categories of Diseases & Indications
PC-9 Zhongchong *Jing-Well Point* ⊥ *superficially 0.1 cun or prick to cause bleeding.* ∂ *is applicable.*	At the center of the tip of the middle finger. 1. Induces resuscitation. 2. Clears heat from heart.	1. The meridian course: Numbness of fingers. 2. Cardiovascular: Cardiac pain, palpitation. 3. Digestive: Epigastric pain, cholera, vomiting, diarrhea. 4. Head and sense organs: Tinnitus, pain and swelling, stiffness of tongue, headache. 5. Mental: Coma, infantile convulsion. 6. Other: High fever, heatstroke, wind stroke.

10. The Points of the Sanjiao Meridian of Hand-Shaoyang (SJ)

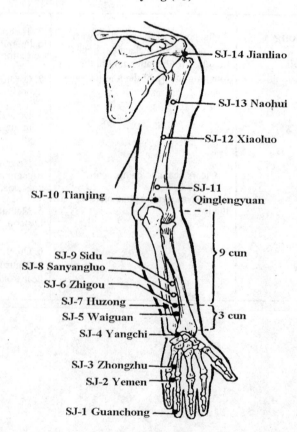

Fig. II-23 Points on the Sanjiao Meridian (1)

Tab. II-11   Points of the Sanjiao Meridian of Hand-Shaoyang (SJ) (Triple Energizer, TE)

Point, Property, Method & Remarks	Location & Action	Categories of Diseases & Indications
SJ-1 Guanchong *Jing-Well Point* ⊥ *superficially 0.1 cun or prick to cause bleeding.* ᵭ *is applicable.*	On the ulnar side of the distal segment of the 4th finger, 0.1 cun from the corner of the nail. 1. Clears heat and relieves exterior. 2. Clears heart and improves hearing acuity.	1. The meridian course: Numbness at tip of fingers, inability to raise limbs. 2. Head and sense organs: Headache, dizziness, tinnitus, deafness, redness and pain of eyes, cataract, stiff tongue, curled tongue, fissured tongue, stiffness of tongue root, dry and fissured lips, sore throat, mumps, submandibular swelling. 3. Digestive: Cholera, vomiting, poor appetite, rectal prolapse. 4. Mental: Apoplexy, sunstroke, coma, loss of consciousness. 5. Other: Febrile disease, malaria.
SJ-2 Yemen *Ying-Spring Point* ⊾ *0.3-0.5 cun toward the interspace of the metacarpal bones.* ᵭ *is applicable.*	On the dorsum of the hand, between the 4th and 5th fingers, at the junction of the red and white skin, proximal to the margin of the web. 1. Clears head and improves hearing acuity. 2. Harmonizes and relieves exterior and interior.	1. The meridian course: Pain in arm and hands, redness and swelling of dorsum of hand, spasms of fingers. 2. Head and sense organs: Headache, dizziness, excessive lacrimation, redness and swelling of eyes, facial edema, deafness, tinnitus, toothache, pain and swelling of gums, aphasia, sore throat. 3. Mental: Timidity, delirium. 4. Other: Febrile diseases, malaria.
SJ-3 Zhongzhu *Shu-Stream Point* ⊥ *0.3-0.5 cun.* ᵭ *is applicable.*	On the dorsum of the hand, proximal to the 4th metacarpophalangeal joint, in the depression between the 4th and 5th metacarpal bones. 1. Clears heat and benefits throat. 2. Improves visual and hearing acuity.	1. The meridian course: Pain in shoulder, back, elbow and arm, limited movement of fingers, torticollis. 2. Head and sense organs: Headache, vertigo, flushed face, redness and pain of eyes, blurring of vision, deafness, tinnitus, sore throat. 3. Other: Febrile disease, malaria, furuncle.

Tab. II-11   Points of the Sanjiao Meridian of Hand-Shaoyang (SJ) (Triple Energizer, TE)

Point, Property, Method & Remarks	Location & Action	Categories of Diseases & Indications
SJ-4 Yangchi *Yuan-Source Point* ⊥ *0.3-0.5 cun.* ᵦ *is applicable.*	At the midpoint of the dorsal crease of the wrist, in the depression on the ulnar side of the tendon of the extensor muscle of the fingers. 1. Benefits throat and improves hearing acuity. 2. Harmonizes and relieves exterior and interior.	1. The meridian course: Pain, weakness, redness and swelling of wrist, motor impairment of wrist or failure to flex wrist, pain in neck, shoulder, elbow and forearm. 2. Head and sense organs: Deafness, redness and swelling of eyes, sore throat. 3. Digestive: Infantile diarrhea, indigestion, malnutrition, diabetes, dry mouth, constipation. 4. Urinary: Enuresis. 5. Other: Febrile disease, malaria, common cold.
SJ-5 Waiguan *Luo-Connecting Point; One of Eight Confluent Points, connecting with Yangwei M.* ⊥ *0.5-1 cun.* ᵦ *is applicable.*	On the dorsal side of the forearm and on the line connecting SJ-4 Yangchi and the tip of the olecranon, 2 cun proximal to the dorsal crease of the wrist, between the radius and ulna. 1. Relieves exterior and clears heat.	1. The meridian course: Difficulty in movement of elbow and arm, pain in upper limbs, shaking of hand, pain in fingers, hemiplegia, hypochondriac pain, torticollis. 2. Head and sense organs: Headache, pain, redness and swelling of eyes, tinnitus, deafness, epistaxis, toothache. 3. Digestive: Abdominal pain, constipation, cholera, appendicitis, poor appetite. 4. Mental: Acute convulsion, irritability and over-susceptibility to anger. 5. Other: Febrile disease, common cold, warts.

Tab. II-11   Points of the Sanjiao Meridian of Hand-Shaoyang (SJ) (Triple Energizer, TE)

Point, Property, Method & Remarks	Location & Action	Categories of Diseases & Indications
SJ-6 Zhigou *Jing-River Point* ⊥ *0.8-1.2 cun.* ᵦ *is applicable.*	On the dorsal side of the forearm and on the line connecting SJ-4 Yangchi and the tip of the olecranon, 3 cun proximal to the dorsal crease of the wrist, between the radius and ulna. 1. Clears heat and improves hearing acuity. 2. Descends large intestine qi and moistens large intestine.	1. The meridian course: Soreness and pain of shoulder, arm and back, pain in hypochondrium, difficulty in movement of neck. 2. Head and sense organs: Deafness, tinnitus, sudden loss of voice, pain and redness of eyes, sore throat. 3. Digestive: Constipation, vomiting, diarrhea. 4. Mental: Irritability, over-susceptibility to anger. 5. Gynecopathies: Amenorrhea, postpartum hemorrhage, dysmenorrhea. 6. Other: Fullness sensation of chest and hypochondrium, febrile disease.
SJ-7 Huizong *Xi-Cleft Point* ⊥ *0.5-1 cun.* ᵦ *is applicable.*	On the dorsal side of the forearm, 3 cun proximal to the dorsal crease of the wrist, on the ulnar side of SJ-6 Zhigou and on the radial border of the ulna. 1. Improves hearing acuity and stops cough.	1. The meridian course: Pain of upper limbs. 2. Head and sense organs: Tinnitus, deafness. 3. Mental: Manic and depressive psychosis.
SJ-8 Sanyangluo ⊥ *0.5-1 cun.* ᵦ *is applicable.*	On the dorsal side of the forearm, 4 cun proximal to the dorsal crease of wrist, between the radius and ulna. 1. Improves hearing acuity and benefits throat.	1. The meridian course: Pain and inability to raise arm. 2. Head and sense organs: Sudden loss of voice, deafness, dental caries, eye problems. 3. Other: Lower back pain due to acute lumbar sprain, aversion to cold, fever without sweating, somnolence.
SJ-9 Sidu ⊥ *0.5-1 cun.* ᵦ *is applicable.*	On the dorsal side of the forearm and on the line connecting SJ-4 Yangchi and the tip of the olecranon, 5 cun distal to the tip of the olecranon, between the radius and ulna. 1. Improves hearing acuity and benefits throat.	1. The meridian course: Pain of forearm. 2. Head and sense organs: Sudden loss of voice, sudden onset of deafness, toothache, globus hystericus.

Tab. II-11   Points of the Sanjiao Meridian of Hand-Shaoyang (SJ) (Triple Energizer, TE)

Point, Property, Method & Remarks	Location & Action	Categories of Diseases & Indications
SJ-10 Tianjing *He-Sea Point* ⊥ *0.3-0.5 cun.* *ᵠ is applicable.*	On the lateral side of the upper arm, in the depression 1 cun proximal to the tip of the olecranon when the elbow is flexed. 1. Improves hearing acuity and calms mind. 2. Regulates qi and transforms phlegm.	1. The meridian course: Pain and numbness of arm and shoulder, elbow pain, hypochondriac pain. 2. Head and sense organs: Migraine, deafness, tinnitus, pain of eyes, sore throat, swelling of cheek. 3. Respiratory: Cough with spitting bloody pus. 4. Cardiovascular: Cardiac pain, palpitation. 5. Mental: Epilepsy, convulsion, apoplexy. 6. Other: Scrofula, goiter, warts, sores, urticaria.
SJ-11 Qinglengyuan ⊥ *0.3-0.5 cun.* *ᵠ is applicable.*	With the elbow flexed, on the lateral side of the upper arm , 2 cun above the tip of the olecranon and 1 cun above SJ-10 Tianjing. 1. Warms the meridian and dispels cold.	1. The meridian course: Motor impairment of shoulder. 2. Head and sense organs: Eye pain, headache. 3. Other: Chills, fever.
SJ-12 Xiaoluo ⊥ *0.5-0.7 cun.* *ᵠ is applicable.*	On the lateral side of the upper arm, at midpoint of line connecting SJ-11 Qinglengyuan and SJ-13 Naohui. 1. Dispels wind and clears heat. 2. Clears heart and calms mind.	1. The meridian course: Stiffness and pain of neck and nape, pain of arm. 2. Head and sense organs: Headache.
SJ-13 Naohui *Crossing Point of SJ & LI; Crossing Point of SJ & Yangwei M.* ⊥ *0.5-0.8 cun.* *ᵠ is applicable.*	On lateral side of upper arm and on the line connecting the olecranon tip and SJ-14 Jianliao, 3 cun below SJ-14 Jianliao, on the posteroinferior border of the deltoid muscle. 1. Regulates qi and transforms phlegm.	1. The meridian course: Pain in scapular region, numbness and pain of arm. 2. Head and sense organs: Eye disorders. 3. Other: Scrofula, goiter.

Tab. II-11   Points of the Sanjiao Meridian of Hand-Shaoyang (SJ) (Triple Energizer, TE)

Point, Property, Method & Remarks	Location & Action	Categories of Diseases & Indications
SJ-14 Jianliao ⊥ *0.7-1 cun.* *ᵟ is applicable.*	On the shoulder, posterior to LI-15 Jianyu, in the depression inferior and posterior to the acromion when the arm is abducted. 1. Stops pain and benefits the joint.	1. The meridian course: Pain and heaviness of arm and inability to raise shoulder.
SJ-15 Tianliao *Crossing Point of SJ & Yangwei M.;* *Crossing Point of Yangwei M. & GB* ⊥ *0.3-0.5 cun.* *ᵟ is applicable.*	On the scapula, at the midpoint between GB-21 Jianjing and SI-13 Quyuan, at the superior angle of the scapula. 1. Clears heat and relieves exterior. 2. Soothes chest oppression and regulates qi.	1. The meridian course: Pain in arm and shoulder, pain in neck. 2. Other: Irritability and fullness in chest, febrile disease without sweating, fever and aversion to cold.
SJ-16 Tianyou ⊥ *0.3-0.5 cun.* *ᵟ is applicable.*	On the lateral side of the neck, directly below the posterior border of the mastoid process, on the level of the mandibular angle, and on the posterior border of the sternocleidomastoid muscle. 1. Opens the orifices in head. 2. Transforms phlegm and stops malaria.	1. Head and sense organs: Headache, dizziness, swelling of face, pain of eyes, blurring of vision, sudden deafness, tinnitus, epistaxis, sore throat. 2. Other: Stiffness of neck, difficulty in movement of neck.
SJ-17 Yifeng *Crossing Point of SJ & GB* ⊥ *0.5-1 cun.* *ᵟ is applicable.*	Posterior to the ear lobe, in the depression between the mastoid process and mandibular angel. 1. Relieves deviation of mouth and eye. 2. Improves hearing acuity and relieves swelling.	1. Head and sense organs: Deviation of eye and mouth, tinnitus, wetness and itching in ear, blurring of vision, cataract, toothache, sore throat, mumps. 2. Mental: Convulsion, mania, stuttering.

Tab. II-11   Points of the Sanjiao Meridian of Hand-Shaoyang (SJ) (Triple Energizer, TE)

Point, Property, Method & Remarks	Location & Action	Categories of Diseases & Indications
SJ-18 Chimai ⊥ *superficially 0.3-0.5 cun or prick to cause bleeding.* ᵟ *is applicable.*	On the head, at the center of the mastoid process, and at the junction of the middle third and lower third of the line connecting SJ-20 Jiaosun and SJ-17 Yifeng along the curve of the ear helix. 1. Improves hearing acuity. 2. Tranquilizes convulsion.	1. Head and sense organs: Tinnitus, deafness, blurring of vision. 2. Digestive: Vomiting, diarrhea, constipation. 3. Mental: Infantile convulsion.
SJ-19 Luxi ⊾ *0.3-0.5 cun.* ᵟ *is applicable.*	On the head, at the junction of the upper third and middle third of line connecting SJ-20 Jiaosun and SJ-17 Yifeng along the curve of ear helix. 1. Dispels wind and clears heat. 2. Tranquilizes convulsion and improves hearing acuity.	1. Head and sense organs: Headache, tinnitus, deafness, swelling and pain of ear, otorrhea. 2. Mental: Infantile convulsion. 3. Other: Asthma, pain in hypochondrium, vomiting, salivation, febrile diseases.
SJ-20 Jiaosun ***Crossing Point of GB & LI*** ⊾ *0.3-0.5 cun.* ᵟ *is applicable.*	On the head, above the ear apex within the hairline. 1. Improves visual acuity and removes nebula.	1. Head and sense organs: Swelling and pain of ear, redness and pain of eyes, blurring of vision, toothache, dry lips, aphthous ulcers, difficulty in chewing, mumps, stiffness of neck and headache.
SJ-21 Ermen ⊥ *0.3-0.5 cun.* ᵟ *is applicable.*	On the face, anterior to the supratragic notch, in the depression behind the posterior border of the condyloid process of the mandible. 1. Improves hearing acuity and relieves swelling.	1. Head and sense organs: Tinnitus, deafness, otorrhea, soreness or pain in ear, toothache, difficulty in chewing, swelling and pain of neck and submandibular region, deviation of mouth and eye.

Tab. II-11   Points of the Sanjiao Meridian of Hand-Shaoyang (SJ) (Triple Energizer, TE)

Point, Property, Method & Remarks	Location & Action	Categories of Diseases & Indications
SJ-22 Erheliao ↘ *0.1-0.3 cun.* *ᵟ is applicable.*	On the lateral side of the head, on the posterior margin of the temples, anterior to the anterior border of the root of the ear auricle and posterior to the superficial temporal artery. 1. Relieves swelling and stops pain. 2. Improves hearing acuity and calms mind.	1. Head and sense organs: Heaviness sensation and pain of head, tetanus, swelling of submandibular region, swelling and pain of tip of nose, running nose, facial paralysis. 2. Mental: Convulsion.
SJ-23 Sizhukong ⊥ *superficially 0.3-0.5 cun.*	On the face, in the depression of the lateral end of the eyebrow. 1. Dispels wind and clears heat. 2. Tranquilizes convulsion and calms mind.	1. Head and sense organs: Headache, vertigo, redness and pain of eyes, excessive lacrimation, twitching of eyelid, toothache. 2. Mental: Manic depression and insanity.

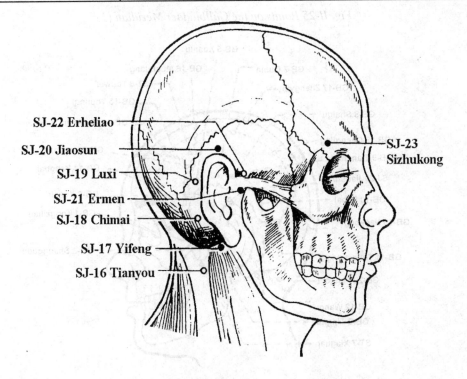

SJ-22 Erheliao
SJ-20 Jiaosun
SJ-19 Luxi
SJ-21 Ermen
SJ-18 Chimai
SJ-17 Yifeng
SJ-16 Tianyou

SJ-23 Sizhukong

Fig. II-24 Points on the Sanjiao Meridian (2)

11. The Points of the Gallbladder Meridian of Foot-Shaoyang (GB)

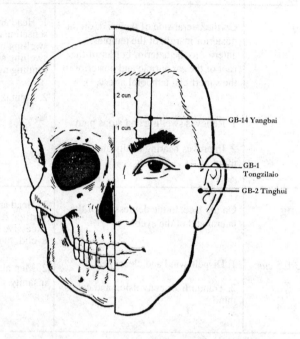

Fig. II-25 Points on the Gallbladder Meridian (1)

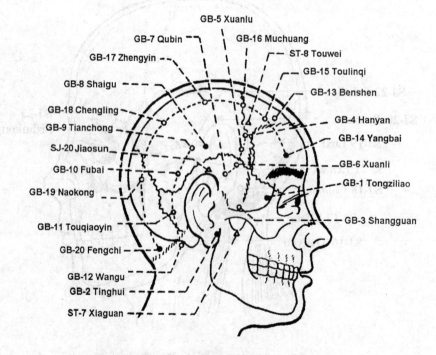

Fig. II-26 Points on the Gallbladder Meridian (2)

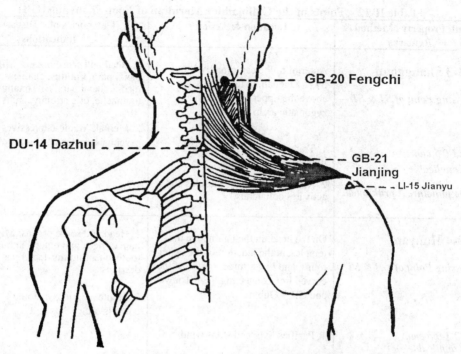

Fig. II-27 Points on the Gallbladder Meridian (3)

Table II-12   Points of the Gallbladder Meridian of Foot-Shaoyang (GB)

Point, Property , Method & Remarks	Location & Action	Categories of Diseases & Indications
GB-1 Tongziliao ***Crossing Point of SI, SJ & GB*** ↳ *0.3-0.5 cun.*	On the face, lateral to the outer canthus, on the lateral border of the orbit. 1. Pacifies liver and stops wind. 2. Improves visual acuity and removes nebula.	1. Head and sense organs: Conjunctival congestion, conjunctivitis, ophthalmalgia, photophobia, epiphora induced by wind, myopia, cataract, blurring of vision, facial paralysis, headache.
GB-2 Tinghui ↧ *0.5-0.7 cun.* *ß is applicable.*	On the face, anterior to the intertragic notch, in the depression posterior to the condyloid process of the mandible when the mouth is open. 1. Induces resuscitation and improves visual acuity. 2. Relieves rigidity of muscles and activates collaterals.	1. Head and sense organs: Headache, mumps, facial pain, tinnitus, deaf-mutism, otitis media, pain of ear, toothache, facial paralysis, mandibular subluxation. 2. Mental: Apoplexy, paralysis of limbs, severe dizziness, salivation, running wildly due to mania, clonic convulsion.

Table II-12   Points of the Gallbladder Meridian of Foot-Shaoyang (GB)

Point, Property , Method & Remarks	Location & Action	Categories of Diseases & Indications
GB-3 Shangguan *Crossing Point of SJ & ST* ⊥ *0.3-0.5 cun.* *ᶿ is applicable.* **Deep puncture is prohibited.**	Anterior to the ear, directly above ST-7 Xiaguan, in the depression above the upper border of the zygomatic arch. 1. Tranquilizes convulsion and improves visual acuity. 2. Relieves rigidity of muscles and activates collaterals.	1. Head and sense organs: Migraine, facial pain, tinnitus, deafness, otitis media, facial paralysis, tetanus, toothache, otic atrophy, arcus senilis. 2. Mental: Manic-depressive psychosis, epilepsy, clonic convulsion.
GB-4 Hanyan *Crossing Point of GB & ST* ↳ *0.3-0.5 cun.* *ᶿ is applicable.*	On the head, in the hair above the temples, at the junction of the upper fourth and lower three fourths of the curved line connecting ST-8 Touwei and GB-7 Qubin. 1. Pacifies liver and stops wind. 2. Tranquilizes convulsion and stops pain.	1. Head and sense organs: Migraine, pain of neck and outer canthus, toothache, tinnitus, facial paralysis, dizziness. 2. Mental: Epilepsy, clonic convulsion.
GB-5 Xuanlu *Crossing Point of SJ, GB & ST* ↳ *0.3-0.5 cun.* *ᶿ is applicable.*	On the head, in the hair above the temples, at the midpoint of the curved line connecting ST-8 Touwei and GB-7 Qubin. 1. Pacifies liver and stops wind. 2. Reduces swelling and alleviates pain.	1. Head and sense organs: Migraine, swelling of face, outer canthus pain, toothache, epistaxis.
GB-6 Xuanli *Crossing Point of SJ, GB & ST* ↳ *0.3-0.5 cun.* *ᶿ is applicable.*	On the head, in the hair above the temples, at the junction of the upper three fourths and lower fourth of the curved line connecting ST-8 Touwei and GB-7 Qubin. 1. Clears heat and relieves exterior. 2. Reduces swelling and alleviates pain.	1. Head and sense organs: Migraine, swelling of face, outer canthus pain, tinnitus, toothache. 2. Digestive: Retching, poor appetite. 3. Mental: Clonic convulsion, irritability. 4. Other: Febrile disease without sweating, over-susceptibility to sneezing.

Table II-12   Points of the Gallbladder Meridian of Foot-Shaoyang (GB)

Point, Property , Method & Remarks	Location & Action	Categories of Diseases & Indications
GB-7 Qubin *Crossing Point of BL & GB* ↳ *0.3-0.5 cun.* ᵷ *is applicable.*	On the head, at a crossing point of the vertical posterior border of the temples and horizontal line through the ear apex. 1. Dispels wind and alleviates pain. 2. Benefits orifices in head.	1. Head and sense organs: Migraine, swelling of submental region and cheek, conjunctival congestion with swelling and pain, neck rigidity, facial paralysis, sudden loss of voice.
GB-8 Shuaigu *Crossing Point of BL & GB* ↳ *0.3-0.5 cun.* ᵷ *is applicable.*	On the head, directly above the ear apex, 1.5 cun above the hairline, directly above SJ-20 Jiaosun. 1. Pacifies liver and stops wind. 2. Calms mind and stops vomiting.	1. Head and sense organs: Migraine and headache, dizziness, conjunctival congestion with swelling and pain, tinnitus, deafness. 2. Digestive: Fullness sensation in epigastrium, restlessness and vomiting, poor appetite. 3. Respiratory: Cough with sputum. 4. Mental: Acute and chronic infantile convulsion.
GB-9 Tianchong *Crossing Point of BL & GB* ↳ *0.3-0.5 cun.* ᵷ *is applicable.*	On the head, directly above the posterior border of the ear root, 2 cun above the hairline and 0.5 cun posterior to GB-8 Shuaigu. 1. Calms mind, reduces swelling and alleviates pain.	1. Head and sense organs: Headache, gingivitis, goiter, tinnitus, deafness. 2. Mental: Depressive psychosis, epilepsy, palpitation due to fright.
GB-10 Fubai *Crossing Point of BL & GB* ↳ *0.3-0.5 cun.* ᵷ *is applicable.*	On the head, posterior and superior to the mastoid process, at the junction of the middle third and upper third of the curved line connecting GB-9 Tianchong and GB-12 Wangu. 1. Dispels wind and transforms phlegm. 2. Regulates qi and alleviates pain.	1. The meridian course: Stiffness of neck, carbuncle, swelling and difficulty in movement of lower limbs, difficulty in walking, paralysis in lower limbs. 2. Head and sense organs: Tinnitus, deafness, toothache, inflammation of throat, ophthalmalgia. 3. Respiratory: Fullness in chest, chest pain, dyspnea, cough, profuse sputum. 4. Other: Scrofula and goiter.

Table II-12   Points of the Gallbladder Meridian of Foot-Shaoyang (GB)

Point, Property , Method & Remarks	Location & Action	Categories of Diseases & Indications
GB-11 Touqiaoyin *Crossing Point of BL & GB* ↳ *0.3-0.5 cun.* ᵰ *is applicable.*	On the head, posterior and superior to the mastoid process, at the junction of the middle third and lower third of the curved line connecting GB-9 Tianchong and GB-12 Wangu. 1. Pacifies liver and stops wind. 2. Benefits the orifices in head.	1. The meridian course: Pain in chest and hypochondrium, limb spasm, feverish sensation of feet and hands, stiffness of neck, paralysis of lower limbs. 2. Head and sense organs: Tinnitus, deafness, pain in ear, ophthalmalgia, inflammation of throat, stiffness of tongue, boils in nose, vertigo, dizziness, headache, bitter taste in mouth.
GB-12 Wangu *Crossing Point of BL & GB* ⬊ *0.3-0.5 cun.* ᵰ *is applicable.*	On the head, in the depression posterior and inferior to the mastoid process. 1. Pacifies liver and stops wind. 2. Relieves epilepsy and calms mind.	1. The meridian course: Foot flaccidity, limited movement of lower limbs. stiffness of neck. 2. Head and sense organs: Headache, edema of face and head, toothache, facial paralysis, inflammation of throat, tetanus, swelling of cheek, pain behind ear. 3. Mental: Epilepsy, insomnia. 4. Other: Malaria.
GB-13 Benshen *Crossing Point of Yangwei M.& GB* ↳ *0.3-0.5 cun.* ᵰ *is applicable.*	On the head, 0.5 cun above the anterior hairline, 3 cun lateral to DU-24 Shenting, at the junction of the medial two thirds and lateral third of the line connecting DU-24 Shenting and ST-8 Touwei. 1. Calms mind. 2. Stops wind and tranquilizes convulsion.	1. The meridian course: Hemiplegia, pain in chest and hypochondrium, stiffness of neck. 2. Head and sense organs: Headache, dizziness, conjunctival congestion, swelling and pain of eyes. 3. Mental: Depressive psychosis, epilepsy, infantile convulsion, coma due to stroke.
GB-14 Yangbai *Crossing Point of Yangwei M. & GB* ↳ *0.3-0.5 cun.* ᵰ *is applicable.*	On the forehead, directly above the pupil, 1 cun above the eyebrow. 1. Clears heat and improves visual acuity.	1. Head and sense organs: Headache, dizziness, eye pain, itching of eye, myopia, nyctalopia, blepharochalsis, twitching of eyelids. 2. Other: Vomiting, neck pain.

Table II-12   Points of the Gallbladder Meridian of Foot-Shaoyang (GB)

Point, Property , Method & Remarks	Location & Action	Categories of Diseases & Indications
GB-15 Toulinqi *Crossing Point of BL, GB & Yangwei M.* ↳ *0.3-0.5 cun.* ᵋ *is applicable.*	On the head, directly above the pupil and 0.5 cun above the anterior hairline, at the midpoint of the line connecting DU-24 Shenting and ST-8 Touwei. 1. Dispels wind and clears heat. 2. Improves visual and hearing acuity.	1. Head and sense organs: Headache, pain on margins of eyelids, pain of outer canthus, blurring of vision, stuffy nose, rhinorrhea with turbid discharge, tinnitus, deafness. 2. Cardiovascular: Sensation of fullness and distention in chest, precordial pain causing difficulty in turning trunk. 3. Mental: Infantile convulsion, apoplexy, coma, epilepsy. 4. Other: Febrile disease, malaria, carbuncle of axilla.
GB-16 Muchuang *Crossing Point of Yangwei M. & GB* ↳ *0.3-0.5 cun.* ᵋ *is applicable.*	On the head, 1.5 cun above the anterior hairline and 2.25 cun lateral to the midline of the head. 1. Stops wind, tranquilizes convulsion and improves visual acuity.	1. Head and sense organs: Headache, vertigo, swelling of face, conjunctival congestion, swelling and pain of eyes, hypermetropia, myopia, optic atrophy, cataract, upper toothache, deafness, stuffy nose. 2. Mental: Child epilepsy induced by terror. 3. Other: Aversion to cold, fever without sweating.
GB-17 Zhengying *Crossing Point of Yangwei M. & GB* ↳ *0.3-0.5 cun.* ᵋ *is applicable.*	On the head, 2.5 cun above the anterior hairline and 2.25 cun lateral to the midline of the head. 1. Pacifies liver and stops wind, relieves rigidity of muscles.	1. Head and sense organs: Headache, vertigo, stiffness of neck, stiffness of lips, toothache. 2. Other: Hemiplegia, aversion to cold.
GB-18 Chengling *Crossing Point of Yangwei M. & GB* ↳ *0.3-0.5 cun.* ᵋ *is applicable.*	On the head, 4 cun above the anterior hairline and 2.25 cun lateral to the midline of the head. 1. Disperses lung and benefits nose. 2. Clears heat and dispels wind.	1. Head and sense organs: Headache, ophthalmalgia, allergic rhinitis, stuffy nose, profuse nasal discharge. 2. Respiratory: Cough, asthma, fever, aversion to cold.

Table II-12   Points of the Gallbladder Meridian of Foot-Shaoyang (GB)

Point, Property , Method & Remarks	Location & Action	Categories of Diseases & Indications
GB-19 Naokong *Crossing Point of Yangwei M. & GB* ↳ *0.3-0.5 cun.* *ᵟ is applicable.*	On the head and on the level of the upper border of the external occipital protuberance or DU-17 Naohu, 2.25 cun lateral to the midline of the head. 1. Clears heat and stops pain. 2. Calms mind and relieves muscular spasms.	1. Head and sense organs: Headache, vertigo, conjunctival congestion and ophthalmalgia, epistaxis and nose pain, tinnitus, deafness, stiffness of neck. 2. Mental: Coma due to high fever, palpitation due to fright, depressive psychosis, mania, epilepsy.
GB-20 Fengchi *Crossing Point of Yangwei M. & GB* ↘ *0.5-1 cun toward the tip of the nose.* *ᵟ is applicable.*	On the nape, below the occipital bone, on the level of DU-16 Fengfu, in the depression between the upper ends of the sternocleidomastoid and trapezius muscles. 1. Pacifies liver and stops wind. 2. Clears heat and relieves exterior.	1. The meridian course: Neck ache and backache, stiff neck, pain of shoulder and arms, pain in back and loins, hemiplegia, flaccidity and arthralgia syndrome of lower limbs. 2. Head and sense organs: Headache and migraine, vertigo, conjunctival congestion, poor vision, excessive lacrimation induced by wind, running nose, epistaxis, rhinorrhea with turbid discharge, tinnitus, deafness, toothache, swelling pain in throat, facial paralysis, difficulty in swallowing. 3. Mental: Apoplexy, coma, insomnia, clonic convulsion. 4. Other: Urticaria, erysipelas, epidemic febrile diesease.
GB-21 Jianjing *Crossing Point of SJ, GB & Yangwei M.* ⊥ *0.3-0.5 cun.* *ᵟ is applicable.* **Puncture with caution in pregnancy.**	On the shoulder, directly above the nipple, at the midpoint of the line connecting DU-14 Dazhui and the acromion. 1. Dispels wind and clears heat. 2. Reduces swelling and alleviates pain.	1. The meridian course: Stiffness of neck, hemiplegia, hysterical paralysis, pain of shoulder and back, stiff neck. 2. Gynecopathies: Difficult labor, retention of placenta, uterine bleeding, cold limbs due to abortion. 3. Other: Hypertension, scrofula, cough with dyspnea, consumptive diesease, hernia, stomachache, acute mastitis, carbuncles, cellulitis, furuncles, boils.

Table II-12 Points of the Gallbladder Meridian of Foot-Shaoyang (GB)

Point, Property , Method & Remarks	Location & Action	Categories of Diseases & Indications
GB-22 Yuanye ↘ *0.3-0.5 cun.* *ᵮ is applicable.*	On the lateral side of the chest, on the midaxillary line when the arm is raised, 3 cun below the axilla, in the 4th intercostal space. 1. Relieves chest oppression and stops pain. 2. Reduces swelling and dredges meridians.	1. Respiratory: Sensation of fullness in chest, cough, fever with chills. 2. Other: Hypochondriac pain, axilla swelling, inability to raise arm.
GB-23 Zhejin ***Crossing Point of BL & GB*** ↘ *0.3-0.5 cun.* *ᵮ is applicable.*	On the lateral side of the chest, 1 cun anterior to GB-22 Yuanye, on the level of the nipple, and in the 4th intercostal space. 1. Subdues rebellious qi and stops asthma. 2. Regulates qi & stops pain.	1. Respiratory: Fullness in sensation in chest leading to difficulty in lying flat, asthma. 2. Digestive: Vomiting, acid regurgitation, excessive salivation, dysentery. 3. Mental: Dysphasia, paralysis of limbs, insomnia.
GB-24 Riyue ***Front-Mu Point of Gallbladder;*** ***Crossing Point of SP & GB*** ↘ *0.3-0.5 cun.* *ᵮ is applicable.*	On the upper abdomen, directly below the nipple, in the 7th intercostal space, 4 cun lateral to the anterior midline. 1. Soothes liver and benefits gallbladder. 2. Strengthens spleen and subdues rebellious qi.	1. Digestive: Stomachache, vomiting, acid regurgitation, hiccups, abdominal distention, salivation, jaundice. 2. Other: Pain in chest and hypochondrium, sighing, over-susceptibility to sorrow.
GB-25 Jingmen ***Front-Mu Point of Kidney*** ⊥ *0.3-0.5 cun.* *ᵮ is applicable.*	On the lateral side of the waist, 1.8 cun posterior to LR-13 Zhangmen, below the free end of the 12th rib. 1. Tonifies kidney and strengthens loins. 2. Strengthens spleen and promotes urination.	1. Digestive: Diarrhea, borborygmus, abdominal distention, vomiting. 2. Urinary: Dysuria, dark urine with face swelling.

Table II-12   Points of the Gallbladder Meridian of Foot-Shaoyang (GB)

Point, Property , Method & Remarks	Location & Action	Categories of Diseases & Indications
GB-26 Daimai *Crossing Point of Dai M. & GB* ⊥ *0.5-0.8 cun.* ᵷ *is applicable.*	On the lateral side of the abdomen, 1.8 cun below LR-13 Zhangmen, at the crossing point of a vertical line through free end of the 11th rib and a horizontal line through umbilicus. 1. Regulates menstruation. 2. Strengthens spleen and arrests leukorrhagia.	1. Gynecopathies: Irregular menstruation, leukorrhea with reddish discharge, prolapse of uterus, pain in lower abdomen. 2. Other: Lumbago, hernia, soreness and weakness of waist, flaccidity of lower limbs.
GB-27 Wushu *Crossing Point of Dai M. & GB* ⊥ *0.5-0.8 cun.* ᵷ *is applicable.*	On the lateral side of the abdomen, anterior to the anteriosuperior iliac spine, 3 cun below the level of the umbilicus. 1. Regulates menstruation and arrests leukorrhagia. 2. Regulates qi and alleviates pain.	1. Digestive: Constipation, tenesmus. 2. Reproductive: Prolapse of uterus, pain in lower abdomen, leukorrhea with reddish discharge, irregular menstruation, hernia, shrinkage of scrotum. 3. Other: Pain in waist and hip, clonic convulsion.
GB-28 Weidao *Crossing Point of Dai M. & GB* ⊥ *0.5-1 cun.* ᵷ *is applicable.*	On the lateral side of the abdomen, anterior and inferior to the anteriosuperior iliac spine, 0.5 cun anterior and inferior to GB-27 Wushu. 1. Regulates menstruation and arrests leukorrhagia. 2. Promotes urination and reduces edema.	1. Digestive: Constipation, acute appendicitis, vomiting and poor appetite. 2. Reproductive: Prolapse of uterus, irregular menstruation, pain in lower abdomen, leukorrhea with reddish discharge. 3. Other: Pain in waist, abdomen and hip, edema, continuous cough with dyspnea, hernia.
GB-29 Juliao *Crossing Point of Yangqiao M. & GB* ⊥ *0.5-1 cun.* ᵷ *is applicable.*	On the hip, at the midpoint of the line connecting the anteriosuperior iliac spine and the prominence of the great trochanter. 1. Dredges meridians and collaterals. 2. Moves qi to stop pain.	1. The meridian course: Pain in waist and legs, paralysis, flaccidity in feet. 2. Reproductive: Irregular menstruation, leukorrhea with reddish discharge. 3. Digestive: Dysentery.

Table II-12   Points of the Gallbladder Meridian of Foot-Shaoyang (GB)

Point, Property , Method & Remarks	Location & Action	Categories of Diseases & Indications
GB-30 Huantiao *Crossing Point of BL & GB* ⊥ *1.5-2.5 cun.* ᶞ *is applicable.*	On the lateral side of the thigh, at the junction of the middle third and lateral third of the line connecting the prominence of the great trochanter and the sacral hiatus when the patient is in a lateral recumbent position with the thigh flexed. 1. Dredges meridians and collaterals. 2. Dispels wind and resolves dampness.	1. The meridian course: Hemiplegia, flaccidity in lower limbs, pain in waist and vertebrae, sprain and contusion of hip. 2. Skin: General rubella, urticaria. 3. Other: Edema, beriberi.
GB-31 Fengshi ⊥ *0.7-1.2 cun.* ᶞ *is applicable.*	On the lateral midline of the thigh, 7 cun above the popliteal crease, or at the place touching the tip of the middle finger when the patient stands erect with the arms hanging down freely. 1. Dredges meridians and collaterals. 2. Dispels wind and resolves dampness.	1. The meridian course: Paralysis of legs, pain in waist and leg. 2. Head and sense organs: Headache, tinnitus, deafness, conjunctival congestion and pain. 3. Other: General pruritis, inflammation of the scrotum, hernia, beriberi.
GB-32 Zhongdu ⊥ *0.7-1 cun.* ᶞ *is applicable.*	On the lateral side of the thigh, 2 cun below GB-31 Fengshi, or 5 cun above the popliteal crease, between the lateral vastus muscle and biceps femoris muscle. 1. Dredges meridians and collaterals. 2. Dispels wind and resolves dampness.	1. The meridian course: Flaccidity and arthralgia in legs, numbness, hemiplegia, pain in waist involving hip and leg, beriberi.
GB-33 Xiyangguan ⊥ *0.5-1 cun.* ᶞ *is applicable.*	On the lateral side of the knee, 3 cun above GB-34 Yanglingquan, in the depression above the external epicondyle of the femur. 1. Dredges meridians and collaterals. 2. Removes dampness and dispels cold.	1. The meridian course: Hemiplegia, swelling pain in knee and knee-cap, contracture or subjective sensation of contraction in regions nearby, numbness in shank, beriberi. 2. Other: Continuously vomiting, excess salivation.

Table II-12   Points of the Gallbladder Meridian of Foot-Shaoyang (GB)

Point, Property , Method & Remarks	Location & Action	Categories of Diseases & Indications
GB-34 Yanglingquan *He-Sea Point;* *Influential Point of Tendons* ⊥ *0.8-1.2 cun.* ᵟ *is applicable.*	On the lateral side of the leg, in the depression anterior and inferior to the head of the fibula. 1. Soothes liver and benefits gallbladder. 2. Comforts sinews and relieves convulsion.	1. The meridian course: Pain in waist and sacrum, hemiplegia, flaccidity, arthralgia and numbness in legs, pain in hypochondrium, shoulder pain. 2. Head and sense organs: Headache, sore throat, swelling, pain and congestion of eyes, tinnitus, deafness. 3. Digestive: Stomachache, abdominal distention, borborygmus, jaundice, constipation. 4. Respiratory: Cough in tuberculosis. 5. Urinary: Enuresis, edema. 6. Mental: Infantile convulsion, tetanus, epilepsy.
GB-35 Yangjiao *Xi-Cleft Point of Yanwei M.* ⊥ *0.5-0.8 cun.* ᵟ *is applicable.*	On the lateral side of the leg, 7 cun above the tip of the external malleolus, on the posterior border of the fibula. 1. Calms heart and spirit. 2. Soothes liver and regulates qi.	1. The meridian course: Flaccidity and arthralgia in legs, hemiplegia, pain in chest and hypochondrium. 2. Respiratory: Dyspnea with fever and chills, inflammation of throat, aphasia. 3. Mental: Terror and mania, depressive psychosis.
GB-36 Waiqiu *Xi-Cleft Point* ⊥ *0.5-0.8 cun.* ᵟ *is applicable.*	On the lateral side of the leg, 7 cun above the tip of the external malleolus, on the anterior border of the fibula and on the level of GB-35 Yangjiao. 1. Calms mind and sedates spirit. 2. Soothes liver and relives chest oppression.	1. The meridian course: Headache, stiffness of neck, flaccidity and numbness of lower limbs, feeling of fullness in chest and hypochondrium. 2. Mental: Depressive psychosis. 3. Other: Infantile pigeon chest and xifosis, chills and fever due to rabies virus.
GB-37 Guangming *Luo-Connecting Point* ⊥ *0.7-1 cun.* ᵟ *is applicable.*	On the lateral side of the leg, 5 cun above the tip of the external malleolus, on the anterior border of the fibula. 1. Clears liver and improves visual acuity. 2. Reduces swelling and alleviates pain.	1. The meridian course: Flaccidity and numbness of lower limbs, hemiplegia, distending pain of breast. 2. Head and sense organs: Itching of eyes, pain of eyes, cataract, night blindness, optic atrophy, migraine. 3. Other: Infantile pigeon chest and xifosis, rabies.

Table II-12   Points of the Gallbladder Meridian of Foot-Shaoyang (GB)

Point, Property , Method & Remarks	Location & Action	Categories of Diseases & Indications
GB-38 Yangfu *Jing-River Point* ⊥ 0.5-0.7 cun. ᵦ is applicable.	On the lateral side of the leg, 4 cun above the tip of the external malleolus, slightly anterior to the anterior border of the fibula. 1. Dredges meridians and collaterals. 2. Dispels wind and clears heat.	1. The meridian course: Hemiplegia, distending pain in chest and hypochondrium, pain in lateral part of lower limbs, lumbago, edema in lower limbs, skin lesions similar to beriberi on limbs. 2. Head and sense organs: Migraine, pain in outer canthus, inflammation of throat. 3. Aversion to cold and fever, scrofula, malaria.
GB-39 Xuanzhong *Influential Point of Marrow* ⊥ 0.3-0.5 cun. ᵦ is applicable.	On the lateral side of the leg, 3 cun above the tip of the external malleolus, on the anterior border of the fibula. 1. Pacifies liver and stops wind. 2. Soothes liver and reinforces kidney.	1. The meridian course: Pain in chest and hypochondrium, hemiplegia, stiffness of neck, lumbosacral pain, pain in lateral side of lower limbs. 2. Head and sense organs: Inflammation of throat, migraine, epistaxis, pain and dryness of nasal cavity. 3. Digestive: Sensation of heat in stomach, poor appetite, constipation. 4. Urinary: Dysuria, stranguria. 5. Respiratory: Cough.
GB-40 Qiuxu *Yuan-Source Point* ⊥ 0.5-0.8 cun. ᵦ is applicable.	Anterior and inferior to the external malleolus, in the depression lateral to the tendon of the long extensor muscle of the toes. 1. Strengthens body resistance and dispels pathogenic factors. 2. Soothes liver and strengthens spleen.	1. The meridian course: Pain in neck, pain and fullness in chest and hypochondrium, pain in waist and lower limbs, hemiplegia, spasm, ankle injury, flaccidity of lower limbs. 2. Head and sense organs: Migraine, red, swollen and painful eyes, blurring of vision. 3. Other: Malaria, cough with dyspnea, over-susceptibility to sighing.
GB-41 Zulinqi *Shu-Stream Point* ⊥ 0.3-0.5 cun. ᵦ is applicable.	On the lateral side of the instep of the foot, posterior to the 4th metatarsophalangeal joint, in the depression lateral to the tendon of the extensor muscle of the little toe. 1. Pacifies liver and stops wind. 2. Transforms phlegm and reduces swelling.	1. Head and sense organs: Migraine, pain in outer canthus, dizziness, feeling of dryness in eyes, deafness, tinnitus. 2. Other: Hemiplegia, irregular menstruation, acute mastitis.

Table II-12   Points of the Gallbladder Meridian of Foot-Shaoyang (GB)

Point, Property , Method & Remarks	Location & Action	Categories of Diseases & Indications
GB-42 Diwuhui ∓ 0.3-0.5 cun. ð is applicable.	On the lateral side of the instep of the foot, posterior to the 4th metatarsophalangeal joint, between the 4th and 5th metatarsal bones, medial to the tendon of the extensor muscle of the little toe. 1. Dispels wind and clears heat. 2. Soothes liver and reduces swelling.	1. The meridian course: Swollen and painful dorsum of foot, fullness and pain in chest and hypochondrium, acute mastitis, lumbago, pain in lower limbs. 2. Head and sense organs: Migraine, red, swollen and painful eyes, deafness, tinnitus. 3. Other: Hemoptysis due to visceral injury.
GB-43 Xiaxi *Ying-Spring Point* ∓ 0.3-0.5 cun. ð is applicable.	On the lateral side of the instep of the foot, between the 4th and 5th toes, at the junction of the red and white skin, proximal to the margin of the web. 1. Pacifies liver and stops wind. 2. Soothes liver and calms heart.	1. The meridian course: Pain in chest and hypochondrium, hemiplegia, pain in lower limbs, acute mastitis, edema of dorsum of foot. 2. Head and sense organs: Migraine, dizziness, deafness, swollen cheek, tinnitus, red and painful outer canthus. 3. Other: Amenorrhea, malaria, exterior syndrome of febrile disease.
GB-44 Zuqiaoyin *Jing-Well Point* ↳ 0.1 cun. ð is applicable.	On the lateral side of the distal segment of the 4th toe, 0.1 cun from the corner of the toenail. 1. Pacifies liver and stops wind. 2. Improves visual and hearing acuity.	1. The meridian course: Hemiplegia, distention and fullness sensation in chest and hypochondrium. 2. Head and sense organs: Migraine, dizziness, red, swollen and painful eyes, tinnitus, deafness, inflammation of throat, stiffness of tongue. 3. Respiratory: Cough, asthma. 4. Gynecopathies: Irregular menstruation, amenorrhea. 5. Surgical: Carbuncle, acute mastitis. 6. Mental: Insomnia, dreamful sleep.

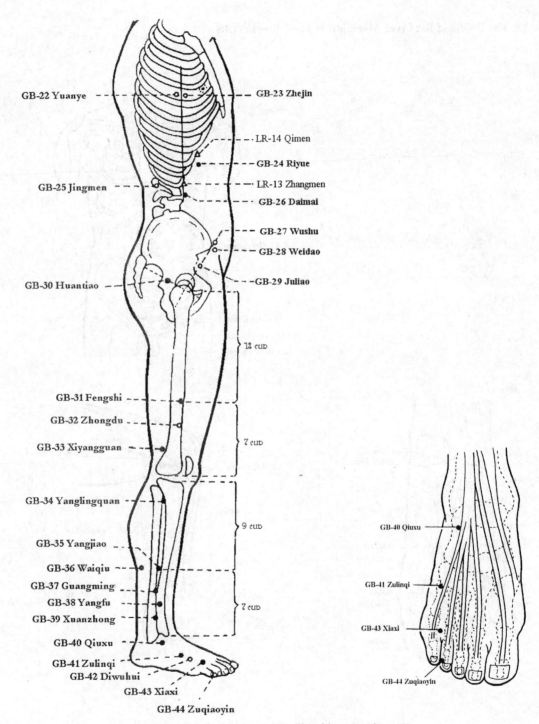

GB-22 Yuanye

GB-23 Zhejin

LR-14 Qimen

GB-24 Riyue

GB-25 Jingmen

LR-13 Zhangmen

GB-26 Daimai

GB-27 Wushu

GB-28 Weidao

GB-29 Juliao

GB-30 Huantiao

12 cun

GB-31 Fengshi

GB-32 Zhongdu

GB-33 Xiyangguan

7 cun

GB-34 Yanglingquan

9 cun

GB-35 Yangjiao

GB-36 Waiqiu

GB-37 Guangming

GB-38 Yangfu

7 cun

GB-39 Xuanzhong

GB-40 Qiuxu

GB-41 Zulinqi

GB-42 Diwuhui

GB-43 Xiaxi

GB-44 Zuqiaoyin

GB-40 Qiuxu

GB-41 Zulinqi

GB-43 Xiaxi

GB-44 Zuqiaoyin

Fig II-28 Points on the Gallbladder Meridian (4)

12. The Points of the Liver Meridian of Foot-Jueyin (LR)

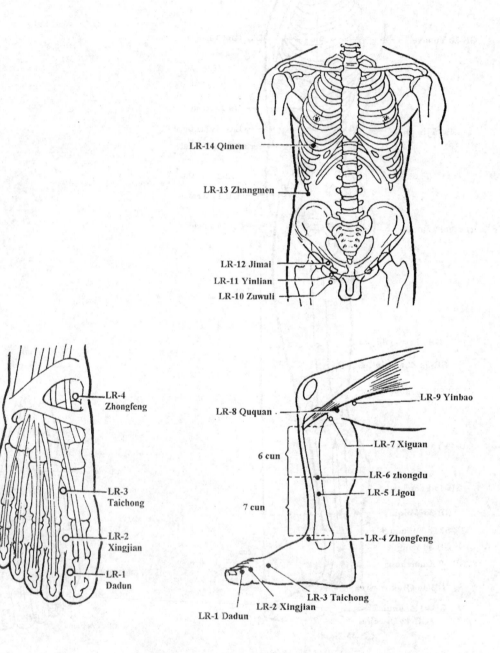

Fig. II-29 Points on the Liver Meridian (1)

Table II-13   Points of the Liver Meridian of Foot-Jueyin (LR)

Point, Property, Method & Remarks	Location & Action	Categories of Diseases & Indications
LR-1 Dadun *Jing-Well Point* ↳ *0.1-0.2 cun.* ß *is applicable.*	On the lateral side of the distal segment of the great toe, 0.1 cun from the corner of the toenail. 1. Regulates liver and regulates qi. 2. Relieves spasm and calms mind.	1. Digestive: Epigastric pain, constipation, hematemesis. 2. Reproductive: Prolapse of uterus, perineal pain, pruritis vulvae, irregular menstruation, metrorrhagia and metrostaxis, amenorrhea, flaccid contraction of penis, pain of glans penis, painful and swollen testis. 3. Urinary: Hematuria, enuresis, stranguria, dysuria, frequent micturition. 4. Mental: Manic-depressive syndrome, epilepsy, apoplexy, drowsiness. 5. Other: Hernia, pain in lower abdomen, blurring of vision.
LR-2 Xingjian *Ying-Spring Point* ⤼ *0.3-0.5 cun.* ß *is applicable.*	On the instep of the foot, between the 1st and 2nd toes, at the junction of the red and white skin proximal to the margin of the web. 1. Pacifies liver and extinguishes wind. 2. Calms heart and spirit.	1. The meridian course: Pain in medial side of knee and thigh, hypochondriac pain, lumbago which causes difficulty in lying flat. 2. Head and sense organs: Headache, vertigo, red, painful and swollen eyes, optic atrophy, bitter taste in mouth, dry and painful throat, toothache. 3. Digestive: Epigastric pain, hiccup, hematemesis, abdominal distention, diarrhea, jaundice. 4. Reproductive: Menorrhagia, dysmenorrhea, amenorrhea, leukorrhea, gonorrhea, pain in perineal area or penis. 5. Urinary: Enuresis, stranguria. 6. Respiratory: Cough, hemoptysis. 7. Mental: Apoplexy, epilepsy, clonic convulsion, hysteria, depressive-syndrome, irritability. 8. Other: Hypertension, hernia, breast abscess.

Table II-13   Points of the Liver Meridian of Foot-Jueyin (LR)

Point, Property, Method & Remarks	Location & Action	Categories of Diseases & Indications
LR-3 Taichong *Shu-Stream Point;* *Yuan-Source Point* $\underline{\perp}$ *0.3-0.5 cun.* *δ is applicable.*	On the instep of the foot, in the depression of the posterior end of the 1st interosseous metatarsal space. 1. Pacifies liver and extinguishes wind. 2. Strengthens spleen and removes dampness.	1. The meridian course: Flaccidity and numbness of lower limbs, hypochondriac pain. 2. Head and sense organs: Headache, dizziness, red, painful and swollen eyes, optic atrophy, dry mouth, dry and painful throat. 3. Digestive: Abdominal distention, borborygmus, epigastric pain, diarrhea, constipation, jaundice. 4. Reproductive: Irregular menstruation, amenorrhea, metrorrhagia and metrostaixs, dysmenorrhea, leukorrhea, persistent sweating after birth, pain of perineal area, shrinkage of external genitals. 5. Urinary: Dysuria, enuresis, stranguria. 6. Respiratory: Cough, oppressive sensation in chest. 7. Mental: Manic-depressive syndrome, epilepsy, infantile convulsion, apoplexy, hysteria, irritability, depression. 8. Other: Hypertension, angina pectoris, hernia.
LR-4 Zhongfeng *Jing-River Point* $\underline{\perp}$ *0.3-0.5 cun.* *δ is applicable.*	On the instep of the foot, anterior to the medial malleolus, on the line connecting SP-5 Shangqiu and ST-41 Jiexi, in the depression medial to the tendon of the anterior tibial muscle. 1. Soothes liver and strengthens spleen. 2. Regulates qi and relieves hernia.	1. The meridian course: Flaccidity and numbness of lower limbs, painful and swollen dorsum of foot, hypochondriac pain. 2. Head and sense organs: Headache, dizziness, wry mouth, painful and swollen throat. 3. Digestive: Tympanites, anorexia, jaundice. 4.Urogenital: Difficulty in urination, stranguria, pain in perineum, nocturnal emission.

Table II-13   Points of the Liver Meridian of Foot-Jueyin (LR)

Point, Property, Method & Remarks	Location & Action	Categories of Diseases & Indications
LR 5-Ligou *Luo-Connecting Point* ↳ *0.3-0.5 cun.* ᵟ *is applicable.*	On the medial side of the leg, 5 cun above the tip of the medial malleolus, on the midline of the medial surface of the tibia. 1. Reinforces liver and regulates menstruation. 2. Clears heat and reduces edema.	1. The meridian course: Pain in tibia, hypochondriac pain. 2. Urogenital: Dysuria, irregular menstruation, metrorrhagia and metrostaxis, leukorrhea with reddish discharge, prolapse of uterus, painful and swollen testis, feeling of fullness and pain in lower abdomen.
LR-6 Zhongdu ↳ *0.5-0.8 cun.* ᵟ *is applicable.*	On the medial side of the leg, 7 cun above the tip of the medial malleolus, on the midline of the medial surface of the tibia. 1. Reinforces liver. 2. Promotes qi flow to stops pain.	1. The meridian course: Flaccidity and numbness of lower limbs, hypochondriac pain. 2. Digestive: Diarrhea, dysentery, abdominal distention. 3. Reproductive: Hernia, pain in lower abdomen, metrorrhagia and metrostaxis, leukorrhea with reddish discharge, fluid retention, pain in perineum.
LR-7 Xiguan ⊥ *0.5-1 cun.* ᵟ *is applicable.*	On the medial side of the leg, posterior and inferior to the medial epicondyle of the tibia, 1 cun posterior to SP-9 Yinlingquan, at the upper end of the medial head of the gastrocnemius muscle. 1. Warms meridians and transforms dampness. 2. Dispels wind and relieves edema.	1. The meridian course: Flaccidity and numbness of lower limbs, hypochondriac pain.

Table II-13   Points of the Liver Meridian of Foot-Jueyin (LR)

Point, Property, Method & Remarks	Location & Action	Categories of Diseases & Indications
LR-8 Ququan *He-Sea Point* ⊥ *0.5-0.8 cun.* ᵷ *is applicable.*	On the medial side of the knee, at the medial end of the popliteal crease when the knee is flexed, posterior to the medial epicondyle of the tibia, in the depression of the anterior border of the insertions of the semimembranous and semitendinous muscles. 1. Soothes liver and relieves restrained qi. 2. Regulates function of external genitalia.	1. The meridian course: Flaccidity and numbness of lower limbs, hypochondriac pain, painful and swollen knee joint. 2. Head and sense organs: Headache, dizziness, painful eyes, epistaxis. 3. Digestive: Diarrhea, dysentery, fullness in stomach, anorexia. 4. Reproductive: Irregular menstruation, dysmenorrhea, leukorrhagia, prolapse of uterus, pruritis and swelling of perineal area, pain in abdomen after delivery, pain in penis, impotence. 5. Urinary: Dysuria, stranguria, retention of urine. 6. Mental: Manic-depressive syndrome.
LR-9 Yinbao ⊥ *0.5-0.7 cun.* ᵷ *is applicable.*	On the medial side of the thigh, 4 cun above the medial epicondyle of the femur, between the medial vastus muscle and sartorius muscle. 1. Tonifies kidney and strengthens spleen. 2. Regulates function of external genitalia.	1. Urogenital: Irregular menstruation, enuresis, dysuria.
LR-10 Zuwuli ⊥ *0.5-1 cun.* ᵷ *is applicable.*	On the medial side of the thigh, 3 cun directly below ST-30 Qichong, at the proximal end of the thigh, below the pubic tubercle and on the lateral border of the long abductor muscle of the thigh. 1. Clears liver and strengthens spleen. 2. Regulates function of external genitalia.	1. Urogenital: Prolapse of uterus, leukorrhagia, painful and swollen testis, eczema and pruritis of scrotum, enuresis, dysuria.

Table II-13   Points of the Liver Meridian of Foot-Jueyin (LR)

Point, Property, Method & Remarks	Location & Action	Categories of Diseases & Indications
LR-11 Yinlian ⊥ *0.5-1 cun.* ᵟ *is applicable.*	On the medial side of the thigh, 2 cun directly below Qichong ST 30, at the proximal end of the thigh, below the pubic tubercle and on the lateral border of the long abductor muscle of the thigh. 1. Regulates menstruation and improves reproductive function. 2. Comforts sinews and activates collaterals.	1. The meridian course: Pain in medial side of thighs, spasm in lower limbs. 2. Reproductive: Irregular. menstruation, leukorrhea with reddish discharge.
LR-12 Jimai ⊥ *0.5-0.8 cun.* ᵟ *is applicable.* ***Avoid puncturing the artery.***	Lateral to the pubic tubercle, lateral and inferior to ST-30 Qichong, in the inguinal groove where the pulsation of the femoral artery is palpable, 2.5 cun lateral to the anterior midline. 1. Regulates liver and stops pain. 2. Regulates qi and relieves hernia.	1. The meridian course: Pain in medial side of thighs. 2. Reproductive: Hernia, pain in lower abdomen, prolapse of uterus, pain in penis.
LR-13 Zhangmen ***Front-Mu Point of Spleen; Influential Point of Zang Organ*** ⊥ *0.5-0.8 cun.* ᵟ *is applicable.*	On the lateral side of the abdomen, below the free end of the 11th rib. 1. Strengthens spleen and relieves abdominal distension. 2. Harmonizes stomach and benefits gallbladder.	1. Respiratory: Cough, dyspnea, shortness of breath. 2. Digestive: Abdominal pain, anorexia, infantile malnutrition, jaundice. 3. Urinary: Polyuria, gonorrhea, retention of urine. 4. Other: Pain in chest and hypochondrium, pain along spinal column, lassitude, emaciation, abdominal masses.

Table II-13   Points of the Liver Meridian of Foot-Jueyin (LR)

Point, Property, Method & Remarks	Location & Action	Categories of Diseases & Indications
LR-14 Qimen *Front-Mu Point of Liver* ⩲ *0.3-0.5 cun.* ᵟ *is applicable.*	On the chest, directly below the nipple, in the 6th intercostal space, 4 cun lateral to the anterior midline. 1. Soothes liver and strengthens spleen. 2. Harmonizes stomach and reverses rebellious qi.	1. Respiratory: Cough, asthma. 2. Digestive: Abdominal distention, stomachache, diarrhea, vomiting, hiccups, acid regurgitation, hunger without appetite. 3. Urinary: Retention of urine, enuresis, dysuria. 4. Other: Feeling of fullness in chest and hypochondrium, malaria, sensation of gas ascending in abdomen.

13. The Points of the Du Meridian (DU)

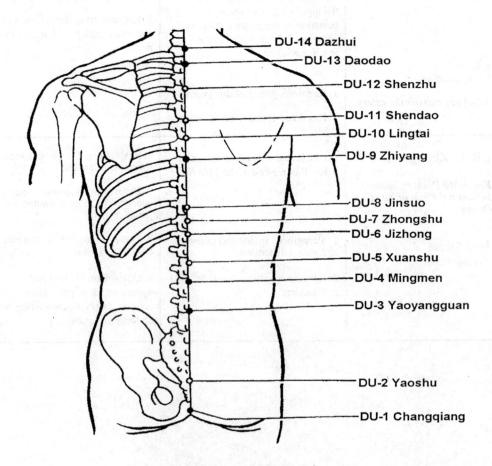

Fig. II-30 Points on the Du Meridian (1)

Table II-14 Points of the Du Meridian (DU) (Governor Vessel, GV)

Point, Property , Method and Remarks	Location & Action	Categories of Diseases & Indications
DU-1 Changqiang *Crossing Point of KI;* *Luo-Connecting Point* ⟍ *0.5-1.2 cun upward along anterior aspect of coccyx.* ᵟ *is applicable.*	Below the tip of the coccyx, at the midpoint of the line connecting the tip of the coccyx and anus. 1. Calms mind and relieves spasm. 2. Facilitates passages of stools and relieves hemorrhoids.	1. Digestive: Diarrhea. constipation, dysentery. 2. Urinary: Dysuria, stranguria. 3. Reproductive: Nocturnal emission, impotence, discharge and pruritis in external vaginal area, pelvic inflammation. 4. Mental: Epilepsy, Mania, epilepsy, convulsion, opisthotonos. 5. Other: Pain in lower back and spine, hernia, hemorrhoids, prolapse of rectum.
DU-2 Yaoshu ⟍ *0.5-1 cun upward.* ᵟ *is applicable.*	On the sacrum and on the posterior midline, at the sacral hiatus. 1. Regulates menstruation and clears heat. 2. Dispels cold and removes dampness.	1. Digestive: Diarrhea. constipation, Bloody stools. 2. Urinary: Dysuria, stranguria, reddish urine, enuresis. 3. Reproductive: Nocturnal emission, irregular menstruation, leukorrhea. 4. Mental: Epilepsy. 5. Other: Malaria, fever without sweating, hemorrhoids, prolapse of rectum, stiffness and pain in lower back and spine, motor impairment and muscular atrophy or numbness in lower limbs.
DU-3 Yaoyangguan ⊥ *0.5-1 cun.* ᵟ *is applicable.*	On the lower back and on the posterior midline, in the depression below the spinous process of the 4th lumbar vertebra. 1. Dispels cold and removes dampness. 2. Comforts sinews and activates collaterals.	1. Digestive: Bloody stools, dysentery, fullness sensation in lower abdomen, vomiting. 2. Reproductive: Irregular menstruation, leukorrhea with reddish discharge, nocturnal emission, impotence, dysuria. 3. Other: Tetanus, hernia, scrofula, pain in lumbar and sacral region, motor impairment and muscular atrophy in lower limbs, pain in knee with motor impairment.

Table II-14   Points of the Du Meridian (DU) (Governor Vessel, GV)

Point, Property , Method and Remarks	Location & Action	Categories of Diseases & Indications
DU-4 Mingmen ⊥ *0.5-1 cun.* ᵟ *is applicable.*	On the low back and on the posterior midline, in the depression below the spinous process of the 2nd lumbar vertebra. 1. Warms and strengthens kidney yang. 2. Relaxes sinews and relieves convulsion.	1. Digestive: Diarrhea, hematochezia. 2. Reproductive: Impotence, nocturnal emission, premature ejaculation, leukorrhagia, dysmenorrhea, habitual abortion. 3. Urinary: Enuresis, frequent urination, dysuria. 4. Mental: Epilepsy, infantile convulsion, fear due to fright, insomnia. 5. Other: General weakness, dizziness, tinnitus, cold limbs, chills, fever without sweating, malaria, headache, hernia, edema, prolapse of rectum, hemorrhoids.
DU-5 Xuanshu ⊥ *0.5-1 cun.* ᵟ *is applicable.*	On the low back and on the posterior midline, in the depression below the spinous process of the 1st lumbar vertebra. 1. Aids in yang qi and strengthens spleen. 2. Regulates intestines and promotes their function.	1. Digestive: Abdominal distention, abdominal pain, indigestion, diarrhea, dysentery, prolapse of rectum. 2. Other: Stiffness, pain and motor impairment in waist and spine.
DU-6 Jizhong ⊥ *0.5-1 cun.* ᵟ *is applicable.*	On the back and on the posterior midline, in the depression below the spinous process of the 11th thoracic vertebra. 1. Strengthens spleen and removes dampness. 2. Calms spirit and relieves spasm.	1. Digestive: Gastric pain, abdominal fullness sensation, diarrhea, dysentery, hematochezia, indigestion in children, poor appetite, jaundice, vomiting, hematemesis, nausea. 2. Other: Hemorrhoids, prolapse of rectum.
DU-7 Zhongshu ⊥ *0.5-1 cun.* ᵟ *is applicable.*	On the back and on the posterior midline, in the depression below the spinous process of the 10th thoracic vertebra. 1. Strengthens spleen and removes dampness. 2.Clears heat and alleviates pain.	1. Digestive: Gastric pain, abdominal fullness sensation, vomiting, poor appetite, jaundice. 2. Other: Aversion to cold with fever, hypopsia, stiffness and pain in lower back and spine with motor impairment.

Table II-14   Points of the Du Meridian (DU) (Governor Vessel, GV)

Point, Property , Method and Remarks	Location & Action	Categories of Diseases & Indications
DU-8 Jinsuo ↧ 0.5-1 cun. ʃ is applicable.	On the back and on the posterior midline, in the depression below the spinous process of the 9th thoracic vertebra. 1. Pacifies liver and extinguishes wind. 2. Calms spirit and relieves spasm.	1. Digestive: Gastric pain, vomiting, jaundice. 2. Mental: Manic-depressive psychosis, infantile epilepsy, convulsion, hysteria. 3. Other: Motor impairment, stiffness and pain in lower back and spine.
DU-9 Zhiyang ↘ upward 0.5-1 cun. ʃ is applicable.	On the back and on the posterior midline, in the depression below the spinous process of the 7th thoracic vertebra. 1. Benefits gallbladder and relieves jaundice. 2. Soothes chest oppression and benefits diaphragm.	1. Respiratory: Cough, asthma, distension and fullness in chest and hypochondrium. 2. Digestive: Gastric pain, abdominal distention, borborygmus, jaundice. 3. Other: Fever, stiffness and pain in back and spine, soreness in leg, general asthenis, shortness of breath with disinclination to talk.
DU-10 Lingtai ↘ upward 0.5-1 cun. ʃ is applicable.	On the back and posterior midline, in the depression below the spinous process of the 6th thoracic vertebra. 1. Clears heat and transforms dampness. 2. Relieves cough and asthma.	1. Respiratory: Cough, asthma. 2. Digestive: Gastric pain, biliary ascariasis. 3. Other: Insomnia, restlessness, stiffness of neck, malaria, furuncle.
DU-11 Shendao ↘ upward 0.5-1 cun. ʃ is applicable.	On the back and posterior midline, in the depression below the spinous process of the 5th thoracic vertebra. 1. Calms heart and mind. 2. Clears heat and relieves asthma.	1. Respiratory: Cough, asthma. 2. Cardiac: Cardiac pain, palpitation. 3. Mental: Apoplexy, epilepsy, insomnia, poor memory, hysteria. 4. Other: Headache, chills and fever.

Table II-14   Points of the Du Meridian (DU) (Governor Vessel, GV)

Point, Property , Method and Remarks	Location & Action	Categories of Diseases & Indications
DU-12 Shenzhu ⤮ *upward 0.5-1 cun.* ᗾ *is applicable.*	On the back and posterior midline, in the depression below the spinous process of the 3rd thoracic vertebra. 1. Disperses lung and clears heat. 2. Calms spirit and relieves convulsion.	1. Respiratory: Cough, asthma, irritable feverish sensation in chest. 2. Mental: Fainting due to emotional upset, manic-depressive psychosis, epilepsy, clonic convulsion, aphasia from apoplexy. 3. Other: Stiffness and pain along spinal column which causes forced sitting position, furuncle, lumbodorsal cellulitis, fever with headache.
DU-13 Taodao ***Crossing Point of DU & BL*** ⤮ *upward 0.5-1 cun.* ᗾ *is applicable.*	On the back and on the posterior midline, in the depression below the spinous process of the 1st thoracic vertebra. 1. Relieves exterior and clears heat. 2. Stops malaria and calms spirit.	1. Respiratory: Cough, asthma. 2. Mental: Manic-depressive psychosis, epilepsy, convulsion, opisthotonos. 3. Other: Stiffness and pain of head and neck, fever, aversion to cold without sweating, malaria, night sweating due to hectic fever, chest pain, soreness along spinal column, inability to raise arm due to pain in shoulder joint, urticaria.
DU-14 Dazhui ***Crossing Point of DU, Three Hand-Yang, and Three Foot-Yang M.*** ⤮ *upward 0.5-1 cun.* ᗾ *is applicable.*	On the posterior midline, in the depression below the 7th cervical vertebra. 1. Relieves exterior and clears heat. 2. Stops malaria and relieves epilepsy. 3. Reinforces yang.	1. Respiratory: Cough, asthma. 2. Conditions of general weakness: Emaciation with weakness due to five kinds of strain, weakness and fatigue due to seven kinds of impairment, spontaneous sweating, night sweating. 3. Mental: Epilepsy, infantile convulsion, opisthotonos, manic-depressive psychosis. 4. Other: Pain shoulder, back and waist, stiffness of spinal column, urticaria, measles, malaria, sunstroke, cholera, jaundice, fever, aversion to wind and cold, headache, stiffness in nape of the neck.

Table II-14   Points of the Du Meridian (DU) (Governor Vessel, GV)

Point, Property , Method and Remarks	Location & Action	Categories of Diseases & Indications
DU-15 Yamen *Crossing Point of DU & Yangwei M.* ⊥ *0.5-0.8 cun.* *Upward puncture or deep puncture is not allowed. It is near the medullary bulb in the deep layer, and strict attention to the depth and angle of insertion should be paid.*	On the nape, 0.5 cun directly above midpoint of the posterior hairline, below the 1st cervical vertebra. 1. Dispels and extinguishes wind. 2. Opens the orifices and induces resuscitation.	1. Head and sense organs: Headache, heaviness of head, stiffness of nape, flaccidity of tongue with aphasia, hoarseness, speaking in a low voice. 2. Mental: Apoplexy, syncope, manic-depressive psychosis, epilepsy, hysteria, clonic convulsion. 3. Other: Epistaxis, vomiting, back rigidity.
DU-16 Fengfu *Crossing Point of DU & Yangwei M.* ⊥ *0.5-0.8 cun.* *Upward puncture or deep puncture is not allowed. It is near the medullary bulb in the deep layer, and strict attention to the depth and angle of insertion should be paid.*	On the nape, 1 cun directly above the midpoint of the posterior hairline, directly below the external occipital protuberance, in the depression between the trapezius muscle of both sides. 1. Dispels and extinguishes wind. 2. Opens the orifices and induces resuscitation.	1. Head and sense organs: Headache, vertigo, stuffy nose, epistaxis, sore throat, stiffness in nape of neck. 2. Mental: Manic-depressive psychosis, epilepsy, hysteria, apoplexy, flaccid tongue with aphasia, dysphoria, palpitation due to sorrow and fright. 3. Other: Flaccidity of lower limbs, numbness of feet, jaundice, common cold, fever.
DU-17 Naohu *Crossing Point of DU & BL* ↳ *0.3-0.5 cun.* ᵟ *is applicable.*	On the head, 2.5 cun directly above the midpoint of the posterior hairline, 1.5 cun above DU-16 Fengfu, in the depression on the upper border of the external occipital protuberance. 1. Opens the orifices and induces resuscitation. 2. Soothes liver and extinguishes wind.	1. Head and sense organs: Heaviness of head, dizziness, headache, flushed face, icteric sclera, opthalamalgia causing myopia, pain and edema of face, stiffness of nape, bleeding in root of tongue. 2. Mental: Manic-depressive psychosis, epilepsy, clonic convulsion, aphasia, apoplexy. 3. Other: Goiter, jaundice.

Table II-14   Points of the Du Meridian (DU) (Governor Vessel, GV)

Point, Property , Method and Remarks	Location & Action	Categories of Diseases & Indications
DU-18 Qiangjian ↳ *0.3-0.5 cun.* *ᵹ is applicable.*	On the head, 4 cun directly above the midpoint of the posterior hairline and 1.5 cun above DU-17 Naohu. 1. Induces resuscitation and calms mind. 2. Soothes liver and extinguishes wind.	1. Head and sense organs: Headache, dizziness, stiffness and pain of neck with inability to turn head. 2. Mental: Manic-depressive psychosis, epilepsy, clonic convulsion. 3. Other:Vomiting, restlessness.
DU-19 Houding ↳ *0.3-0.5 cun.* *ᵹ is applicable.*	On the head, 5.5 cun directly above the midpoint of the posterior hairline and 3 cun above DU-17 Naohu. 1. Induces resuscitation and calms mind. 2. Extinguishes wind and relieves convulsion.	1. Head and sense organs: Vertex pain, migraine, vertigo, blurred vision, stiffness and pain of neck. 2. Mental: Manic-depressive psychosis, restlessness, insomnia, clonic convulsion. 3. Other: Epidemic febrile disease due to exopathogen.
DU-20 Baihui *Crossing Point of DU & BL* ↳ *0.3-0.5 cun.* *ᵹ is applicable.*	On the head, 5 cun directly above the midpoint of the anterior hairline, at the midpoint of the line connecting the apexes of both ears. 1. Extinguishes wind and induces resuscitation. 2. Raises yang and restores prolapse.	1. Head and sense organs: Headache, dizziness, tinnitus, deafness, dizziness due to wind pathogen, heaviness in head, blurred vision, conjunctival congestion, nasal obstruction. 2. Mental: Amnesia, syncope, shock, aphasia due to apoplexy, tetanus, hemiplegia, epilepsy, hysteria, clonic convulsion. 3. Digestive: Poor appetite, epistaxis, rectal prolapse, protracted diarrhea, dysentery, gastroptosis. 4. Urogenital: Nephroptosis, enuresis, prolapse of uterus, impotence. 5. Other: Hypertension, palpitation.

Table II-14 Points of the Du Meridian (DU) (Governor Vessel, GV)

Point, Property , Method and Remarks	Location & Action	Categories of Diseases & Indications
DU-21 Qianding ↳ 0.3-0.5 cun. ℰ is applicable.	On the head, 3.5 cun directly above the midpoint of the anterior hairline and 1.5 cun anterior to DU-20 Baihui. 1. Extinguishes wind and induces resuscitation. 2. Calms mind and relieves spasm.	1. Head and sense organs: Vertigo, stuffy nose with clear discharge, rhinorrhea with turbid discharge, epistaxis, conjunctival congestion, blurred vision, flushed and swollen face. 2. Mental: Manic-depressive psychosis, clonic convulsion, apoplexy. 3. Other: Hypertension, edema.
DU-22 Xinhui ↳ 0.3-0.5 cun. ℰ is applicable. **Prohibited in infants with metropism (uncovered fontanelle).**	On the head, 2 cun directly above the midpoint of the anterior hairline and 3 cun anterior to DU-20 Baihui. 1. Induces resuscitation and calms mind. 2. Clears heat and reduces swelling.	1. Head and sense organs: Headache, vertigo, flushed and swollen face, rhinorrhea with turbid discharge, epistaxis, nasal polyp, carbuncle of nose, cold sensation and pain in head, itching of scalp with much scurf. 2. Mental: Epilepsy, infantile convulsion, apoplexy, insomnia, lethargy. 3. Other: Hypertension.
DU-23 Shangxing ↳ 0.3-0.5 cun or prick to cause bleeding. ℰ is applicable. **It is prohibited in infants with metropism.**	On the head, 1 cun directly above the midpoint of the anterior hairline. 1. Extinguishes wind and clears heat. 2. Calms mind and clears obstruction from nose.	1. Head and sense organs: Headache, vertigo, edema of face, conjunctival congestion, excessive lacrimation induced by wind, myopia, epistaxis, rhinorrhea with turbid discharge, nasal polyp, carbuncle of nose. 2. Mental: Manic-depressive psychosis, epilepsy, infantile convulsion, apoplexy. 3. Other: Malaria, febrile disease, anhidrosis, vomiting.
DU-24 Shenting **Crossing Point of DU, BL & ST** ↳ 0.3-0.5 cun or prick to cause bleeding. ℰ is applicable.	On the head, 0.5 cun directly above the midpoint of the anterior hairline. 1. Induces resuscitation and calms mind. 2. Reverses rebellious qi and relieves asthma.	1. Head and sense organs: Headache, vertigo, conjunctival congestion, nebula, night blindness, rhinorrhea with turbid discharge, running nose, stuffy nose, epistaxis. 2. Mental: Manic-depressive psychosis, epilepsy, infantile convulsion, apoplexy, opisthotonos, neurogenic vomiting. 3. Other: Involuntary movement of the tongue, dyspnea with thirst.

Table II-14   Points of the Du Meridian (DU) (Governor Vessel, GV)

Point, Property , Method and Remarks	Location & Action	Categories of Diseases & Indications
DU-25 Suliao ⊥ *0.2-0.3 cun or prick to cause bleeding.*	On the face, at the center of the nose apex. 1. Clears heat and reduces swelling. 2. Benefits and removes obstruction from nose.	1. Head and sense organs: Stuffy nose, epistaxis, running nose, rhinorrhea with turbid discharge, nasal polyp, carbuncle of nose, epidemic hemorrhagic conjunctivitis. 2. Digestive: Cholera, vomiting. 3. Mental: Convulsion, coma, shock, infantile convulsion, irritability.
DU-26 Shuigou ***Crossing Point of DU, LI & ST*** ↘ *upward 0.3-0.5 cun.*	On the face, at the junction of the upper third and middle third of the philtrum. 1. Opens the orifices to induce resuscitation. 2. Clears heat and extinguishes wind.	1. Head and sense organs: Facial paralysis, toothache, stuffy nose, epistaxis, edema of face due to wind, tetanus. 2. Mental: Coma, syncope, manic-depressive psychosis, epilepsy, acute and chronic convulsion, sunstroke, opisthotonos, hysteria. 3. Other: Jaundice, diabetes, plague, stuffiness and pain of spinal column, lumbago due to sprain and contusion, stiff neck.
DU-27 Duiduan ↘ *upward 0.2-0.3 cun.*	On the face, on the labial tubercle of the upper lip, at the vermilion border between the philtrum and upper lip. 1. Induces resuscitation and calms mind. 2. Generates fluids to relieve thirst.	1. Head and sense organs: Lip tremor, aphthous ulcers and halitosis, toothache, gingivitis, tetanus, nebula, stuffy nose, epistaxis, extreme thirst, dry tongue. 2. Mental: Coma, syncope, manic-depressive psychosis, hysteria. 3. Digestive: Jaundice, deep yellow urine. 4. Other: Coccydynia.
DU-28 Yinjiao ***Crossing Point of DU & RN*** ↘ *upward 0.1-0.2 cun or prick to cause bleeding.*	Inside of the upper lip, at the junction of the labial frenum and upper gum. 1. Calms spirit and relieves spasm. 2. Clears heat and reduces swelling.	1. Head and sense organs: Gingivitis, deviation of mouth, tetanus, halitosis, gingival bleeding, sinusitis, flushed face, swollen cheek, sores or tinea on face, sores on cheeks. 2. Mental: Manic-depressive psychosis. 3. Other: Stiff neck.

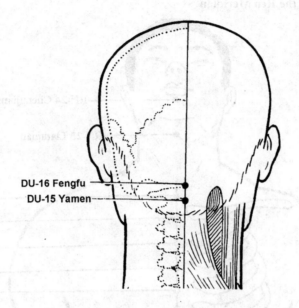

Fig, II-31 Points on the Du Meridian (2)

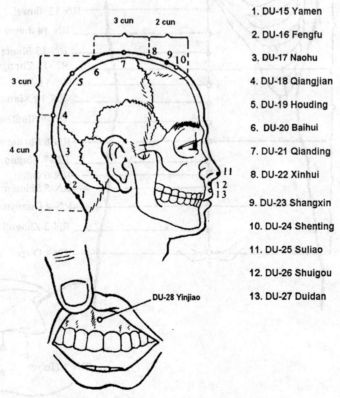

1. DU-15 Yamen

2. DU-16 Fengfu

3. DU-17 Naohu

4. DU-18 Qiangjian

5. DU-19 Houding

6. DU-20 Baihui

7. DU-21 Qianding

8. DU-22 Xinhui

9. DU-23 Shangxin

10. DU-24 Shenting

11. DU-25 Suliao

12. DU-26 Shuigou

13. DU-27 Duidan

Fig. II-32 Points on the Du Meridian (3)

14. The Points of the Ren Meridian

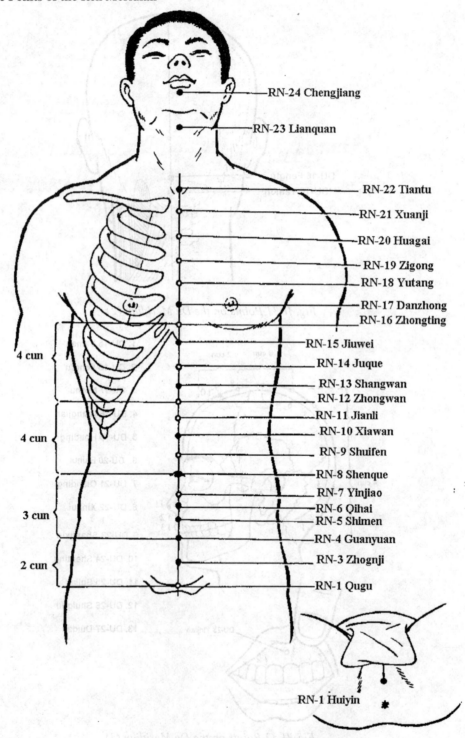

RN-24 Chengjiang

RN-23 Lianquan

RN-22 Tiantu

RN-21 Xuanji

RN-20 Huagai

RN-19 Zigong

RN-18 Yutang

RN-17 Danzhong

RN-16 Zhongting

RN-15 Jiuwei

RN-14 Juque

RN-13 Shangwan

RN-12 Zhongwan

RN-11 Jianli

RN-10 Xiawan

RN-9 Shuifen

RN-8 Shenque

RN-7 Yinjiao

RN-6 Qihai

RN-5 Shimen

RN-4 Guanyuan

RN-3 Zhognji

RN-1 Qugu

4 cun

4 cun

3 cun

2 cun

RN-1 Huiyin

Fig. II-33 Points on the Ren Meridian (1)

Table II-15 Points of the Ren Meridian (RN) (Conception Vessel, CV)

Point, Property , Method & Remarks	Location & Action	Categories of Diseases & Indications
RN-1 Huiyin *Crossing Point of RN, DU & Chong M.* ⊥ *0.5-1 cun.* ϐ *is applicable.*	On the perineum, at the midpoint between the posterior border of the scrotum and anus in male, and between the posterior commissure of the labia major and anus in female. 1. Induces resuscitation and relieves spasm. 2. Regulates function of external genitalia and anus.	1. Urinary: Difficult urination, enuresis. 2. Reproductive: Vulvar pain, pruritis vulvae, vulval eczema, uterus prolapse, nocturnal emission, irregular menstruation. 3. Mental: Coma, manic-depressive psychosis, epilepsy. 4. Other: First aid for asphyxia due to near-drowning, hernia, hemorrhoids, prolapse of rectum.
RN-2 Qugu *Crossing Point of RN & LR* ⊥ *0.5-1 cun.* ϐ *is applicable.* *Puncture with caution in pregnancy.*	On the lower abdomen and on the anterior midline, at the midpoint of the upper border of the pubic symphysis. 1. Promotes urination. 2. Regulates menstruation and alleviates pain.	1. Urinary: Lower abdominal distension, dribbling of urine, retention of urine, enuresis. 2. Reproductive: Nocturnal emission, impotence, irregular menstruation, leukorrhagia with reddish discharge, sterility, vulvar eczema. 3. Mental: Depressive disorders. 4. Other: Lower abdominal pain, hernia, edema, cramps in severe cholera.
RN-3 Zhongji *Front-Mu Point of Urinary Bladder;* *Crossing Point of RN & Three Foot-Yin M.* ⊥ *0.5-1 cun.* ϐ *is applicable.* *Puncture with caution in pregnancy.*	On the lower abdomen and on the anterior midline, 4 cun below the center of the umbilicus. 1. Reinforces kidney and strengthens yang. 2. Regulates menstruation and arrests leukorrhagia.	1. Urinary: Dysuria, frequent micturition, urgent urination, stranguria, enuresis. 2. Reproductive: Nocturnal emission, impotence, sterility, premature ejaculation, irregular menstruation, dysmenorrhea, uterine bleeding, prolapse of uterus, postpartum persistent lochia, retention of placenta, infertility. 3. Mental: Corpse-like syncope. 4. Other: Hernia, abdominal masses, sensation of gas rising in abdomen.

Table II-15   Points of the Ren Meridian (RN) (Conception Vessel, CV)

Point, Property , Method & Remarks	Location & Action	Categories of Diseases & Indications
RN-4 Guanyuan *Front-Mu Point of Small Intestine* ⊥ *0.8-1.2 cun.* ᵟ *is applicable.* *Puncture with caution in pregnancy.*	On the lower abdomen and on the anterior midline, 3 cun below the center of the umbilicus. 1. Tonifies original qi. 2. Promotes urination.	1. Urinary: Frequent micturition, retention of urine, hematuria, dribbling of urine, enuresis. 2. Reproductive: Nocturnal emission, impotence, premature ejaculation, gonorrhea, irregular menstruation, amenorrhea, uterine bleeding, leukorrhagia with reddish discharge, prolapse of uterus, pruritis vulvae, postpartum persistent lochia, retained placenta. 3. Mental: Prostration syndrome due to apoplexy, syncope, insomnia, dreaminess, poor memory. 4. Respiratory: Cough, asthma, hemoptoic cough, lack of strength in speaking, tuberculosis of lung. 5. Digestive: Cholera morbus, vomiting, diarrhea, abdominal pain, dysentery, bloody stools, chronic diarrhea and dysentery, jaundice, diabetes. 6. Other: Consumptive disease, weakness and asthenia in waist and legs, palpitation, shortness of breath, apoplexy, furuncle.
RN-5 Shimen *Front-Mu Point of Sanjiao* ⊥ *0.5-1 cun.* ᵟ *is applicable.* *Puncture with caution in pregnancy.*	On the lower abdomen and on the anterior midline, 2 cun below the center of the umbilicus. 1. Regulates qi and alleviates pain. 2. Dredges water passage.	1. Urinary: Dribbling of urine, frequent micturition, urgency of urination, stranguria, hematuria, enuresis, retention of urine. 2. Reproductive: Nocturnal emission, impotence, premature ejaculation, sterility, irregular menstruation, postpartum persistent lochia, retention of placenta. 3. Digestive : Abdominal distention, diarrhea, dysentery, constipation, indigestion, vomiting. 4. Other: Feeling of gas ascending in abdomen, hernia, retraction of penis.

Table II-15   Points of the Ren Meridian (RN) (Conception Vessel, CV)

Point, Property , Method & Remarks	Location & Action	Categories of Diseases & Indications
RN-6 Qihai ⊥ *0.8-1.2 cun.* *ß is applicable.* ***Puncture with caution in pregnancy.***	On the lower abdomen and on the anterior midline, 1.5 cun below the center of the umbilicus. 1. Reinforces qi and strengthens yang. 2. Regulates menstruation and consolidates essence.	1. Reproductive: Nocturnal emission, impotence, premature ejaculation, sterility, irregular menstruation, dysmenorrhea, amenorrhea, metrorrhagia and metrostaxis, leukorrhagia with reddish discharge, prolapse of uterus, postpartum persistent lochia, retention of placenta. 2. Mental: Collapse syndrome of apoplexy, acute infantile omphalitis. 3. Respiratory: Cough, asthma, shortness of breath. 4. Digestive: Pain and distention of stomach, hiccup, vomiting, indigestion, constipation, dysentery, acute diarrhea. 5. Other: Hernia, lumbago, pain around umbilicus, cold limbs, shortness of breath due to qi deficiency of five zang organs, emaciation, acratia, infantile metropism.
RN-7 Yinjiao ***Crossing Point of RN & Chong M.*** ⊥ *0.8-1.2 cun.* *ß is applicable.* ***Puncture with caution in pregnancy.***	On the lower abdomen and on the anterior midline, 1 cun below the center of the umbilicus. 1. Regulates menstruation and arrests leukorrhagia. 2. Promotes urination to reduce edema.	1. Urinary: Retention of urine, edema. 2. Reproductive: Irregular menstruation, leukorrhagia with reddish discharge, postpartum persistent lochia, retention of placenta. 3. Digestive: Diarrhea, borborygmus, abdominal distention, chronic dysentery. 4. Other: Hernia, lumbago.

Table II-15   Points of the Ren Meridian (RN) (Conception Vessel, CV)

Point, Property , Method & Remarks	Location & Action	Categories of Diseases & Indications
RM-8 Shenque *ᵹ is applicable.* ***Puncture is prohibited.***	At the center of the umbilicus. 1. Warms yang and restores devastated yang. 2. Promotes urination and relieves edema.	1. Urinary: Enuresis, retention of urine, edema, stranguria. 2. Reproductive: Irregular menstruation, metrorrhagia and metrostaxis, sterility. 3. Mental: Collapse syndrome of apoplexy, syncope, loss of consciousness, opisthotonos, exhaustion syndrome. 4. Other: Cold in lower limbs, tidal fever and night sweating, anaphylaxis, allergic urticaria, allergic bronchial asthma, allergic enteritis, hernia, pain around umbilicus, general acratia.
RN-9 Shuifen ⊥ *0.5-1 cun.* *ᵹ is applicable.*	On the upper abdomen and on the anterior midline, 1 cun above the center of the umbilicus. 1. Dredges water passage. 2. Regulates qi to stop pain.	1. Urinary: Retention of urine, edema. 2. Digestive: Pain around umbilicus, borborygmus, diarrhea, regurgitation, anorexia, prolapse of rectum, difficult defecation. 3. Other: Hernia, stiffness and pain along the spinal column.
RN-10 Xiawan ***Crossing Point of RN & SP M.*** ⊥ *0.5-1.2 cun.* *ᵹ is applicable.*	On the upper abdomen and on the anterior midline, 2 cun above the center of the umbilicus. 1. Strengthens spleen and harmonizes stomach. 2. Reverses rebellious qi and stops vomiting.	1. Digestive: Stomachache, abdominal distention and pain, vomiting, borborygmus, hiccup, indigestion, diarrhea. 2. Urinary: Dark urine.
RN-11 Jianli ⊥ *0.5-1.2 cun.* *ᵹ is applicable.*	On the upper abdomen and on the anterior midline, 3 cun above the center of the umbilicus. 1. Strengthens spleen and harmonizes stomach. 2. Reverses rebellious qi and removes water.	1. Digestive: Stomachache, abdominal distention and pain, vomiting, borborygmus, poor appetite, cholera morbus.

Table II-15   Points of the Ren Meridian (RN) (Conception Vessel, CV)

Point, Property , Method & Remarks	Location & Action	Categories of Diseases & Indications
RN-12 Zhongwan *Front-Mu Point of Stomach;* *Influential Point of Fu Organs;* *Crossing Point of SI, SJ& ST* ⊥ *0.5-1.2 cun.* ᵝ *is applicable.*	On the upper abdomen and on the anterior midline, 4 cun above the center of the umbilicus. 1. Strengthens spleen and harmonizes stomach. 2. Descends stomach and large intestine qi.	1. Respiratory: Asthma, profuse phlegm, emaciation with weakness, hematemesis. 2. Cardiovascular: Palpitation, cardiac pain. 3. Digestive: Stomachache, abdominal distention, vomiting, hiccup, nausea, acid-regurgitation, anorexia, indigestion, infantile malnutrition, abdominal pain, borborygmus, diarrhea, cholera morbus, bloody stools, constipation, edema, jaundice. 4. Gynecopathies: Hysteroptosis, pernicious vomiting. 5. Mental: Insomnia, hysteria, manic-depressive psychosis, epilepsy, apoplexy, syncope, acute or chronic infantile convulsion. 6. Other: Urticaria, dark sallow complexion, lassitude, fever, dark urine, burning sensation and foul smell in nose.
RN-13 Shangwan *Crossing Point of RN, ST & SI* ⊥ *0.5-1.2 cun.* ᵝ *is applicable.*	On the upper abdomen and on the anterior midline, 5 cun above the center of the umbilicus. 1. Harmonizes stomach and reverses rebellious qi. 2. Transforms phlegm and calms mind.	1. Respiratory: Cough, asthma, profuse phlegm, hemoptysis. 2. Cardiovascular: Angina pectoris, restlessness, palpitation. 3. Digestive: Stomachache, abdominal distention and pain, borborygmus, diarrhea, cholera morbus, vomiting, hiccup, anorexia, jaundice. 4. Mental: Manic-depressive psychosis, epilepsy. 5. Other: Fever with anhidrosis, dizziness and blurred vision.

Table II-15   Points of the Ren Meridian (RN) (Conception Vessel, CV)

Point, Property , Method & Remarks	Location & Action	Categories of Diseases & Indications
RN-14 Juque *Front-Mu Point of Heart* ⊥ *0.3-0.8 cun.* ᵷ *is applicable.*	On the upper abdomen and on the anterior midline, 6 cun above the center of the umbilicus. 1. Calms mind. 2. Soothes chest oppression and alleviates pain.	1. Respiratory: Fullness of chest, shortness of breath, cough, asthma, hemoptysis. 2. Cardiovascular: Feeling of oppression in chest, pain of chest, restlessness, palpitation. 3. Digestive: Stomachache, upper abdominal distention, cholera morbus, vomiting, dysphagia, acid regurgitation, diarrhea, dysentery, pain of chest due to ascariasis, jaundice. 4. Mental: Syncope, manic-depressive psychosis, epilepsy, poor memory, insomnia. 5. Other: Beriberi, hernia.
RN-15 Jiuwei *Luo-Connecting Point* ↘ *downward 0.4-0.6 cun.* ᵷ *is applicable.*	On the upper abdomen and on the anterior midline, 1 cun below the xiphisternal synchondrosis. 1. Calms mind. 2. Soothes chest oppression and relieves asthma.	1. Head and sense organs: Migraine, sore throat. 2. Cardiovascular: Cardiac pain, palpitation, restlessness, oppressive feeling in chest, pain in chest, shortness of breath, listlessness. 3. Digestive: Vomiting, hiccups, regurgitation, pain in stomach, abdominal distention. 4. Mental: Manic-depressive psychosis, epilepsy, hysteria. 5. Other: Prolapse of rectum, sexual excess, exhaustion of spirit, sunken fontanelle in infant.
RN-16 Zhongting ↳ *0.3-0.5 cun.* ᵷ *is applicable.*	On the chest and on the anterior midline at the 5th intercostal space, on the xiphosternal synchondrosis. 1. Soothes chest oppression and relieves distention. 2. Reverses rebellious qi and relieves vomiting.	1. Cardiovascular: Cardiac pain, palpitation, feeling of oppression in chest, pain of chest. 2. Digestive: Abdominal distention, dysphagia, vomiting, anorexia. 3. Other: Globus hystericus, pain in pharynx.

Table II-15 Points of the Ren Meridian (RN) (Conception Vessel, CV)

Point, Property , Method & Remarks	Location & Action	Categories of Diseases & Indications
RN-17 Danzhong *Front-Mu Point of Pericardium;* *Influential Point of Qi* ↳ *0.3-0.5 cun.* ∂ *is applicable.*	On the chest and on the anterior midline at the 4th intercostal space, at the midpoint of the line connecting both nipples. 1. Regulates qi and alleviates pain. 2. Generates body fluids.	1. Respiratory: Cough, asthma, shortness of breath. 2. Cardiovascular: Cardiac pain, pain chest, palpitation, irritability. 3. Digestive: Dysphagia, abdominal distention, vomiting with salvia and spittle. 4. Other: Postpartum lactation deficiency, goiter, cramp in cholera morbus, syncope.
RN-18 Yutang ↳ *0.3-0.5 cun.* ∂ *is applicable.*	On the chest and on the anterior midline at the 3rd intercostal space. 1. Soothes chest oppression and alleviates pain. 2. Relieves cough and asthma.	1. Respiratory: Pain in chest, cough, asthma, inflammation of throat, swelling of pharynx. 2. Digestive: Vomiting. 3. Other: Swelling and pain in breasts.
RN-19 Zigong ↳ *0.3-0.5 cun.* ∂ *is applicable.*	On the chest and on the anterior midline at the 2nd intercostal space. 1. Soothes chest oppression and regulates qi. 2. Relieves cough and asthma.	1. Respiratory: Pain in chest, cough, asthma, sore throat. 2. Digestive: Vomiting, indigestion, dysphagia. 3. Other: Pain in breasts.
RN-20 Huagai ↳ *0.3-0.5 cun.* ∂ *is applicable.*	On the chest and on the anterior midline at the 1st intercostal space. 1. Soothes chest oppression and benefits diaphragm. 2. Relieves cough and asthma.	1. Respiratory: Cough, asthma, hematemesis, pain in chest, sore throat. 2. Digestive: Vomiting, dysphagia.
RN-21 Xuanji ↳ *0.3-0.5 cun.* ∂ *is applicable.*	On the chest and on the anterior midline, 1 cun below RN-22 Tiantu. 1. Soothes chest oppression and benefits lung. 2. Relieves cough and asthma.	1. Respiratory: Cough, asthma, pain in chest, throat redness, swelling and pain on swallowing, wheezing sounds in throat of infants. 2. Digestive: Dyspepsia.

Table II-15   Points of the Ren Meridian (RN) (Conception Vessel, CV)

Point, Property , Method & Remarks	Location & Action	Categories of Diseases & Indications
RN-22 Tiantu *First ± 0.2 cun, then insert the needle downward along the posterior aspect of sternum 0.5-1 cun.* *Ɵ is applicable.*	On the neck and on the anterior midline, at the center of the suprasternal fossa. 1. Disperse lung qi. 2. Transforms phlegm to relieve cough and asthma.	1. Respiratory: Cough, asthma, sensation of gas ascending in chest, pulmonary abscess, pain of throat on swallowing, sudden hoarseness of voice. 2. Digestive: Dysphagia, vomiting. 3. Cardiovascular: Cardiac pain. 4. Other: Subglossal spasm, goiter, globus hystericus, swelling of nape of neck and shoulder pain.
RN-23 Lianquan ***Crossing Point of RN & Yinwei M.*** *↘ 0.5-1 cun toward the tongue root.* *Ɵ is applicable.*	On the neck and on the anterior midline, above the laryngeal protuberance, in the depression above the upper border of the hyoid bone. 1. Benefits throat and tongue. 2. Reduces swelling and alleviates pain.	1. Head and sense organs: Subglossal swelling and pain, spasmodic pain at root of tongue, involuntary protrusion of tongue, stiff tongue, dry tongue and mouth, sore tongue, sudden loss of voice, redness, sore throat, difficulty in swallowing. 2. Digestive: Dyspepsia, diabetes. 3. Mental: Aphasia due to apoplexy, infantile convulsion, manic-depressive psychosis, epilepsy.
RN-24 Chengjiang ***Crossing Point of RN & ST*** *↘ upward 0.2-0.3 cun.* *Ɵ is applicable.*	On the face, in the depression at the midpoint of the mentolabial sulcus. 1. Generates body fluids and arrests salivation. 2. Comforts sinews and activates collaterals.	1. Head and sense organs: Deviation of mouth and eye, spasm of lips, swelling of face, toothache, gingival bleeding, gingivitis, salivation, sore tongue. 2. Digestive: Diabetes, thirst. 3. Urinary: Enuresis. 4. Mental: Epilepsy, infantile convulsion. 5. Other: Hemiplegia.

V. LOCATION, ACTION & INDICATIONS OF THE EXTRA POINTS, EX

1. Commonly-Used Extra Points of the Head and Neck (EX-HN)

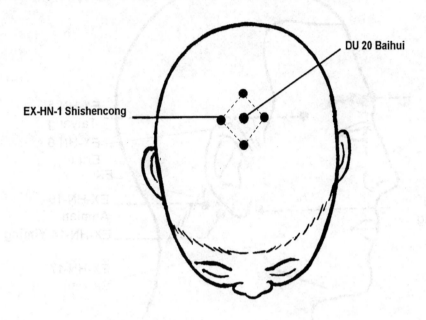

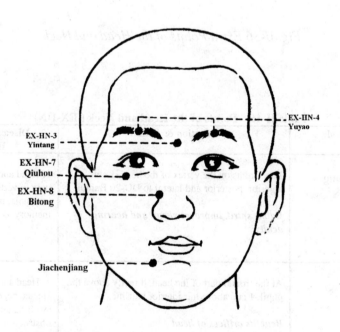

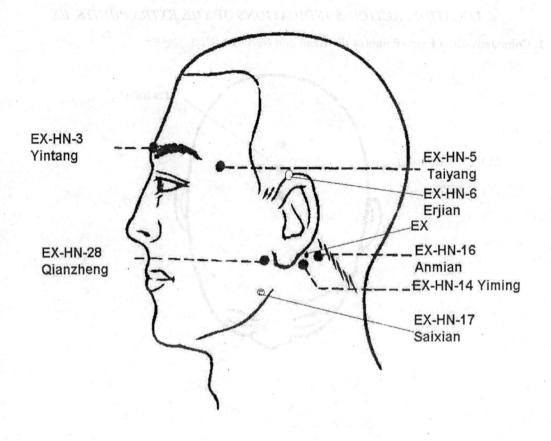

EX-HN-3
Yintang

EX-HN-5
Taiyang

EX-HN-6
Erjian

EX

EX-HN-28
Qianzheng

EX-HN-16
Anmian

EX-HN-14 Yiming

EX-HN-17
Saixian

Fig. II-36 Extra Points of the Head and Neck

Table II-16   Points of the Head and Neck (EX-HN)

Point & Method	Location & Action	Disease Categories & Indications
EX-HN-1 Sishencong ↳ 0.5-1 cun. ᵝ is applicable.	Four points on the vertex of the head, 1 cun anterior, posterior and lateral to DU-20 Baihui. *Calms spirit, improves visual and hearing acuity.*	1. Head and mental: Distending pain in vertex of head, vertigo, insomnia, neurasthenia, poor memory, epilepsy.
EX-HN-2 Dangyang ↳ 0.5-1 cun. ᵝ is applicable.	At the frontal part of the head, directly above the pupil, 1 cun above the anterior hairline. *Benefits orifices of head.*	1. Head and sense organ: Headache, dizziness, redness, swelling and pain in eye, nasal obstruction

Table II-16 Points of the Head and Neck (EX-HN)

Point & Method	Location & Action	Disease Categories & Indications
EX-HN-3 Yintang ↳ 0.3-0.5 cun. ठ is applicable.	On the forehead, at the midpoint between the eyebrows. *Calms mind, improves visual acuity, unobstructs nose.*	1. Head and Nose: Headache, vertigo, rhinorrhea, insomnia, pain in forehead, heaviness in head. 2. Other: Anxiety, infantile convulsion.
EX-HN-4 Yuyao ↳ 0.3-0.5 cun. ठ is applicable.	On the forehead, directly above the pupil, in the eyebrow. *Improves visual acuity, reduces swelling, comforts sinews & activates collaterals.*	1. Eye: Pain in supraorbital region, twitching of eyelids, ptosis of eyelid, cloudiness of cornea, redness, swelling and pain in the eye.
EX-HN-5 Taiyang ⊥ 0.3-0.5 cun, or prick to cause bleeding.	At the temporal part of the head, between the lateral end of the eyebrow and the outer canthus, in the depression one finger breadth behind them. *Clears heat, reduces swelling, activates collaterals, stops pain.*	1. Head and face: Headache, migraine, facial paralysis, trigeminal neuralgia, deviation of eye and mouth.
EX-HN-6 Erjian ⊥ 0.1-0.2 cun, or prick to cause bleeding. ठ is applicable.	Above the apex of the ear auricle, at the tip of the auricle when the ear is folded forward. *Clears heat, reduces swelling, brightens eyes and benefits throat.*	1. Eye: Redness, swelling and pain in the eyes, nebula 2. Headache, sore throat.
EX-HN-7 Qiuhou Push eyeball upward gently, ⊥ 0.5-1.2 cun along the orbital margin slowly without any lifting, thrusting, twisting or rotating manipulation.	On the face, at the junction of the lateral fourth and medial three fourths of infraorbital margin. *Improves visual acuity.*	1. Eye: Myopia, optic neuritis, optic atrophy, pigmentary degeneration of retina.
EX-HN-8 Bitong (Shangyingxiang) ↘ upward 0.3-0.5 cun. ठ is applicable.	On the face, at the junction of the alar cartilage of the nose and the nasal concha, near the upper end of the nasolabial groove. *Clears heat, dispels wind, brightens eyes, unobstructs nose.*	1. Nasal: Nasal obstruction, allergic rhinitis, hypertrophied rhinitis, atrophic rhinitis, sinusitis. 2. Headache.
EX-HN-9 Neiyingxiang Prick to bleed.	In the nostril, at the junction between the mucous of the alar cartilage of the nose and the nasal concha. *Clears heat, reduces swelling, improves visual acuity, unobstructs nose.*	1. Eye: Redness, swelling and pain of eyes. 2. Nasal: Any nasal disorder. 3. Other: Sore throat, febrile diseases, sunstroke, vertigo.

Table II-16   Points of the Head and Neck (EX-HN)

Point & Method	Location & Action	Disease Categories & Indications
EX-HN-10 Juquan ⊥ 0.1-0.2 cun, or prick to cause bleeding.	In the mouth, at the midpoint of the dorsal midline of the tongue. *Relieves cough and asthma, activates collaterals.*	1. Tongue: Stiff tongue, flaccid tongue. 2. Other: Diabetes, asthma, cough.
EX-HN-11 Haiquan Prick to bleed.	In the mouth, at the midpoint of the frenulum of the tongue. *1. Clears heat, generates fluids.* *2. Tranquilizes mind.*	1. Diabetes. 2. Spasm of diaphragm. 3. Glossitis. 4. Psychoses.
EX-HN-12 Jinjin Prick to bleed.	In the mouth, on the vein in the left side of the frenulum of the tongue. *Clears heat, reduces swelling, clears heart, reverses rebellious qi.*	1. Tongue and speech: Stiff tongue, swelling of tongue, aphasia. 2. Other: Diabetes, vomiting, diarrhea, sore throat.
EX-HN-13 Yuye Prick to bleed.	In the mouth, on the vein in the right side of the frenulum of the tongue. *Clears heat, reduces swelling, clears heart, reverses rebellious qi.*	1. Tongue and speech: Stiff tongue, swelling of tongue, aphasia. 2. Other: Diabetes, vomiting, diarrhea, sore throat.
EX-HN-14 Yiming ↘ or ↪ 0.5-1 cun. ᵦ is applicable.	On the nape, 1 cun posterior to SJ-17 Yifeng. *Improves visual acuity and relieves nebula, extinguishes wind and calms mind.*	1. Eye: Near sight, night blindness, optic atrophy, cataract. 2. Other: Tinnitus, vertigo, parotitis, headache, insomnia.
EX-HN-15 Jingbailao ⊥ 0.5-1 cun. ᵦ is applicable.	On the nape, 2 cun directly above Dazhui DU 14 and 1 cun lateral to the posterior midline. *Transforms phlegm and relieves swelling, relieves cough and asthma.*	1. Neck: Stiffness and pain in the neck. 2. Other: Hectic fever, spontaneous sweating, night sweating, scrofula, cough, asthma.
EX-HN-16 Anmiang ⊥ 0.5-1 cun. ᵦ is applicable.	On the nape, at the midpoint of the line connecting GB-20 Fengchi and SJ-17 Yifeng. *Pacifies liver, extinguishes wind, calms mind.*	1. Insomnia.
EX-H-17 Saixian ⊥ 0.3-0.7 cun. ᵦ is applicable.	On the cheek, at the midpoint of the line connecting the lower border of the ear lobe and the angle of the mandible. *Clears heat, dispels wind, and reduces swelling in cheek.*	1. Mumps.

Table II-16   Points of the Head and Neck (EX-HN)

Point & Method	Location & Action	Disease Categories & Indications
EX-HN-18 Pressure-Lowering Point ⊥ 0.5-1 cun.	At the midpoint of the line connecting BL-1 Jingming and BL-2Cuanzhu. *Pacifies liver, suppresses yang.*	1. Hypertension.
EX-HN-19 Neijiache Prick to bleed.	On the mucosa of the mouth, opposite to SJ-6 Jiache. *Clears heat, dispels wind and activates collaterals.*	1. Facial paralysis.
EX-HN-20 Yemen ↳ 0.5-1 cun.	On the surface of the tongue, 1 cm from the tongue tip. *Opens the orifice to improve speech.*	1. Aphasia due to cerebrovascular accident.
EX-HN-21 Tousanjiao ↳ 0.5-1 cun.	Three points in total, located on forehead, respectively at the crossing points of the perpendicular line from the inner canthus and the front hairline, and DU-23 Shangxing. *Improves blood circulation and calms mind.*	1. Insomnia with headache.
EX-HN-22 Shangtianzhu ⊥ 0.3-0.5 cun. ß is applicable.	0.5 cun directly above BL-10 Tianzhu. *Pacifies liver, suppresses yang, benefits eyes.*	1. Exophthalmus due to hyperthyroidism.
EX-HN-23 Xinming 1 ↘ or ↳ 0.5-1 cun. ß is applicable.	On the joint of the ear lobe and cheek, 0.5 cun anterior and superior to SJ-17 Yifeng. *Improves visual acuity.*	1. Optic atrophy.
EX-HN-24 Xinming 2 ↘ or ↳ 0.5-1 cun. ß is applicable.	On the forehead, 1 cun above and 0.5 cun lateral to the lateral end of the eyebrow. *Improves visual acuity.*	1. Optic atrophy.
EX-HN-25 Jiaozhong ↘ or ↳ 0.5-1 cun. ß is applicable.	On the midpoint of the line connecting ST-7 Xiaguan and ST-6 Jiache. *Improves circulation of qi and blood.*	1. Temporomandibular joint disease.

Table II-16   Points of the Head and Neck (EX-HN)

Point & Method	Location & Action	Disease Categories & Indications
EX-HN-26 Neidicang Prick to bleed.	On the mucus of the mouth, opposite to ST-4 Dicang. *Descends rebellious qi of stomach to stop vomiting.*	1. Vomiting.
EX-HN-27 Liyan ↘ or ↪ 0.5-1 cun. ʃ is applicable.	On the face, at the midpoint of the line connecting the lowest point of the ear lobe and the angle of the mandible. *Promotes flow of qi and blood, clears heat and benefits throat.*	1. Throat diseases.

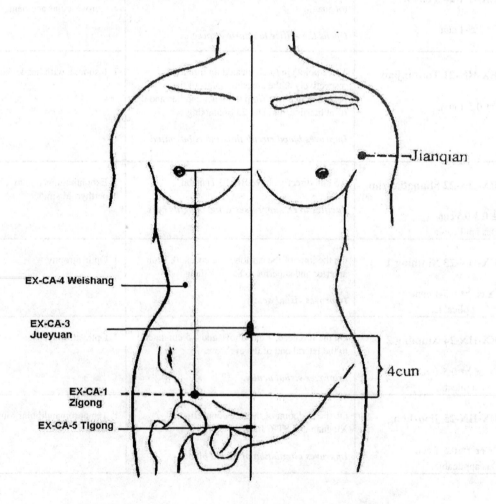

Fig. II-37   Extra Points of the Chest and Abdomen

2. Commonly-Used Extra Points of the Chest and Abdomen (EX-CA)

Table II-17   Points of the Chest and Abdomen, EX-CA

Point & Method	Location & Action	Disease Categories & Indications
EX-CA-1 Zigong ⊥ 1-1.2 cun. δ is applicable.	On the lower abdomen, 4 cun below the center of the umbilicus and 3 cun lateral to RN-3 Zhongji. *Regulates menstruation, improves reproductive function, regulates qi and alleviates pain.*	1. Gynecopathies: Prolapse of uterus, irregular menstruation, menorrhagia, pelvic inflammation, infertility in women, cystitis, orchitis. 2. Other: Appendicitis.
EX-CA-2 Huiyinhou ⊥ 1-1.2 cun. δ is applicable.	On the midpoint of the line connecting the perineum and anus. *Promotes qi and blood circulation and reduces swelling.*	1. Chronic prostatitis.
EX-AC-3 Jueyuan ⊥ 1-1.2 cun. δ is applicable.	On the upper border of RN-8 Shenque. *Clears heat, removes dampness, arrests diarrhea.*	1. Acute infantile diarrhea.
EX-AC-4 Weishang ↳ 1.5-2 cun. δ is applicable.	On the abdomen, 4 cun lateral to RN-10 Xiawan. *Strengthens spleen and harmonizes stomach.*	1. Gastroptosis.
EX-CA-5 Tigong ⊥ 1-1.5 cun. δ is applicable.	On the abdomen, 2 finger breadth directly below the midpoint of the anterior border of the pubic area. *Raises yang to restore normal position of uterus.*	1. Prolapse of uterus.
EX-CA-6 Yumen ⊥ 0.2-0.4 cun.	On the female external genetalia, at the center of the clitoris. *Tranquilizes mind.*	1. Psychoses characterized by dreaming of having sexual action with ghost.

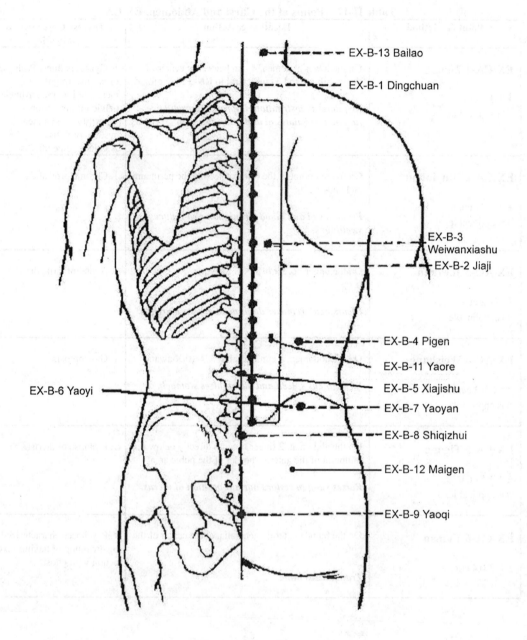

Fig. II-38 Extra Points of the Back

3. Commonly-Used Extra Points of the Back (EX-B)

Table II-18   Points of the Back, EX-B

Point & Method	Location & Action	Disease Categories & Indications
EX-B-1 Dingchuan ⊥ 0.5-1 cun. β is applicable.	On the back, below the spinous process of the 7th cervical vertebra, 0.5 cun lateral to the posterior midline. *Relieves cough and asthma.*	1. Respiratory: Cough, bronchitis, asthma. 2. Other: Neck rigidity, urticaria.
EX-B-2 Jiaji ⊥ 0.5-1 cun in cervical and chest region and 1-1.5 cun in lumbar region. β is applicable.	On the back and low back, 17 points on each side, below the spinous processes from the 1st thoracic to the 5th lumbar vertebrae, 0.5 cun lateral to the posterior midline. Customally named after the related vertebra and according to the vertebra order, such as T1, the point level to the interspaxe of the first and 2nd end vertebrae. *Promotes qi and blood circulation, regulates yin and yang, improves internal organs' function.*	1. T1-3 for diseases in upper limbs. 2. T1-8 for diseases in chest region. 3. T6-L5 for diseases in abdominal region. 4. L1-5 for diseases in lower limbs.
EX-B-3 Weiwanxiashu ↘ 0.5-0.7 cun. β is applicable.	On the back, below the spinous process of the 8th thoracic vertebra, 1.5 cun lateral to the posterior midline. *Strengthens spleen and harmonizes stomach.*	1. Digestive: Diabetes, stomach problems, abdominal pain, vomiting. 2. Other: Intercostal neuralgia.
EX-B-4 Pigen ↘ 0.5-0.8 cun. β is applicable.	On the lower back, below the spinous process of the 1st lumbar vertebra, 3.5 cun lateral to the posterior midline. *Regulates spleen and stomach, strengthens kidney.*	1. Digestive: Gastritis, enteritis. 2. Other: Ptosis of kidney, lower back pain, hypochondriac pain.
EX-B-5 Xiajishu ↘ 0.5-0.8 cun. β is applicable.	On the midline of the low back, below the spinous process of the third lumbar vertebra. *Strengthens spleen and reinforces kidney.*	1. Lower back pain, diarrhea, dysuria, enuresis, paralysis of lower limbs.
EX-B-6 Yaoyi ↘ 0.5-0.8 cun. β is applicable.	On the lower back, below the spinous process of the 4th lumbar vertebra, 3 cun lateral to the posterior midline. *Strengthens kidney.*	1. Lower back pain, dysfunctional uterine bleeding.

Table II-18   Points of the Back, EX-B

Point & Method	Location & Action	Disease Categories & Indications
EX-B-7 Yaoyan ↘ 0.5-0.8 cun. ⊘ is applicable.	On the low back, below the spinous process of the 4th lumbar vertebra, in the depression 3.5 cun lateral to posterior midline. *Strengthens kidney.*	1. Injury of waist, ptosis of kidney, orchitis, frequent urination, irregular menstruation.
EX-B-8 Shiqizhui ↘ upward 0.5-1.5 cun. ⊘ is applicable.	On the low back and on the posterior midline, below the spinous of the 5th lumbar vertebra. *Strengthens kidney and promotes urination.*	1. Pain in lumbosacral region, sciatica, dysfunctional uterine bleeding, menorrhagia, disorders of anus, paraplegia, retention of urine.
EX-B-9 Yaoqi ↪ upward 1-1.5 cun. ⊘ is applicable.	On the low back, 2 cun directly above the tip of the coccyx, in the depression between the sacral horns. *Tranquilizes convulsion and stops epilepsy, strengthens kidney.*	1. Epilepsy, headache, insomnia, constipation.
EX-B-10 Herpes Zoster Point ↓ or ↘ upward 0.5-0.8 cun. ⊘ is applicable.	On the midline of the back, at the point where the ends of a thread, which is as long as the patient's head circumference, reach when the line circles the neck with its ends at the midline of the back. *Clears heat, removes dampness, reduces swelling and alleviates pain.*	1. Herpes zoster.
EX-B-11 Yaoer ↘ 0.5-0.8 cun. ⊘ is applicable.	Below the spinous process of the 2nd lumbar vertebra, and 1 cun lateral to the midline of the back, on the diseased side. *Comforts sinews, activates collaterals, alleviates pain.*	1. Sciatica.
EX-B-12 Maigen ↓ 0.5-1.5 cun. ⊘ is applicable.	On lower back, 0.5 cun below the level of the second spinal process of the sacrum and 3 cun lateral to the spinal column. *Moves qi and activates blood.*	1. Thromboangitis obliterans.

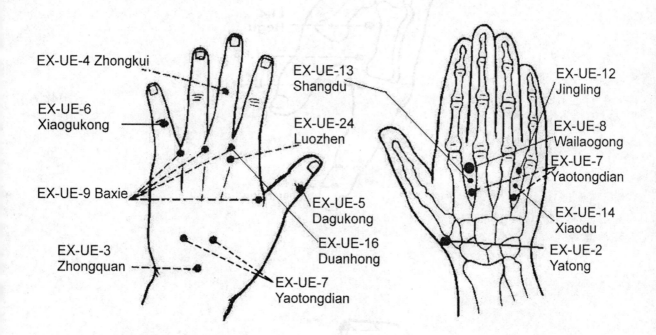

EX-UE-4 Zhongkui

EX-UE-6
Xiaogukong

EX-UE-9 Baxie

EX-UE-3
Zhongquan

EX-UE-13
Shangdu

EX-UE-24
Luozhen

EX-UE-5
Dagukong

EX-UE-16
Duanhong

EX-UE-7
Yaotongdian

EX-UE-12
Jingling

EX-UE-8
Wailaogong

EX-UE-7
Yaotongdian

EX-UE-14
Xiaodu

EX-UE-2
Yatong

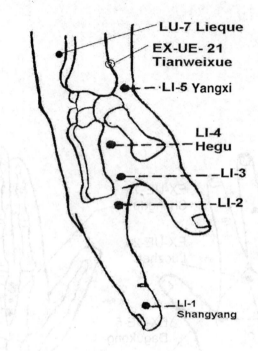

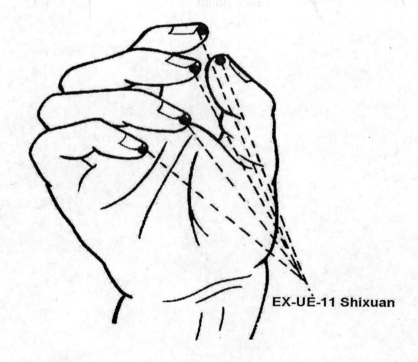

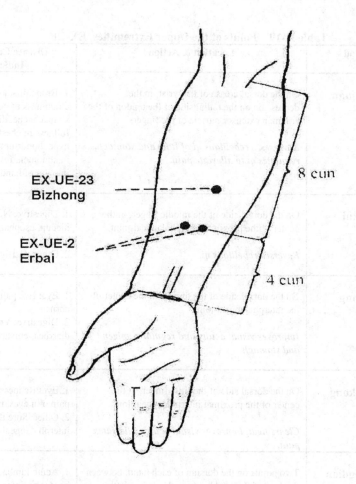

EX-UE-23
Bizhong

EX-UE-2
Erbai

8 cun

4 cun

Fig. II- 39 Extra Points of the Upper Extremities

4. Commonly-Used Extra Points of the Upper Extremities (EX-UE)

Table II-19   Points of the Upper Extremities, EX-UE

Point & Method	Location & Action	Disease Categories & Indications
EX-UE-1 Zhoujian ꝑ is applicable.	On the posterior side of the elbow, at the tip of the olecranon when the elbow is flexed. ***Transforms phlegm, reduces swelling, clears heat.***	1. Scrofula, furuncle, carbuncle, appendicitis, cholera morbus.
EX-UE-2 Erbai ⊥ 0.5-0.7 cun. ꝑ is applicable.	Two points on the palmar side of each forearm, 4 cun proximal to the crease of the wrist, on each side of the tendon of the radial flexor muscle of the wrist. ***Relieves hemorrhoids, raises prolapsed rectum, activates collaterals to alleviate pain.***	1. Hemorrhoids, prolapse of rectum, neuralgia in forearm, pain in chest and hypochondrium.

Table II-19   Points of the Upper Extremities, EX-UE

Point & Method	Location & Action	Disease Categories & Indications
EX-UE-3 Zhongquan ⊥ 0.2-0.3 cun. ∂ is applicable.	On the dorsal crease of the wrist, in the depression on the radial side of the tendon of the common extensor muscle of the fingers. *Reverses rebellious qi of lung and stomach, regulates qi to alleviate pain.*	1. Bronchitis, asthma, cloudiness of cornea, stomachache, distention and fullness in chest and hypochondrium, distending pain in abdomen, feverish sensation in palm of hand.
EX-UE-4 Zhongkui ⊥ 0.2-0.3 cun. ∂ is applicable.	On the dorsal side of the middle finger, at the center of the proximal interphalangeal joint. *Reverses rebellious qi.*	1. Digestive: Nausea, vomiting, hiccup, esophageal spasm, epistaxis. 2. Other: Vertigo.
EX-UE-5 Dagukong ∂ is applicable.	On the dorsal side of the thumb, at the center of the interphalangeal joint. *Improves visual acuity and regulates spleen and stomach.*	1. Eye: Eye pain, cloudiness of cornea. 2. Digestive: Vomiting, diarrhea, epistaxis.
EX-UE-6 Xiaogukong ∂ is applicable.	On the dorsal side of the little finger, at the center of the proximal interphalangeal joint. *Clears heat, improves visual acuity, alleviates pain.*	1. Eye: Redness, swelling and pain o in eyes, nebula. 2. Other: Sore throat, pain in interphalangeal joints.
EX-UE-7 Yaotongdian ↘ 0.3-0.5 toward the middle of metacarpus.	Two points on the dorsum of each hand, between the 1st and 2nd and between the 3rd and 4th metacarpal bones, and at the midpoint between the dorsal crease of the wrist and the metacarpophalangeal joint. *Moves qi, activates blood, removes blood stasis.*	1. Acute lumbar sprain, headache, infantile convulsion, redness, swelling and pain of dorsum of hand.
EX-UE-8 Wailaogong ⊥ 0.5-0.8 cun.	On the dorsum of the hand, between the 2nd and 3rd metacarpal bones, and 0.5 cun proximal to the metacarpophalangeal joint. *Reduces swelling, alleviates pain, strengthens spleen and dissolves accumulation.*	1. Stiff neck, migraine, motor impairment of fingers, infantile maldigestion, stomachache, sore throat, pain in shoulder & arm.
EX-UE-9 Baxie ↘ 0.5-0.8 cun or prick to bleed. ∂ is applicable.	Four points on the dorsum of each hand, at the junction of the red and white skin proximal to the margin of the webs between each two of the five fingers of a hand. *Clears heat and reduces swelling.*	1. Joints of fingers. 2. Pain syndromes: Pain in vertex of head, sore throat, toothache, pain in eye.

Table II-19   Points of the Upper Extremities, EX-UE

Point & Method	Location & Action	Disease Categories & Indications
EX-UE-10 Sifeng Prick to bleed and squeeze out some yellowish fluid.	Four points on each hand, on the palmar side of the 2nd to 5th fingers and at the center of the proximal interphalangeal joints. *Strengthens spleen and dissolves food accumulation.*	1. Respiratory: Cough, asthma. 2. Digestive: Infantile. maldigestion, infantile diarrhea.
EX-UE-11 Shixuan ↳ 0.1-0.2 cun or prick to bleed.	Ten points on both hands, at the tips of the ten fingers, 0.1 cun from the free margin of the nails. *Opens the orifice to induce resuscitation, clears heat and relieves convulsion.*	1. Shock, coma, high fever, sunstroke, epilepsy, infantile convulsion, sore throat, numbness of ends of fingers.
EX-UE-12 Jinling ⊥ 0.5-0.7 cun.	On the dorsum of the hand, at the proximal border of the interspace of the 4th and 5th metacarpal bones, in the depression at the midpoint between the transverse crease of the wrist and the small head of the metacarpal bone. *Tranquilizes spasm, reduces swelling, calms spirit.*	1. Biliary ascariasis.
EX-UE-13 Shangdu ⊥ 0.5-0.7 cun.	On the dorsum of the hand, between the second and third metacarpophalangeal joints. *Moves qi, activates blood, alleviates pain.*	1. Acute lumbar sprain.
EX-UE-14 Xiadu ⊥ 0.5-0.7 cun.	On the dorsum of the hand, between the 4th and 5th metacarpal bones, and proximal to the joint of the metacarpophalangeal joint. *Moves qi, activates blood, alleviates pain.*	1. Acute lumbar sprain, tinnitus, arrhythmic disorder, cutaneous pruritis.
EX-UE-15 Shanyao ⊥ 0.5-1.2 cun.	Three points in total on the arm. At the three points of an equilateral triangle, in which LI-11 Quchi is its upper point, the point 1 cun radial to the midpoint of the line connecting LI-11 Quchi and LI-10 Shousanli is one of the bottom points, and the point on the line connecting the olecranon, which is 1 cun from the others is the other bottom point. *Moves qi, activates blood, alleviates pain.*	1. Pain of lower back, lumbar sprain.

Table II-19   Points of the Upper Extremities, EX-UE

Point & Method	Location & Action	Disease Categories & Indications
EX-UE-16 Duanhong ⊥ 0.5-0.7 cun.	On the dorsum of the palm, between and distal to the second and third phalangeal-carpal joints, namely, one of the EX-UE-9 Baxie. *Strengthens spleen and liver and raises yang to stop bleeding.*	1. Dysfunctional uterine bleeding.
EX-UE-17 Urine-Controlling Point ⊥ 0.5-0.7 cun.	On the palmar surface of the hand, at the midpoint of the first transverse crease of the small finger. *Strengthens kidney to relieve enuresis.*	1. Enuresis.
EX-UE-18 Yatongling ⊥ 0.5-0.7 cun.	On the palmar aspect of the hand, between the 3rd and 4th metacarpophalangeal joints. *Dispels wind, clears fire, reduces swelling and pain of tooth.*	1. Toothache.
EX-UE-19 Zitu ⊥ 0.5-0.7 cun.	On the medial aspect of the hand, 0.5 cun distal to the midpoint of the transverse crease of the wrist. *Descends stomach qi to relieve vomiting.*	1. Vomiting.
EX-UE-20 Shouni ⊥ 0.7-1.5 cun. ℬ is applicable.	On the midline of the medial aspect of the arm, at the midpoint of the line connecting the transverse crease of the wrist and elbow. *Warms yang, moves qi and activates blood.*	1. Thromboangitis obliterans at the early or middle stage.
EX-UE-21 Tianweixue ⊥ 0.5-0.7 cun.	On the hand, at the midpoint of the line connecting LU-7 Lieque and LI-5 Yangxi. *Calms mind, detoxifies poison, relieves addiction to smoking.*	1. Addiction to smoking.
EX-UE-22 Yatong ⊥ 0.5-0.7 cun.	On the dorsal aspect of the hand, at the center of the 1st metacarpophalangeal joint. *Dispels wind, clears fire, reduces swelling and pain of tooth.*	1. Toothache.

5. **Commonly-Used Extra Points of the Lower Extremities (EX-LE)**

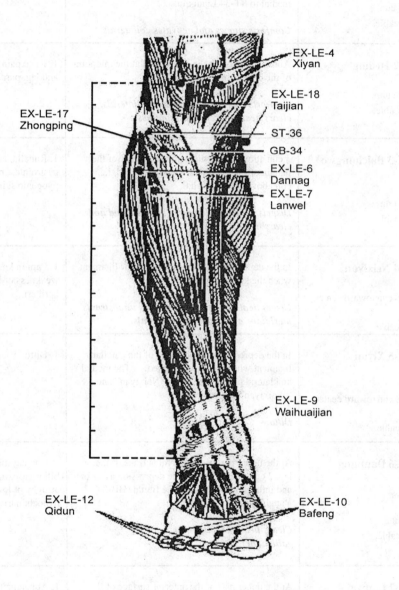

EX-LE-4
Xiyan

EX-LE-18
Taijian

EX-LE-17
Zhongping

ST-36

GB-34

EX-LE-6
Dannag

EX-LE-7
Lanwel

EX-LE-9
Waihuaijian

EX-LE-12
Qidun

EX-LE-10
Bafeng

Fig, II-40 Extra Points of the Lower Extremities

Table II-20   Points of the Lower Extremities, EX-LE

Point & Method	Location & Action	Disease Categories & Indications
EX-LE-1 Kuangu ⊥ 0.7-1.5 cun. ᵹ is applicable.	Two points on each thigh, in the lower part of the anterior surface of the thigh, 1.5 cun lateral and medial to ST-34 Liangqiu. ***Comforts sinews and activates collaterals.***	1. Pain in knee, thigh and leg, paralysis of lower limb.
EX-LE-2 Heding ⊥ 0.7-0.8 cun. ᵹ is applicable.	Above the knee, in the depression at the midpoint of the upper border of the patella. ***Comforts sinews and activates collaterals, clears heat and removes dampness.***	1. Knee pain, weakness of foot and leg, paralysis of lower limb.
EX-LE-3 Baichongwo ⊥ 0.7-1.5 cun. ᵹ is applicable.	3 cun above the medial superior corner of the patella of the thigh with the knee flexed, i.e. 1 cun above SP-10 Xuehai. ***Dispels wind and dampness, cools blood and clears heat.***	1. Rubella, eczema, gastrointestinal parasites, pyogenic skin infection of leg.
EX-LE-4 Neixiyan ↘ 0.7-0.8 cun toward center of knee. ᵹ is applicable.	In the depression medial to the patellar ligament when the knee is flexed. ***Clears heat and reduces swelling, unobstructs meridians and activates collaterals.***	1. Pain in knee joint, aching and weakness of lower limbs, beriberi.
EX-LE-5 Xiyan ↘ 0.7-0.8 cun toward center of knee. ᵹ is applicable.	In the depression on both sides of the patellar ligament when the knee is flexed The medial and lateral points are named "Neixiyan" and "Waixiyan" respectively. ***Ditto.***	1. Ditto.
EX-LE-6 Dannang ⊥ 1-1.5 cun. ᵹ is applicable.	At the upper part of the lateral surface of the leg, 2 cun directly below the depression anterior and inferior to the head of the fibula (GB-34 Yanglingquan). ***Clears heat and dampness, benefits gallbladder.***	1. Cholecystitis, cholelithiasis, biliary ascariasis, paralysis and atrophy of lower limbs, hypochondriac pain.
EX-LE-7 Lanwei ⊥ 0.7-1.5 cun. ᵹ is applicable.	At the upper part of the anterior surface of the leg, 5 cun below ST-35 Dubi, one finger breadth lateral to the anterior crest of the tibia. ***Descends qi of stomach and large intestine, clears heat and alleviates pain.***	1. Appendicitis, maldigestion, epigastric pain, numbness and muscular atrophy of lower limbs.

Table II-20   Points of the Lower Extremities, EX-LE

Point & Method	Location & Action	Disease Categories & Indications
EX-LE-8 Neihuaijian Prick to bleed. ᵰ is applicable.	On the medial side of the foot, at the tip of the medial malleolus. *Clears heat, reduces swelling, activates collaterals.*	1. Toothache, sore throat, spasm of medial side of leg.
EX-LE-9 Waihuaijian Prick to bleed. ᵰ is applicable.	On the lateral side of the foot, at the tip of the lateral malleolus. *Clears heat, reduces swelling, activates collaterals.*	1. Toothache, beriberi, spasm of toes, hemiplegia.
EX-LE-10 Bafeng ↘ 0.5-0.8 cun, or prick to bleed. ᵰ is applicable.	Eight points on both feet, at the junction of the red and white skin proximal to the margin of the webs between each two neighboring toes. *Relieves malaria and reduces swelling, regulates menstruation.*	1. Swelling and pain in back and feet, weakness of leg, beriberi, headache, toothache, toe pain, snake-bite, cyanosis of toes, irregular menstruation.
EX-LE-11 Duyin ↓ 0.1-0.2 cun. ᵰ is applicable.	On the plantar side of the 2nd toe, at the center of the distal interphalangeal joint. *Reverses rebellious qi and harmonizes stomach, regulates menstruation.*	1. Irregular menstruation, retention of placenta, epigastric pain, pain in chest and hypochondrium, hernia, vomiting, hematemesis.
EX-LE-12 Qiduan ↓ 0.1-0.2 cun. ᵰ is applicable.	Ten points at the tips of the 10 toes, 0.1 cun from the free margin of each toenail. *Clears heat, opens orifices to induce rseuscitation.*	1. Coma, numbness of toes, redness, swelling and pain of dorsum of foot.
EX-LE-13 Huanzhong ↓ 1.2-2 cun. ᵰ is applicable.	On the posterio-superior aspect of the buttock, at the midpoint of the line connecting the prominence of the great trochanter and the sacral hiatus. *Removes dampness and activates collaterals.*	1. Sciatica, prolapse of uterus.
EX-LE-14 Huanshang ↓ 1.2-2 cun. ᵰ is applicable.	At the point 0.5 cun superior and lateral to EX-LE-13 Huanzhong which is at the midpoint of the line connecting the prominence of the great trochanter and the hiatus of the sacrum. *Removes dampness and activates collaterals.*	1. Sciatica, prolapse of uterus.
EX-LE-15 Huanzhongshang ↓ 1.2-2 cun. ᵰ is applicable.	On the point 2 cun above and 0.5 cun lateral to the midpoint of the line connecting the end of the coccyx and the pertrochantery. *Removes dampness and activates collaterals.*	1. Sciatica.

Table II-20   Points of the Lower Extremities, EX-LE

Point & Method	Location & Action	Disease Categories & Indications
EX-LE-16 Tongmai ⊥ 0.7-1.5 cun. 𝛿 is applicable.	On the supero-bacterior aspect of the buttock, at the crossing point of the line starting from BL-30 Baihuanshu and going down perpendicularly and the line starting from EX-LE-13 Huanzhong and going horizontally. *Warms yang, moves qi and activates blood.*	1. Thromboangitis obliterans at the early stage or middle stage.
EX-LE-17 Zhongping ⊥ 0.7-1.5 cun. 𝛿 is applicable.	On the leg, 1 cun directly below ST-36 Zusanli. *Comforts sinews and activates collaterals.*	1. Scapulohumeral periarthritis.
EX-LE-18 Taijian ⊥ 0.7-1.5 cun. 𝛿 is applicable.	On the leg, 0.8 cun directly below SP-9 Yinglingquan. *Comforts sinews and activates collaterals.*	1. Acute neck sprain, scapulohumeral periarthritis.
EX-LE-19 Yiniao ⊥ 0.2-0.3 cun. 𝛿 is applicable.	On the bottom of the foot, at the midpoint of the interphalangeal transverse crease. *Strengthens kidney to arrest enuresis.*	1. Enuresis.
EX-LE-20 Fuxietexiaoxue ⊥ 0.2-0.3 cun. 𝛿 is applicable.	On the lateral aspect of the foot, directly below the tip of the external malleolus, at the junction of the red and white skin. *Strengthens spleen, removes dampness and arrests diarrhea.*	1. Enteritis.
EX-LE-21 Shimian ⊥ 0.5-0.7 cun. 𝛿 is applicable.	On the bottom of the foot, at the crossing point of the perpendicular line from the tip of the external malleolus and the midline of the foot bottom. *Calms mind.*	1. Insomnia.
EX-LE-22 Shangququan ⊥ 0.7-1.5 cun. 𝛿 is applicable.	On the posterior border of the thigh and 3 cun directly above LR-8 Ququan. *Warms yang, moves qi and activates blood.*	1. Thromboangitis obliterans.
EX-LE-23 Zigongjing ⊥ 0.7-1.5 cun. 𝛿 is applicable.	On the leg, 3 cun above the tip of the internal malleolus, one finger-breadth prior to the tendon calcaneus., slightly posterior to SP-6 Sanyinjiao. *Clears damp-heat.*	1. Cervical vaginal erosion.

VI. SPECIFIC POINTS & THEIR CLINICAL APPLICATION

Among the acupoints of the fourteen meridians, certain points have their specific functions and clinical indications in the treatment. Moreover, they respectively have their additional specific names. They are called specific points and very frequently selected in clinics. Traditionally, the specific points mainly include the Five Shu Points, Yuan-Source Points, Luo-Connecting Points, Xi-Cleft Points, Back-Shu Points, Front-Mu Points, Eight Influential Points, Eight Confluence Points, Lower He-Sea Points, Crossing Points, Four General Points, Four Gate Points, Ma Danyang Twelve Points and Thirteen Ghost Points, etc.

1. Five Shu Points

1). General introduction

The Five Shu Points refer to the five important points of each of the twelve meridians. They are situated distal to the elbow or knee of the limbs, and named Jing-Well, Ying-Spring, Shu-Stream, Jing-River and He-Sea Points. They are arranged from the distal end of the limbs to the elbow or knee, in the order of Jing, Ying, Shu, Jing and He, and the qi in them increases one by one. The ancient writers compared the flow of qi in the meridians to that of water in the nature and used the terms for description of the natural course of

the water flowing in a river from the small to the large, and from the shallow to the deep to designate the volume of qi in the meridians and particular acupoints of the different sites along the courses of the meridians. The Jing-Well Point is situated in the place where the meridian qi starts to bubble. The Ying-Spring Point is where the meridians qi starts to gush. The Shu-Stream Point is where the meridian qi flourishes. The Jing-River Point is where the meridian qi is pouring abundantly. Finally, the He-Sea Point signifies the confluence of rivers in the sea, where the meridian qi is the most flourishing.

As coordinated with the five elements, they are also named "the acupoints of the five elements". The five elements refer to metal, wood, water, fire and earth. The Chinese Ancients thought that these five kinds of material were the indispensable and most fundamental elements in constituting the Universe. There exist enhancing, inhibiting and restraining relationships among them. They are also in constant motion and change. In TCM, the theory of five elements is used to explain and expand a series of medical problems by comparing with and deducing from such properties and mutual relationships. Additionally, it can be used to explain and expand the properties of the Five Shu Points and twelve meridians, so the Five Shu Points and twelve meridians can be termed under the five elements (Seen in the Tab. II-21 and II-22).

Tab. II-21 Five Shu Points & Their Matching with the Five Elements in the Yin Meridians

Meridians	Jing-Well (Wood)	Ying-Spring (Fire)	Shu-Stream (Earth)	Jing-River (Metal)	He-Sea (Water)
LU	LU-11 Shaoshang	LU-10 Yuji	LU-9 Taiyuan	LU-8 Jingqu	LU-5 Chize
PC	PC-9 Zhongchong	PC-8 Laogong	PC-7 Daling	PC-5 Jianshi	PC-3 Quze
HT	HT-9 Shaochong	HT-8 Shaofu	HT-7 Shenmen	HT-4 Lingdao	HT-3 Shaohai
SP	SP-1 Yinbai	SP-2 Dadu	SP-3 Taibai	SP-5 Shangqiu	SP-9 Yinlingquan
LR	LR-1 Dadun	LR-2 Xingjian	LR-3 Taichong	LR-4 Zhongfeng	LR-8 Ququan
KI	KI-1 Yongquan	KI-2 Rangu	KI-3 Taixi	KI-7 Fuliu	KI-10 Yingu

Tab. II-22 Five Shu Points & Their Matching with the Five Elements in the Yang Meridians

Meridians	Jing-Well (Metal)	Ying-Spring (Water)	Shu-Stream (Wood)	Jing-River (Fire)	He-Sea (Earth)
LI	LI-1 Shangyang	LI-2 Erjian	LI-3 Sanjian	LI-5 Yangxi	LI-11 Quchi
SJ	SJ-1 Guanchong	SJ-2 Yemen	SJ-3 Zhongzhu	SJ-6 Zhigou	SJ-10 Tianjing
SI	SI-1 Shaoze	SI-2 Qiangu	SI-3 Houxi	SI-5 Yanggu	SI-8 Xiaohai
ST	ST-45 Lidui	ST-44 Neiting	ST-43 Xiangu	ST-41 Jiexi	ST-36 Zusanli
GB	GB-44 Zuqiaoyin	GB-43 Xiaxi	GB-41 Zulinqi	GB-38 Yangfu	GB-34 Yanglingquan
BL	BL-67 Zhiyin	BL-66 Zutonggu	BL-65 Shugu	BL-60 Kunlun	BL-40 Weizhong

2). Clinical application

a. General application

The Five Shu Points can be indicated in diseases of the five zang organs. The indications of Five Shu Points in general are as the follows:

- Jing-Well Points — liver diseases, including mental illness, high fever and loss of consciousness, because they have the actions of soothing the liver, extinguishing wind, relieving depression, inducing resuscitation and clearing heat;

- Ying-Spring Points—heart diseases, including febrile diseases, because they have the action of clearing the heart, calming spirit, purging heat and cooling blood;

- Shu-Stream Points — spleen diseases, including painful disorders and heavy sensation of the body, because they have the action of strengthening spleen and harmonizing stomach, transforming dampness, and promoting circulation of qi and blood;

- Jing-River Points—lung diseases, including asthma, cough, chills with fever, and problems of the related meridians, because they have the action of promoting dispersing function of the lung, relieving exterior syndrome, arresting cough and asthma and descending qi;

- He-Sea Points — kidney diseases, including adverse flow of qi, diarrhea, enuresis and spermatorrhea, because they have the actions of reinforcing the kidney.

b. Special application — Applying reinforcing-reducing method based on five elements theory

See "10. Combining Among the Specific Points" (Page 281) for details.

Tab. II-23   Main Specific Points in Addition to Five Shu Points

Meridians	Yuan-ource	Luo-Connecting	Xi-Cleft	Front-Mu	Back-Shu	Lower He-Sea
LU	LU-9 Taiyuan	LU-7 Lieque	LU-6 Kongzui	LU-1 Zhongfu	BL-13 Feishu	
LI	LI-4 Hegu	LI-6 Pianli	LI-7 Wenliu	ST-25 Tianshu	BL-25 Dachangshu	ST-37 Shangjuxu
HT	HT-7 Shenmen	HT-5 Tongli	HT-6 Yinxi	RN-14 Juque	BL-15 Xinshu	
SI	SI-4 Wangu	SI-7 Zhizheng	SI-6 Yanglao	RN-4 Guanyuan	BL-27 Xiaochangshu	ST-39 Xiajuxu
PC	PC-7 Daling	PC-6 Neiguan	PC-4 Ximen	RN-17 Danzhong	BL-14 Jueyinshu	
SJ	SJ-4 Yangchi	SJ-5 Waiguan	SJ-7 Huizong	RN-5 Shimen	BL-22 Sanjiaoshu	BL-39 Weiyang
SP	SP-3 Taibai	SP-4 Gongsun	SP-8 Diji	LR-13 Zhangmen	BL-20 Pishu	
ST	ST-42 Chongyang	ST-40 Fenglong	ST-43 Liangqiu	RN-12 Zhongwan	BL-21 Weishu	ST-36 Zusanli
KI	KI-3 Taixi	KI-4 Dazhong	KI-5 Shuiquan	GB-25 Jingmen	BL-23 Shenshu	
BL	BL-64 Jinggu	BL-58 Feiyang	BL-63 Jinmen	RN-3 Zhongji	BL-28 Pangguanshu	BL-40 Weizhong
LR	LR-3 Taichong	LR-5 Ligou	LR-6 Zhongdu	LR-14 Qimen	BL-18 Ganshu	
GB	GB-40 Qiuxu	GB-37 Guangming	GB-36 Waiqiu	GB-24 Riyue	BL-19 Danshu	GB-34 Yanglingquan
RN		RN-15 Jiuwei				
DU		DU-1 Changqiang				
Yangwei			GB-35 Yangjiao			
Yinwei			KI-9 Zhubin			
Yangqiao			BL-59 Fuyang			
Yinqiao			KI-8 Jiaoxin			

2. Back-Shu Points

1). General introduction
The Back-Shu Points are the sites where the qi of the zang and fu organs is infused at the back of the body.   Each of the zang-fu organs has a Back-Shu Point. They are named in accordance with their corresponding zang-fu organs, such as the Back-Shu Point of the heart is called BL-13 Xinshu (Xin means the heart and Shu means the Back-Shu); the Back-Shu Point of the kidney is called BL-23 Shenshu (Shen means the kidney and Shu means Back-Shu) and so on. There are 12 Back-Shu Points in total. (See Tab. II-23)

2). Clinical application
a. Diagnosis significance
When the zang-fu organs are diseased, there may appear a tenderness in the corresponding Back-Shu Point.

b. Treatment significance
The Back-Shu Points are frequently selected for treatment of diseases of the corresponding zang-fu organs and their related orifices. For example, BL-13 Feishu, the Back-Shu Point of the lung, may be chosen for cough and oppressed feeling in the chest which are diagnosed as the disorder of the lung, BL-23 Shenshu, the Back-Shu Point of the kidney, is frequently selected for treatment of deafness as the ear is the opening of the kidney. See Tab. VI-3 (page 282) in details.

3. Front-Mu Points

1). General introduction
The Front-Mu Points are the sites where the qi of the zang and fu organs is infused at the chest and abdomen of the body.   Each of the zang-fu organs has a Front-Mu Point. They are situated closely to their respectively related zang-fu organs. There are 12 Front-Mu Points in total. (See Tab. II-23)

2). Clinical application
a. Diagnosis significance
When a zang or fu organ is diseased, there may appear a tenderness in the corresponding Front-Mu Point.

b. Treatment significance

The Front-Mu Points are mainly applied to treat disorders of the corresponding zang-fu organs and in the local areas. For example, disorders of the large intestine such as borborygmus and diarrhoea may be relieved by needling ST-25 Tianshu, the Front-Mu Point of the large intestine, and liver disorders associated with hypochondriac pain may be relieved by needling LR-14 Qimen, the Front-Mu Point of the liver. See Tab. VI-3 in details.

4. Yuan-Source Points

1). General introduction
Yuan means "original". The Yuan-Source Points are located in the vicinity of the wrist and ankle. Each of the Twelve Regular Meridians has a Yuan-Source Point. The twelve Yuan-Source Points are closely related to the five zang and the six fu organs, and they are the points where the original qi of zang and fu organs infuses and retains. The original qi originates from the kidney, distributing over the whole body and concerning the qi activities. It travels over each yang meridian through Sanjiao. The place where the original qi is centered is the location of the Yuan-Source Point. Therefore, Yuan-Source Points are closely related to Sanjiao and primary qi. In the yin meridians, the Yuan-Source Point and Shu-Stream Point of the same meridian overlap each other, in an other word, the Yuan-Source Points are replaced by the Shu-Stream Points in the yin meridians. (See Tab.II-23)

2). Clinical application
Disorders of the zang-fu organs may usually be relieved by treating the twelve Yuan-Source Points.

5. Luo-Connecting Points

1). General introduction
Luo means connecting. The Luo-Connecting Points are the emerging areas of the fifteen collaterals from the fourteen meridians. Each of the twelve regular meridians has a Luo-Connecting Point on the limb to link its exteriorly-internally related meridian. Each of the Du and Ren Meridians, and the Major Collateral of the Spleen has its Luo-Connecting Point on the trunk. They are termed "the Fifteen Luo-Connecting Points", and belong to the fifteen collaterals and their pertaining meridians respectively. (See Tab. II-24)

2). Clinical application

a. The Luo-Connecting Points may be indicated in disorders of the fifteen collaterals and their pertaining meridians. For example, HT-5 Tongli, the Luo-Connecting Point of the Heart Meridian is selected for the treatment of fullness and distressed feeling in the chest due to excess of the Heart Meridian, or aphasia due to deficiency of the Heart Meridian.

b. The Luo-Connecting Points may be indicated in simultaneous disorders of the two exteriorly-internally related meridians. For example, LU-7 Lieque, the Luo-Connecting Point of the Lung Meridian, can be selected for the treatment of cough and asthma, which are disorders of the Lung Meridian, accompanied with toothache and headache which are disorders of the Large Intestine Meridian.

c. The Luo-Connecting Points may be indicated in course-prolonged disorders. According to TCM, a fresh disorder always attacks the meridians, but a prolonged disease may affect the collaterals and the pathogen may retain in the collaterals. This is why accumulation of stagnant blood, stagnant qi, retention of phlegm and retention of dampness for long term always transmit from the meridians to the collaterals, retaining in the collaterals. Therefore, stimulating the corresponding Luo-Connecting Points is frequently selected for long-term or obstinate diseases. For example, ST-40 Fenglong, the Luo-Connecting Point of the Stomach Meridian, is often selected for epilepsy and manic or depressive diseases, and SP-21 Dabao, the Luo-Connecting Point of the Major Collaterals of the Spleen, is usually pricked to treat blood stasis syndromes. See Tab. II-23 & 24 in detail.

Tab. II-24 Luo-Connecting Points

Collaterals	Luo-Connecting Points	Meridians Pertained to	Chief Indications
Hand Taiyin	LU-7 Lieque	LU	Heat sensation in the palms
Hand Shaoyin Collateral	HT-5 Tongli	HT	Hiccup
Hand Jueyin Collateral	PC-6 Neiguan	PC	Heart pain
Hand Taiyang Collateral	SI-7 Zhizheng	SI	Loose elbow
Hand Yangming Collateral	LI-6 Pianli	LI	Toothache & deafness
Hand Shaoyang Collateral	SJ-5 Waiguan	SJ	Elbow spasm
Foot Taiyang Collateral	BL-58 Feiyang	BL	Nasal obstruction
Foot Yangming Collateral	ST-40 Fenglong	ST	Manic-depressive psychosis
Foot Shaoyang Collateral	GB-37 Guangming	GB	Qi-syncope
Foot Taiyin Collateral	SP-4 Gongsun	SP	Intestine colic
Foot Shaoyin Collateral	KI-4 Dazhong	KI	Uroschesis
Foot Jueyin Collateral	LR-5 Ligou	LR	Orchitis, hernia
Du Collateral	DU-1 Changqiang	DU	Acute abdominal pain
Ren Collateral	RN-15 Jiuwei	RN	Spinal pain
Large Collateral of Spleen	SP-21 Dabao	SP	General aches

6. Xi-Cleft Points

1). General introduction

The Xi-Cleft Points are those located at the sites where qi and blood in the meridians are converged and accumulated. Each of the twelve regular meridians has a Xi-Cleft Point on the limbs and, in addition, each of Yangqiao, Yinqiao, Yangwei and Yinwei Meridians has a Xi-Cleft Point on the limbs as well, sixteen Xi-Cleft Points in total. They respectively pertain to the meridians where they are located at. (See Tab. II-23 and II-25)

Tab. II-25 Chief Indications of Sixteen Xi-Cleft Points

Meridians	Xi-Cleft Points	Chief Indications
Lung	LU-6 Kongzui	Hemoptysis, hemorrhoids, dyspnea, tuberculosis, tracheitis.
Large Intestine	LI-7 Wenliu	Toothache, cold, hemorrhoids.
Stomach	ST-34 Liangqiu	Gastric neuralgia, acute or chronic gastritis.
Spleen	SP-8 Diji	Acute diarrhea, edema.
Small Intestine	SI-6 Yanglao	Eye diseases, pain in the shoulder and arm.
Heart	HT-6 Yinxi	Cardiac pain, epilepsy, night sweating, insomnia.
Urinary Bladder	BL-63 Jinmen	Systremma, infantile convulsion.
Kidney	KI-5 Shuiquan	Dysmenorrhea, hysteroptosis.
Pericardium	PC-4 Ximen	Heart diseases, cardiac pain intercostal neuralgia.
Sanjiao	SJ-7 Huizong	Angina pectoris, appendicitis.
Gallbladder	GB-36 Waiqiu	Epilepsy, rabies.
Liver	LR-6 Zhongdu	Hernia, metrorrhagia.
Yangqiao	BL-59 Fuyang	Redness and swelling of the lateral malleolus, paralysis atrophy, waist pain.
Yinqiao	KI-8 Jiaoxin	Irregular menstruation, dribbling urination, metrorrhagia, constipation, dysentery, psychosis.
Yangwei	GB-35 Yangjiao	Facial edema, sore throat, fullness of the chest, swollen knees, weakness of foot.
Yinwei	KI-9 Zhubin	Hernia in children, psychosis, pain in the feet.

2). Clinical application

a. The Xi-Cleft Points of the Yang Meridians are mainly indicated in painful syndromes and acute syndromes of the meridians and zang-fu organs which they pertain to. For example, LI-7 Wenliu, the Xi-Cleft Point of the Large Intestine Meridian, may be selected for borborygmus and acute abdominal pain.

b. The Xi-Cleft Points of the Yin Meridians are mainly indicated in bleeding syndromes and acute syndromes of the meridians and zang-fu organs which they pertain to. For example, LU-6 Kongzui, the Xi-Cleft Point of the Lung Meridian, is frequently used for the treatment of hemoptysis. (See Tab. II-25 in details)

7. Lower He-Sea Points

1). General introduction
The Lower He-Sea Points refer to the six He-Sea Points pertaining to the six fu organs along the three yang meridians of foot. The Lower He-Sea Points of the stomach, gallbladder and bladder, whose meridians run along the foot and are named after the foot, are respectively overlapped with the He-Sea Points of the Stomach, Gallbladder and Bladder Meridians. But the large intestine, small intestine and Sanjiao have their Lower He-Sea Points different from the He-Sea Points of the meridians pertaining to them. Their Lower He-Sea Points are respectively ST-37 Shangjuxu, ST-39 Xiajuxu and BL-31 Weiyang, all of them locating at the lower limbs. (See Tab. II-26)

2). Clinical application
The Lower He-Sea Points are frequently used for the treatment of disorders of the six fu organs. For example, ST-36 Zusanli, the Lower He-Sea Point of the stomach, is indicated in epigastric pain due to dysfunction of the stomach, and ST-37 Shangjuxu, the Lower He-Sea Point of the large intestine, is used to treat appendicitis and dysentery due to dysfunction of the large intestine.

Tab. II-26 Lower He-Sea Points

Fu Organs	Meridians	Points
Stomach	ST	ST-36 Zusanli
Gallbladder	GB	GB-34 Yanglingquan
Urinary Bladder	BL	BL-40 Weizhong
Large Intestine	LI	ST-37 Shangjuxu
Sanjiao	SJ	BL-39 Weiyang
Small Intestine	SI	ST-39 Xiajuxu

8. Eight Influential Points

1). General introduction
The Eight Influential Points are eight important acupoints which are closely related to the zang organs, fu organs, qi, blood, tendon, vessels, bones and marrow respectively. (See Tab. II-27)

2). Clinical application
The Eight Influential Points are frequently selected for the treatment of diseases of zang organs, fu organs, qi, blood, tendons, vessels, bones and marrow. (See Tab. II-28)

Tab. II-27 Eight Influential Points

Confluent Parts	Points
Zang organs	LR-13 Zhangmen
Fu organs	RN-12 Zhongwan
Qi	RN-17 Danzhong
Blood	BL-17 Geshu
Tendons	GB-34 Yanglingquan
Vessels & Pulse	LU-9 Taiyuan
Bone	BL-11 Dazhu
Marrow	GB-39 Xuanzhong

Tab. II-28 Chief Indications of Eight Influential Points

Points	Confluent Parts	Disease Categories & Chief Indications
LR-13 Zhangmen	Zang organs	Chest, liver, spleen & kidney
RN-12 Zhongwan	Fu organs	Stomach & intestines
RN-17 Danzhong	Qi	Fullness feeling in chest, dyspnea, asthma
BL-17 Geshu	Blood	Blood stagnation, boils, heart problems
GB-34 Yanglingquan	Tendons	Joint pain, muscular spasm, paralysis
LU-9 Taiyuan	Vessels & Pulse	Cold limbs, heart failure, no pulse
BL-11 Dazhu	Bone	Back pain, emaciation with weakness
GB-39 Xuanzhong	Marrow	Bone pain, aversion to cold, tiredness

9. Eight Confluent Points

1). General introduction

The Eight Confluent Points are eight important points located on the limbs and connecting the eight extraordinary meridians with the twelve regular meridians. They are the points of the twelve meridians. Only two of them can directly connect with the eight extra meridians, namely, KI-6 Zhaohai connects Yinqiao Meridian and BL-62 Shenmai connects Yangqiao Meridian directly. The others connect the eight extra meridians only through meeting of their pertaining meridians with the certain extra meridians in the trunk. Due to meeting of the Chong and Spleen Meridians, and Yinwei and Pericardium Meridians in the stomach, heart and chest, SP-4 Gongsun of the Spleen Meridian connects with the Chong Meridian, and PC-6 Neiguan of the Pericardium Meridian connects with the Yinwei Meridian. Due to meeting of the Small Intestine Meridian and Du Meridian, and the Bladder Meridian and Yangqiao Meridian at the inner canthus and scapular region, SI-3 Houxi of the Small Intestine Meridian connects with the Du Meridian, and BL-62 Shenmai of the Bladder Meridian connects with Yangqiao Meridian. Due to meeting of the Gallbladder and Dai Meridians, and Sanjiao and Yangwei Meridians at the outer canthus and scapular region, GB-41 Zulinqi of the Gallbladder Meridian connects with the Dai Meridian, and SJ-5 Waiguan of the Sanjiao Meridian connects with the Yangwei Meridian. Due to the meeting of the Lung and Ren Meridians, and the Kidney and Yinqiao Meridians at the throat, lung, chest and diaphragm, LU-7 Lieque of the Lung Meridian connects with the Ren Meridian, and KI-6 Zhaohai of the Kidney Meridian connects with the Yinqiao Meridian. (See Tab. II-29)

2). Clinical application

The Eight Confluent Points are frequently selected in the treatment of disorders of the eight extra meridians and problems in the area distributed by the eight extra meridians. Usually, they are used in a pair as the following:

- SP-4 Gongsun connecting the Chong Meridian and PC-6 Neiguan Connecting the Yinwei Meridian are a pair;

- SI-3 Houxi connecting the Du Meridian and BL-62 Shenmai connecting the Yangqiao Meridian are a pair;

- GB-41 Zulinqi connecting the Dai Meridian and SJ-5 Waiguan connecting the Yangwei Meridian are a pair;

- LU-7 Lieque connecting the Ren Meridian and KI-6 Zhaohai connecting the Yinqiao Meridian are a pair.

Tab. II-29 The Eight Confluent Points

Eight Extra Meridians	Confluent Points	Twelve Regular Meridians
Chong	SP-4 Gongsun	SP
Yinwei	PC-6 Neiguan	PC
Dai	GB-41 Zulinqi	GB
Yangwei	SJ-5 Waiguan	SJ
Du	SI-3 Houxi	SI
Yangqiao	BL-62 Shenmai	BL
Ren	LU-7 Lieque	LU
Yinqiao	KI-6 Zhaohai	KI

Tab. II-30 Indications of Coordination of the Eight Confluent Points

Meridians	Points	Disease Categories
Chong- SP Yinwei- PC	SP-4 Gongsun PC-6 Neiguan	Heart, chest & stomach
Dai -GB Yangwei-SJ	GB-41 Zulinqi SJ-5 Waiguan	Neck, shoulder, back & inner canthus
DU-SI Yangqiao	SI-3 Houxi BL-62 Shenmai	Inner canthus, neck, nape, ear & shoulder
RN-LU Yinqiao-KI	LU-7 Lieque KI-6 Zhaohai	Throat, chest & lung

10. Crossing Points

1). General introduction

The Crossing Points refer to those located at the intersection of two or more meridians , including the twelve meridians and eight extra meridians. There are about one hundred or more crossing points and most of them are distributed on the trunk, the head and the face. (See Tab. II-31 & 32)

2). Clinical application

The Crossing Points are often used to treat the diseases appearing simultaneously in meridians intersecting each other. For example, DU-14 Dazhui located at the intersection of the three hand yang meridians and Du Meridian may be used to treat diseases of the three hand yang meridians. SP-6 Sanyinjiao, a crossing point in the three foot yin meridians is frequently used for diseases of the Liver, Spleen and Kidney Meridians.

Tab. II-31 The Crossing Points of the Yang Meridians

	DU	BL	SI	GB	SJ	ST	LI	Yang Wei	Yang Qiao	Dai	Remarks
DU-24 Shenting	0	X				X					
DU-26 Shuigou	0					X	X				
DU-20 Baihui	0	X									
DU-17 Naohu	0										
DU-16 Fengfu	0							X			
DU-15 Yamen	0							X			
DU-14 Dazhui	0	X		X		X					
DU-13 Taodao	0										
DU-1 Changqiang	0										Knotting at Shaoyin
BL-1 Jingming		0	X			X					

BL-11 Dazhu		0	X							
BL-12 Fengmen	X	0								
BL-41 Fufen		0	X							
BL-59 Fuyang		0					X	X		Xi-Cleft of Yangqiao
BL-62 Shenmai		0					X	X		Promoted by Yangqiao
BL-61 Pucan		0					X	X		Root of Yangqiao
BL-63 Jinmen		0					X	X		Collateral of Yangwei
SI-10 Naoshu			0				X	X		
SI-12 Bingfeng			0	X	X	X	X			
SI-18 Quanliao			0		X					
SI-19 Tinggong			0	X	X					
GB-1 Tongziliao			X	0	X					
GB-3 Shangguan				0	X	X				
GB-4 Hanyan				0						
GB-6 Xuanli		X		0						
GB-7 Qubin		X		0						
GB-8 Shuaigu		X		0						
GB-10 Fubai		X		0						
GB-11 Touqiaoyin		X		0						
GB-12 Wangu		X		0						
GB-13 Benshen				0			X			
GB-14 Yangbai				0			X			
GB-15 Toulinqi		X		0			X			
GB-16 Muchuang				0			X			
GB-17 Zhengying				0			X			
GB-18 Chengling				0	.		X			
GB-19 Naokong				0			X			
GB-20 Fengchi				0			X			

GB-21 Jianjing			*0*			*X*				
GB-24 Riyue			*0*							*Meeting with SP*
GB-30 Huantiao	*X*		*0*							
GB-26 Daimai			*0*					*X*		
GB-27 Wuchu			*0*					*X*		
GB-28 Weidao			*0*					*X*		
GB-29 Juliao			*0*							
GB-35 Yangjiao			*0*			*X*				*Xi-Cleft of Yangwei*
SJ-15 Tianliao				*0*						
SJ-17 Yifeng			*X*	*0*						
SJ-20 Jiaosun			*X*	*0*		*X*				
SJ-22 Erheliao		*X*	*X*	*0*						
ST-1 Chengqi					*0*		*X*			*Meeting with RN*
ST-3 Juliao					*0*		*X*			
ST-4 Dicang					*0*	*X*	*X*			
ST-7 Xiaguan				*X*	*0*					
ST-8 Touwei				*X*	*0*		*X*			
ST-39 Qichong					*0*					*Starting point of Chong Meridian*
LI-14 Binao						*0*				*Meeting with collateral of LI*
LI-15 Jianyu						*0*		*X*		
LI-16 Jugu						*0*		*X*		
LI-20 Yingxiang						*X*	*0*			

Tab. II-32 The Crossing Points of the Yin Meridians

	RN	SP	LU	LR	PC	KI	HT	Yin-wei	Yin-qiao	Cho-ng	Remarks
RN-24 Chengjiang	*0*										*Meeting with ST*
RN-23 Lianquan	*0*							*X*			
RN-22 Tiantu	*0*							*X*			

RN-13 Shangwan	0								Meeting with ST & LU
RN-12 Zhongwan	0								Promoted by SI, SJ & ST
RN-10 Xiawan	0	X						X	
RN-7 Yinjiao	0								
RN-4 Guanyuan	0	X		X		X			
RN-3 Zhongji	0	X		X		X			
RN-2 Qugu	0			X					
RN-1 Huiyin	0							X	Along with DU & Chong
SP-6 Sanyinjiao		0		X		X			
SP-12 Chongmen		0		X					
SP-13 Fushe		0		X			X		
SP-15 Daheng		0					X		
SP-16 Fuai		0					X		
LU-1 Zhongfu		X	0						
LR-13 Zhangmen				0					Meeting with GB
LR-14 Qimen		X		0			X		
PC-1 Tianchi					0				Meeting with GB
KI-11					0			X	
KI-12					0			X	
KI-13					0			X	
KI-14					0			X	
KI-15					0			X	
KI-16					0			X	

KI-17						*O*			*X*	
KI-18						*O*			*X*	
KI-19						*O*			*X*	
KI-20						*O.*			*X*	
KI-21						*O*			*X*	
KI-6						*O*		*X*		*Promoted by Yinqiao*
KI-8						*O*		*X*		*Xi-Cleft of Yinqiao*
KI-9						*O*	*X*			*Xi-Cleft of Yinwei*

11. Four General Points

1). General introduction

The Four General Points refer to the most frequently used four acupoints. They are ST-36 Zusanli, BL-40 Weizhong, LU-7 Lieque and LI-4 Hegu. They are listed into the Danyang Ma's Twelve Points by Dr. Danyang Ma as well. (See Tab. II-34)

2). Clinical application

In Great Compendium of Acupuncture and Moxibustion, there is a Song of Four General Points, which sums up the general indications of the Four General Points. It is, "In treating disorders of the abdomen, ST-36 Zusanli should be punctured with the needle retained. In treating disorders of the waist and back, BL-40 Weizhong should be selected. In treating disorders in the head and neck, LU-7 Lieque should be used. In treating disorders of the face and mouth, LI-4 Hegu can achieve the effect." Their indications in detail can be seen in Tab. II-33.

12. Four Gate Points

1). General introduction

In Great Compendium of Acupuncture and Moxibustion, the Four Gate Points are initially recorded. But it should be pointed out that the Four Gate Points actually refer to two points only, i.e., LI-11 Hegu and LR-3 Taichong. As these two points are located at the both sides of the body, and usually, the points of the both sides should be selected simultaneously, four treatment points in total, they are named as "four".

2). Clinical application

If LI-11 Hegu and LR-3 Taichong of both sides are used simultaneously, namely, the Four Gate Points are employed, it will have the actions of soothing the liver and calming the spirit. Also it has the actions of treating cold limbs with trembling and treating aphasia.

13. Thirteen Ghost Points

1). General introduction

In Great Compendium of Acupuncture and Moxibustion, Dr. Simiao Sun's Thirteen Ghost Points are recorded. Dr. Sun is a very famous doctor in Tang Dynasty (618-907AD). These thirteen points are named as "ghost" because they can be used to treat severe mental diseases (including psychosis illness), which were considered as the result of interfere of the human being by ghost in ancient China. Each of the points takes a part, a place or an action of the ghost as its special and additional name, although it has its own ordinary name and most of them are points of the Fourteen Meridians. (See Tab. II-33)

2). Clinical application

The Thirteen Ghost Points are indicated in severe mental diseases, including psychosis, severe hysteria and   severe emotional depression.

The Thirteen Ghost Points are usually punctured shallowly, 0.1-0.2 cun deep, when they are used to severe mental diseases.

Tab. II-33 The Thirteen Ghost Points

Names with Ghost	Points
Ghost Palace	DU-26 Shuigou
Ghost Sign	LU-11 Shaoshang
Ghost Building	SP-1 Yinbai
Ghost Heart	PC-7 Daling
Ghost Road	BL-62 Shenmai
Ghost Pillow	DU-16 Fengfu
Ghost Bed	ST-6 Jiache
Ghost Market	RN-24 Chengjiang
Ghost Den	PC-8 Laogong
Ghost Hall	DU-23 Shangxing
Ghost Viscera	RN-1 Huiyin in male, EX-CA-7 Yumen in female
Ghost Leg	LI-11 Quchi
Ghost Sealing	EX-HN-29 Haiquan

14. Danyang Ma's Twelve Points

1). General introduction
Danyang Ma was a famous Chinese acupuncturist in the Jin Dynasty (265-420 AD). The Danyang Ma's Twelve Points refer to the most frequently used twelve points recommended by him (See Tab. II-34). The Twelve Points include the Four General Points. The clinical applications of these twelve acupoints were summarised by him as well.

2). Clinical application
The indications of the Danyang Ma's Twelve Points (including the Four General Points) are seen in Tab. II-34.

Tab. II-34 Indications of Danyang Ma's Twelve Points (Including the Four General Points)

Points	Chief Indications
ST-36* Zusanli	Stomach pain, abdominal distention, indigestion, vomiting, diarrhea, constipation, dysentery, asthma, breast pain, dizziness, apoplexy, paralysis, edema, pain in the lower limbs, malnutrition.
ST-44 Neiting	Toothache, facial paralysis, sore throat, nasal bleeding, abdominal pain, diarrhea, dysentery, swelling and pain of foot, fever, vomiting.
LI-11 Quchi	Sore throat, swelling and pain in the arm, hand paralysis, irregular menstruation, abdominal pain with vomiting and diarrhea, dysentery, fever, erysipelas.
LI-4* Hegu	Headache, red and painful eyes, nasal bleeding, nasal sinusitis, toothache, deafness, facial edema, boil, sore throat, cough, toe spasm, arm pain, closed teeth, facial paralysis, profuse sweating, amenorrhea, dystocia with pain, constipation, dysentery, high fever in children, urticaria, mumps.
BL-40 * **Weizhong**	Lower back pain, stuffy hip joint, popliteal spasm, paralysis of lower limbs, abdominal pain, diarrhea and vomiting, erysipelas.
BL-57 Chengshan	Lower back pain, leg pain with spasm, constipation, beriberi, systremma, hemorrhoids.
BL-60 Kunlun	Headache, stiffness of the neck, dizziness, nasal bleeding, contraction of shoulder and arm, lower back pain, dystocia, neck pain, heel pain, epilepsy, difficult labor.
LR-3 Taichong	Metrorrhagia, hernia, difficult urination, enuresis, hypochondriac pain, facial paralysis, high fever in children, epilepsy, headache, redness and swelling of eyes, dizziness, hepatitis.
GB-30 Huantiao	Lower back pain, muscular atrophy of the lower limbs, hemiplegia, urticaria, urticaria, arthritis, sciatica.
GB-34 Yanglingquan	Hemiplegia, muscular atrophy and numbness of the lower limbs, swollen knees, beriberi, hypochondria pain, bitter taste in the mouth, vomiting, jaundice, infantile convulsion.
HT-5 Tongli	Palpitation, dizziness, sore throat, sudden lose of voice, stiff tongue without speech, forearm pain, insomnia.
LU-7* Lieque	Headache, cough, sore throat, asthma, hemiplegia, facial paralysis, lockjaw, toothache, loose wrist, arthritis with numbness.

"*" means the point is one of the Four General Points as well.

CHAPTER THREE
ZHENJIU MANIPULATIONS

1. Filiform Needle Manipulations

The filiform needle manipulation refers to a Zhenjiu manner of handling a filiform needle after insertion. The purpose of needle manipulation is to induce a needling sensation (arrival of qi), and to induce a reinforcing, reducing, or an even reinforcing-reducing effect. Based on summarization of needling manipulations recorded in traditional Chinese medical literature, such as *Elementary Courses for Medicine, The Rhymes for Golden Needle, Compendium of Acupuncture and Moxibustion, The Questions and Answers on Classics of Miraculous Cures*, and on references to the manipulations of famous acupuncture and moxibustion doctors in modern times, the needle manipulations can be classified into four types: The basic manipulation, the reinforcing-reducing manipulation, the auxiliary manipulation and the other manipulations.

I. BASIC MANIPULATIONS

1. Lifting and Thrusting

1). Manipulation:
Lifting and thrusting manipulation refers to the lifting up and thrusting down of the needle in the acupoint after inserting it to a certain depth. The "thrusting" refers to making the needle move from the superficial to the deep and the "lifting" refers to making the needle move from the deep to the superficial. Repeated thrusting and lifting movements are taken as the lifting-thrusting manipulation. The amplitude, frequency and duration of this movement depend on the patient's physical constitution, pathological condition, location of the acupoint, and the therapeutic purpose.

2). Actions & Indications:
This manipulation is a main method to induce arrival of qi, and cause a reinforcing or reducing result. Generally, lifting and thrusting the needle with great amplitude, slow frequency and strong force, also termed the "pounding method", functions to induce arrival of qi and to causes a

reducing result. It is suitable to patients with excess syndrome, a strong physical constitution, poor needling sensitivity, or in situations of short disease course. That with less amplitude, quicker frequency and milder force, also termed "vibrating method", functions to promote arrival of qi and to induce a reinforcing result. It is suitable to patients with a deficiency syndrome, a weak physical constitution, or high needling sensitivity.

2. Twirling and Rotating

1). Manipulation:
Twirling and rotating manipulation refers to the manner in which the needle is alternately rotated clockwise and counter-clockwise after the needle is inserted to a certain depth. The duration and frequency of twirling movement should depend on the patient's physical constitution, their pathological condition and the desired therapeutic purpose.

2). Actions & Indications:
This manipulation is a main method to induce arrival of qi, and cause a reinforcing or reducing result. Generally, twirling or rotating the needle with great amplitude, quick frequency and strong force functions to induce arrival of qi and to cause a reducing result. It is suitable to patients with an excess syndrome, a strong physical constitution, and poor needling sensitivity or in situations of short disease course. That with less amplitude, slower frequency and milder force functions to promote arrival of qi and to induce a reinforcing results. It is suitable to patients with a deficiency syndrome, a weak physical constitution, or high needling sensitivity.

II. AUXILIARY MANIPULATIONS

1. Massaging Along the Meridian

1). Manipulation:
Massaging along the meridian refers to the method by which, after insertion of the needle into the acupoint to a certain depth, the skin along the course of the meridian upon which the acupoint locates is gently pressed, with the

finger bellies moving upwards and downwards, or side to side.

2). Actions & Indications:
This method may be conducive to induce the circulation of the channel-qi, to diagnose the meridian condition (deficient or excessive), and to promote circulation of qi and blood. It exerts a dominantly reinforcing effect (i.e. an effect of reinforcing and nourishing a deficiency of qi, blood, yin or yang).

2. Pinching Along the Meridian

1). Manipulation:
Pinching along the meridian refers to the manner in which, after insertion of a needle into an acupoint to a certain depth, the body tissue is pinched and pressed with the nails of the thumb, index and middle fingers, upwards and downwards along the meridian of the acupoint.

2). Actions & Indications:
This method may promote the circulation of qi and blood and expel the pathogenic factor. This is because it is a comparatively heavy manipulation, which induces a predominately reducing effect (i.e. an effect of purging and dispelling pathogenic factors).

3. Flicking Method

1). Manipulation:
Flicking method refers to the manner by which, after inserting a needle into an acupoint to a certain depth, the needle tail is gently flicked with the thumb or index finger, causing a mild vibration of the needle.

2). Actions & Indications:
It acts to quicken the circulation of channel-qi, or aid in arrival of qi.

4. Scraping Method

1). Manipulation:
Scraping method refers to the manner in which, after inserting a needle into an acupoint to certain depth, and by resisting the needle tail with the thumb belly, the needle handle is

scraped from the lower to upper portion with the nail of the index and middle fingers. It can also be achieved by resisting the needle tail with the belly of the index finger and scraping the needle handle from the lower to upper portion with the nail of the thumb frequently and gently.

2). Actions & Indications:
This method acts to induce the arrival of qi or strengthen the needling sensation.

5. Flying Method

1). Manipulation:
Flying method refers to the manner in which, after inserting a needle into an acupoint to a certain depth, the needle handle is held with the index, middle finger and thumb (which is opposite to the first two fingers), and the needle is rotated at a great speed. It is twirled clockwise by an introflexion of the index and middle fingers, then released by moving it counter-clockwise via the abduction of the index and middle fingers. The alternate movements of twirling and releasing the fingers make them appear like the spreading wings of a flying bird, thus giving this method the name "flying".

2). Actions & Indications:
This method functions to promote circulation of qi and to induce arrival of qi, thereby increasing and transmitting the needling sensation.

6. Shaking Method

1). Manipulation:
Shaking method refers to a manner in which, after insertion of the needle into an acupoint to a certain depth, the needle tail is held with the hand and is shaken to the left and right.

2). Actions & Indications:
It acts to increase the needling sensation and induce the needling sensation radiating to a certain part of the body. If the needle shaft is perpendicular to the skin, the needling sensation may be enhanced. If the needle is at a horizontal or oblique angle, the needling sensation may spread in a certain direction.

7. Circling Method

1). Manipulation:
Circling method refers to a manner in which, after insertion of the needle into an acupoint to a certain depth, the needle tail is held with the hand and moved in a circle; or, after the arrival of qi, the needle is lifted to the superficial portion of the acupoint, the needle shaft is inclined, then moved in a circle or a half circle at an angle of 15-40 degrees to the skin.

2). Actions & Indications:
This method acts to induce a reinforcing or reducing result. It may be used in cooperation with other reinforcing and reducing methods. As a rule, circling the needle clockwise with thrusting is taken as reinforcing, while counter-clockwise circling with lifting is considered reducing. This method is suitable for acupuncture on the abdomen.

8. Pressing Method

1). Manipulation:
Pressing method refers to a manner in which, after arrival of qi at an acupoint, the needle is held with the hand tightly without inserting or withdrawing. The needle shaft is then steadied and pressed with the middle finger, making the shaft bend like a bow.

2). Actions & Indications:
The function of this method is to induce arrival of qi as well as maintain and increase the needling sensation.

Another form of this method may be seen in clinic, that is, to hold and press the needle handle tightly with the fingers. The thumb is positioned below, and the index, middle and ring fingers feel and press the needle handle as if feeling the cunkou pulse (the location at both wrists that is medial to the head of the radius, where pulse diagnosis is performed in TCM). If the needling sensation is required to spread upwards, press the needle shaft downwards. Otherwise, press the needle shaft upwards to make the needling sensation move downwards.

9. Earth to Heaven Lifting Method

1). Manipulation:
Withdrawing method refers to a manner in which the needle is quickly removed from the "earth" position (the deepest portion of a point) to the "heaven" position (the shallowest portion of a point), moving the thumb backward and the index finger forwards along the shaft to rotate the needle, reinserting the needle to the "earth" portion, and moving the thumb forwards and the index finger backward. When withdrawing, a mild force should be used, but a heavier force should be used during insertion.

2). Actions & Indications:
This method is used when qi does not arrive, or arrives, but fails to circulate further after a comparatively long time has passed.

10. Tapping Method

1). Manipulation:
Tapping method refers to a manner in which, after the arrival of qi is induced by needle manipulation, the needle tail is tapped vertically and frequently, making the needle move gradually deeper until it reaches a certain depth, then, lifting the needle upwards about 1 cun and tapping the tail again. This movement is repeated several times.

2). Actions & Indications:
The manipulation can serve to prevent qi around the needle from being interrupted or it can promote qi flow.

11. Pushing Method

1). Manipulation:
Pushing method refers to a manner in which, when a needling sensation does not spread far enough, the needle is gently lifted from where the needling sensation is induced with the thumb and index finger. The needle tip is then directed towards the area, in which the operator wants the needling sensation to spread, by evenly and forcefully twisting and pushing the needle handle forwards with the thumb and index finger until the distal transverse crease of the thumb touches the needle. Then, the needle is gently lifted to the original place. This movement is repeated several times or even several dozen times, until the needling sensation reaches the designated area. Note: during the operation, the needle handle should be twisted and pushed slowly, evenly and forcefully.

2). Actions & Indications:
The manipulation can serve to make the needling sensation radiate, or to guide the needling sensation transmitting to a designed part.

III. REINFORCING & REDUCING MANIPULATIONS

After occurrence of needling sensation, some reinforcing or reducing manipulations should be carried out according to the patient's physical constitution and pathological condition. For example, it should be determined whether the condition belongs to exterior or interior, yin or yang, cold or heat, deficiency or excess. This can be determined by proper syndrome differentiation. Deficiency syndromes (referring to a morbid condition showing deficiency of primary qi, lowered body resistance and decline of function, such as yin or yang deficiency) should be treated with reinforcing, and excess syndromes should be treated with reducing manipulations. What we seek to reinforce by needling manipulation is the constructive qi (Zheng qi) of the body. This refers to inborn resistance, the defensive mechanisms and the adaptive capability of the body. Reduction manipulations by needling are meant to decrease the evil qi, which includes such pathogenic factors as the six excessive atmospheric interference, stagnancy of undigested food in the digestive tract, blood stagnation, retention of phlegm, etc. Therefore, reinforcing manipulation is meant to reinforce bodily resistance and reducing manipulation to dispel the pathogenic factors. Therefore, the meaning of reinforcement and reduction are the same as in the other branches of TCM.

1. The Basic Reinforcing and Reducing Methods

1). Reinforcing and reducing by twirling and rotating the needle:

After arrival of the needling sensation, if the needle is twisted clockwise, the manipulation is taken as reinforcing. If the needle is twisted counter-clockwise it is considered reducing. In fact, reinforcing or reducing by twirling and rotating manipulations, and puncturing along or against the running direction of the meridian can be used in combination.

It is said that the reducing or reinforcing effect of this method depends on whether the needle tip twists along or against the channel course. Reinforcing method is distinguished by right (clockwise) rotation of the needle along the acupoint of the three Yang Meridians of hand, three Yin Meridians of foot and the Ren Meridian, and conversely, left (counter-clockwise) rotation of the needle at the three Yin Meridians of hand, three Yang Meridians of foot and the Du Meridian. Reducing method is distinguished by the reverse of the above.

In recent years, some doctors have suggested that twirling the needle to a small extent, at a lower frequency and with milder force, for a short period of time, should be taken as reinforcing. Conversely, twirling with greater extent and force and at a higher frequency, for a comparatively long period of time, should be considered as reducing. This method has become widely accepted and is the most commonly used.

2). Reinforcing and reducing by lifting and thrusting the needle:

After arrival of qi, the reinforcing effect is obtained by thrusting heavily and lifting the needle gently. This is repeated with small amplitude, and at a lower frequency. On the contrary, a reducing effect is obtained by thrusting the needle gently and lifting it heavily, at great amplitude and with a quicker frequency.

3). Reinforcing and reducing achieved by rapid and slow insertion and withdrawal of the needle:

Reinforcing is achieved by inserting the needle slowly and with less rotation, then withdrawing the needle swiftly. A reducing effect is achieved by inserting the needle rapidly and with frequent rotation, then withdrawing it slowly.

4). Reinforcing and reducing achieved by puncturing along and against the direction of the meridian:

Inserting a needle with its tip pointing to the running direction of the course of the meridian is reinforcing. Puncturing with the needle tip against the running direction of the meridian is reducing. For example, when needling the three Yang Meridians which run from the hand upwards to the head, puncturing with the needle tip pointing downwards (against the course) is known as the reducing method, while insertion with the needle tip facing upwards (along the course) is a reinforcing method.

5). Reinforcing and reducing achieved by manipulating the needle in cooperation with the patient's respiration:

Reinforcing effect is achieved by inserting the needle during the patient's exhalation and withdrawing it during the patient's inhalation. Reducing is achieved by inserting the needle during the inhalation and withdrawing it during the exhalation.

6). Reinforcing and reducing achieved by keeping the needle hole open or closed:

For reinforcing, the puncture hole is pressed immediately upon the withdrawal of the needle. For a reducing effect, shake the needle as it is being withdrawn to increase the size of the puncture hole.

2. Uniform Reinforcing and Reducing Method

Uniform reinforcing and reducing manipulation is a method achieved by twirling, lifting and thrusting the needle evenly after arrival of qi. Or following the needle insertion, reinforcing succeeds reducing. Needle manipulation is performed evenly with a proper amplitude and favorable angle during lifting, thrusting and twirling. Following the needle sensation the needle may be retained or withdrawn immediately.

In recent years, it has been pointed out that by twirling and rotating the needle between the angles of 180-360°, at a rate of about 100 turns per minute creates a uniform reducing and reinforcing effect. Generally, the lifting and thrusting method and the twirling and rotating method are combined to achieve a uniform reinforcing and reducing effect.

3. The Commonly-Used Comprehensive Reinforcing and Reducing Methods

The comprehensive reinforcing and reducing manipulation refers to the use of two or more reinforcing and reducing manipulations in coordination. The most commonly used ones are as follows:

1). Burning the mountain, cooling the sky (Heat-producing puncture and cool-producing puncture)

a. Burning the mountain:
Manipulation:
First, determine the desired puncture depth, and then divide it into shallow, middle and deep portions. After inserting a needle into the skin, thrust it forcefully and lift it gently several times at the shallow portion. Then, insert the needle deeper into the middle portion, thrust it forcefully and lift it gently at this layer several times. Finally, insert the needle to the deep portion, thrust it forcefully and lift it gently at this layer several times. Repeat this course until the patient complains of hot sensations at the punctured area. Then, leave the needle at the deep portion until it is withdrawn. During the operation, reinforcement can be achieved by twirling and rotating the needle or by manipulating the needle in coordination with the patient's respiration. In this operation, the puncture hole should be pressed as soon as the needle is withdrawn.

Actions & Indications:
Heat-producing needling is a warm reinforcing method used to make yang qi enter into the body, and to induce a warmer sensation at the local area or throughout the whole body of the patient. This method is suitable in treatment of cold disorders of deficiency type, such as intractable numbness, coldness and pain of limbs. It is usually applied to the acupoints located at areas with thick muscle.

b. Cooling the sky
Manipulation:
As with the heat-producing method, determine the deep, middle and upper portion of the needling site prior to insertion. First, insert the needle into the deep portion, gently thrust and forcefully lift several times. Next, lift the needle to the middle portion, and again, thrust gently and lift forcefully several times. Finally, withdraw the needle to the shallow portion, and again gently thrust and forcefully lift several times. Repeat this course of action several times, finishing with the needle in the shallow portion, leaving it there until removal of the needle. During the operation, reduction can be obtained by twirling the needle or manipulating the needle in coordination with the patient's respiration. The puncture hole should not be pressed after withdrawing the needle.

Actions & Indications:
Cool-producing needling is a reducing and cooling method, which makes yin qi go outwards, thus inducing cool sensations in the patient. It is applied to heat syndromes.

2). Fire (yang)-producing needling and water (yin)-producing needling

a. Fire (yang)-producing:
Manipulation:
In this needling manipulation the reinforcing method of rapid-slow insertion and withdrawal, the reinforcing method of needling in coordination with respiration and the reinforcing method by lifting and thrusting the needle are combined. To undertake the operation, ask the patient to breathe out with the mouth and, during his/her exhalation, quickly insert the needle 0.1 cun deep, aided by the pressure of the fingers of the pressing hand. When the needling sensation has been induced, rapidly thrust and then slowly lift the needle continuously three times, with the needle tip towards the area in which the needling sensation is felt by the patient. Insert the needle

0.1 cun at a time, until the needle tip reaches the designated depth. Repeat the previous course three times after every 0.1 cun insertion to make the hot sensation spread. If no hot sensation is induced, ask the patient to breathe in through the nose and out through the mouth naturally three times, or, scrape the needle handle to make the needle tip tremble and promote the arrival of qi. When the hot sensation has been induced in the patient, slowly pull out the needle and immediately press the puncture hole.

Actions & Indications:
Reinforcing method by fire (yang)-producing needling is a comprehensive warm-reinforcing manipulation formed by simplifying and developing the heat-producing needling. It was first described in the Compendium of Acupuncture and Moxibustion. It is applicable to cold syndromes and yin syndromes, and is frequently used in treatment of wind-cold-dampness, wind-dampness or cold-dampness type of Bi syndrome.

b. Water (yin)-producing:
Manipulation:
In this method, the reducing methods by rapid and slow insertion and withdrawal, by manipulation in conjunction with respiration, and by lifting and thrusting the needle, are combined. Ask the patient to breathe in through the mouth and, during inhalation, insert the needle into the acupoint to the earth (deep) portion with the fingers stretching the skin and without twirling or rotating the needle. After the arrival of the needling sensation, withdraw the needle 0.1 cun. Then, in three 0.1 cun steps, slowly thrust and rapidly lift the needle 3 times per step. The patient should experience a cool sensation. If there is no cool sensation, ask the patient to breathe out through the nose and in through the mouth naturally for three times, or, shake the needle handle to promote the needling sensation. When numbness, coldness or electrifying sensation are induced in the patient, pull out the needle quickly and give no pressure over the puncture hole.

Actions & Indications:
Reducing method by water (yin)-producing

needling is a comprehensive method formed from simplifying and developing the cool-producing needling. It was also first recorded in the Compendium of Acupuncture and Moxibustion. It is applicable to heat syndromes and yang syndromes, and is frequently used in treatment of heat Bi syndrome turning from wind-cold-dampness Bi syndrome.

3). Yin occluding in yang and yang occluding in yin

a. Yin occluding in yang:
Manipulation:
Yin occluding in yang refers to a needling method beginning with reinforcing manipulation followed by reducing manipulation. Begin by determining the appropriate depth of the acupoint and then divide it into the shallow and deep portions. Insert the needle into the shallow portion. At this layer, forcefully thrust and gently lift the needle nine times. Then, insert the needle to the deep portion, forcefully lift and gently thrust it for six times. Repeat this course several times before withdrawal of the needle.

Actions & Indications:
This method is applicable to syndromes of cold followed by heat, or deficiency complicated with excess.

b. Yang occluding in yin:
Manipulation:
It refers to a method beginning with a reducing manner and following with a reinforcing manipulation. First insert the needle to the deep portion of the point, gently thrust and forcefully lift the needle six times. Then, withdraw the needle to the shallow portion, forcefully thrust and gently lift the needle nine times. Repeat this course several times before withdrawal of the needle.

Actions & Indications:
This method is applicable to syndromes of heat followed by cold, or excess complicated by deficiency.

IV. RETAINING AND WITHDRAWING THE NEEDLE

1.   Retaining the Needle

After the needle is inserted into the selected acupoint and the required manipulation is performed, the needle may be kept in place. This is in order to strengthen the needling sensation, to allow for continued manipulation of the needle, or to wait for the needling sensation which should be, but has not yet been induced by the manipulations. Generally, the period of needle retention is 20-40 minutes at one session of treatment, but in treating specific disorders such as acute abdominal pain, stubborn numbness or spasm, it may be retained for 1-2 hours or more.

2. Withdrawing the Needle

This is the last step in acupuncture manipulation. In withdrawing a needle, press the skin around the needle with the thumb and index finger of the left hand, hold the needle with the other hand and twirl it gently, then lift it to the area beneath the skin and finally take it out. According to the patient's condition and the therapeutic purpose, massage and press the punctured hole or enlarge it by shaking the needle during withdrawal. However, the puncture hole which is located in an area with many blood vessels is required to be pressed with a dry, sterilized swab for a moment so as to prevent bleeding (except the cases which need the treatment to cause bleeding by acupuncture.)

2. Acupuncture with the Three-Edged Needle

The three-edged needle was called the sharp needle in ancient times. Acupuncture with this device is a method of treatment where the acupoint or superficial blood vessel is pricked to obtain minor bloodletting. This method functions to promote the blood circulation for reducing swelling, causing resuscitation, reducing heat, cleaning and activating the meridian and collateral (i.e. dredging the meridians and collaterals and ensuring the flow of qi and blood through them).

I. ACTIONS

1. Clears Heat

Acupuncture with the three-edged needle has a good action to eliminate excessive heat.

2. Promotes Flow of Qi and Blood and Removes Blood Stasis

Acupuncture with the three-edged needle has a good action to promote the smooth flow of qi and blood in meridians, activate collaterals and remove blood stasis.

II. INDICATIONS

Acupuncture with the three-edged needle is applicable to various heat syndromes, excess syndromes and pain syndromes. It is usually employed in treating high fever, heat stroke, acute tonsillitis, sore and swollen throat, conjunctivitis, sprain, furuncle, lymphangitis, neurodermatitis, etc.

III. MANIPULATIONS

The following are the methods of puncture with the three-edged needle. All these methods are carried out with routine local sterilization indicated at the beginning of the procedure.

1. Spot Pricking

Spot pricking is a method that was known as collateral pricking in ancient times. Press and push the site to be pricked in order to create local congestion. Hold the needle with the right hand, the thumb and index finger gripping the handle, and the belly of the middle finger supporting the lower portion of its shaft, leaving 0.3 cm from the tip of the needle exposed. Direct the tip of the needle precisely to the acupoint and swiftly prick it to a depth of 0.1-0.2 cm, and withdraw immediately. Squeeze out a few drops of blood by pressing the skin around the punctured hole, and press over the hole with a sterilized swab for a moment. This method is mainly applicable for high fever, convulsion, apoplexy with coma, heat stroke, acute tonsillitis and acute lumbar sprain. It is extremely applicable when there is little or no other medical aid available.

2. Scattering Pricking

Scattering pricking method is also called "surrounding needling". To begin, use the fingers of the left hand and stretch the skin to be punctured. Hold the needle with the right hand as in spot pricking and prick the skin around the associated focus perpendicularly and rapidly. Then, gently press the skin to obtain mild bloodletting. This method is mainly applicable for traumatic pain due to stagnant blood, erysipelas, carbuncle, sore, etc.

3. Fibrous-Tissue-Broken Pricking

This method is also termed "breaking". To start, press the skin at two sides of the acupoint or sensitive spot (like a rush, 2-4 mm in diameter, usually with dark-yellow, green, reddish, of white color which disappears if pressed) with the left hand; this will fix the skin. Hold the needle with the right hand, the thumb above the middle, index and ring fingers, leaving 0.3-0.5 cm of the needle tip exposed. Then quickly prick and break the skin of the acupoint or selected spot at an angle of 15-30 degrees (from the surface of the skin). Insert the needle to the subcutaneous tissue, tilt the shaft of the needle

and then gently move it upwards to break some of the fibrous tissue. It is advisable to use the force formed by a combination of the left-right movement of the wrist joint, and that of the fingers for this procedure. It is applicable at acupoints to treat redness, swelling, pain in the eye, erysipelas, hemorrhoids, etc.

IV. PRECAUTIONS

1. Strictly observe the aseptic operation rule to prevent infection.

2. It is advisable to manipulate gently and swiftly. No more than a few drops of blood should be squeezed out. Never injure the deep, big artery.

3. This method should never be used on patients with hemorrhaged diseases, such as thrombocytopenia or hemophilia. It should be used with a great deal of care when treating patients who are pregnant, postpartum, famished, full from over-eating, or over-fatigued.

4. Generally, this method is carried out once every three days, once every other day, or once per 3-7 days, depending on the therapeutic intent. One therapeutic course needs 3-5 treatments.

3. Acupuncture with the Intradermal Needle

Acupuncture with the intradermal needle, also called "needle-embedding therapy", involves the insertion and long term retention of a small needle beneath the skin so as to give the body a long-lasting, continuous stimulation for regulating the visceral functions.

I. ACTIONS

1. Provides A Stimulation Effect of Long Time Retaining of the Needle

Acupuncture with the intradermal needle can exert the continuous needling stimulation to the patient.

2. Regulates the Functions of the Zang-Fu Organs

Acupuncture with the intradermal needle in the ear has a good action to regulate the functions of the zang-fu organs.

II. INDICATIONS

It is applicable to chronic and painful disorders in which prolonged retention of the needle is needed for treatment purposes. Disorders for which intradermal needle use is applicable include: headache, trigeminal neuralgia, toothache, stomachache, asthma, insomnia, irregular menstruation, dysmenorrhea, enuresis and other painful disorders.

III. MANIPULATIONS

Sterilize the intradermal needle, forceps and skin area to be punctured. If the acupoint is located on the trunk or limbs, the intradermal needle with wheat-granule or circle shape is selected. To begin, push the skin at the acupoint area in two opposite directions with the thumb and index finger of the left hand. Hold the needle handle with a pair of forceps with the right hand. Insert the needle perpendicularly, directly into the dermis of the acupoint. Then, horizontally

puncture in a direction crossing the meridian course, and embed the needle shaft 0.5-0.1 cm inside the skin. Finally, fix the handle of the needle left outside onto the skin with a piece of adhesive plaster. If the acupoint is located at the auricle, use the needle with a thumbtack, or thumb-pin, shape. Using a pair of forceps, direct the needle tip to the acupoint, making the flat, expanded handle of the needle lie flat on the skin. Then, fix the handle with a piece of adhesive tape, or place adhesive paste onto the needle handle before insertion and then proceed as outlined above. The duration of embedment varies with the season. Generally 1-2 days in the summer or 3-5 days in the fall or winter. During the embedding period, the patient should press the thumbtack needle several times daily, each time lasting 1-2 minutes, so as to strengthen the stimulation and increase the therapeutic effect.

IV. PRECAUTIONS

1. No needle embedment is allowed over a joint as movement might then cause pain.

2. It is not suitable to embed the needle in purulent, infected skin or in broken and ulcerated skin.

3. In order to prevent infection, the needle apparatus and the site to be punctured should be sterilized strictly, and the puncture site should not be allowed to get wet. It is inadvisable to have the needle imbedded for too long in the summer because during that time the patient may be liable to profuse sweating.

4. If the patient feels pain or has disorders of body movement after embedment, the embedded needle should be taken out and then re-embedded.

4. Acupuncture with the Skin Needle

Acupuncture with the skin needle, also known as plum-blossom, seven-star, or cutaneous needling, uses several small needles to tap on the skin of the corresponding area shallowly.

I. ACTIONS

1. Promotes Flow of Qi and Blood and Removes Blood Stasis

Acupuncture with the plum-blossom needle has a good action to promote the smooth flow of qi and blood in meridians, activate collaterals and remove blood stasis.

2. Regulates the Functions of the Zang-Fu Organs

Acupuncture with the plum-blossom needle has some actions to regulate the functions of the zang-fu organs.

II. INDICATIONS

Plum-blossom needling is applicable for hypertension, headache, myopia, neurasthenia, gastrointestinal disorder, alopecia areata, dysmenorrhea, arthralgia, pain of back and loin, numbness of skin, intercostal neuralgia, facial paralysis, neurodermatitis, etc.

III. MANIPULATIONS

After routine and local sterilization, fix the end of the needle handle with the ring and small fingers of the right hand at the small thenar eminence of the palm. Hold the needle handle with the middle finger of the right hand, the index finger pressing over the middle of the handle, then tap quickly and perpendicularly on the skin with a flexible movement of the wrist, like a chicken pecking at rice, causing the short sound "da". The tapping force should be focused, and no oblique or slipping puncture should occur. If a gentle tapping is needed, tap until the area appears red and congested. If a

heavy tapping is required, tap until the local area appears to be bleeding. The tapping manipulation depends on the pathological condition and the patient's physical constitution. Generally, in one treatment session 5-7 sets of tapping are done with a frequency of approximately 80 times per minute, and within an interval space of 1-2 cm.

This method may be combined with electro-acupuncture. To operate, connect one of a pair of output leads from a transistor electro-acupuncture unit to the skin needle and the other to a copper stick. Usually, select 100-120 volts as the peak output, 16-300 cycles per minute as the frequency of output of an irregular wave, and a fry battery with 9-volt output supplying a current below 5 mA (direct current) as the power. During this operation, the patient is asked to hold the copper stick and the operator holds the skin needle to tap in the way mentioned above.

IV. STIMULATING AREAS

1. The Routine Area

The routine area of the skin needling includes the posterior median line on the spinal column. Specifically, the course of the Du Meridian on the spinal column, and the four lines respectively 1.5 cun and 3 cun lateral to the posterior median line on the back (i.e. the branches of the Bladder Meridian on the back), five lines in total.

2. The Corresponding Meridian Area

Take the corresponding meridian course as the stimulating area, based on the differentiation of the syndromes. Collect and analyze the patient's symptoms and signs, and summarize under the guidance of TCM theories so as to identify the etiology, the location of the disease, the pathologic changes, the body condition, etc. Determine which organ or meridian the disease is closely related to and tap the skin along the corresponding meridian course. For example, tap the skin along the course of the Lung Meridian of Hand-Taiyin for asthma and cough; tap the skin at the head and nape along the courses of the Gallbladder Meridian of Foot-Shaoyang and the Triple Energizer Meridian of Hand-Shaoyang for migraine.

3. The Corresponding Points

Based on differentiation of syndromes and chief indications of the acupoint, choose some acupoints (mainly referring to the special acupoints) as tapping areas. For example, asthma and cough due to failure of the kidney in receiving air may be treated by tapping on LU-1 Zhongfu, BL-13 Feishu, BL-43 Gaohuang, BL-12 Fengmen, BL-23 Shenshu, K-13 Taixi, and K-17 Fuliu.

4. The Affected Area

Take the diseased area as the tapping area. Usually, line-puncture or circle-puncture is given to the area. For example, in treating pain of the shoulder joint, a circle-puncture over the shoulder joint is given; in alopecia areata, the local diseased area and the area around it may be selected in combination. In order to meet the need of the treatment, 2-3 tapping methods may be used in coordination. In treating neurasthenia, for example, the routine stimulating area is tapped first, then some related acupoints such as BL-15 Xinshu, BL-23 Shenmen, BL-18 Ganshu are tapped. In treating intercostal neuralgia, some areas along the course of the liver Meridian are tapped in combination with tapping the painful intercostal area from the middle side to the lateral side.

V. PRECAUTIONS

1. Pay attention to sterilization before and after operation so as to prevent infection.

2. Check the needle apparatus prior to operation. It is required that the tips of the needles be even and free of any hook.

3. Tapping is not allowed at local trauma and ulcers. It is also contraindicated when treating patients with hemorrhagic diseases.

5. Acupuncture with the Dull Needle

This acupuncture method uses the dull needle, one of the nine ancient needles, to press the meridian and acupoint. This method has the merit of simplicity and requires no insertion, making it acceptable for children, the aged or weak persons. The patients themselves after instructions from the doctor can apply it.

I. ACTIONS

Like the other acupuncture methods, acupuncture with the dull needle can promote qi and blood flow and regulate the functions of the zang-fu organs. It acts to replace the filiform needle in treatment of children or adults who are afraid of needling.

II. INDICATIONS

This method is applicable for disorders caused by deficiency of the qi of the channel such as stomachache, abdominal pain, indigestion, neurogenic vomiting, vomiting related to pregnancy and enuresis.

III. MANIPULATIONS

Hold the needle with the thumb, middle and ring fingers with the index finger resisting the needle tail. Alternatively, hold the needle handle with the thumb, index and middle fingers with the ring finger resisting the needle shaft. Then, press the needle tip over the acupoint or meridian. When pressing, scraping the needle handle with the nail of the finger may strengthen the needling sensation. The manipulation of the dull needle may be classified, according to the intensity of the pressing force, into two types: Gentle pressing and heavy pressing. The type of pressing is chosen based on the patient's constitution and pathological condition. The gentle method, suitable for syndromes of the deficiency type, is employed by gently pressing the needle on the meridian or acupoint. After the appearance of local red areola or upon relief of symptoms, the needle is slowly taken away and the local area is massaged for a while. In the heavy pressing method, suitable for syndromes of excess, the needle is heavily pressed on the acupoint or meridian. After the patient has a feeling of pain, soreness or distention spreading upwards, the needle is quickly taken away.

A therapeutic course requires ten treatments, but in milder disorders, only one or two treatments may be required. If the dull needle method doesn't work after ten sessions, it is suggested that it be combined or replaced with some other therapeutic methods.

Additionally, the dull needle technique may be used to treat disorders of the nervous system and various types of inflammation by using it to conduct pulse wave current at a low frequency through the needle to the acupoint of the body. This induces qi of the channel to circulate and spread. In China, the ZKC-2 type electric dull-needling unit (made in the Beijing Motomation Equipment Factory) is frequently employed. To operate this unit, connect the negative potential wristband to one arm and the probe (i.e. dull needle) to the positive line. Set the frequency and amplitude to the lowest degrees, then turn on the power and probe the acupoint with the needle. During probing and pressing, the strength of stimulation should be chosen according to the patient's sensitivity. The controls should be adjusted until the patient feels a scorching sensation and a beating sensation at the acupoint being pressed by the electric needle.

One or two times of treatment are needed daily with two to five acupoints selected for each treatment. Two to ten minutes of stimulation are required for each point. One therapeutic course consists of ten treatments.

6. Acupuncture with the Hot Needle

Acupuncture with a hot needle is an ancient treatment that employs the insertion of a thick, warm needle into a particular area of the body. This method serves to warm the meridian and to clear and activate the channel and collateral.

I. ACTIONS

1. Warms the Meridians, Dispels Cold and Alleviates Pain

Acupuncture with the hot needle can directly warm the meridians and collaterals, dispel coldness from the meridian, promote the smooth flow of qi and blood, activate collaterals and relieve pain.

2. Removes Toxic Materials

Acupuncture with the hot needle can directly remove toxic materials or accumulation of phlegm and blood stasis, such as pus and nodules, from the local region.

II. INDICATIONS

It is usually indicated in arthralgia due to wind-cold-dampness (wind, cold and dampness combined as a pathogen), and swelling and pain due to cold of deficiency type. Additionally, it can be used in the treatment of scrofula, neurodermatitis, flat wart, nevus, elephantiasis crus and filaria infection.

III. MANIPULATIONS

Sterilize the skin of the selected acupoint or area with 2% iodine, then swab the iodine away with 75% alcohol. Then, according to the patient's adaptability, infiltration anesthesia with 1% procaine (or combined with 0.1% adrenaline hydrochloride to prevent bleeding) may be given to minimize patient's pain and apprehension. Two minutes later the puncture can be carried out. The manipulation of the hot needle may be classified, according to the patient's constitution and pathological condition, into deep puncture and shallow puncture.

1. Deep Puncture

It is suitable for the treatment of external diseases such as carbuncle, cellulitis, scrofula and elephantiasis crus. Usually a thicker needle is selected for expelling pus while a comparatively thin needle is selected for treating Yin syndromes such as scrofula. To perform puncture, fix the acupoint with the left hand, the fingers pressing, stretching or pinching the skin at the acupoint. Hold the needle with the right hand and heat its tip and lower portion of the needle shaft until red-hot. Then, insert the needle into the acupoint or required area accurately and quickly and remove it immediately. Then press the needle hole with a sterilized cotton ball.

2. Shallow Puncture

This is mainly used in the treatment of arthralgia due to wind-dampness, cold-dampness, numbness of the skin and neurodermatitis. To apply treatment, hold the needle with the right hand and warm the lower portion of the needle over the flame until red-hot. Then gently tap on the skin surface with the needle. In the treatment of neurodermatitis, shallow puncture may be carried out with a skin needle (i.e. seven-star needle), which replaces the hot needle and is classified as shallow puncture with multi-needles.

Generally, the treatment is given once per 3-6 days, and a therapeutic course may be long or short according to the pathological condition.

IV. PRECAUTIONS

1. The hot needling should be used with great care and is even contraindicated when treating patients with a weak constitution. This applies in pregnancy as well because the stimulation caused by hot needling is very strong. It is also contraindicated on the face.

2. In applying deep puncture, the operator should be careful to manipulate the needle swiftly, inserting it in one motion and avoiding the blood vessels, muscular tendons, nerve trunks and internal organs.

3. In applying shallow puncture, the operator should not tap too forcefully or with uneven force. The tapping should be even and loosely spaced so as to prevent incidents such as epidermal desquamation during needle removal.

4. After puncture, the patient should not bathe or scratch the skin until the local redness and swelling disappear. If tapping too deep, the needle hole should be covered with a sterile dressing fixed with an adhesive plaster for one or two days to prevent infection.

7. Electro-Acupuncture

Electro-acupuncture is a therapeutic technique in which an electric current, almost as weak as bioelectric current, is supplied to the needle inserted into the acupoint to strengthen the stimulation.

The way to apply treatment and select points in electro-acupuncture is similar to that of filiform needling. Generally, 1-3 pairs of acupoints on both sides (namely 1-3 pair of lines) are a suitable number. Too many acupoints used at once may induce too strong a stimulation for the patient to endure.

I. ACTIONS

Electro-acupuncture can act to adjust the functions of the zang-fu organs, increase analgesic and sedative effects, promote blood circulation and adjust muscular tension.

II. MANIPULATION

After needling sensation is induced, a suitable electro-acupuncture unit is selected. The output is set to "0" and the negative electrode is connected to the main acupoint and the positive electrode attaches to the corresponding acupoint. It is permissible to attach the electrodes without considering the polarity. Generally, two output electrodes of a pair should be connected to the same side of the body. Moreover, when the electro-acupuncture is applied to the back and chest, it is forbidden to connect a pair of output electrodes to opposite sides of the body, otherwise serious complications may occur.

When the power is turned on and the electrodes are attached, the designed wave mode and frequency are selected and the output of current is gradually increased until tolerable soreness and numbness are induced in the patient. The duration of electric stimulation is usually 10-20 minutes. At the end of treatment, the device is set back to "0", the power is turned off, the output leads are disconnected and the filiform needles are withdrawn. The patient who has experienced electro-acupuncture many times may gradually become tolerant to this kind of stimulation. For this kind of patient, an increase in the electric current and a change of frequency are necessary in maintaining continuous stimulation.

If only one acupoint is needed in treatment, one lead is connected to the handle of the needle and the other is connected to a thin, electrically conductive skin patch about 2cm x 3cm in size which is then wrapped in several layers of wet cloth and laid on the skin somewhat remote to the needle (usually on DU-14 Dazhui, SP-6 Sanyinjiao or PC-6 Neiguan). The rest of the procedure is carried out the same way as is mentioned above.

III. SELECTION AND INDICATIONS OF THE WAVE FORMS

The functions and indications of the electroacupuncture vary with the wave and frequency of a low frequent pulse current. In clinical practice, the proper wave and frequency should be selected based on the patient's condition so as to enhance the therapeutic effect.

High Frequency: Also termed dense wave. Its frequency is high, usually 50-100 pulses per second (PPS). It is useful to lower nerve irritability by inhibiting the sensory nerve at first, then the motor nerve. This frequency is usually selected to induce analgesic and sedative effects, to reduce muscle or blood vessel spasm, for treatment of painful syndromes and for anesthesia, etc.

Low Frequency: Also termed sparse wave. Its frequency is low, generally around 2-5 PPS and its stimulation is comparatively strong. It may induce contracture of muscle and increase tension of muscle and ligament. Its result of inhibiting the sensory and motor nerves occurs comparatively late. This frequency is usually indicated in atrophy, impairment of the joint, muscle and ligament, etc.

Irregular Wave: Also termed alternately dense and sparse wave. This wave is formed by spontaneously alternating the appearance of low and high waves. It has the merit of avoiding the build up of tolerance that is usually caused by applying only one kind of wave. Since its excitation function is predominant it can serve to promote metabolism and circulation of qi and blood, improve tissue nutrition, and subdue inflammatory swelling. It is usually applied to painful syndromes, injuries due to sprain and contusion, arthritis, disorders of circulation of qi and blood, sciatic neuralgia, facial paralysis, amyostenia, local cold injury, etc.

Intermittent Wave: This is a special kind of low frequency, appearing regularly and intermittently. It can serve to enhance the irritability of muscle tissue and provide a good stimulation to a strained muscle. It is selected for atrophy and paralysis.

Sawtooth Wave: This wave appears on the oscilloscope in the shape of a sawtooth. Its frequency is almost like that of a person's respiration; therefore, it is also termed a respiratory wave. It may serve to stimulate the phrenic nerve and is useful as an electric spirophorus to salvage a person with respiratory failure. It may also serve to enhance the irritability of nerve and muscle, adjust channel function and improve the circulation of qi and blood.

IV. PRECAUTIONS

1. If the output current is discontinuous, it may be due to a poor lead connection. Repair it as necessary.

2. In the patient with heart disease, the back-flow of current should be prevented from passing through the heart. In the area near the medullar bulb and spinal cord, the output current should be low to prevent accident. It should also be given with great care to pregnant women.

3. The increase of the electric current should be graduated for the comfort of the patient. Sudden increases of current may cause broken or bent needles, or needling fainting due to possible sudden contracture of muscles.

4. The direct current or direct pulse current of electrolysis is liable to cause fracture of the needle and burning of tissue. Therefore it should not be used as the output current of the electro-acupuncture unit.

5. If the electro-acupuncture unit has its output voltage higher than 40 volts, the current should be limited to below one mA in order to avoid electric shock.

6. Do not connect electrodes to a needle handle, which is oxidized and thus rendered as a poor conductor. Instead, connect the lead to the needle shaft. Oxidation may occur from moxibustion or the warm needle technique.

8. Moxibustion

Moxibustion is a therapeutic method that uses the burning of specific combustible materials or the application of a drug-compress or drug-plaster over the acupoint or affected area in order to produce a warm-hot stimulation to the patient. This heat acts on the acupoint and is conducted through the channel so that the equilibrium of the physical function of the body can be adjusted.

I. GENERAL ACTIONS & INDICATIONS

Moxibustion can produce the effect of warming qi and promoting blood circulation, strengthening the body resistance to eliminate pathogenic factors. It is widely applied to treat or prevent diseases.

1. Actions

1). Warms meridians and expels cold
Moxibustion provides direct warm stimulation to the meridians of the body. Warmth can conquer coldness, and warmth can dispel cold. Moreover, moxibustion has a good effect to warm yang and restore collapsed yang, recuperate yang and rescue patient from collapse.

2). Promotes qi and blood circulation and relieve pain
Qi and blood like warmth and hate cold. Cold may obstruct the circulation of qi and blood in the meridians, while warmth can remove the obstruction and promote the flow of qi and blood. Thus moxibustion can promote qi and blood flows, relieve obstruction of qi and blood, cause an analgesic effect.

3) Subdues swelling and resolves masses
Moxibustion has some effect to subdue swelling and resolve masses.

2.   Indications

Moxibustion may be employed in the treatment of either acute diseases, cold syndromes, diseases of the channel and exterior syndromes, or chronic syndromes and diseases of the viscera. Additionally, it may work in health maintenance and disease prevention. In clinical practice, moxibustion is frequently applied in treatment of the following diseases:

- Arthralgia due to wind-cold-dampness;
- Yang collapse syndrome;
- Diseases of the zang-fu organs due to yang deficiency or retention of cold, such as chronic diarrhea, chronic dysentery, asthma, phlegm retention and flaccidity syndrome, etc.;
- Qi sinking syndrome, such as visceroptosis;
- Some gynecological diseases, such as dysmenorrhea, prolapse of uterus, abnormal fetal position and leukorrhea, etc.;
- Some infantile diseases, such as enuresis and diarrhea;
- Some external diseases, such as carbuncle in the first stage or with intractable ulcer;
- Some exterior syndromes, such as common cold.

Additionally, acupuncture and moxibustion can be applied at the same time, and in treatment of many diseases, a result induced by combining these two therapies will be better than that induced by using either singly.

II. COMMONLY-USED MOXIBUSTION TECHNIQUES

1. Moxibustion with Moxa Cone

Moxa cone consists of moxa wool made into a cone shape by the rolling of the moxa wool with the hand. The moxa cone may be small, medium or large in size. The large one is 1cm high, with a bottom of 0.8cm diameter; the medium one is one half as big as the large one, like a jubepit; the small one is as big as a grain of wheat. They are referred to as cones or "zhuang", a unit of measurement that pertains to the number of moxa cones used.

There are two kinds of moxibustion that usecones: Direct and indirect moxibustion

1). Direct Moxibustion
It means that a moxa cone of pertinent size is placed upon the skin and ignited. This type of moxibustion is subdivided into scarring and non-scarring types, depending on whether or not a scar is formed after receiving treatment.

a. Non-scarring moxibustion:
Also termed non-pulsated moxibustion, so named because it will not cause a blister, scar or pus after application. In clinical practice a medium or small moxa cone is placed on the acupoint and then ignited. When it is 1/5 burnt or the patient feels discomfort, remove the cone and replace it with another one. Continue this until the appropriate number of cones has been used. At this time, erythema of the skin may be seen. This method is applicable in cases of cold-deficiency syndrome such as chronic diarrhea or asthma.

Sometimes this method may cause the skin to blister. If this occurs, do not break the blister but leave it to heal on its own accord.

b. Scarring moxibustion:
Also termed pulsated or festering moxibustion. It refers to a procedure that the moxa cone is placed directly on the acupoint and ignited. In this case, moxibustion is continued until a blister appears by which local purulence and crust will be formed. After decrustation a scar will be left. Generally, 2-6 moxa cones are employed on each acupoint for a treatment. If the moxa cones are smaller, it is better. The number of cones may be reduced for children and for weak persons according to their condition. To perform this type of moxibustion, smear some garlic juice on the skin at the acupoint, place a moxa cone on it and ignite the cone. After it is completely burnt out, take away the ashes, swab some more garlic juice and apply another moxa cone. Repeat this course until the designed number of cones has been used up. After moxibustion, there is a local blister on the skin that should become purulent in about a week and will heal with decrustation about 45 days later. A scar will be left. This treatment must have the informed consent of the patient because it is painful and leaves scars. The scorching pain caused by the operation can be relieved by gently tapping on the skin around the moxa cone or by giving an intradermic or subcutaneous injection of 2-3 ml of 0.2% procaine hydrochloride to the acupoint area. In clinic, this type of moxibustion is usually applied to chronic intractable diseases such as asthma, pulmonary tuberculosis, epilepsy, etc.

2). Indirect Moxibustion
Indirect moxibustion is performed by placing a substance between the smoldering moxa cone and the skin. In this way, moxa and drug treatment can be carried out at the same time. It is also more appealing for the patient because there is no blistering or purulence. It has a wide range of indications in the sphere of internal medicine, surgery, pediatrics, gynecology, otolaryngology, opthamology and stomatology. Its commonly used methods are as follows:

a.   Ginger (sheng jiang) moxibustion:
This is a method that uses a slice of ginger (raw) placed between the moxa cone and the acupoint. To perform the operation, cut a slice of ginger 2-3 mm thick with a diameter the same as the moxa cone, poke several holes through its center and place it on the selected acupoint. Then place the moxa cone on the ginger and ignite it. When the patient feels a burning sensation, slightly lift the ginger and moxa cone for a short period of time and then put them on the skin again, or if needed, replace the finished cone with a new one. Repeat this until there is a local erythema of the skin. Generally 5-10 cones are used on each point selected during a treatment session.

Ginger has the property of regulating the ying and wei. (Ying refers to the material foundation of the body's function while wei refers to the defensive mechanism or yang principle for defense at the body's surface.) Its other important properties are dispelling cold to relieve exterior syndrome, regulating the middle-jiao to comfort the stomach, dispelling the accumulation of qi and regulating qi, ventilating the lung, removing water and promoting digestion. Therefore, this method can produce good therapeutic results in treating disorders of cold syndrome of a deficiency type, such as vomiting, diarrhea, stomachache, abdominal pain and arthritis due to wind-cold-dampness.

b. *Garlic moxibustion:*

This is a method that uses a slice of raw garlic placed between the moxa cone and the acupoint. To perform the operation, cut a slice of raw garlic 2-3 mm thick, punch several holes in the center and place it on the selected acupoint. Then place the moxa cone on the garlic and ignite it. After 2-3 cones have burnt down, replace the garlic with a fresh piece and continue the operation until there is an erythema of the skin. Generally, 5-10 cones are used for each point in a treatment session.

Garlic can serve to dispel a cold-damp factor and expel the pathogen. It strengthens the spleen and stomach, relieves swelling and resolves masses. Because of this it may be employed in the treatment of disease in the field of surgery and traumatology such as carbuncle, deep-rooted carbuncle, sores, furuncle (boil) and snakebite, as well as some internal diseases such as pulmonary tuberculosis and abdominal masses.

c. *Salt moxibustion:*

This is a method of moxibustion that uses salt between the moxa cone and the acupoint. It is also termed moxibustion at RN-8 Shenque point because it is applied only on the umbilicus. To perform the operation, fill the umbilicus with dry salt (or fried hot salt) to the level of the skin, a piece of ginger may be placed between the salt and the moxa cone. The ginger serves to protect the patient from scalding that may be caused by explosion of salt crystals coming in direct contact with the fire. If the patient's umbilicus is not concave in shape, a piece of wet noodle or similar material may be placed around the umbilicus and then filled with salt. This method is applicable for acute gastroenteritis, pain around the umbilicus, dysentery, hernia and prostration syndrome with profuse sweating and cold limbs, etc.

d. *Monkshood (fu zi) moxibustion:*

There are two commonly used types in clinic. One is to place a slice of monkshood (aconite) root between a moxa cone and the acupoint; the other is to place a cake of monkshood between a moxa cone and the acupoint. To perform the operation, cut a slice of monkshood or select a monkshood cake, punch numerous holes in it and place it on the acupoint selected. Then place a moxa cone on top and ignite it. The moxibustion continues until there is a slight burning sensation and erythema of the local skin. Generally 5-10 cones are burnt out on each point selected during a treatment session.

Aconite root has the property of dispelling wind and cold and it reinforces the kidney yang. Therefore, this method is applicable for various syndromes of insufficiency of yang including impotence, diarrhea at dawn, cold limbs, etc.

2. Moxibustion with Moxa Stick

This method applies the ignited end of a moxa stick or drug stick. It is classified into mild-warm moxibustion, rounding moxibustion and sparrow-pecking moxibustion.

1). Mild-Warming Moxibustion

Ignite one of the ends of the moxa stick and hold the burning end in a fixed position above the acupoint. When the patient indicates the heat from the moxa is too strong, quickly and properly lift the end of the moxa stick. Apply moxibustion until there is erythema of the skin. This method has the property of promoting flow of qi by warming the channel, as well as dispelling wind, cold and damp pathogens.

2). Rounding Moxibustion

Also termed circling moxibustion. To perform the operation, hold the lighted end of a moxa stick above the acupoint. Then move the stick horizontally in a circular motion above the acupoint to cause a warming sensation to the patient.

3). Sparrow-Pecking Moxibustion

Keep the burning end of a moxa stick over the acupoint and move it up and down, like a sparrow pecking at its food.

The three methods mentioned above could be used in diseases that can be treated with moxibustion. However, the mild warming and rounding moxibustion methods are mainly applied in chronic diseases such as arthritis due to wind-cold-dampness; and the sparrow-pecking moxibustion is mainly employed when treating acute diseases such as coma and syncope as well as in certain childhood diseases.

3. Moxibustion with Warming Needle

This type of moxibustion is also termed warm needling and is a form of acupuncture combined with moxibustion. It is the most commonly used moxibustion method in clinic. After arrival of qi and with the needle retained in the point, a segment of moxa stick about 2cm long is pierced through by the needle handle, or the handle is pinched with some moxa wool and then the moxa is ignited.

The purpose of this type of moxibustion is to conduct heat energy through the needle shaft into the punctured point thus producing a therapeutic effect of combination of acupuncture and moxibustion. Therefore, it is used very frequently in clinic. For example, it can be applicable to wind-cold-damp bi syndrome (arthralgia) and flaccidity syndrome, etc. In this method, it is possible for the skin to be injured by moxa fire or the fall of ashes from the stick. As a precaution, place a piece of thick paper with a small hole in its center, through which the needle pierces, on the skin prior to attaching the moxa medium.

4. Rush-Burning Moxibustion

Rush-burning moxibustion, also termed limpwick moxibustion, or moxibustion with medulla junci, is a method performed by pressing a burning oiled rush directly over an acupoint and then immediately moving it away. To apply, make a mark on the selected acupoint, then select a segment of rush pith 4-5cm long and put one end in vegetable oil approximately 1-2cm deep. Then remove and dry the pith slightly with a paper towel. Hold the rush with the thumb and index finger of the right hand, expose the oiled end of the rush about 1cm, and ignite the end. Quickly press it over the acupoint and immediately take away. If a sound "pa" is heard when the rush touches the skin, it indicates that the technique is successfully applied. If the sound is not heard repeat the procedure one more

time. Be careful to keep the local area clean after moxibustion so as to prevent infection. This method may serve to dispel wind for relieving exterior syndrome, to promote the flow of qi for dispelling phlegm, to relieve stagnant qi to relieve chest oppression, to clear heat for removing toxin, and to induce resuscitation for calming endogenous wind. It is mainly indicated in mumps, infantile clonic convulsion, coma, stomachache, abdominal pain, etc.

5. Crude Herb Moxibustion

This therapy is applied by pasting irritant medicines on the skin at certain acupoints to cause local congestion and blistering. The commonly used methods are as follows:

1). Mashed Garlic Moxibustion
Mash some garlic to a pulp and place 3-5 g on the skin. Then cover it with a piece of plastic film and secure with adhesive tape. Keep the garlic on the skin until there is itching, redness or blistering. Usually the duration is 1-3 hours. Various diseases may be treated by this method. For example, hemoptysis and epistaxis may be treated by placing the garlic on KI-1 Yongquan and tonsillitis is treated by applying the garlic to LU-10 Yuji.

2). Castor Seed Moxibustion
Remove the shell of a castor seed, mash it and plaster the mashed seed over the acupoint in the same fashion as above. This may be used to treat prolonged labor by applying plaster to KI-1 Yongquan, and prolapse of the uterus, gastroptosis and prolapse of the rectum are treated by applying the treatment on DU-20 Baihui.

3). Fructus Euodiae (wu zhu yu) Moxibustion
Grind a proper amount of fructus euodiae into powder and make it into a paste by using vinegar. Use the same method as above to apply. This is performed once daily and may be used to treat certain diseases. For example, hypertension, canker sore and infantile edema are treated by applying this type of moxibustion to KI-1 Yongquan.

Additionally, moxibustion with folium

ranunculus japonucus applied to PC-6 Neiguan and DU-14 Dazhui can be used for malaria. Apply it over the affected area for pain due to cold-dampness. Moxibustion by using semen cleomis may be applied in the above manner to BL-13 Feishu and BL-43 Gaohuang for treating asthma and pulmonary tuberculosis.

III. REINFORCING AND REDUCING IN MOXIBUSTION THERAPY

This mainly applies to the use of the moxa stick. In clinical applications of moxibustion, reducing is used when the pathogen is dominant; reinforcing is used when the vital qi is weak. To perform the reinforcing method, the moxa stick is lit and directed at the acupoint and allowed to burn of its own accord until extinguished. In this way a milder heat is produced and it lasts for a comparatively long time. The area to which moxibustion is applied is pressed with the hand as soon as the process is over. This is in order to keep the genuine qi, also known as vital qi, inside, thus preventing its escape. Genuine qi is the dynamic force of all vital functions. It arises from the combination of inherited original qi and acquired energy derived from food and air.

To perform the reducing method, the glowing end of the moxa stick is blown upon by the breath so as to quicken its burning speed and to produce greater heat. When the patient feels heat and a burning sensation, the moxa stick is quickly replaced with another one. The duration of the treatment is relatively short, fewer moxa sticks are used, and after moxibustion the acupoint is not pressed. This makes the pathogen removed from the body.

IV. CONTRAINDICATIONS AND PRECAUTIONS

1. It is inadvisable to apply moxibustion and forbidden to apply scarring moxibustion to the face, to areas near the important viscera, large vessels and tendons. In pregnant women, it is inadvisable to apply moxibustion to the lumbar-sacral region, lower abdomen, nipple and lower orifice region.

2. In general, it is inadvisable to apply moxibustion for treatment of febrile disease due to exogenous pathogen, interior-heat syndrome due to yin deficiency and excess-heat syndrome.

3. It is inadvisable to apply moxibustion to patients who are over fatigued, famished, full from over eating, tipsy, very thirsty, nervous, angry or frightened.

4. In weak patients, it is inadvisable to apply moxibustion with too large moxa cone and stimulate too strongly.

5. Generally, relatively few moxa cones should be used on the chest and limbs; fewer on the head and neck; but more may be applied to the loin, back and abdomen. Use only a few moxa cones and shorten the duration of moxibustion for the aged and children. For the young, more cones may be used and the duration may be lengthened.

6. After using the scarring type of moxibustion, advise the patient to refrain from heavy physical labor during the purulence period. If the local area becomes inflamed due to infection, give anti-inflammatory treatment and cover the area with a sterilized dressing to prevent further contamination.

7. Do not treat the reddish color and burning sensation of local skin that appear after treatment, but rather, wait for them to disappear of their own accord. When blisters appear due to excessive or prolonged moxibustion, do not break the small ones but allow them to disappear of their own accord. If the blister is large, break it with a sterilized needle to drain the fluid, cover with a sterile dressing and fix the dressing on the skin.

8. To patients suffering from coma, numbness of limbs or dysesthesia, excessive moxibustion is contraindicated and close attention should be paid to prevent the local skin from being burnt.

9.   Cupping Method

Cupping is a therapeutic method in which a jar or cup is attached to the surface of the skin to cause local congestion. This is achieved by the creation of a negative pressure inside the cup via the introduction of ignited material into the jar.

Commonly used cupping apparatus are made of bamboo, glass or pottery.

I. ACTIONS

This method serves to promote the circulation of qi and blood, induce an analgesic effect, subdue swelling and expel wind, cold and damp pathogens.

II. INDICATIONS

Indications for cupping include arthritis due to wind-cold-dampness, acute sprain, facial paralysis, hemiplegia, common cold, cough, stomachache, abdominal pain, furuncle, carbuncle, deep-rooted carbuncle, early stages of ulcer, etc.

III. MANIPULATIONS

1. Cup-Placing Method

1). Fire-Throwing Method
Throw an ignited alcohol ball or a piece of ignited paper into a cup or jar, then immediately place the mouth of the container firmly against the skin on the desired location thus causing, through the vacuum principle, a firm attachment to the skin. This method is only applied when the jar is attached horizontally; otherwise, the burning material may fall onto the skin, causing a scalding to the patient.

2). Fire-Twinkling Method
Clamp an alcohol ball with a pair of forceps, ignite and put it into the cup. Then immediately withdraw it and place the cup on the selected area of the skin. This method is frequently applied because it is safe for the patient.

3). Cotton-Attaching Method
Attach a cotton ball that has been soaked with a small amount of alcohol to the internal wall of the cup, ignite it and immediately place the jar on the selected point. Be very careful to avoid using too much alcohol to wet the cotton during this procedure as some burning liquid may drip onto the skin and cause a scalding to the patient.

4). Material-Placing Method
Place a circle-shaped hard rubber or bakelite stopper over the skin of the selected area, and then place a cotton ball soaked with 95% alcohol on the stopper. Ignite the ball and immediately cover with a cup (preferably glass). This method is safe for the patient and causes the cup to adhere firmly to the skin.

2. Cup-Manipulating Method

1). Retaining Cupping
After the cup or jar is attached to the skin, leave it in place for 10-20 minutes. One jar is often employed, but for the area with abundant muscles, 2-5 jars may be employed. This method is applicable for most diseases that are treated with cupping.

2). Successive Flash Cupping (Quick Cupping)
Attach cup to the skin by using the fire-twinkling method and immediately remove it. Repeat this course several times. This method is suitable for treating numbness of the local skin or deficiency type syndrome due to hypofunction.

3). Moving Cupping
Also termed pushing cupping. This method is suitable for cupping on the area with abundant muscle such as the back, loin, buttock and thigh. To perform this operation, smear Vaseline over the selected area of skin and attach a jar. Then, hold the jar with the right hand while drawing it downwards with the left hand for a certain distance. Then forcefully press the skin below the jar with the left hand and slide it upwards with the right hand for a certain distance. Repeat this course several times. After erythema appears on the local area, take the jar away and wipe off the Vaseline. This method is mainly used in treating obstruction of the channel or

wandering pain.

4). Cupping with the Needle Inside the Jar

This method combines both cupping and acupuncture. To perform this operation, insert a filiform needle into a selected acupoint and induce a needling sensation. Retain the needle. Then quickly place a jar by using the fire-twinkling method over the skin where the needle is positioned, the needle being inside the jar. This method is used mainly for treating intractable diseases of the deep layer, such as internal organ diseases.

5). Blood-Letting Puncture and Cupping

After pricking the selected area with a three-edged needle or plum-blossomed needle, apply cupping over that spot immediately to cause bleeding. Generally, retain the jar for 10-15 minutes. Then take away the jar and wipe away the blood print. This method is used in treating various diseases due to stagnation of qi and blood such as sprain and snakebite.

As well as the methods mentioned above, drug cupping and aspiration cupping have been employed in recent years.

Drug Cupping: Make a prescription of Chinese herbal drugs, boil the drugs with water to the proper consistency and add a bamboo jar or cup to the mixture and boil for 1 minute. Take the jar out with a pair of forceps, eliminate the fluid in the jar and press the hot jar over the selected area of skin until it adheres via the vacuum effect. This method is usually used to treat painful syndromes due to wind-dampness.

The common drug prescription is 6 g each of Herba Ephedrae, Folium Artemisiae Argyi, Notopterygium, Radix Angelicae Pubescentis, Radix Ledebouriellae, Radix Gantianae Macrophyllae, Fructus Chaenomelis, Pericripium Zanthoxyli, Fresh Radix Aconiti, Flos Stramonii, Herba Serissae, Resina Boswelliae Carterii, and Myrrha.

Aspirating Cupping: Select specially designed aspirating jars for the size required by the cupping area. Then attach the mouth of the jar to the skin of the selected area, hold the pistil hand with the hand and withdraw it upwards a little. The jar should become attached to the skin through a vacuum effect. As an alternative, select a special serum bottle (with no bottom) and using a syringe draw the air from the bottle.

IV. PRECAUTIONS

1. The mouth of the jar or cup should be round and smooth and without break otherwise the skin may be injured.

2. A site with abundant muscular mass should be selected and the patient should be in a comfortable position.

3. The duration of cup retention is usually 15 minutes. Longer duration may cause blistering.

4. The hand maneuver to remove the jar should be gentle and slow. When removing the jar, press the skin around the mouth to break the seal, thus allowing air to enter the vacuum. The cup may then be easily removed. It is forbidden to use strong force to draw and turn the jar, otherwise the skin may be injured.

5. When the fire-twinkling method is used, the fire flame should be moved around inside of the jar but not near the mouth so as to prevent scalding.

6. Jars and cups of different sizes are used according to the area being treated.

7. There may be local blood stasis after cupping and this is considered normal. It will most likely disappear of its own accord. However, when the stasis is severe, cupping should be discontinued from use on that area temporarily. If there are blisters after cupping, the small ones will be absolved on their own accord. Large ones should be treated by piercing through the bottom with a sterilized needle and then covering with a sterile dressing after the fluid has been drained.

8. It is inadvisable to apply cupping to a patient with fever, clonic convulsion or spasm, and it should be avoided on the lumbo-sacral region of women who are pregnant and areas with leptochroa or broken ulcer.

10. Precautions & Management of Possible Accidents in Zhenjiu Treatment

I. GENERAL PRECAUTIONS

1. For the person who is weak, nervous, or at a first visit, chose the recumbent position.

2. It is contraindicated to puncture acupoints on the lower abdomen of women within the first three months of pregnancy. In addition, to those beyond the first trimester it is also contraindicated to puncture acupoints on the abdomen and lumbo-sacral region. SP-6 Sanyinjiao, LI-4 Hegu, BL-67 Zhiyin and BL-60 Kunlun should not be punctured in pregnant women and in women who have a normal menstruation and are now at the menstruation period.

3. Retention of the needle should not be given to children who may not be in cooperation. Acupoints on the vertex of infants should not be punctured when the fontanel is not closed.

4. It is contraindicated to apply puncture to patients suffering from spontaneous bleeding or those with poor blood coagulation.

5. Special attention must be paid when puncturing acupoints on the chest, hypochondria, back and loin, where the important viscera are located. Puncturing too deeply at these areas may injure the corresponding internal viscera, leading to trauma and poor results. An operator must know the anatomy of acupoints well and strictly control the angle and depth of insertion.

6. In acupoints at the area around the orbital region where the blood vessels are rich, the needle should not be rotated, lifted or thrust in large amplitude so as to prevent bleeding.

7. Skin that is infected, ulcerated, scarred or with tumor should not be punctured.

II. CAUSES, MANIFESTATIONS, MANAGEMENT AND PREVENTION OF POSSIBLE ACCIDENTS

1. Stuck Needle
1). Cause and Management:
This may be due to too strong manipulation or from rotating the needle in a single direction only, resulting in entanglement of the needle with the muscle fibers. When this happens, withdraw the needle while rotating it in the opposite direction, then twirl it left and right gently to cause its release from the entanglement. If it is caused by muscular spasm due to nervousness, advise the patient to relax his or her muscles, prolong the period of retention of the needle and massage the area close to the acupoint to relieve the spasm. If it is caused by changing of patient's posture, move the patient to the original position and then withdraw the needle.

2). Prevention:
Speak some words to the first-time patient or the nervous patient in order to relax him / her and make him / her more cooperative prior to the operation. Avoid twirling the needle in too large amplitude or in a single direction with too much force, and avoid changing the patient's posture after insertion of the needle.

2. Bent Needle
1). Cause and Management:
This may be due to unskillful manipulation or over-violent manipulation, or changing of the patient's posture. If the bend is slight, withdraw the needle by following the course of the bend slowly. If pronounced, shake the needle shaft slightly while withdrawing it by following the course of the bend. If the needle is bent in several places, withdraw it section by section, following the course of bends. Never withdraw the bent needle suddenly and forcefully, otherwise, the needle may be broken. If it is caused by changing of the patient's posture, move the patient to the original position to relax the local muscle and then withdraw the needle.

2). Prevention:
Only qualified needles are selected for treatment. The manipulation should be gentle and skillful, and the area to be punctured as well as the needle shaft should not be impacted or pressed by an external force. A comfortable posture that is suitable for the patient to accept during the length of the treatment should be chosen.

3. Broken Needle

1). Cause and Management:
This occurs occasionally due to a poor quality needle, corrosion of the needle shaft, violent manipulation, changing of the patient's posture, improper management of insertion or bent needle, or a sudden increase of electric current in electric acupuncture. Once a needle is broken, ask the patient not to change the posture so as to prevent the distal broken fragment of the needle from going deeper into the muscle. If the end of the broken fragment of the needle is above the skin, immediately press the skin around it with the thumb and index finger of one hand to expose the end. Then pull it out with a pair of forceps held with the other hand. If the broken fragment end is completely under the skin surface or in an organ of the body, perform a surgical operation to take it out and, if necessary, do the operation under X-ray examination.

2). Prevention:
A dependable method of preventing a needle from being broken is to make an inspection of the quality of the needle prior to treatment and to use only a smooth and flexible needle with its root fixed. The complete insertion of the needle shaft is not allowed. There should be 0.2-0.3 cun (6-9 mm) left above the skin in order to the broken needle can be easily removed if it happens.

4. Needling Fainting

1). Cause and Management:
This may be due to the patient's receiving acupuncture at the first time, nervous tension, fatigue, hunger, overreacting, prolonged illness, over-sweating, improper posture, or the operator's over-violent manipulation. It is manifested by a sudden feeling of oppression in the chest, nausea, dizziness and vertigo, followed by pallor complexion, cold extremities, sweating and deep and thready pulse. In extreme cases there may even be a lowering of blood pressure, unconsciousness or coma, cyanosis of the lips and finger nails, incontinence of urine and stools, etc. If the phenomena mentioned above happens, take the needle out immediately, keep the patient in a recumbent position, help them lie with the head lower and the feet higher, loosen the collar and the waistband, and give them fresh air.

For a milder case, advise the patient to take a short rest and drink some warm water or sugar solution. This should result in the disappearance of the patient's symptoms. For severe cases, it is necessary to press DU-26 Renzhong with the fingernail, puncture PC-6 Neiguan and apply moxibustion on ST-36 Zusanli, RN-17 Danzhong, RN-6 Qihai, DU-20 Baihui, etc. Through this treatment the patient, generally, will revive. If the patient has faint respiration, faint pulse and loss of consciousness, help the patient smell ammonia water, apply artificial respiration and inject cardiac stimulant. In a case with lowered blood pressure, administer per oral ephedrine and inject 50% glucose into to him / her, or give other emergency treatments according to conditions.

2). Prevention:
Give some assurance to the patient prior to treatment to help relieve his/her nervousness. Place him/her in a recumbent position if possible, avoid violent manipulation of the needle and advise the patient to have a short rest prior to treatment. If the patient is hungry, ask him or her to take some food before acupuncture. During manipulation of the needle, pay close attention to the patient's facial expression, and apply the management immediately whenever the prodromal symptoms and signs of fainting appear.

5. Hematoma

1). Cause and Management:
This may be due to injury of some small blood vessels by needling, which is sometimes unavoidable, especially when the tip of the needle is hooked. If there is a little oozing of blood or subcutaneous bleeding, give no treatment to it, but allow it to abate of its own accord. If there is a local, larger hematoma with distention that disturbs bodily activity, apply cold compress or press the punctured area to stop bleeding at first. Then, apply hot compress and massage to promote absorption of the extravasated blood.

2). Prevention:
In order to reduce the possibility of inducing hematoma due to acupuncture, strictly select the needle to be used, avoid blood vessels during insertion, and avoid twirling, lifting and thrusting the needle with large amplitude in areas having a rich distribution of blood vessels.

6. Sequel

1). Cause and Management:
After withdrawal of the needle, there may still remain an uncomfortable feeling such as soreness, pain, heaviness, distention and numbness, which are known as sequel. The sequel in acupuncture treatment is mainly due to violent manipulation or overly forceful stimulation. In milder cases, apply no management because it should disappear of its own accord within several ten minutes. For severe cases, massage the local area in co-ordination with moxibustion. This should result in its disappearance within 1-3 days.

2). Prevention:
Choose proper stimulation intensity and avoid shaking, lifting and thrusting the needle with large amplitude in areas containing nerve trunk distribution.

7. Traumatic Pneumothorax

1). Causes:
It is usually due to incorrect angle, depth and direction of puncture at points on the anterior or lateral chest, on the supraclavicular fossa, or on the upper border of the costal incisures of the sternum. This results in broken visceral pleura causing air to enter the thoracic cavity.

Possible common acupoints relating to injury of the lung by puncture: RN-22 Tiantu, KI-27 Shufu, ST-18 Rugen, LU-1 Zhonfu, SP-21 Dabao, HT-1 Jiquan, GB-21 Jianjing, SI-14 Jianwaishu, LR-14 Qimen, BL-11 Dashu, BL-12 Fengmen, BL-13 Feishu, BL-14 Jueyinshu, BL-15 Xinshu, BL-17 Geshu, BL-18 Ganshu, BL-19 Danshu, BL-20 Pishu, BL-43 Gaohuanshu, and EX-B-1 Dingchuan.

2). Manifestations:
Sudden occurrence of depressed feeling in the chest, chest pain, or even such shock manifestations as dysgenic respiration, tachycardia, cyanosis, sweating, and lowered blood pressure. Percussion and auscultation will find that the percussion note of the diseased side of the chest increases and the vesicular breath sound of the diseased side largely decreases or even disappears as compared with the healthy side. In severe cases, tracheal displacement to the healthy side of the chest may be found. X-ray examination of the chest helps the diagnosis. The manifestations usually occur just a short time after the puncture. However, in a few cases, they may occur several hours after the puncture.

3). Management:
Immediately upon finding the manifestations of traumatic pneumothorax, help the patient lie at a semi-reclining position. A mild case with only a small amount of air entering the thoracic cavity may be absolved of its own accord. In this case, observe the patient closely, administer some antiseptic to prevent infection, and prescribe some antitussive if the patient has cough. However, in severe cases with dyspnea, cyanosis or even shock, first aid measurement should be applied immediately. At first, insert a sterilized, thick and short syringe needle into the thoracic cavity through the 2nd intercostal space at the midclavicular line of the diseased side of the chest to make the air automatically leave the cavity. Alternatively, insert a pneumothorax

puncture needle which, through a flexible plastic line, is connected to a sterilized 50-100 ml syringe. Aspire the air, or apply some other exsufflation methods. Then, send the patient to the emergency room for further treatment.

4). Prevention:
The rule of correct depth, angle and direction of puncture should be obeyed strictly. Generally, the depth of perpendicular puncture at points at the anterior or lateral chest should not be more than 0.2-0.3 cun (referring to the proportional unit of the body). The depth of perpendicular puncture at points at the upper back should be less than 0.8 cun (referring to the proportional unit of the body compared with the middle finger). It is advisable to keep the depth of puncture at 0.3-0.5 cun (0.5-1 cm). For safety, all of these points should be punctured obliquely.

8. Injury to the Heart, Liver, Spleen, Kidney and Other Internal Organs

1). Cause:
It may be due to puncturing too deeply at the points on the body surface corresponding to the internal organs. Especially, when the patient has epitomegoly, splenomegaly or a full bladder, the liver, spleen or bladder is more easily injured by improper puncture.

Possible common acupoints relating to injury of the heart, liver, spleen, kidney, gallbladder, stomach, large and small intestines, and bladder: RN-15 Jiuwei, RN-14 Juque, RN-12 Zhongwan, RN-10 Xiawan, RN-6 Qihai, RN-5 Shimen, RN-4 Guanyuan, ST-25 Tianshu, ST-28 Shuidao, ST-29 Guilai, SP-15 Daheng, GB-24 Riyue, GB-25 Jingmen, GB-26 Daimai, LR-13 Zhangmen, BL-22 Sanjiaoshu, BL-23 Shenshu, BL-25 Dachangshu and BL-52 Zhishi.

2). Manifestations:
Impairment of the heart by puncture: Symptoms and signs due to bleeding from the heart may be caused and, in severe cases, manifestations caused by the filling of the pericardium with blood can be seen which may result in death.

Impairment of the liver or spleen by puncture: Heptalgia due to bleeding of the liver or the spleen which can sometimes spread to the back. If the bleeding is not stopped, abdominal pain, tension of the abdominal muscles, abdominal tenderness and rebounding pain may accompany.

Impairment of the kidney by puncture: Lumbago, tenderness over the kidney region during percussion or pressing, hematuria, or lowering of blood pressure or even shock due to profuse bleeding in severe cases.

Impairment of the gallbladder, bladder, stomach or intestines due to puncture: Signs of peritoneal irritation or even the manifestation of acute abdominal pain may be due to the leakage of some of the contents of these organs.

3). Management:
For mild case, apply expectant treatment and advise the patient to rest, allowing the impairment to be cured of its own accord. In severe cases, surgical operation may be needed.

4). Prevention:
Before giving puncture, you must have a sound knowledge of human anatomy as well as of the locations of internal organ projection on the body surface. You should also obey the manipulation rules, control the puncture depth, direction and angle strictly. When puncture points which are below the xiphoid process and near the epigastric region, it is proper to select needles about 1 cun long and pay attention to the patient's position. For example, when puncturing RN-15 Jiuwei, ask the patient to raise his or her chest. When puncturing points around the umbilicus and points at the lower abdomen, select 1.5-cun long needles and push the needle less than 1.5 cun. In cases with liver enlargement, gallbladder enlargement, or spleen enlargement, deep insertion is forbidden at LR-14 Qimen, GB-24 Riyue, LR-13 Zhangmen and ST-21 Liangmen. In cases of urine retention, deep insertion is forbidden when puncturing RN-2 Qugu, RN-3 Zhongji and RN-4 Guanyuan. If the stomach is enlarged due to overeating, it is forbidden to apply deep puncture at RN-13

Shangwan, RN-12 Zhongwan, and RN-10 Xiawan, as well as the points around them. In cases of intestinal adhesion or obstruction, it is forbidden to insert the needle through the abdominal wall into the abdominal cavity when puncturing points on the abdomen, such as ST-25 Tianshu, SP-15 Daheng, ST-28 Shuidao and ST-29 Guilai.

9. Injury of the Brain and Spinal Cord

1). Causes:
The bulb, pons and cerebellum can be injured when a needle enters the cranial cavity through the great occipital foramen. This condition is usually due to incorrect angle, direction, depth of puncture of the points on the region below the occiput along the posterior median line of the neck, such as DU-15 Yamen and DU-16 Fengfu, or of the points lateral to the line, such as GB-20 Fengchi and BL-10 Tianzhu. The spinal cord may be injured by deep puncture at the points located between the spinous process above the first lumbar vertebra, or by deep puncture at EX-B-2 Jiaji with the needle directed towards the inter-spinal area.

2). Manifestation and Treatment:
Injury of the brain: Headache, nausea and vomiting in mild cases, or loss of consciousness and even death in severe cases. Take out the needle immediately whenever finding a manifestation of the above symptoms and carefully check the condition of the patient. If the patient has gone into a coma, apply emergency treatment at once.

Injury of the spinal cord: Electrifying sensation radiating to the distal ends of the extremities in mild cases and temporary paralysis of the extremities in severe cases. Remove the needle immediately if any of the above symptoms manifest. Advise rest to the patient and give some expectant treatment to the patient. Usually the injury will be cured of its own accord.

3). Prevention:
When puncturing the points at the area mentioned above, strictly control the angle, direction and depth of needle insertion. In case

of electrifying sensations in the patient due to puncturing of these areas, never take it as a sign of good needling sensation and never apply a thrusting-lifting manipulation further, but remove the needle immediately.

CHAPTER FOUR
EAR ACUPUNCTURE, SCALP ACUPUNCTURE, & WRIST-ANKLE ACUPUNCTURE

1. Ear Acupuncture

I. ANATOMICAL NOMENCLATURE OF THE AURICULAR SURFACE

1. Helix: The portion of the auricular border that bends inward.
2. Helix crus: A part of the helix which transverses in the auricular cavity and extends into the auricular concha.
3. Auricular tubercle: The small tubercle on the posterior-superior aspect of the helix.
4. Helix cauda: The lower end of the helix, at the junction of the helix and earlobe.
5. Antihelix: The prominence opposite the helix.
6. Superior crus of the antihelix: The superior branch of the upper portion of the antihelix.
7. Interior crus of the antihelix: The inferior branch of the upper portion of the antihelix.
8. Triangular fossa: The triangular depression between the two crura of the antihelix.
9. Scapha: The groove between the helix and the antihelix.
10. Tragus: The valviform prominence in front of the auricle.
11. Supratragic notch: The notch between the superior border of the tragus and the crus of the helix.
12. Antitragus: The prominence on the lower part of the antihelix and opposite to the tragus.
13. Intertragic notch: The depression between the tragus and the antitragus.
14. Notch between antitragus and antihelix: The depression between antitragus and antihelix.
15. Ear lobe: The lowest portion of the auricle, containing no cartilage.
16. Cavum concha: The part of the auricular cavity, which is below the helix crus.
17. Cymba concha: The part of the auricular cavity, which is above the helix crus.
18. Orifice of the external auditory meatus: The orifice lying in the cavity of the conchae and covered by the tragus.

II. THE DISTRIBUTION RULE AND NOMENCLATURE OF THE EAR POINTS

1. The Distribution Rule

The auricle is a miniature of the entire human body; each part of the body has a corresponding auricular point or area. These points and areas reflect the physiological and pathological condition of the body, and can be stimulated to regulate dysfunction of their corresponding body parts. The distribution of the ear points and areas resembles an upside-down fetus in shape, and each part of the body has a corresponding ear point or area:

- The lobe corresponds to the head and face.
- The antitragus corresponds to the head and brain.
- The tragus corresponds to the throat and internal nose.
- The antihelix corresponds to the trunk.
- The superior crus of the antihelix corresponds to the lower limbs.
- The inferior crus of the antihelix corresponds to the buttocks.
- The scaphoid fossa corresponds to the upper limbs.
- The triangular fossa corresponds to the pelvic cavity and the internal genitals.
- The helix crus corresponds to the diaphragm.
- The peripheral crus of the helix corresponds to the digestive tract.
- The superior concha corresponds to the abdominal cavity.
- The inferior concha corresponds to the thoracic cavity.

2. Nomenclature of the Ear Points & Its Relation with Indications

There are 90 ear points listed in the International Standard of Auricular Points. They are classified into 4 types according to their nomenclature:

1). Sixty-one points named according to gross anatomy
These include points corresponding to the trunk, limbs, sensory organs, and internal organs. They are frequently used in the treatment of diseases of their corresponding body parts. For example, ear point Nose is used to rhinitis. Additionally, points among them corresponding to the zang-fu organs can also be used to treat diseases of the organs and tissues, which the zang-fu organs are closely related to. For example, the liver opens in the eye so ear point Liver can be used to treat eye disorders.

2). Twenty points named according to auricular anatomy
Indications of these points are usually determined according to clinical experience. For example, ear point Ear Apex is frequently used to clear heat, and ear point Groove of Dorsal Surface, to lower blood pressure.

3). Five points according to modern medicine
Indications of these points are determined according to modern medicine theory. For example, ear point Adrenal Gland can be used to allergic diseases.

4).Four points named according to TCM
Indications of these points are closely related to their names. For example, ear point Liver Yang can be used to disorders due to hyperactivity of liver yang.

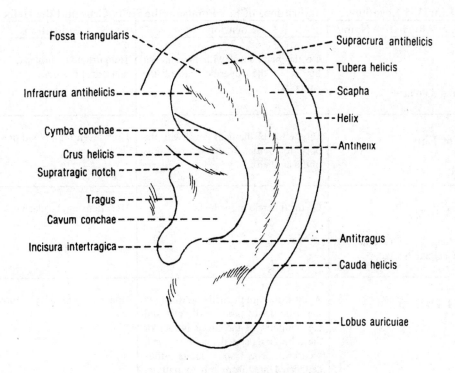

Fig. IV-1 Ear Geography

III.   LOCATIONS & INDICATIONS OF THE EAR POINTS

1. Locations and Indications of Ear Points on the Helix Crus and the Helix

Tab. IV-1 Locations and Indications of Ear Points on the Helix Crus and the Helix

Name & Alternative Name	Location	Indications
Cater of Ear Zero Point, Diaphragm, Neurosis	On the helix crus.	Hiccup, urticaria, cutaneous pruritis, infantile enuresis, and hemoptysis.
Rectum Lower Part of Rectum	On the helix close to the notch superior to the tragus and level with Large Intestine.	Constipation, diarrhea, prolapse of the anus, hemorrhoids.
Urethra	On the helix superior to Rectum, level with Urinary Bladder.	Frequent, painful, or dripping urination, retention of urine.
External Genitals	On the helix superior to Urethra, level with Sympathesis.	Testitis, ovaritis, epididymitis, vulvar or scrotal pruritis.

Tab. IV-1 Locations and Indications of Ear Points on the Helix Crus and the Helix

Name & Alternative Name	Location	Indications
Anus Hemorrhoid Point	On the helix level with the anterior border of the superior crus of the antihelix.	Hemorrhoids, prolapse of the anus, anal fissure.
Apex of Ear Tonsil 1	On the top of the helix level with the posterior border of the superior crus of the antihelix.	High fever, high blood pressure.
Liver Yang Liver Yang 1, Liver Yang 2, Lesser Occipital Nerve	On the tubercle of the helix.	Hypertension, headache.
Helix 1-Helix 6	A line drawn on the helix between the lower border of tubercle of helix and the midpoint of the lower border of the lobe is separated into five equal sections. The six points thus delineated are, from top to bottom, Helix 1, Helix 2, Helix 3, Helix 4, Helix 5, and Helix 6.	Upper respiratory infection, fever.

2.   Locations and Indications of Ear Points on the Scaphoid Fossa

Tab. IV-2   Locations and Indications of Ear Points on the Scaphoid Fossa

Name & Alternative Name	Location	Indications
Fingers Appendix 1	At the most upper section when the scaphoid fossa is separated into six equal horizontal sections.	Paronychia, pain and numbness of the fingers.
Wind Stream Allergy Area, Urticaria Point, Internal Tubercle	Between Fingers and Wrist.	Urticaria, cutaneous pruritis, allergic rhinitis.
Wrist	On the second section from the top of the scaphoid fossa.	Wrist pain or numbness.
Elbow Sleep Inducing Point	On the third section from the top of the scaphoid fossa.	Tennis elbow, elbow pain, insomnia.

Shoulder Appendix 2	On the fourth and fifth sections from the top of the scaphoid fossa.	Scapulohumeral periarthritis, shoulder pain.
Clavicle Nephritis Point, Appendix 3	On the lowest section from the top of the scaphoid fossa.	Scapulohumeral periarthritis.

3. Locations and Indications of Ear Points on the Antihelix

Tab. IV-3 Locations and Indications of Ear Points on the Antihelix

Name & Alternative Name	Location	Indications
Toes	On the posteriosuperior portion of the superior crus of the antihelix, close to the upper portion of the triangular fossa, posterior to Heel.	Paronychia, pain in the toes.
Heel	On the posteriosuperior portion of the superior crus of the antihelix, close to the upper portion of the triangular fossa, anterior to Toes.	Heel pain.
Ankle	Between Heel and Knee.	Pain of strain of the ankle joint.
Knee	On the middle one-third of the superior crus of the antihelix.	Swelling and pain of the knee joint.
Hip	On the lower one-third of the superior crus of the antihelix.	Sciatica, pain of the hip joint.
Buttock	On the posterior one-third of the inferior crus of the antihelix.	Sciatica, gluteal fasciitis.
Sciatic Nerve	On the anterior one-third of the inferior crus of the antihelix.	Sciatica.
Sympathesis	On the juncture between the terminus of the inferior crus of the antihelix and the helix.	Angina pectoris, gastrointestinal spasm, biliary colic, ureterolith, functional disturbance of the autonomic nervous system.

Tab. IV-3 Locations and Indications of Ear Points on the Antihelix

Name & Alternative Name	Location	Indications
Cervical Vertebrae Thyroid	At the lowest section when the body of the antihelix is separated into five equal horizontal sections.	Stiff neck, cervical spondylopathy.
Thoracic Vertebrae Mammary Gland	On the upper middle two sections when the body of the antihelix is separated into five equal horizontal sections.	Mastitis, chest pain, premenstrual swelling of the breasts.
Lumbosacral Vertebrae	On the upper two sections when the body of the antihelix is separated into five equal horizontal sections.	Pain in the lumbosacral region.
Neck	On the border of the concha anterior to Cervical Vertebrae.	Pain or swelling of the neck, stiff neck.
Chest	On the border of the concha anterior to Thoracic Vertebrae.	Pain in the chest, hypochondriac pain, fullness in the chest, mastitis.
Abdomen	On the border of the concha anterior to Lumbosacral Vertebrae.	Abdominal pain or distention, diarrhea, acute lumbar strain.

4. Locations and Indications of Ear Points on the Triangular Fossa

Tab. IV-4   Locations and Indications of Ear Points on the Triangular Fossa

Name & Alternative Name	Location	Indications
Shenmen	On the triangular fossa superior to the origin of the superior and inferior crura of the antihelix.	Insomnia, nightmares, pain, irritability, restlessness.
Pelvis Lumbago Point	On the triangular fossa inferior to the origin of the superior and inferior crura of the antihelix.	Pelvic inflammation, lumbago.
Middle Triangular Fossa Asthma Point, Hepatitis Point	On the middle one-third of the triangular fossa.	Asthma, hepatitis.

Internal Genitals Uterus, Essence Palace, Tian Gui	On the anterior one-third of the triangular fossa.	Dysmenorrhea, irregular menstruation, leukorrhagia, dysfunctional uterine bleeding, seminal emission, premature ejaculation, impotence.
Superior Triangular Fossa Blood Pressure Lowering Point	Anteriosuperior to the triangular fossa.	Hypertension.

5. Locations and Indications of Ear Points on the Tragus

Tab. IV-5 Locations and Indications of Ear Points on the Tragus

Name & Alternative Name	Location	Indications
External Ear Ear	Anterior to the notch superior to the tragus and close to the helix.	Tinnitus, deafness, pain of the ear.
External Nose Nose and Eye Cleaning Point, Hunger Point	Slightly anterior to the center of the external side of the tragus.	Rhinitis, nasal stuffiness, obesity.
Apex of Tragus Top of Tragus, Thirst Point	On the top of the upper eminence of the tragus.	Thirst, fever, toothache.
Adrenal Gland	On the top of the lower eminence of the tragus.	Hypotension, rheumatic arthritis, mumps, intermittent malaria, vertigo.
Throat	On the upper half of the medial side of the tragus.	Hoarseness, laryngalpharyngitis, tonsillitis.
Internal Nose	On lower half of the medial side of the tragus.	Rhinitis, paranasal sinusitis, epistaxis.

6.   Locations and Indications of Ear Points on the Antitragus

Tab. IV-6   Locations and Indications of Points on the Antitragus

Name & Alternative Name	Location	Indications
Apex of Antitragus Asthma-relieving Point, Parotid Gland	On the upper portion of the antitragus.	Asthma, parotitis, cutaneous pruritis, testitis, ovaritis, epididymitis.
Midpoint of Rim Brain Point, Brain Stem, Enuresis Point	On the midpoint between Apex of Antitragus and the notch between the antitragus and the antihelix.	Enuresis, Meniree's disease.
Occiput Dizziness Point	On the posteriosuperior portion of the external side of the antitragus.	Dizziness, headache, asthma, epilepsy, neurosis.
Temple Taiyang	On the middle portion of the external side of the antitragus.	Migraine.
Forehead	On the anteriosuperior portion of the external side of the antitragus.	Headache, dizziness, insomnia, nightmares.
Subcortex Ovary, Testicle, Excitation Point	On the medial side of the antitragus.	Pain, neurosis, testitis, ovaritis.

7.   Locations and Indications of Ear Points on the Cavum Concha

Tab. IV-7   Locations and Indications of Ear Points on the Cavum Concha

Name & Alternative Name	Location	Indications
Heart	On the center of the cavum concha.	Tachycardia, arrhythmia, angina pectoris, pulselessness, neurosis, hysteria, stomatoglossitis.
Lung Lung Point, Tuberculosis Point, Pulmonary Emphysema Point	On the cavum concha, peripheral to Heart.	Cough, asthma, fullness in chest, hoarseness, flat wart, constipation, cutaneous pruritis, urticaria, acne, and addiction to smoking or drinking.

Tab. IV-7   Locations and Indications of Ear Points on the Cavum Concha

Name & Alternative Name	Location	Indications
Trachea	On the cavum concha, between the foramen of the external auditory canal and Heart.	Cough, asthma.
Spleen	On the posteriosuperior portion of the cavum concha.	Abdominal pain, distention, diarrhea, constipation, poor appetite, dysfunctional uterine bleeding, leukorrhagia, and Meniere's disease.
Endocrine	On the base of the cavum concha, close to the notch between the tragus and the antitragus.	Dysmenorrhea, irregular menstruation, menopausal syndrome, acne.
Sanjiao	On the base of the cavum concha, superior to Endocrine.	Abdominal distention and pain, constipation.

8.   Locations and Indications of Ear Points on the Cymba Concha

Tab. IV-8   Locations and Indications of Ear Points on the Cymba Concha

Name & Alternative Name	Location	Indications
Liver	On the posterioinferior portion of the cymba concha.	Hypochondriac pain, vertigo, premenstrual syndrome, irregular menstruation, and hypertension.
Pancreas & Gallbladder	Between Liver and Kidney.	Gallstones, cholecystitis, biliary ascariasis, migraine, herpes zoster, otitis media, tinnitus, deafness, acute pancreatitis.
Kidney	On the cymba concha, inferior to the origin of the superior and inferior crura of the helix.	Lumbago, tinnitus, neurosis, asthma, enuresis, irregular menstruation, seminal emission, premature ejaculation.
Ureter	Between Kidney and Urinary Bladder.	Uretheral colic.

Tab. IV-8   Locations and Indications of Ear Points on the Cymba Concha

Name & Alternative Name	Location	Indications
Urinary Bladder	Between Kidney and Angle of Cymba Concha.	Urocystitis, enuresis, retention of urine, lumbago, sciatica, occipital headache.
Angle of Cymba Concha Prostate	On the anteriorsuperior angle of the cymba concha.	Prostatitis, urethritis.
Middle Cymba Concha Center of Umbilicus, Ascites, Drunk Point, Anterior Peritoneum, Posterior Peritoneum	On the center of the cymba concha.	Abdominal pain or distention, biliary ascariasis, parotitis.

9. Locations and Indications of Ear Points on the Peripheral Crus of the Helix

Tab. IV-9 Locations and Indications of Ear Points on the Peripheral Crus of the Helix

Name & Alternative Name	Location	Indications
Mouth	The anterior one-third of the area, inferior to the crus of the helix.	Facial paralysis, stomatitis, cholecystitis, gallstones, withdrawal syndrome.
Esophagus	The middle one-third of the area, inferior to the crus of the helix.	Esophagitis, esophagospasm, globus hystericus.
Cardiac	The posterior one-third of the area, inferior to the crus of the helix.	Cardiaospasm, neurogenic vomiting.
Stomach Pylorus, Gastroptosis Point	On the terminus of the crus of the helix.	Gastrospasm, gastritis, gastric ulcer, insomnia, toothache, indigestion.
Duodenum	The posterior one-third of the area superior to the curs of the helix.	Duodenal ulcer, cholecystitis, gallstones, pylorospasm.
Small Intestine	The middle one-third of the area superior to the curs of the helix.	Indigestion, abdominal distention or pain, tachycardia, arrhythmia.

Tab. IV-9 Locations and Indications of Ear Points on the Peripheral Crus of the Helix

Name & Alternative Name	Location	Indications
Large Intestine	The anterior one-third of the area superior to the curs of the helix.	Abdominal distention or pain, constipation, cough, acne.
Appendix	Between Small Intestine and Large Intestine.	Simple appendicitis, diarrhea.

10. Locations and Indications of Ear Points on the Earlobe

Tab. IV-10   Locations and Indications of Ear Points on the Earlobe

Name & Alternative Name	Location	Indications
Eye 1 Glaucoma Point	On the frontal surface of the earlobe, anterioinferior to the notch between the tragus and the antitragus.	Psuedomyopia.
Eye 2 Astigma Point	On the frontal surface of the earlobe, posterioinferior to the notch between the tragus and the antitragus.	Psuedomyopia.
Teeth Anesthesia Point for Dental Extraction, Toothache Point, Blood Pressure Raising Point	A grid of nine equal sections is delineated on the frontal surface of the earlobe by drawing three equidistant horizontal lines below the lower border of the cartilage of the notch between the tragus and the antitragus, and two equidistant vertical lines. The sections are numbered from anterior to posterior and from top to bottom. Teeth is located on the first section of the earlobe grid.	Toothache, periodontitis, hypotension.
Tongue Palate, Lower Palate	On the second section of the earlobe grid.	Glossitis, stomatitis.
Jaw Upper Jaw, Mandible	On the third section of the earlobe grid.	Toothache, dysfunction of the temperomandibular joints.
Anterior Lobe Anesthesia Point for Dental Extraction, Neurosis Point	On the fourth section of the earlobe grid.	Toothache, neurosis.

Tab. IV-10   Locations and Indications of Ear Points on the Earlobe

Name & Alternative Name	Location	Indications
Eye	On the fifth section of the earlobe grid.	Acute conjunctivitis, electric opthalmitis, psuedomyopia.
Internal Ear	On the sixth section of the earlobe grid.	Meniere's disease, tinnitus, deafness.
Cheek	On the border between the fifth and sixth section of the earlobe grid.	Peripheral facial paralysis, trigeminal neuralgia, acne, flat wart.
Tonsil Tonsil 4	On the eighth section of the earlobe grid.	Tonsillitis, pharyngitis.

11. Locations and Indications of Ear Points on the Dorsal Surface of the Auricle

Tab. IV-11   Locations and Indications of Ear Points on the Dorsal Surface of the Auricle

Name & Alternative Name	Location	Indications
Upper Ear Root Spinal Cord 1, Stagnation in the Interior	On the upper portion of the ear root.	Epistaxis.
Root of Ear Vagus	On the juncture of the dorsal surface of the auricle and the mastoid process, corresponding to the crus of the helix.	Cholecystitis, gallstones, biliary ascariasis, nasal obstruction, tachycardia, abdominal pain, diarrhea.
Lower Ear Root	On the lower portion of the ear root.	Hypotension.
Groove of Dorsal Surface Blood Pressure Lowering Point	The groove formed by the antihelix and its two branches on the dorsal surface of the auricle.	Hypertension, cutaneous pruritis.
Heart of Dorsal Surface	On the upper portion of the dorsal surface of the auricle.	Palpitation, insomnia, nightmares.
Spleen of Dorsal Surface	On the dorsal surface of the auricle, close to the teminus of the crus of the helix.	Epigastric pain, indigestion, poor appetite.

Tab. IV-11   Locations and Indications of Ear Points on the Dorsal Surface of the Auricle

Name & Alternative Name	Location	Indications
Liver of Dorsal Surface	On the dorsal surface of the auricle, lateral to Spleen of Dorsal Surface.	Cholecystitis, gallstones, hypochondriac pain.
Lung of Dorsal Surface	On the dorsal surface of the auricle, medial to Spleen of Dorsal Surface.	Cough, asthma, cutaneous pruritis.
Kidney of Dorsal Surface	On the lower portion of the dorsal surface of the auricle.	Dizziness, headache, neurosis.

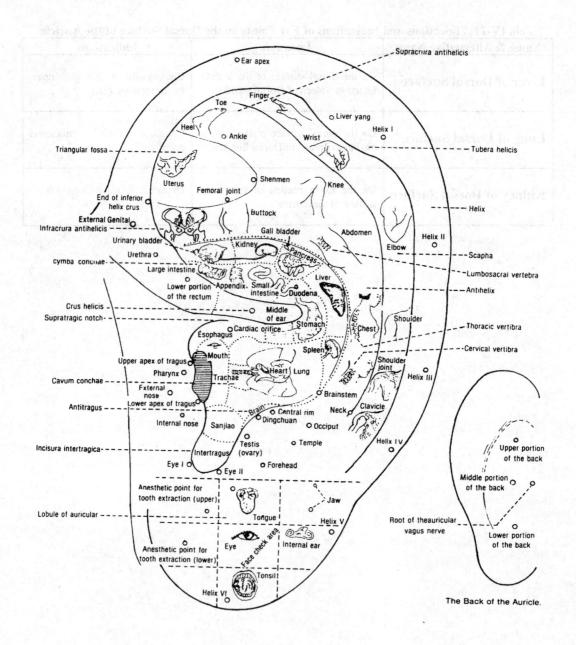

Fig. IV-2 Map of the Otopoints (1)

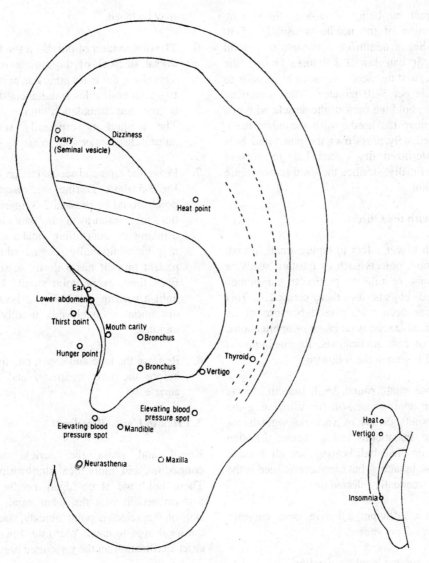

Fig. IV-3 Map of the Otopoints (2)

IV. COMMONLY-USED EAR THERAPEUTIC METHODS

1. Puncture with the Filiform Needle

Press the selected point with a needle handle or match stick to make a mark on it, and perform a routine local sterilization. Then, fix the auricle with the thumb and index finger of the one hand, and hold back the opposite aspect of the puncture area with the middle finger of the same

hand in order to control the depth of insertion of the needle and to relieve pain due to insertion. Then, hold the needle with the thumb, index and middle fingers of the other hand, and insert it into the marked spot as twirling it. The depth of insertion is just deep enough to piece through the cartilage but not through the skin of the opposite surface. Usually, manipulation of the needle is performed by twisting the needle but without lifting or thrusting. The stimulation intensity depends upon the patient's condition, inducing arrival of qi including heat, distention or mild pain but being tolerable to the patient. The retention of the needle is usually 15-30 minutes, but in treatment of chronic or painful diseases, it can last 1-2 hours. During the retention, twist the needle for several seconds to one minute per 5-10 minutes. When removing the needle, hold the back of the auricle with one hand, remove the needle with the other hand, and immediately press over the punctured hole with a sterilized dry cotton ball to prevent bleeding. Finally, sterilize the local region again with alcohol.

2. Tape with the Object

Tape with object refers to taping small, round, hard, smooth objects such as mustard seeds or small beans, or pills to particular ear points. The taped objects are then pressed.   This method has been widely used because of its safety, effectiveness, wide range of applications, and lack of contraindications. Its manipulation procedure is seen in the following:

1. Choose small, round, hard, smooth objects of the appropriate size for stimulating the ear points. Seeds of vaccaria segetalis or semen impatientis, mung beans, Liushen pills, or small ball bearings are all suitable for use in taping, but the vaccaria seed is the most frequently selected one.

2. Prepare sufficient adhesive tape, cut into pieces 0.5 cm square.

3. Apply routine local sterilization.

4. Hold the auricle with one hand, with the other hand use a detection probe (any instrument with a blunt point with the size of a match head) to press the auricular points hard enough to leave depressions. Tape the seeds, etc. to the positive points and press for several minutes until a needling sensation of heat, pain, or distention is achieved.

5. Tape the points in the order of upper to lower and frontal to dorsal, mainly tape the affected side.   Bilateral auricular points may be taped.

6. The distribution of points on the frontal and dorsal surfaces of the auricle is identical. Therefore, the main auricular points may be taped on both sides simultaneously in order to increase stimulation and effectiveness. The method is especially suitable for painful diseases or sore joints.

7. Leave the tape and seeds, etc. on the auricle for 3-5 days. During the retention, each point should be pressed 2-3 times each day, but for withdrawal of smoking, drug, drinking or controlling intake of food, it may be additionally pressed whenever the patient himself has a desire to smoke, etc. Each time, every point should be pressed until a needling sensation of heat, pain, or distention is achieved, usually for 3-5 minutes.

8. Remove the tape and seeds, etc. the evening before the next treatment and clean the auricle.

3. Prick to Cause Bleeding

Knead and press the auricle to induce congestion, and apply local sterilization strictly. Then, hold the three-edged needle or thick filiform needle with the other hand, prick the skin of the selected point quickly, and squeeze the local area to cause bleeding. Finally, apply strict sterilization on the punctured area again.

V. PRECAUTIONS

1. Strict sterilization should be given to prevent infection of the auricle, as severe infection in the auricle is very difficult to be controlled, and may lead to very bad outcome. In case of redness around the needle hole, or distention or pain in the auricle after puncture, which may be due to mild infection, timely and appropriate measures should be taken for it, such as applying 2.5% iodine or oral administration of anti-inflammation medicine. During summer, it is not advisable to embed the

skin needle for a long period, usually, within 1-3 days. The area with inflammation or cold injury is forbidden to be punctured, otherwise, chondric infection may occur.

2. In treatment of sprain or motor function impairment of the limbs, the therapeutic effect may be enhanced by patient's movement of the diseased limb during the treatment procedure in cooperation.

3. Otopuncture has various indications, which can be applied to treat any disease, which can be treated with the body puncture. But it still has its limitation. Therefore, in treating patients, usually, it is combined with other therapeutic methods in order to improve the effect.

4. Pay attention to preventing needling fainting because the stimulation caused by otopuncture may lead to serious pain. If the fainting occurs, it may be treated with the same way as in body puncture. It should be carefully applied or even forbidden temporally to the pregnant, the aged, or the very weak patients.

2. Scalp Acupuncture

Scalp acupuncture is a therapeutic method by needling the specific areas or lines of the scalp. There are many schools about it. Out of them, the acupuncture method based on combination of the acupuncture method of TCM and the theory of location of corticocerebral function of modern medicine is more popular in clinics.

I. THE CHARACTERISTICS & GENERAL INDICATIONS

1. The selected puncture area is not acupoints, but the stimulation lines on the scalp.

2. The manipulation is usually quick and constant twisting method without many changes.

3. The area or line to be punctured is usually at the side opposite to that with clinical signs and symptoms.

4. It is mainly indicated in diseases originated at the brain, such as paralysis due to apoplexy, numbness, aphonia, dizziness, chorea, and Parkinson's disease, as well as lumbago, pain of the leg, nocturia, or various neuralgia.

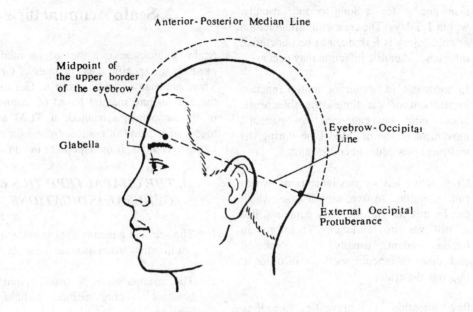

Fig. IV-4 the Reference Line on the Scalp

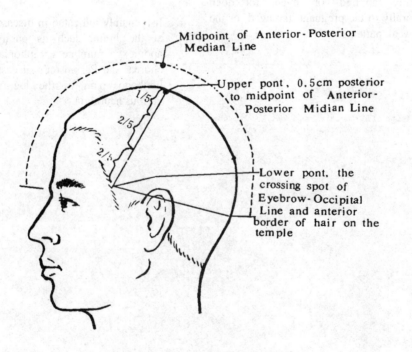

Fig. IV-5 The Motor Area

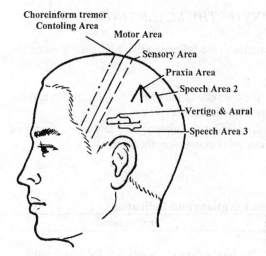

Fig. IV-6 In Lateral View

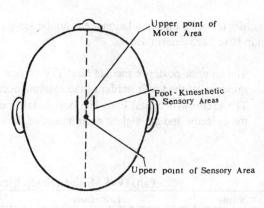

Fig. IV-7 In Vertex View

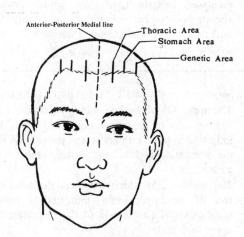

Fig.IV-8 In Anterior View

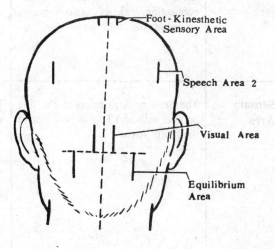

Fig. IV-9 In Posterior View

II. LOCATIONS & INDICATIONS OF THE SCALP LINES

In order to locate the stimulation areas on the scalp precisely, the following two reference lines on the scalp have been determined:

- The anterior-posterior median line: The vertical line connecting the center of the glabella and the midpoint of the lower border of the external occipital protuberance.
- The eyebrow-occipital line: The horizontal line connecting the midpoint of the upper border of the eyebrow and the highest prominence of the external occipital protuberance.

Tab. IV-6 Modern Scalp Lines: Locations and Indications

Name	Location	Indications
Motor Area	Its upper point is 0.5 cm posterior to the midpoint of the anterioposteior median line, and its lower point at the junction of the eyebrow-occipital line and the temporal hair line (if the temporal hair line is not obvious, the point 0.5 cm anterior to the junction of the eyebrow-occipital line and the line ascending vertically from the midpoint of the zygomatic arch is taken as the lower point). The line connecting these two points represents the motor area.	The Motor Area is equally divided into 5 parts: • The upper 1/5 of the line, which represents the motor area of the lower limbs and trunk, is indicated in paralysis of the contralateral lower limb; • The middle 2/5, which represent the motor area of the upper limbs, indicated in paralysis of the contralateral upper limb and: • The lower 2/5, which represent the motor area of the face (also termed Speech Area), indicated in central contrallateral facial paralysis, aphasia (partly or whole losing speech ability, but remaining the ability to understand the language), salivation, and dysphonia.
Sensory Area	The Sensory Area refers to the line parallel with and 1.5 cm posterior to the Motor Area.	The Sensory Area is equally divided into 5 parts too: • The upper 1/5 of the line, which represents the sensory area of the lower limbs and trunk, is indicated in pain, numbness and paresthesia of the contralateral loin and lower limb, and vertex pain; • The middle 2/5, which represent the sensory area of the upper limbs, indicated in pain, numbness and paresthesia of the contralateral upper limb and; • The lower 2/5, which represent the sensory area of the face, indicated in numbness of the contralateral face, and migraine, trigeminal neuralgia, and arthritis of the temporomandibular joint of the opposite side.

Tab. IV-6 Modern Scalp Lines: Locations and Indications

Name	Location	Indications
Choreiform Tremor Control Area	The line parallel with and 1.5 cm anterior to the Motor Area.	Chorea, Parkinson's disease.
Vertigo & Aural Area	The line with its midpoint 1.5 cm above the apex of the auricle, extending horizontally 2 cm forward and backward.	Vertigo, tinnitus, decrease of the hearing ability.
Speech Area 2	The straight line beginning at the point 2 cm inferioposterior to the parietal eminence and extending 3 cm backward, parallel with the anteroposterior median line.	Anemia aphasia.
Speech Area 3	The line extending from the midpoint of the Vertigo & Aural Area, extending horizontally 4 cm backward.	Sensory aphasia (disorder in comprehension of speech).
Praxia Area	The three lines beginning from the parietal eminence, of the them extending vertically downward 3 cm and the others extending respectively anteriorly and posteriorly 3 cm at an angle of 40 degree with the former line.	Apraxia (the muscular power and tension and basic motor are normal but there is disturbance in skill ability such as disability to undo a button and tie a bootlace).
Foot-Kinesthetic Sensory Area	The straight lines, beginning from the points 1 cm respectively lateral to the midpoint of the anteroposterior median line, extending 3 cm backward, parallel with the anteroposterior median line.	Paralysis, pain and numbness of the contrallateral lower limb, acute sprain in the lumbar region, nocturnal enuresis, prolapse of the uterus, cortical polyuria.
Visual Area	The two straight lines, beginning from the point 1 cm lateral to the external occipital protuberance and extending 4 cm upward, parallel with the anteroposterior median line.	Cortical disturbance of vision.

Tab. IV-6 Modern Scalp Lines: Locations and Indications

Name	Location	Indications
Equi-librium Area	The two straight lines, beginning from the point 3.5 cm lateral to the occipital protuberance and extending 4 cm downward, parallel with the anterioposterior median line.	Cerebellar disturbance of equilibrium.
Stomach Area	The two lines, respectively beginning from the cross point of the straight line ascending vertically from the pupil and the hair line, extending 2 cm upward, and parallel with the anterioposterior median line.	Stomachache, uncomfortable feeling in the upper abdomen.
Thoracic Area	The two lines, respectively between the Stomach Area and anteriorposterior median line, extending from the hair line upward 2 cm and downward 2 cm, parallel with the anteriorposterior median line.	Bronchial asthma, oppressed feeling in the chest, pain in the chest, palpitation.
Genetic Area	The two lines, respectively beginning from the corner of the forehead and extending upward 2 cm, parallel with the anteiorposterior median line.	Functional metrorrhagia, pelvic inflammation, leukorrhagia, prolapse of uterus.

Appendix: STANDARD NOMENCLATURE OF CHINESE SCALP ACUPUNCTURE LINES

(Put forward in The Complete Works on Chinese Acupuncture & Moxibustion, complied by Wang Xuetai, et al.)

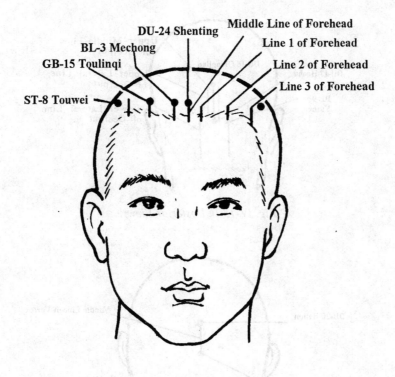

DU-24 Shenting
Middle Line of Forehead
BL-3 Mechong
Line 1 of Forehead
GB-15 Toulinqi
Line 2 of Forehead
Line 3 of Forehead
ST-8 Touwei

Fig. IV-10 In Anterior View

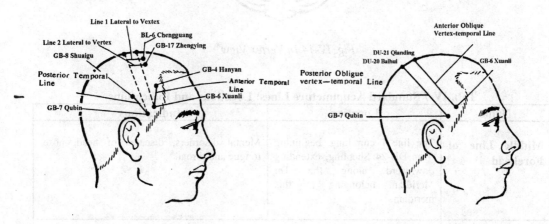

Line 1 Lateral to Vextex
BL-6 Chengguang
Line 2 Lateral to Vertex
GB-17 Zhengying
GB-8 Shuaigu
GB-4 Hanyan
Posterior Temporal Line
Anterior Temporal Line
GB-6 Xuanli
GB-7 Qubin

Anterior Oblique Vertex-temporal Line
DU-21 Qianding
DU-20 Baihui
GB-6 Xuanli
Posterior Obligue vertex—temporal Line
GB-7 Qubin

Fig.IV-11In Lateral View A

Fig. IV-12 In Lateral View B

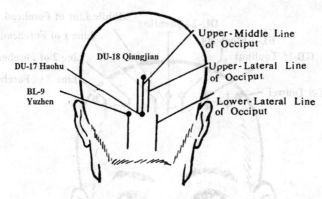

Fig. IV-13 In Posterior View

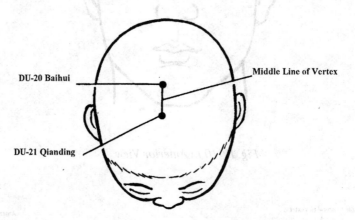

Fig. IV-14 In Vertex View

Tab. IV-7 Standard Acupuncture Lines: Locations and Indications

Name	Location	Indications
Middle Line of Forehead	The line 1 cun long, beginning from DU-24 Shenting, extending downward along the Du Meridian, belonging to this meridian.	Mental disorders, diseases of head, nose, tongue and throat.
Line 1 Lateral to Forehead	The line 1 cun long, beginning from BL-3 Meichong, extending downward along the Bladder Meridian, belonging to this meridian.	Disorders of the Upper Jiao, including lung, bronchus, and heart.

Tab. IV-7 Standard Acupuncture Lines: Locations and Indications

Name	Location	Indications
Line 2 Lateral to Forehead	The line 1 cun long, beginning from GB-15 Toulinqi, extending sprightly downward along the Gallbladder Meridian, belonging this meridian.	Disorders of the middle-jiao including spleen, stomach, liver, gallbladder and pancreas.
Line 3 Lateral to Forehead	The line 1 cun long, beginning from the 0.75 cun medial to ST-8 Touwei, extending straightway downward, belonging to the Gallbladder and Stomach Meridians.	Disorders of the lower-jiao, including kidney, urinary bladder, and genetic system.
Middle Line of Vertex	The line beginning from DU-20 Baihui to DU-21 Qianding, belonging to the Du Meridian.	Disorders of waist and lower limbs, such as paralysis, numbness and pain, cortical polyuria, prolapse of anus, infantile nocturnal enuresis, hypertension, and pain in the vertex.
Anterior Oblique Line of Vertex-Temporal	The line beginning from DU-21 Qianding obliquely to GB-6 Xuanli, passing across the Du, Bladder and Gallbladder Meridians.	When the line is divided equally into 5 portions, the upper 1/5 for dyskinesia of the lower limb such as paralysis and arthralgia; the middle 2/5, for dyskinesia of the upper limbs, such as paralysis, asthenia and arthralgia; and the lower 2/5, for disorders of head and face such as cortical paralysis, aphasia, salivation and cerebral arteriosclerosis.
Posterior Oblique Line of Vertex-Temporal	The line beginning from DU-20 Baihui oblique to GB-7 Qubin, 1 cun posterior to and parallel with the Anterior Oblique Line of Vertex-Temporal, passing across the DU, Bladder and Gallbladder Meridians.	When the line is equally divided into 5 portions, the upper 1/5 for sensory disorders of the lower limbs; the middle 5/2, for sensory problems of the upper limbs; and the lower 2/5, for sensory troubles of face.
Line 1 Lateral to Vertex	The line, 1.5 cun long, 1.5 cun lateral to Middle Line of Vertex, beginning from BL-6 Chengguang, extending backward along the Bladder Meridian, and belonging to the Meridian.	Disorders of waist and legs such as paralysis, numbness, and pain.

Tab. IV-7 Standard Acupuncture Lines: Locations and Indications

Name	Location	Indications
Line 2 Lateral to Vertex	The line 1.5 cun long, 0.75 cun lateral the Line 1 Lateral to Vertex, beginning from GB-17 Zhengying backwards along the Gallbladder meridian, and belonging to this Meridian.	Disorders of shoulder, upper arm, and hand, including paralysis, numbness and pain.
Anterior Temporal Line	The line from GB-4 Hanyan to GB-6 Xuanli, belonging to the Gallbladder Meridian.	Migraine, aphasia, Bell's palsy, disorders of the mouth.
Posterior Temporal Line	The from GB-8 Shaigu to GB-7 Qubin, belonging to the Gallbladder Meridian.	Migraine, vertigo, deafness, tinnitus.
Upper-Middle Line of Occiput	The line from DU-18 Qiangjian to DU-17 Haohu, belonging to the Du Meridian.	Eye problems, pain in the back.
Upper-Lateral Line of Occiput	The line 0.5 cun lateral and parallel to the Upper-Middle Line of Occiput, belonging to the Bladder Meridian.	Cortical disturbance of vision, cataract, myopia, some other eye disorders, Hong Kong foot, lumbar muscle strain.
Lower-Lateral Line of Occiput	The line from BL-9 Yuzhen to BL-10 Tianzhu, belonging to the Bladder Meridian.	Disorders due to problems of cerebellum, such as disequilibrium, and pain of the back and head.

III. MANIPULATION

1. Insertion of the Needle

Select a sterilized filiform needle 1.5-2.5 cun long and at the gauge No. 26-28. Insert the needle obliquely at an angle of 30 degree into the scalp. Then, push the needle horizontally under the scalp along the direction of stimulation to the depth needed. In pushing, if the patient feels pain or there is resistance feeling around the needle, the needle should be withdrawn to the subcutaneous layer for another try in different angle.

2. Manipulating the Needle

After the needle is inserted to a certain depth, make the joints of shoulder, elbow and wrist and the thumb at the fixed position, keep the index finger at half flexion, and hold the needle handle with the palmar side of the tip portion of the thumb and radial side of the tip portion of the index finger, twirl the needle by continuous and alternate flexion and extension of the metacarpal phalangeal joint of the index finger at sequence of about 200 times per minute, every time having about two clockwise and anti-clockwise turns, for 0.5-1 minute. Then, retain the needle for 30 minutes. During the retention, twirl the needle in the way mentioned above once per 5-10 minutes.

For treatment of motor function impairment, during twirling or retaining the needle, ask the patient's relative to help the patient move his/her affected limb or ask the patient to do so by himself so as to enhance the therapeutic effect by strengthening functional exercise of the affected limbs. Generally, through the stimulation for 3-5 minutes, if the patient has reaction at the affected area, including heat, numbness, distention, cold or trembling, the patient may get a good therapeutic effect.

The following manipulation method is welcome by some acupuncture specialists. After insertion of the needle, various reinforcing and reducing manipulations, including those by lifting and thrusting the needle, twirling and rotating the needle, puncturing along and against the direction of the course of the meridian, rapid and slow insertion and withdrawal of the needle, and keeping the needle hole open or close, as well as the qi-entering reinforcing manner and the qi-withdrawing reducing manner, are applied. All manipulations mentioned above, except qi-withdrawing reducing manner and qi entering reinforcing manner, is the same as in body puncture.

Qi-withdrawing method in scalp puncture refers to the following needling manipulation. The needle is inserted to the selected line at an angle of 15 degree to the subfascial layer, and push horizontally along the layer about 1 cun. Then, thrust the needle quickly for about 0.1 cun and lift it slowly to the original place. Repeat this course for several times to induce and strengthen needling sensation.

Generally, scalp acupuncture is done once every other day or every 3-5 days, 10 treatments are taken as a therapeutic course, and next course can be done after an interval of 5-7 days.

IV. PRECAUTIONS

1. As the hair on the head makes difficulty in sterilization, a strict sterilization should be given so as to prevent infection.

2. As the stimulation caused by scalp puncture is strong, special attention should be paid to preventing needling fainting. The patient's expression or reaction to the puncture should be closely observed, and the needle should be withdrawn immediately if the patient feels nausea and discomfort in chest, has sweating, and his/her complexion turns pale. In case of fainting, it should be treated in the same way as in the body puncture.

3. To patients with cerebral vascular hemorrhage, scalp puncture should not be done until the patient's condition and blood pressure are improved. It is not advisable to do scalp puncture to patients who have high fever or heart failure.

3. Wrist-Ankle Acupuncture

Wrist-ankle acupuncture is a therapeutic method based on channel theory and neurology, in which six pairs of points proximal to the wrist and ankle are punctured in order to treat disease of the corresponding areas. It is characterized by relatively few puncture points, a wide range of applications and simplicity in operation.

I. LOCATION & INDICATIONS OF WRIST-ANKLE ACUPUNCTURE

There are 12 stimulating points in the wrist-ankle acupuncture in total. The points of the wrist acupuncture are located at the circle about two finger-breadths proximal to the transverse crease of the wrist, which are, in order, termed upper 1-6 from the ulnar side to the radial side of the palmar surface and then from the radial side to the ulnar side of the dorsal surface; the points of the ankle acupuncture are located at the circle about 3 finger-breadths proximal to the highest points of the internal and external condyles, which are termed lower 1-6 in the order circling the ankle from the internal side of the Achilles tendon. (See Fig. IV-15 & 16)

Tab. IV-8 Wrist and Ankle Acupuncture: Locations and Indications

Name	Location	Indications
Upper 1	Between the internal side of the ulna and the tendon of ulnar flexor muscle of wrist, two fingerbreadths proximal to the transverse crease of the wrist.	Foreheadache, eye disorders, nasal disorder, facial swelling, toothache, trigeminal neuralgia, bronchitis, gastrointestinal disorders, heart diseases, dizziness, insomnia, hypertension.
Upper 2	Between the tendon palmaris longus and tendon of radial flexor muscle, two fingerbreadths proximal to the transverse crease of the wrist.	Pain of temple, toothache, submandibular swelling and pain, chest distress and pain, asthma, pain in the center of palm, numbness of fingertip.
Upper 3	At palmar surface, radial to the radial artery, two fingerbreadths proximal to the transverse crease of the wrist.	Hypertension, chest pains.
Upper 4	At radial border of the radius with the palm facing inward, two fingerbreadths proximal to the transverse crease of the wrist.	Headache, ear disorder, functional disorder of mandibular articulation, shoulder joint pain, chest pain.
Upper 5	At center of dorsal wrist, between the radius and ulna, two fingerbreadths proximal to the transverse crease of the wrist.	Pain of the temple, shoulder pain, numbness of upper limb, paralysis, tremble, chorea, pain of joints of elbow, wrist and finger.

Tab. IV-8 Wrist and Ankle Acupuncture: Locations and Indications

Name	Location	Indications
Upper 6	At lateral border of the ulna, two fingerbreadths proximal to the transverse crease of the wrist.	Pain of back, occipital pain and vertex pain, pain of neck, chest, spinal column and the area near it.
Lower 1	At interior border of the Achilles tendon, 3 fingerbreadths proximal to the highest points of the internal and external condyles.	Pain and distention of upper abdomen, pain around umbilicus, dysmenorrhea, leukorrhagia, enuresis, pruritus vulvae, pain in heel.
Lower 2	At posterior border of interior side of the shinbone, 3 fingerbreadths proximal to the highest points of the internal and external condyles.	Heptalgia, pain in lateral side of the abdomen, allergic enteritis.
Lower 3	1 cm medial to the anterior spine of the tibia, 3 fingerbreadths proximal to the highest points of the internal and external condyles.	Pain in the medial border of knee joint.
Lower 4	At posterior border of the tibia and anterior border of the fibula, 3 fingerbreadths proximal to the highest points of the internal and external condyles.	Pain in knee joint, pain of quadriceps femoralis, numbness of lower limbs, hypersensitivity, paralysis, tremor, chorea, pain of toe joint.
Lower 5	At posterior border the fibula, 3 fingerbreadths proximal to the highest points of the internal and external condyles.	Pain of the hip joint, sprain of the ankle joint.
Lower 6	At lateral border of Achilles tendon, 3 fingerbreadths proximal to the highest points of the internal and external condyles.	Acute lumbar sprain, lumbar muscle strain, sciatic neuralgia, pain of gastrocnemius, pain of anterior planta.

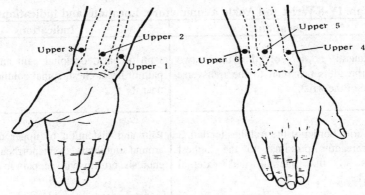

Fig IV-15 Wrist Acupuncture Points

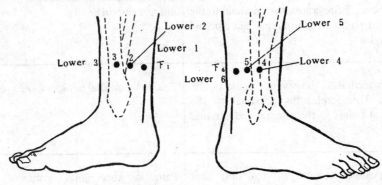

Fig. IV-16 Ankle Acupuncture Points

II. MANIPULATION

Select 1.5-2 cun No. 28-30 filiform needles. Sterilize the point to be punctured in the routine way, fix the skin around the area with the left hand, and hold the needle handle with the thumb, index and middle fingers of the right hand, the thumb being lower than the other fingers. Then, swiftly insert the needle at a 30-degree angle formed by the skin surface and the needle shaft, through the skin. Then, horizontally push the needle along the superficial layer of subcutaneous tissue. If soft sensation under the needle is felt and no pain is caused to the patient, this manipulation is better. If the patient complains of soreness, numbness, distention or pain, it indicates that the needle has been inserted too deeply into the deeper layer of the subcutaneous tissue or the needle is along a vertical straight line. In this case, the needle should be withdrawn to the superficial layer of the subcutaneous tissue and pushed shallowly for another try, or, the direction of insertion should be changed slightly for another try. Generally, the needle is pushed for about 1.2 cun and the direction of the needle tip is upward in puncture. However, if the disease is located at the wrist, ankle or the part distal to the wrist or ankle, the direction of needling may be downward. Never twirl, rotate, lift or thrust the needle after insertion. Retain the needle for 30 minutes, but in chronic cases, retention of the needle may be prolonged properly. This acupuncture is done once daily or every other day. One therapeutic course requires ten treatments.

CHAPTER FIVE
TREATMENT PRINCIPLES

Zhenjiu therapy takes the theories of TCM as guidance to treat patients with acupuncture and moxibustion based on differentiation of syndromes. The general principles of treatment are worked out under the guidance of the holistic concept and differentiation of syndromes. They are of universal significance in decision of treating methods and point prescriptions.

I. REGULATION OF YIN AND YANG

The occurrence of any disease is, fundamentally speaking, due to the relative imbalance of yin and yang. Namely, either preponderance or discomfiture of yin and yang disturbs the normal inter-consuming-supporting relationship between them. Regulation of yin and yang is therefore a fundamental principle in clinical treatment. It is well known that how to regulate yin and yang is most important in Zhenjiu treatment.

Yang in excess makes yin suffer and yin in excess makes yang suffer. Excessive heat (yang) is likely to injure yin essence, while excessive cold (yin) is likely to damage yang qi. In treatment, we should reduce excessive heat or expel cold through the methods of "eliminating the excess" and "reducing the preponderance". On regulating the preponderance of yin or yang, attention should be paid to the condition whether a corresponding yin or yang deficiency exists. If one is deficient, consideration should be given to yang reduction and yin reinforcement, yin reduction and yang reinforcement, or both dispelling cold (yin) and warming yang simultaneously.

Yin in deficiency fails to control yang, manifested by deficiency heat syndrome and yang hyperactivity due to yin deficiency. Yang in deficiency fails to control yin, as shown in deficiency cold syndrome and excess of yin due to yang deficiency. Therefore, hyperactivity of yang due to yin deficiency should be treated by strengthening yin to control yang, while cold (yin) due to yang deficiency should be treated by reinforcing yang to control yin. If they are both deficient, yin and yang should be reinforced simultaneously. In treatment of diseases marked by yin or yang deficiency, try to achieve yang from yin and achieve yin from yang, because they are interdependent. For example, RN-4 Guanyuan, a point of the yin meridian and one of the Front-Mu Points (belonging to yin due to their location on the front of the trunk) is frequently used to treat yang deficiency. BL-18 Ganshu, a point of the yang meridian and one of the Back-Shu Points (belonging to yang due to their location on the back of the trunk) is often used to replenish liver yin deficiency.

Yin and yang are conferred the general principle for differentiation of syndromes. In a broad sense, "relieving deficiency by the tonifying method, reducing excess, dispelling cold by the warming method, nutrient and defensive qi regulation, and qi and blood promotion" all fall into the aspect of regulation of yin and yang. Zhenjiu therapy is to apply different techniques of manipulations to points to treat diseases by means of regulating yin and yang.

II. STRENGTHENING THE BODY RESISTANCE & ELIMINATING THE PATHOGENIC FACTORS

The course of a disease is actually the process of struggle between the antipathogenic factors (Zheng qi) and pathogenic factors (Xie qi). Mobilizing the antipathogenic factors to defeat the pathogenic factors is the right way to cure the disease. Therefore, strengthening the body resistance is to reinforce the antipathogenic qi and build up health. Once the body resistance against disease is strengthened, the pathogenic factors are eliminated. Once the pathogenic factors are removed, the body resistance will be reinforced. Since they are closely related to each other, strengthening the body resistance is baneful to dispelling the pathogenic factors and vice versa.

Clinically, the condition of the pathogenic factors and antipathogenic factors should be carefully observed, upon which, strengthening the body resistance first or dispelling the pathogenic first can be determined. For patients with weak body resistance, strengthening antipathogenic factor is considered first. For patients with excessive pathogenic factors but

body resistance not yet damaged, the prime task is to eliminate the pathogenic factors. But for patients with weak body resistance and excessive pathogenic factors as well, both methods should be employed simultaneously. Try to distinguish what is primary from what is secondary. For those with weak body resistance priority should be placed on building body resistance and do something to get rid of the pathogenic factors, and vice versa.   When the patient is in a relatively critical condition attacked by excessive pathogenic factors, and the body resistance is too weak, even the pathogenic factors are not eliminated, the body resistance should be strengthened first and then consideration is given to remove the pathogenic factor. If the patient is in a very poor condition with excessive pathogenic factors but with weak body resistance, eliminate the pathogenic factors first, and then strengthen the body resistance.

III. DISTINGUISHING THE PRIMARY FROM THE SECONDARY

The conception of the primary and the secondary are relative to each other involving different meanings. In terms of the antipathogenic factors and pathogenic factors, the former is the primary, and the latter is the secondary. Judged by the etiology and manifestation, the etiology is the primary, and the manifestation is the secondary. As to the localisation of a lesion, the internal portion is the primary, and the external is the secondary. As for the clinical course of a disease the original is the primary, while the complication is the secondary. This concept represents the two opposite aspects of one entity during the course of a disease. The symptom is generally the phenomenon and the secondary aspect; the root cause is generally the nature and the primary aspect.

Clinically, a disease should be assessed according to such different situations of the primary, the secondary, the root cause, the symptoms, the acute, and the chronic so as to ascertain the main aspect of the contradictions, and thus treated accordingly. Under general circumstances, the primary or root cause should be found first, but if the symptoms are acute, they should be treated first. If the symptoms and root cause are both serious, they should be taken into account at the same time.

Trying to find out the primary or root cause is of importance. In clinic, the nature and the primary aspect of a disease should be well commanded so as to treat the root cause. Some diseases, although their symptoms are different, the etiology and pathogenesis are the same, so they can be treated by the same method. For example, in case of sore throat due to yin deficiency of the kidney and low back pain due to yin deficiency of the kidney, the treatment to nourish the kidney yin is adopted. This is called "treating different diseases with the same method". For some other diseases, although their symptoms are alike, the etiology and pathogenesis are different, different methods therefore should be used to treat the root cause. For example, headache due to liver yang hyperactivity should be treated by nourishing yin to reduce yang, but headache caused by both qi and blood deficiency should be treated by reinforcing qi and blood. However, headache caused by invasion of the meridians by wind-cold must be treated by diminishing wind and cold. This is called "treating the same disease with different methods".

Under certain circumstances, symptoms may be critical, if not treated immediately, they shall affect the treatment of the root cause or perhaps cause death. In this case it is necessary to observe the principle of "treating the symptoms first when they are acute, and treating the root cause when these symptoms are relieved". For example, if a patient with chronic cough and asthma catches common cold, accompanied with fever and aversion to cold, his/her common cold should be treated first because it is the acute aspect. After the common cold is relieved, chronic cough and asthma should be treated because they are the primary aspects. But if the primary and secondary aspects both are serious or urgent, they must be treated at the same time.

It is also important to pay attention to prevention principle. It includes prevention before the attack of a disease and prevention from deterioration after occurrence of a disease. For example,

regular moxibustion on ST-36 Zusanli, an important tonifying point, can strengthen one's constitution and body resistance, and help him/her keep from diseases, thus moxibustion to ST-36 Zusanli is often recommended for prevention of many diseases. Moreover, importance is attached to early diagnosis and treatment of a disease for fear of its negative development. During the prevention and treatment of diseases, doctors are required to know the laws of their occurrence and development, and the ways of their transmission. If a patient has liver qi stagnation, for example, ST-36 Zusanli is frequently employed because the liver disease may transmit to the spleen and ST-36 Zusanli has the function of strengthening the spleen, preventing it from attack by pathogenic factors from the liver.

IV. CONSIDERING CLIMATIC & SEASONAL CONDITIONS, GEOGRAPHICAL LOCATIONS & THE INDIVIDUAL CONDITIONS

The climatic and seasonal conditions, geographical locations, patient's age, constitution and others must be taken into consideration to determine an appropriate method in Zhenjiu treatment.

1. Climatic and Seasonal Conditions

In accordance with the characteristics of climate and seasons, appropriate therapeutic methods are used. For example, in the treatment of wind-cold syndrome of common cold, long time and strong force of moxibustion may be applicable in winter, but only mild moxibustion with short course may be applicable in summer. Generally, in spring and summer, shallow acupuncture is applied, and in autumn and winter, deep puncture is preferred.

In addition, the acupuncture time is also important. For example, treatment of irregular menstruation and dysmenorrhea is usually given 5~7 days before the menstrual period.

2. Geographical Locations

The appropriate therapeutic methods should be determined according to different geographical locations. Climate and life style vary in different regions, so do the physiological activities and pathological changes, therefore, the methods of treatment should be different. For example, more attention should be paid to removing dampness in treating patients in the region with big humidity, especially, if they were used to live in the region with dry whether.

3. Individual Conditions

Treatment is also based on age, sex, constitution and sensitivity to Zhenjiu treatment.

1). Pay attention to sex
Men and women are different in physiology; women have menstruation, pregnancy and puerperal problems, so the points may be different when treatment is given to different sexes.   For example, in treatment of vomiting, LI-4 Hegu is frequently selected in men, but it is prohibited in pregnant women.

2). Pay attention to age
People of different ages are different in physiology and pathology, so treatment methods may be different when treatment is given to people of different ages. For example, in treatment of poor appetite, soothing the liver is often employed as an assistant method for adults, because poor appetite, a kind of spleen disorder, may be induced by liver qi stagnation due to emotional depression, but it is not employed for infantile because infantile are usually free from emotional depression.

3). Pay attention to body constitution
People of different constitutions are different in physiology and pathology, so treatment methods may be different when treatment is given to people of different constitutions. For example, in treatment of diarrhea, moxibustion is frequently used in patients with yang deficiency constitution, but it is not used in patients with the constitution of yin deficiency with fire.

4). Pay attention to sensitivity to Zhenjiu treatment
People may have different sensitivities to Zhenjiu treatment, so treatment methods may be different when treatment is given to people of different sensitivities. For example, in treatment of patients with high sensitivity to needling stimulation, a few needles, mild manipulations and short period of retaining of needles are recommended, while in treatment of patients with lower sensitivity to needling stimulation, more needles, strong manipulations and long period of retaining of the needles are recommended.

CHAPTER SIX
SELECTION OF POINTS

I. PRINCIPLES OF SELECTION OF POINTS

Usually, 3-6 points are used at each treatment and, generally, selecting a point means selecting both the left and the right ones if the point is located on the both sides of the body. In this book, if there is no specific explanation, applying treatment on a point always means applying treatment on the point in both sides. Generally, selection of points should be based on the treatment principle and point therapeutic properties such as actions and indications. This is the general principle of selection of points. Based on it, the following principles of selection of points are most frequently used in clinics.

1. Selection of Points According to Their Therapeutic Properties

The therapeutic properties of the points are the basis of selection of points. They mainly include local or adjacent therapeutic properties, remote therapeutic properties and special therapeutic properties. Each point has its own feature in these properties, suggesting whether it is effective or good for treatment of a certain disease. Generally, a point should be selected according to its feature in the therapeutic properties. This principle includes the following three aspects.

1). Selection of Nearby Points

Selection of nearby acupoints refers to selection of the points on the diseased area or the adjacent area of the disease. This principle is applicable in most acupoints. Generally speaking, in the treatment of diseases of the internal organs, meridians, tendons and joints, which are manifested by marked local symptoms and signs, the points on the diseased region or near the region may be selected. For example, BL-1 Jingming and EX-HN-5 Taiyang are frequently selected in the treatment of eye disorders, LI-20 Yingxiang and EX-HN-3 Yintang are selected in the treatment of nasal disorders, and LI-15 Jianyu and SI-11 Tianzong are selected for pain in the shoulder.

2). Selection of Distant Points

Selection of distant points refers to selection of points on the area far from the diseased region, usually the points locating along the affected meridian or the meridian, which is exteriorly-interiorly related with the affected meridian. This principle is applicable mainly in the acupoints of the fourteen meridians. Generally, among the points of the fourteen meridians, those located on the limbs, especially below the elbow and knee joints, are frequently selected in the treatment of diseases of the internal organs and tissues which are related to their pertaining meridians or the meridians which are exteriorly-interiorly related to their pertaining meridians. For example, in the treatment of epigastric pain, a disorder of the stomach or the Stomach Meridian, ST-36 Zusanli is selected, which belongs to the Stomach Meridian but is located on the leg, far away from the epigastric region, or SP-4 Gongsun is selected, which belongs to the Spleen Meridian which is exteriorly-interiorly related with the Stomach Meridian and is located on the leg, far away from the epigastric region too.

3). Selection of Symptomatic Points

Selection of symptomatic points refers to selection of the points according to their special prominent effect in the treatment of a certain symptom or disorder.   This principle is applicable in most acupoints, although it is more often seen in selection of extra points or points in the extraordinary acupuncture. For example, LI-4 Hegu is selected in the treatment of pain of the lower tooth, PC-6 Neiguan is selected for nausea and vomiting, and ear point Ear Apex is selected for high fever.

2. Selection of Points According to the Specific Point Theory

Selection of points according to the specific point theory refers to applying the specific point theory and selecting the specific points in the treatment. This principle is applicable only in specific acupoints. Among the acupoints of the fourteen meridians, specific points have special properties and are grouped under special names. They are very frequently used in clinics. Selection of points according to the specific

point theory is one of the most important ways in point selection.

3. Selection of Points According to Theories of TCM

Selection of points should be based on differentiation of syndromes and the point actions according to the theories of TCM. This principle is applicable in most acupoints. For example, in the treatment of dizziness, KI-7 Fuliu is selected if the syndrome belongs to kidney yin deficiency; while LR-3 Taichong is selected if the syndrome belongs to hyperactivity of liver yang.

4. Selection of Points According to Modern Medical Theories

Selection of points may depend upon the knowledge of physiology and pathology of the modern medical science. For example, EX-LE-7 Lanwei (Appendix) is selected for appendicitis. But this principle is more frequently used in extraordinary acupuncture. For example, ear point Endocrine is selected for irregular menstruation; and scalp point Motor Area is selected for paralysis.

5. Selection of Points According to Clinical Experiences

Selection of points according to clinical experiences refers to the principle that attention should be paid to selection of experiential points in the treatment. In the long-term clinical practice, new points or new functions of the old points, which are more effective in the treatment of certain diseases comparing to the traditional points or traditional functions of the points, have being discovered successively. If utilising the achievement of these discoveries properly, you may improve your treatment result greatly. For example, SJ-3 Yemen is selected in the treatment of common cold at the early stage.

II. METHODS OF COMBINATION OF POINTS

Combining points means selecting two or more points with the same or similar indications to bring about the cooperation action, so as to get good clinical effect. The points selected should be less but effective. There are many point-combining methods. They mainly include "combining points on the same meridians", "combining points on the exteriorly-interiorly related meridians", "combining points on the meridians sharing the same name", "combining points on the anterior and posterior aspects of the body", "combining points on the superior and inferior portions of the body", "combining points having correspondence in location", "combining points on the distal and local regions of the body".

1. Combining Points on the Same Meridians

When there is a disease in a certain meridian or the zang-fu organ, which belongs to, the points on this meridian can be chosen for the treatment. For example, LR-3 Taichong and LR-14 Qimen are selected for liver qi stagnation with hypochondriac pain.

Usually, the start-stop points of a certain meridian are used together for treating the meridian disease and disorders of the head, face, and five sense organs. For example, LI-1 Shangyang and LI-20 Yingxiang are selected for nasal bleeding due to heat.

2. Combining Points on the Exteriorly-Interiorly Related Meridians

Also known as yin-yang point combination. This form of combining points is frequently seen in clinics. It is based on the exterior-interior relationship of the three Yin and three Yang Meridians of the body. For example, LU-7 Lieque and LI-4 Hegu are often used as a group to common cold with cough.

In the application of the specific points, combination of the Yuan-Source and Luo-Connecting Points belongs to this method.

3. Combining Points on the Meridians Sharing the Same Name

It is a method of combining points by selecting the points respectively on a Hand and a Foot Meridians which have the same type of yin or yang name, namely, Taiyang, Shaoyang, Taiyin, Shaoyin, and so on. For example, SJ-3 Zhongzhu, a point of the Hand-Shaoyang, and GB-43 Xiaxi, a point of the Foot-Shaoyang, are used together for tinnitus and deafness.

The following combinations are effective to treat certain disorders and frequently applied in clinics:

- LI-4 Hegu and ST-41, points of the Hand and Foot Yangming Meridians, are used for pain in the forehead;

- ST-5 Waiguan and GB-41 Zulinqi, points of the Hand and Foot Shaoyang Meridians, are used for pain in the lateral side of the head;

- SI-3 Houxi and BL-62 Shenmai, points of the Hand and Foot Taiyang Meridians, are used for pain in the back of the head;

- LU-11 Shaoshang and SP-1 Yinbai, points of the Hand and Foot Taiyin Meridians, are used for manic of depressive psychosis;

- PC-6 Neiguan and LR-3 Taichong, points of the Hand and Foot Jueyin Meridians, are used for Epilepsy;

- HT-7 Shenmen and KI-6 Zhaohai, points of the Hand and Foot Shaoyin Meridians, are used for insomnia.

4. Combining Points on the Anterior and Posterior Aspects of the Body

It refers to selecting the points on the chest and abdomen (anterior) and the points on the back (posterior) simultaneously. For example, RN-4 Guanyuan and BL-23 Shenshu are frequently selected together for emission or enuresis.

Combining points on the anterior and posterior aspects of the body is usually for treating diseases of the zang-fu organs. Combination of the Back-Shu and Front-Mu Points is a good example.

5. Combining Points on the Superior and Inferior Portions of the Body

It refers to selecting the points on the upper and lower parts of the body simultaneously. For example, GB-20 Fengchi and LR-3 Taichong are frequently used to dizziness and headache due to overactivity of liver yang, and ST-6 Jiache and ST-44 Neiting are selected for toothache due to stomach fire.

Generally, the points on the upper portion of the body have the action of ascending, and the points on the lower portion of the body have the action of descending. Therefore, combining superior-inferior points can be beneficial in regulating the ascending-descending activities of the qi.

Combining the Eight Confluent Points belongs to this method.

6. Combining Points Having Correspondence in Location

It refers to selecting a point on the diseased side and another point on the healthy side, which is in correspondence to the former in location. For example, ST-7 Jiache of both sides is selected for facial paralysis. This method is mainly used for treatment of painful syndromes and paralysis.

7. Combining Points on the Distal and Local Regions of the Body

Combining distal-local points refers the application of points, which are distant and adjacent to the diseased area according to the local and adjacent therapeutic properties and the remote therapeutic properties of the points, and differentiation of the syndromes. Generally, the local points are used for promoting qi and blood circulation and dredging the meridian and collaterals in the diseased region, while the distal point for regulating the diseased meridian and

internal organ, and treating the pathogenesis of the syndrome, in order to meet the requirement that treatment should be based on differentiation of syndromes. The method is the most commonly seen one in combination point conditions. Examples are seen in the Tab. VI-1.

Tab. VI-1 Common Combination Conditions of Local & Distal Points

Diseased Area	Local Points	Distal Points
Heart	BL-15 Xinshu, BL-14 Jueyinshu, RN-22 Tiantu	PC-6 Neiguan, HT-7 Shenmen, PC-5 Jianshi, HT-6 Yinxi
Liver	BL-18 Ganshu, LR-14 Qimen	LR-3 Taichong
Spleen	BL-20 Pishu	ST-36 Zusanli, SP-4 Gongsun
Lung	BL-13 Feishu, RN-17 Danzhong, RN-22 Tiantu	LU-7 Lieque, LU-5 Chize
Kidney	BL-23 Shenshu, BL-52 Zhishi	KI-3 Taixi
Stomach	BL-21 Weishu, RN-12 Zhongwan	ST-36 Zusanli, PC-6 Neiguan
Gallbladder	BL-19 Danshu	GB-34 Yanglingquan
Urinary Bladder	BL-28 Pangguanshu, BL-32 Ciliao, RN-3 Zhongji	SP-6 Sanyinjiao
Large Intestine	BL-25 Dachangshu, ST-25 Tianshu	ST-37 Shangjuxu, ST-44 Neiting
Small Intestine	BL-27 Xiaochangshu, RN-4 Guanyuan	ST-36 Zusanli
Uterus	RN-4 Guanyuan, ST-29 Guilai	SP-6 Sanyinjiao
Vertex	DU-20 Baihui, EX-HN-1 Sishencong	LR-3 Taichong
Temple	EX-HN-5 Taiyang, GB-8 Shuaigu	SJ-3 Zhongzhu, GB-41 Zulinqi, GB-43 Xiaxi, SJ-5 Waiguan
Forehead	EX-HN-3 Yintang, GB-14 Yangbai	LI-4 Hegu, ST-44 Neiting
Eye	BL-1 Jingming, ST-1 Chengqi, EX-HN-7 Qiuhou	GB-37 Guangming, SI-6 Yanglao
Nose	LI-20 Yingxiang, EX-HN-3 Yintang	LI-4 Hegu, ST-45 Lidui
Mouth & Teeth	ST-4 Dicang, ST-6 Jiache, ST-7 Xiaguan	LI-4 Hegu, ST-44 Neiting
Ear	SJ-17 Yifeng, SI-19 Tinggong, SJ-21 Ermen, GB-2 Tinghui	SJ-5 Waiguan, SJ-3 Zhongzhu

Neck	GB-20 Fengchi, BL-10 Tianzhu	LU-7 Lieque, SI-3 Houxi, BL-65 Shugu
Throat	RN-22 Tiantu, RN-23 Lianquan	LU-11 Shaoshang, KI-6 Zhaohai
Chest	RN-22 Tiantu, RN-17 Danzhong	LU-7 Lieque, PC-6 Neiguan, BL-13 Feishu
Costal & Hyphochodrium	BL-18 Ganshu, LR-14 Qimen	SJ-6 Zhigou, GB-34 Yanglingquan, PC-6 Neiguan
Upper Abdomen	RN-12 Zhongwan, BL-21 Weishu	PC-6 Neiguan, ST-36 Zusanli
Lower Abdomen	RN-4 Guanyuan, RN-6 Qihai, ST-25 Tianshu	SP-6 Sanyinjiao, SP-1 Yinbai
Upper Back	EX-B-2 Jiaji (TV 1-8)	SI-3 Houxi
Lower Back	BL-23 Shenshu, BL-25 Dachangshu	BL-40 Weizhong, BL-60 Kunlun
Anus	DU-1 Changqiang, BL-54 Zhibian	BL-57 Chengshan
Rectum	BL-30 Baihuangshu, DU-1 Changqiang	BL-57 Chengshan, DU-20 Baihui
Genital Organ	RN-3 Zhongji, RN-4 Guanyuan, RN-2 Qugu	SP-6 Sanyinjiao, LR-3 Taichong
Upper Limbs	LI-15 Jianyu, LI-11 Quchi, LI-4 Hegu	EX-B-2 Jiaji (CV5-TV1)
Lower Limbs	GB-30 Huantiao, BL-40 Weizhong, GB-34 Yanglingquan	EX-B-2 Jiaji (LV3-SV1)

8. Combining Points on the Lateral and Medial Aspects of the Limbs

It refers to selection of a lateral point and a medial point simultaneously. The lateral points refer to those on the lateral side of the Yin Meridians of hand and foot, while the medial points to those on the medial side of the Yang Meridians of hand and foot. Generally, to diseases of the Yang Meridians, lateral points are taken as the main while medial ones as the assistant, and to diseases of the Yin Meridians, medial points are taken as the main while lateral ones as the assistant. For example, BL-62 Shenmai and KI-6 Zhaohai are frequently used together in treatment of strephenopodia or strephexopodia. In the following pairs of the points, each of them has the action of regulating and communicating the corresponding Yin and Yang Meridians if penetration needling (point-to-point puncturing) is applied, namely, puncture the point with the needle tip arriving at the tissue below the skin of its counterpart point:

- SP-9 Yinlingquan and GB-34 Yanglingquan
- GB-40 Qiuxu and KI-6 Zhaohai
- PC-6 Neiguan and SJ-5 Waiguan

These combination conditions are just examples of combining lateral-medial points.

9. Combining Points on the Left and Right Sides of the Body

This method is based on the theory that the meridians cross each other. Generally, this method is mainly used in treating disorders of the head and face. For example, facial paralysis of the left side can be treated by puncturing LI-4 Hegu of the right side; headache of the right side by puncturing GB-34 Yanglingquan and GB-43 Xiaxi of the left side.

As a rule, stimulation is always given to points of the both sides in treatment of diseases of the internal organs, because the meridians are distributed over the body symmetrically.

Additionally, it may induce some effective result in treating paralysis and painful syndromes of the limbs by only selecting points of the healthy side.

10. Combining Among the Specific Points

1). Combining among the Five Shu Points
Combination of points among the Five Shu Points is based on the actions and indications of the points and the five-element theory, and used to achieve a reinforcing or reducing effect in treatment. According to the five elements theory, the Five Shu Points are correlated respectively to the five elements and the zang-fu organs (seen in Tab.II-2 & 3). Thus, the Five Shu Points can be selected for reinforcing and reducing in treatment diseases of zang-fu organs according to their relations with the Five Elements and the zang-fu organs. As the zang-fu organs belong to five elements, and the Twelve Meridians pertain to zang-fu organs, reinforcing-reducing effect, according to the five element theory, can be achieved not only by selecting the points of the diseased meridian, but also by selecting points of the meridian which is the mother or son comparing to the diseased meridian and points of the meridian which has action of restraining the diseased meridian. Generally, it includes following two aspects.

Tab. VI-2 Selection of Five Shu Points for Reinforcing & Reducing Based on Deficiency-Excess

	EXCESS SYNDROME				DEFICIENCY SYNDROME			
	REINFORCING *Ke (restraining) cycle*		*REDUCING* *Sheng (promoting) cycle*		*REINFORCING* *Sheng (promoting) cycle*		*REDUCING* *Ke (restraining) cycle*	
	Ke point of the Ke meridian	*Ke point of the diseased meridian*	*Son point of the Son meridian*	*Son point of the diseased meridian*	*Mother point of diseased meridian*	*Mother point of Mother meridian*	*Ke point of the Ke meridian*	*Ke point of the diseased meridian*
LU	HT-8 Shaofu	LU-10 Yuji	KI-10 Yingu	LU-5 Chize	LU-9 Taiyuan	SP-3 Taibai	HT-8 Shaofu	LU-10 Yuji
KI	SP-3 Taibai	KI-3 Taixi	LR-1 Dadun	KI-1 Yong-quan	KI-7 Fuliu	LU-8 Jingqu	SP-3 Taibai	KI-3 Taixi
LR	LU-8 Jingqu	LR-4 Zhong-feng	HT-8 Shaofu	LR-2 Xingjian	LR-8 Ququan	KI-10 Yingu	LU-8 Jingqu	LR-4 Zhong-feng
HT	KI-10 Yingu	HT-3 Shaohai	SP-3 Taibai	HT-7 Shenmen	HT-9 Shao-chong	LR-1 Dadun	KI-10 Yingu	HT-3 Shaohai
SP	LR-1 Dadun	SP-1 Yinbai	LU-8 Jingqu	SP-5 Shangqiu	SP-2 Dadu	HT-8 Shaofu	LR-1 Dadun	SP-1 Yinbai
LI	SI-5 Yanggu	LI-5 Yangxi	KI-2 Rangu	LI-2 Erjian	LI-11 Quchi	ST-36 Zusanli	SI-5 Yanggu	LI-5 Yangxi
BL	ST-36 Zusanli	BL-40 Wei-zhong	GB-41 Zulinqi	BL-65 Shugu	BL-67 Zhiyin	LI-1 Shang-yang	ST-36 Zusanli	BL-40 Wei-zhong
GB	LI-1 Shang-yang	GB-44 Zuqiao-yin	SI-5 Yingu	GB-38 Yangfu	GB-43 Xiaxi	BL-66 Zutong-gu	LI-1 Shang-yang	GB-44 Zuqiao-yin
SI	BL-66 Zutonggu	SI-2 Qiangu	ST-36 Zusanli	SI-8 Xiaohai	SI-3 Houxi	GB-45 Zulinqi	BL-66 Zutonggu	SI-2 Qiangu
ST	GB-41 Zulinqi	ST-43 Xiangu	LI-1 Shang-yang	ST-45 Lidui	ST-41 Jiexi	SI-5 Yanggu	GB-41 Zulinqi	ST-43 Xiangu
PC	KI-10 Yingu	PC-3 Quze	ST-36 Zusanli	PC-7 Daling	PC-9 Zhong-chong	GB-41 Zulinqi	KI-10 Yingu	PC-3 Quze
SJ	BL-66 Zutong-gu	SJ-2 Yemen	ST-36 Zusanli	SJ-10 Tianjing	SJ-3 Zhong-zhu	GB-41 Zulinqi	BL-66 Zutong-gu	SJ-2 Yemen

a. Reinforcing-reducing effect achieved based on the "mother-son" (Sheng cycle) relation theory

According to the five-element theory, in every two elements between which there is the "mother-son relation", the element promoting the other is known as "mother" and the element being promoted as "son".

Generally, "deficiency should be treated by tonifying the mother, while excess by reducing the son". Namely, deficiency should be treated by tonifying the point which is the "mother element" of the diseased meridian and the meridian which is the "mother element" comparing to the diseased meridian, while excess by reducing the "son element" of the diseased meridian and the meridian which the "son element" comparing to the diseased meridian. Also "the mother can become stronger by treating its son, while the pathogen in the son can become weak by treating the mother". Here, "mother" and "son" are named to two specific Five Shu Points, the zang-fu organs and meridians according to their promoting-promoted relationship based on the five-element theory. The following procedure shows how to combine the Five Shu Points to achieve a reinforcing or reducing effect based on the mother-son relation theory (taking deficiency and excess of the lung Meridian or lung as example):

1. Determine which meridian (zang-fu organ) is diseased and whether the syndrome belongs to deficiency or excess.

2. Determine the treatment principle, i.e., reinforcing or reducing a meridian (zang-fu organ).

3. Determine which does the diseased meridian (zang-fu organ) belong to in the Five Element properties. For example, the Lung Meridian belongs to metal. Based on it, determine which meridian is the "son" or "mother" comparing to the diseased meridian. For example, the Spleen Meridian is the mother and the Kidney

Meridian is the son comparing to the Lung Meridian.

4. Determine which point of the diseased meridian and which point of the "son" or "mother" meridian belongs to the "son" or "mother" element. For example, LU-9 Taiyuan belonging to earth and LU-5 Chize belonging to water are respectively the mother point and son point of the diseased meridian (the Lung Meridian), SP-3 Taibai belonging to earth is the mother point of the mother meridian (Spleen Meridian) comparing to the diseased meridian (the Lung Meridian), and KI-10 Yingu belonging to water is the son point of the son meridian comparing to the Lung Meridian.

5. Select the point, which is the mother element of the diseased meridian, and the point, which is the mother element of the meridian, which is the mother, comparing to the diseased meridian, and perform reinforcing manipulation in treatment of deficiency syndrome of the diseased meridian. Select the point, which is the son element of the diseased meridian, and the point, which is the son element of the meridian which is the son comparing to the diseased meridian, and apply reducing manipulation in treatment of excess syndrome of the diseased meridian. For example, in treatment of deficiency of the lung or the Lung Meridian, LU-9 Taiyuan, which belongs to earth of the diseased meridian (Lung Meridian) and SP-3 Taibai, which belongs to earth of the mother meridian (Spleen Meridian) of the Lung Meridian should be selected and reinforcing manipulation be performed. While in treatment of excess of the lung or the Lung Meridian, LU-5 Chize, which belongs to water of the Lung Meridian, and KI-10 Yingu, which belongs to water of the mother meridian (Kidney Meridian) of the Lung Meridian should be selected and reducing manipulation be performed.

b. Reinforcing-reducing effect achieved based on "restraining-being restrained' (Ke cycle) relation theory

Additionally, in every two elements between which there is a "restraining-being restrained relation", the element restraining the other is known as the restraining (Ke) element, while that being restrained by the other is known as the restrained (Bei Ke) element. Therefore, releasing the restraining from the restraining element, namely, reducing the restraining element, can make the restrained element stronger, namely, having the effect of reinforcing the restrained element, while strengthening the restraining element can have the effect of reducing excess of the restrained element.

According to restraining-being restrained relation, deficiency of a zang-fu organ or meridian should be treated by reducing the point which is the "restraining element" of the diseased meridian or of the meridian which acts as the "restraining element" comparing to the diseased meridian, while excess of a zang-fu organ or meridian should be treated by tonifying the point which is the "restraining element" of the diseased meridian and of the meridian which is the "restraining element" comparing to the diseased meridian. Here, "restraining element" and "restrained element" are named to two specific Five Shu Points and the zang-fu organs or meridians according to their restraining-restrained relationship based on the five-element theory. The following procedure shows how to combine the Five Shu Points to achieve a reinforcing or reducing effect based on the restraining-restrained relation theory (taking deficiency and excess of the lung Meridian or lung as example):

1. Determine which meridian (zang-fu organ) is diseased and whether the syndrome belongs to deficiency or excess.

2. Determine the treatment principle, i.e., reinforcing or reducing a meridian (zang-fu organ).

3. Determine which does the diseased meridian (zang-fu organ) belong to in the Five Element properties. For example, the Lung Meridian belongs to metal. Based on it, determine which meridian is the "restraining" or "restrained" comparing to the diseased meridian. For example, the Heart Meridian is the restraining and the Liver Meridian is the restrained comparing to the Lung Meridian.

4. Determine which point of the diseased meridian and which point of the "restraining" meridian belong to the restraining. For example, LU-10 Yuji, belonging to fire, is the restraining point of the Lung Meridian, and HT-8 Shaofu, belonging to fire, is the restraining point of the restraining meridian (the Heart Meridian which belongs to fire) comparing to the Lung Meridian.

5. Select the point, which is the restraining element of the diseased meridian, and the point, which is the restraining element of the meridian, which is the restraining comparing to the diseased meridian. In treatment of excess syndrome of the diseased meridian, apply reinforcing manipulation on the selected points, while to deficiency syndrome, and perform reducing manipulation on the selected points. For example, in treatment of deficiency of the lung or the Lung Meridian, LU-10 Yuji, which belongs to fire of the Lung Meridian and HT-8 Shaofu, which belongs to fire of the restraining meridian (Heart Meridian) of the Lung Meridian should be selected and reducing manipulation be performed. While in treatment of excess of the lung or the Lung Meridian, LU-10 Yuji, which belongs to fire of the Lung Meridian, and HT-8 Shaofu, which belongs to fire of the restraining meridian (Heart Meridian) of the Lung Meridian should be selected and reinforcing manipulation be performed.

See Tab. VI-2 for details.

2). Combining Back-Shu and Front-Mu Points
The Back-Shu Points and the Front-Mu Points may be used independently or in combination. Whenever an internal organ is affected, the Back-Shu Point or the Front-Mu Point pertaining to that organ may be prescribed. The application of both may strengthen the therapeutic effects. For example, BL-21 Weishu and RN-12 Zhongwan, the Back-Shu and Front Points of the stomach, is frequently used together for digestive disorders. See Tab. IV-3 for details.

3). Combining Yuan-Source and Luo-Connecting Points
The Yuan-Source Points and Luo-Connecting Points may be used independently or in combination. The combination of them is called the "host and guest combination", which is applied according to the occurring order of the disease on a pair of exteriorly-interiorly related meridians. When a meridian is first affected, called "host", its Yuan-Source Point is used, while for second affected meridian, called "guest", its Luo-Connecting Point is used. Namely, it is a way by simultaneously selecting the Yuan-Source Point of the host meridian (first affected meridian) and the Luo-Connecting Point of the guest meridian (second affected meridian) in treatment of diseases occurring in a pair of interiorly-exteriorly related meridians. For instance, both the Lung Meridian and the Large Intestine Meridians are diseased, but the former is affected first, LU-9 Taiyuan, its Yuan-Source Point is selected as a main point, and LI-6 Pianli, the Luo-Connecting, is used as a combining point. On the contrary, if the Large Intestine Meridian is diseased first and then the Lung Meridian, LI-4 Hegu, the Yuan-Source Point of the Large Intestine Meridian should be prescribed as a main point, while LU-7 Lieque, the Luo-Connecting Point of the Lung Meridian as a combining point. This method is adopted when the exteriorly-interiorly related meridians are affected. Therefore it is also known as the combination of the exterior-interior points. See Tab. VI-4 for details.

Tab. VI- 3 Chief Indications of Back-Shu & Front-Mu Points in Combination

Zang-Fu organs	Back-Shu	Front-Mu	Chief Disease Category & Indication Examples
Lung	BL-13 Feishu	LU-1 Zhongfu	Respiratory: cough, dyspnea, difficult breath
Pericardium	BL-14 Jueyinshu	RN-17 Danzhong	Cardiac: Chest pain, palpitation.
Heart	BL-15 Xinshu	RN-14 Juque	Cardiac & gastric: Palpitation, stomach pain, and neurosis.
Liver	BL-18 Ganshu	LR-14 Qimen	Digestive: Liver & stomach problems, such as pain in the liver region, vomiting, acid regurgitation
Gallbladder	BL-19 Danshu	GB-24 Riyue	Digestive: Liver & spleen problems, such as enlarged liver & spleen, abdominal pain, indigestion.
Spleen	BL-20 Pishu	LR-13 Zhangmen	Digestive: Liver & stomach problems, such as pain in hypochondriac region, poor appetite, abdominal distention or/and pain.
Stomach	BL-21 Weishu	RN-12 Zhongwan	Digestive: Gastric pain or fullness, poor appetite.
Sanjiao	BL-22 Sanjiaoshu	RN-5 Shimen	Water metabolism: Edema, diarrhea.
Kidney	BL-23 Shenshu	GB-25 Jingmen	Reproductive & urinary: Pain in the waist, seminal emission, impotence, and irregular menstruation.
Large Intestine	BL-25 Dachangshu	Tianshu ST-25	Digestive: Constipation, diarrhea, and abdominal pain.
Small Intestine	BL-27 Xiaochangshu	RN-4 Guanyuan	Digestive, urinary & reproductive: Intestinal colic, emission, and enuresis.
Urinary Bladder	BL-28 Pangguanshu	RN-3 Zhongji	Reproductive & urinary: Enuresis, emission, absence of urine, irregular menstruation.

Tab. VI-4 Chief Indications of Yuan-Source and Luo-Connecting Points in Combination

Host/Guest Meridians	Source/Connecting Points	Indications
LU/LI	LU-9 Taiyuan/LI-6 Pianli	Trachitis, sore throat, shortness of breath with phlegm, sweating, fever in the palms, shoulder pain on the lateral side, pain in both breasts.
LI/LU	LI-4 Hegu/LU-7 Lieque	Toothache, lymphadenitis, parotitis, sore throat, dry mouth, jaundice, nasal watery discharge, pain in the anterior shoulder.
SP/ST	SP-3 Taibai/ST-40 Fenglong	Stiff tongue, abdominal pain, vomiting, heaviness and weakness of the body, constipation, pain in the medial side of the foot, malaria.
ST/SP	ST-42 Chongyang/SP-4 Gongsun	Nasal bleeding, facial paralysis, neurosis, malaria, abdominal fullness, pain in the anterior side of the foot.
HT/SI	HT-7 Shenmen/SI-7 Zhizheng	Angina pectoris, tachycardia, dry mouth, jaundice, pain in the ulnar side of the upper extremities.
SI/HT	SI-4 Wangu/HT-5 Tongli	Swelling and pain of the check, shoulder pain, neck pain, deafness, pain in the exterior-posterior side of the upper extremities.
KI/BL	KI-3 Taixi/BL-58 Feiyang	Neurosis, lassitude, anorexia, pain in the waist.
BL/KI	BL-64 Jinggu/KI-4 Dazhong	Pain in the eyes, neck, back, waist and legs, epilepsy, psychoses, opisthotonus, supraorbital neuralgia, nasal bleeding, proctoptosis, haemorrhoids.
PC/SJ	PC-7 Daling/SJ-5 Waiguan	Spasm or pain of the forearm and fingers, pain in the chest and hypochondrium, palpitation, restlessness, cardiac pain, fever in the palms, psychoses.

SJ /PC	SJ-4 Yangchi/PC-6 Neiguan	Deafness, sore throat, shoulder and back pain, spinal pain, constipation, conjunctivitis, anuresis, and enuresis.
LR /GB	LR-3 Taichong/GB-37 Guangming	Hernia, orchitis, waist pain, fullness in the chest, vomiting, abdominal pain, diarrhoea, anuresis, enuresis.
GB/LR	GB-40 Qiuxu/LR-5 Ligou	Hypochondriac pain, headache, eye disorders, malaria, lymph nodes due to tuberculosis, goiter.

PART TWO

TREATMENT OF
COMMON DISEASES

CHAPTER ONE
INTERNAL DISEASES

1. Common Cold and Influenza

Common cold is an acute catarrhal inflammation of the upper respiratory tract caused by bacteria or virus. Clinically, it is marked by fever, chills, stuffy nose, sneezing, rhinorrhea, and sore throat. Influenza is an infectious disease of the respiratory tract, caused by the influenza viruses. Clinically, it is marked by abrupt onset of fever, chills, headache and myalgia, or even high fever, chest pain, and dyspnea in severe cases. It usually spreads to a large number of persons within a short period. According to TCM, common cold belongs to the category of Shang Feng (attack by pathogenic wind) or Shang Feng Gan Mao (common cold due to attack by wind); while influenza, belongs to Shi Xing Gan Mao (epidemic common cold). They are usually discussed together.

I. STANDARD TREATMENT

Common cold and influenza are generally divided into three types — wind-cold, wind-heat, qi deficiency. Points of the Lung, Large Intestine and Bladder Meridians are frequently selected in their treatment.

1. Wind-Cold

Manifestations: Nasal stuffiness with clear discharge, sneezing, itching in the throat, coarse voice, coughing with thin and white sputum, aversion to cold, fever, headache, general aching, absence of sweating in severe cases.

Tongue: Thin and white coating.

Pulse: Superficial or superficial and tense.

Treatment Principle: Relieve exterior syndrome and dispel wind-cold.

Point Prescription & Manipulation:
Primary points:
　　GB-20 Fengchi　　- ^
　　SJ-5 Waiguan　　- ^
　　LU-7 Lieque　　- ^

Explanation:
- GB-20 Fengchi and SJ-5 Waiguan dispel external pathogen and relieve exterior syndrome, and LU-7 Lieque disperses Lung qi. Moxibustion on these three points disperses cold pathogen;
- LI-20 Yingxiang opens the orifice of the nose.

Secondary points according to conditions:
1️⃣ Severe nasal congestion —LI-20 Yingxiang [-];
2️⃣ Severe cases—LI-4 Hegu [-] and BL-12 Fengmen and BL-13 Feishu which are applied with cupping.

2. Wind-Heat

Manifestations: Fever, slight aversion to cold, sweating, headache, nasal stuffiness with turbid discharge, thirst, congested and sore throat, coughing with thick, yellow sputum.

Tongue: Thin and yellow coating.

Pulse: Superficial and rapid.

Treatment Principle: Relieve exterior syndrome, disperse wind-heat.

Point Prescription & Manipulation:
Primary points:
    GB-20 Fengchi   -
    DU-17 Dazhui 17 -
    LI-4 Hegu   -
    LU-5 Chize   -

Explanation:
- GB-20 Fengchi, DU-14 Dazhui and LI-4 Hegu dispel pathogenic wind, relieve exterior syndrome and clear heat;
- LU-5 Chize clears heat in the lung.

Secondary points according to conditions:
1️⃣ High fever — LI-11 Quchi [-];
2️⃣ Sore throat — LI-1 Shangyang [-];
3️⃣ Nasal congestion — LU-11 Shaoshang [-];
4️⃣ Severe headache — EX-HN-5 Taiyang [-] and EX-HN-3 Yintang [-]

3. Qi Deficiency

Manifestations: Chilliness, fever, headache, nasal stuffiness, cough with white and thin sputum, lassitude, disinclination to talk.

Tongue: Thin and white coating.

Pulse: Superficial and weak.

Treatment Principle: Reinforce qi and relieve exterior syndrome.

Point Prescription & Manipulation:
Primary points:
    RN-6 Qihai   + ^
    ST-36 Zusanli   + ^
    LI-4 Hegu   /
    GB-20 Fengchi   -

Explanation:
- LI-4 Hegu and LI-11 Quchi dispel external pathogen and relieve exterior syndrome;
- ST-36 Zusanli and RN-6 Qihai tonify qi and reinforce body resistance. Moxibustion on these points warms yang qi for consolidating the exterior.

Secondary points according to conditions:
1️⃣ If there is accompanying blood deficiency— SP-6 Sanyinjiao [+] and SP-10 Xuehai [+];
2️⃣ Severe cases—BL-12 Fengmen and BL-13 Feishu which are applied with cupping.

II. EXPERIENTIAL TREATMENT

1. Puncturing SJ-2 Yemen

Indication: Various types of common cold.

Point Prescription:
Primary points:
    SI-2 Yemen of one side.

Secondary points according to conditions:
1️⃣ Severe case—SJ-2 Yemen of the other side.

Manipulation: Select a 1.2-cun filiform needle, insert it into the point obliquely upward

0.5-1.0 cun and twist it several times. If the arrival of qi has not been induced in 10 minutes, the opposite point should be punctured with the same manipulation. The needles are retained for 15-30 minutes. The treatment is given once a day, and within 3-5 days, common cold will be cured.

2. Puncturing DU-14 Dazhui

Indication: Common cold with high temperature or common cold at the early stage.

Point Prescription:
DU-14 Dazhui

Manipulation: Ask the patient to lie on the side with legs bent. Hold the head at the occiput region firmly with the hands to make the neck bend forward in the largest possible angle. Insert a 2-cun needle into DU-14 Dazhui. After thrusting through the skin, insert a 2-cun needle horizontally 15 degrees downward along the spinal column to a depth of 1.5-2.0 cun. Then, press the spinal column from the place below DU-14 Dazhui downward to the coccyx and rotate the needle 5-15 minutes to induce a cooling sensation to the patient. The treatment is given once only.

3. Acupressure with Fingers

Indication: Common cold at the beginning stage with no complications or cases in children.

Point Prescription:
The posterior border of the middle segment of the sternocleidomastoid.

Manipulation: Ask the patient to sit upright and loose the collar button. Stand behind the patient, press and knead the selected region by using the thumb and the other four fingers of the right hand, which are separated. Apply the manipulation from the mild to heavy, from slow to quick. Change the hands to manipulation to press and knead 100-200 times until the patient feels unobstructed in the nose, slight sweating, milder headache and a comfortable sensation in whole body. The treatment is given 2-3 times a day.

4. Acupuncture and Moxibustion on ST-36 Zusanli

Indication: Prevention of common cold or influenza.

Point Prescription:
ST-36 Zusanli

Manipulation: Applying mild-warm moxibustion or bird-pecking moxibustion on ST-36 Zusanli of both sides with moxa stick 10-20 minutes. If the patient feels heat in the body and has slight sweating, it is better. The treatment is given once a day and for 2-3 days. Alternatively, insert a filiform needle into ST-36 Zusanli of one side and use a twisting, lifting and thrusting manipulation to gently induce soreness, numbness and distending sensation radiating to the dorsum of the foot. Then, remove the needle. The treatment is given once only.

Comment:

Acupuncture and moxibustion (Zhenjiu) are effective in the treatment of common cold and influenza, especially if they are given at the first day or the second day of onset. In addition, given to healthy people at the common cold or influenza epidemic period, the treatment will have good preventive effect. In clinic, acupuncture is usually the first choice in treatment of common cold or influenza, but massage or moxibustion is selected for prevention more frequently than acupuncture.

Notes:

2. Mumps

Mumps is an acute communicable disease caused by the mumps virus. Clinically, it is marked by fever and pain and swelling of the parotid glands. The prognosis is generally good, but if appropriate and timely treatment is not given there may be complications including meningitis, orchitis or ovaritis with possible subsequent sterility. According to TCM, mumps, called Za Sai in Chinese, is due to attack of the wind, damp and pernicious factor which are accompanied with phlegm-fire, leading to obstruction of Shaoyang Meridian by the pathogen.

I. STANDARD TREATMENT

Mumps is usually divided into three types—wind-heat, stomach fire and stagnant heat in the Liver Meridian. Points of the Sanjiao and Large Intestine Meridians are frequently selected.

1. Wind-Heat

Manifestations: Fever, aversion to cold, headache, aching pain of the parotid region, difficulty in chewing followed by diffuse swelling and pain at one or both sides of the parotid glands.

Tongue: Red body tip with thin and yellow coating.

Pulse: Floating and rapid.

Treatment Principle: Dispel wind, clear heat, subdue swelling.

Point Prescription & Manipulation:
Primary points:
    LI-4 Hegu   -
    SJ-5Waiguan   -
    ST-6 Jiache   -
    SJ-17 Yifeng   -

Explanation:

On the local points such as ST-6 Jiache and SJ-17 Yifeng, insert the needle with its tip toward the center of the swelling parotid gland.
- LI-4 Hegu and SJ-5 Waiguan relieve exterior syndrome and clear heat from Shaoyang and Yangming Meridians;
- ST-6 Jiache and SJ-17 Yifeng, the local points, clear heat from the Shaoyang and Yangming Meridians and disperse accumulation to relieve swelling.

Secondary points according to conditions:
1〕 High fever —GB-43 Xiaxi [-] and LI-11 Quchi[-];
2〕 Sore throat —LU-11 Shaoshang and LI-1 Shangyang are pricked to bleed.

2. Fire in the Stomach

Manifestations: Persistent high fever, restlessness, thirst, headache, swelling and pain of the parotid gland with burning sensation and aggravated by pressing, difficulty in chewing, constipation, scanty dark urine.

Tongue: Red body with yellow coating.

Pulse: Slippery and rapid.

Treatment Principle: Remove heat and resolve hard mass.

Point Prescription & Manipulation:
Primary points:
    DU-14 Dazhui   -
    LI-11 Quchi   -
    LI-4 Hegu   -
    SJ-3 Zhongzhu   -
    ST-6 Jiache   -
    SJ-17 Yifeng   -
    GB-41 Zulinqi   -

Explanation:
Manipulation of the needles in the local points is the same as above.

- LI-11 Quchi and LI-4 Hegu clear heat from the Yangming Meridian;

- SJ-3 Zhongzhu clears heat from the Shaoyang Meridian;
- DU-14 Dazhui clears heat and relieves fever;
- GB-41 Zulinqi leads heat downward and removes it;
- ST-6 Jiache and SJ-17 Yifeng, the local points, clear heat from the Shaoyang and Yangming Meridians and disperse accumulation to relieve swelling.

Secondary points according to conditions:
1] Sore throat—LU-11 Shaoshang and LI-1 Shangyang are pricked to bleed.
2] Constipation — ST-44 Neiting [-];
3] Severe headache — GB-20 Fengchi [-] and ST-8 Touwei [-].

3. Stagnant Heat in the Liver Meridian

Manifestations: Swelling and distending pain of the testis which radiates to the lower abdomen following diffuse swelling and pain at one or both sides of the parotid, high fever, chills, restlessness, thirst.

Tongue: Red body with yellow coating.

Pulse: Wiry and rapid.

Treatment Principle: Clear heat, regulate gallbladder and resolve hard mass.

Point Prescription & Manipulation:
Primary points:
 LR-1 Dadun -
 GB-41 Zulinqi -
 ST-29 Guilai -
 LR-8 Ququan -

Explanation:
- LR-1 Dadun, the Jing-Well Point of the Liver Meridian, dredges the Liver Meridian and resolves hardness for stopping pain;
- GB-41 Zulinqi and LR-8 Ququan clear heat from the Liver Meridian;
- ST-29 Guilai, local point, regulates qi and stops lower abdominal pain.

Secondary points according to conditions:

1] Severe pain of the testis — GB-34 Yanglingquan [-] and LR-2 Xingjian [-];
2] High fever — DU-14 Dazhui [-] and LI-11 Quchi [-].

II. EXPERIENTIAL TREATMENT

1. Moxibustion with Match Stick

Indication: Mumps with wind-heat syndrome or fire in stomach.

Point Prescription:
 SJ-20 Jiaosun of the diseased side.

Manipulation: Cut out the hair at SJ-20 Jiaosun of the diseased side, face the point with the ignited matchstick, and poke the point with the lit end to induce a sound "ca". If there is no the sound, repeat this course to induce it. Generally, only one treatment is needed to cure this disease. In case the first time fails in curing it, repeat the treatment on the next day.

2. Puncturing EX-HN-17 Saixian

Indication: Mumps without complications.

Point Prescription:
 EX-HN-17 Saixian (Parotid Gland) of the diseased side, located on the cheek, at the midpoint of the line connecting the lower border of the ear lobe and the angle of the mandible.

Manipulation: Insert a needle into the point with its tip toward the center of the parotid gland, push the needle deep until its tip reaches the center, rotate the needle 2-5 minutes, and take out the needle. The treatment is given once daily and usually, only 2-3 treatments are needed in curing this disease.

Comment:
As mumps is very infectious, the patient should be isolated. Moxibustion on SJ-20 Jiaosun with matchstick is quite effective in treatment of mumps. However, in severe cases with complications, other treatments are suggested in cooperation.

Notes:

3. Viral Hepatitis

Viral hepatitis refers to an infectious disease of the liver caused by hepatitis virus. Clinically, it is marked by poor appetite, hepatalgia and fatigue. According to TCM, hepatitis belongs to the categories of Huang Dan (jaundice), Gan Yu (stagnation of liver qi), Xie Tong (hypochondriac pain), and Zheng Jia (mass in the abdomen), and is caused mainly by accumulation of damp-heat in the middle-jiao.

I. STANDARD TREATMENT

Viral hepatitis is usually divided into four type— accumulation of damp-heat, accumulation of damp-cold, stagnation of liver qi, and impairment of yin fluid by pathogen. Points of the Stomach, Liver and Gallbladder Meridians are frequently selected in its treatment.

1. Accumulation of Damp-Heat

Manifestations: Bright yellow coloration of the skin and sclera, fever, feeling of fullness and distention in the epigastrium, poor appetite, abdominal fullness and distention, hypochondriac distending pain, fatigue.

Tongue: Red body with yellow and sticky coating.

Pulse: Rapid and wiry or soft and rapid.

Treatment Principle: Clear heat and promote diuresis.

Point Prescription & Manipulation:
Primary points:
    DU-14 Dazhui   -
    GB-34 Yanglingquan   -
    ST-36 Zusanli   /
    LR-3 Taichong   -
    BL-48 Yanggang   -

Explanation:
- DU-14Dazhui clears heat;

- GB-34 Yanglingquan, LR-3 Taichong and BL-48 Yanggang   clear damp-heat from the liver and gallbladder, and relieve jaundice;
- ST-36 Zusanli strengthens the spleen and stomach for prevention and treatment of attack of pathogenic qi from the liver.

Secondary points according to conditions:
1️⃣ Severe jaundice — BL-19 Danshu [-], DU-9 Zhiyang [-] and SP-4 Gongsun [-];
2️⃣ High fever — LI-11 Quchi[-] and LI-4 Hegu [-];
3️⃣ Loose stool and severe abdominal fullness and distention — SP-9 Yinlingquan [/];
4️⃣ Severe hypochondriac pain —LR-14 Qimen [-], PC-4 Neiguan [-] and SJ-6 Zhigou [-].

2. Stagnation of Liver Qi

Manifestations: Hypochondriac distending pain, abdominal fullness and distention, nausea, regurgitation, poor appetite, fatigue.

Tongue: White or thin, yellow coating.

Pulse: Thready and wiry.

Treatment Principle: Soothe the liver, promote qi circulation, and regulate the spleen and stomach.

Point Prescription & Manipulation:
Primary points:
    LR-3 Taichong   -
    BL-18 Ganshu   -
    BL-20 Pishu   /
    ST-36 Zusanli ST   +
    GB-34 Yanglingquan   -

Explanation:
- LR-3 Taichong, PC-6 Neiguan, BL-18 Ganshu and GB-34 Yanglingquan soothe the liver and promote qi circulation;
- BL-20 Pishu, RN-12 Zhongwan and ST-36 Zusanli reinforce the spleen and stomach for prevention and treatment of attack of pathogenic qi of the liver.

Secondary points according to conditions:

1. Hypochondriac pain — GB-24 Riyue [-] and LR-14 Qimen [-];
2. Anorexia — RN-12 Zhongwan [/];
3. Chest oppression and nausea—PC-6 Neiguan [-].

3. Accumulation of Cold-Dampness in Spleen

Manifestations: Dark yellow coloration of the skin and sclera, listlessness, fatigue, poor appetite, abdominal distention and fullness, loose stool, aversion to cold

Tongue: Pale body with white and sticky coating.

Pulse: Soft and slow.

Treatment Principle: Reinforce the function of the spleen, remove dampness, and warm yang.

Point Prescription & Manipulation:
Primary points:

> RN-12 Zhongwan + ^
> BL-20 Pishu + ^
> BL-48 Yanggang + ^
> ST-36 Zusanli + ^
> SP-6 Sanyinjiao + ^
> SP-9 Yinlingquan + ^
> BL-19 Danshu + ^

Explanation:

- RN-12 Zhongwan, BL-20 Pishu and ST-36 Zusanli warm the middle-jiao and reinforce its function to dispel cold and remove dampness;
- SP-6 Sanyinjiao and SP-9 Yinlingquan reinforce the spleen to drain dampness;
- BL-19 Danshu relieves jaundice.

Secondary points according to conditions:

1. Severe jaundice — BL-19 Danshu [^ -] and BL-21 Weishu [^ -];
2. Severe abdominal distention—RN-6 Qihai [+ ^];
3. Chills — DU-14 Dazhui [+ ^] and DU-9 Zhiyang [+ ^].

4. Impairment of Yin by Pathogen

Manifestations: Intermittent low fever, heat sensation of the palms and soles, hypochondriac pain, bitter taste, dryness of the throat.

Tongue: Red body with little coating.

Pulse: Thready, wiry and rapid.

Treatment Principle: Nourish yin, clear heat.

Point Prescription & Manipulation:
Primary points:

> DU-14 Dazhui /
> KI-1 Taixi +
> PC-5 Jianshi /
> BL-18 Ganshu +
> BL-23 Shenshu +
> PC-6 Neiguan /

Explanation:

- KI-3 Taixi, BL-18 Ganshu and BL-23 Shenshu reinforce the kidney and liver and nourish yin;
- DU-14 Dazhui and PC-5 Jianshi clear heat;
- PC-6 Neiguan promotes qi circulation and clears heat.

Secondary points according to conditions:

1. Hypochondriac pain—LR-3 Taichong [/] and GB-34 Yanglingquan [/].

II. EXPERIENTIAL TREATMENT

1. Puncturing GB-34 Yanglingquan, etc.

Indication: Chronic hepatitis.

Point Prescription:
Primary points:

> GB-34 Yanglingquan
> LR-3 Taichong
> ST-36 Zusanli
> SP-6 Sanyinjiao

Secondary points according to conditions:

1. High fever — LI-11 Quchi;
2. Severe jaundice — BL-48 Yanggang and

BL-19 Danshu.

Manipulation: For mild cases, acupuncture is performed on the points of one side each time, and the two sides are selected alternatively; for severe cases, the points of both sides are punctured each time. Acupuncture is applied with reducing or uniform reinforcing and reducing manipulation. The treatment is given once daily, with 10 treatments as a course. Generally, persistent treatments for 3 months are needed.

2. Puncturing through BL-18 Ganshu to BL-19 Danshu

Indication: Acute hepatitis.

Point Prescription:
Primary point:
   BL-18 Ganshu

Secondary points according to conditions:
1 Jaundice—ST-36 Zusanli   and GB-34
   Yanglingquan;
2 Abdominal pain and diarrhea—ST-25
   Tianshu and SP-4 Gongsun;
3 Constipation — BL-25 Dachangshu;
4 Abdominal distention and poor appetite—
   RN-12 Zhongwan.

Manipulation: Ask the patient to lie on the stomach. On BL-18 Ganshu, inset a 3-cun needle horizontally at an angle of 15 degrees, with the needle tip toward to BL-19 Danshu. Lift, thrust and rotate the needle while inserting it deep. On ST-36 Zusanli and SP-9 Yinlingquan, puncture 2 cun deep; On SP-6 Sanyinjiao, puncture 1.5 cun deep. On all of the points, perform a strong stimulation, retain the needles for 30-40 minutes and manipulate them every 10 minutes. The treatment is given once daily until the disease is cured.

3. Puncturing Two Groups of the Points

Indication: Chronic hepatitis.

Point Prescription:
Primary points:

Group 1: DU-9 Zhiyang, BL-18 Ganshu, GB-34 Yanglingquan, ST-36 Zusanli;

Group 2: DU-14 Dazhui, BL-20 Pishu, RN-6 Qihai, SP-6 Sanyinjiao.

Secondary points according to conditions:
1 Damp-heat syndrome—LR-2 Xingjian   and
   SP-9 Yinlingquan;
2 Yin deficiency syndrome — KI-3 Taixi;
3 Positive HBsAg—The inguinal lymph nodes.

Manipulation: On DU-9 Zhiyang, puncture obliquely upward 1 cun deep; on BL-19 Ganshu, puncture obliquely toward the spinal column 0.5-0.8 cun deep; on GB-34 Yanglingquan and ST-36 Zusanli, puncture perpendicularly 1.5 cun deep; on DU-14 Dazhui, puncture obliquely upward 1 cun deep; on BL-20 Pishu, puncture obliquely toward the spinal column 1 cun deep; On RN-6 Qihai and SP-6 Sanyinjiao, puncture perpendicularly 1 cun deep. When puncturing the inguinal lymph nodes, fix the node with the thumb and index finger of one hand, insert the needle quickly into the node with the other hand, and take out the needle when the patient feels the needling sensation radiating downward to the leg. The other points are punctured in a regular way. Group 1 and group 2 are selected alternatively. The treatment is given once daily to patients with obvious symptoms and once every other day to patients without obvious symptoms. Two months of the treatment are taken as one course.

Comment:
Virus hepatitis is very infectious during some stage of its course, and very severe in some cases. Generally, the patients need comprehensive treatments, and acupuncture is only taken as one of them. In chronic hepatitis, acupuncture treatment should be applied for about 3 months.

Notes:

4. Hypertension

Hypertension is a common complaint in clinical practice. It is characterized by rising of the arterial pressure (systolic pressure greater than 21.2 Kpa or 160 mm Hg, or diastolic pressure greater than 12.5 Kpa or 95 mm Hg), and is classified into primary and second types. Primary hypertension refers to high blood pressure with no clear cause. It is an independent disease marked by high blood pressure of the arterial system; other manifestations include headache, dizziness, numbness of the limbs, insomnia and irritability. Secondary hypertension refers to hypertension occurring secondary to organic problems, such as nephritic, cardiac, or endocrine disorder. In these cases, hypertension is a symptom of the disease. According to TCM, essential hypertension belongs to the categories of Xuan Yun (vertigo) and Tou Tong (headache). It is caused mainly by mental injury resulting in stagnation of the liver qi and subsequent flaring-up of the liver yang with deficiency of kidney yin, and by improper diet resulting in deficiency of the spleen and accumulation of phlegm in the interior.

I. STANDARD TREATMENT

Essential hypertension is generally divided into four types — overactivity of liver fire, accumulation of turbid phlegm, over-activity of yang with yin deficiency, and deficiency of yin and yang. Points of the Urinary Bladder, Liver, Kidney, Gallbladder Meridians are frequently selected in its treatment.

1. Over-Activity of Liver Fire

Manifestations: High blood pressure, headache, dizziness, flushed face, red eyes, bitter taste, irritability, constipation.

Tongue: Red body with yellow coating.

Pulse: Wiry and rapid.

Treatment Principle: Clear liver and reduce fire.

Point Prescription & Manipulation:

Primary points:
　　GB-20 Fengchi　　-
　　LR-3 Taichong　　-
　　LR-2 Xingjian　　-
　　LI-11 Quchi　　-
　　LI-4 Hegu　　-

Explanation:
- GB-20 Fengchi, the Crossing Point of the Gallbladder and Yangwei Meridians, clears fire in the head and eyes and tranquilizes pain in the head;
- LR-2 Xingjian and LR-3 Taichong reduce liver fire;
- LI-11 Quchi and LI-4 Hegu clear heat and lower high blood pressure.

Secondary points according to conditions:
1〕 Irritability and insomnia — HT-7 Shenmen [-], GB-43 Xiaxi [-] and GB-13 Benshen [-];
2〕 Constipation — SJ-6 Zhigou [-].

2. Accumulation of Turbid Phlegm

Manipulations: High blood pressure, dizziness, pain and distention in the head, distressing sensation of the chest and epigastric region, poor appetite, heaviness of the limbs.

Tongue: White and sticky coating.

Pulse: Wiry and smooth.

Treatment Principle: Resolve turbid phlegm.

Point Prescription & Manipulation:
Primary points:
　　GB-20 Fengchi　　/
　　RN-12 Zhongwan　　/
　　ST-40 Fenglong　　-
　　LI-11 Quchi　　-
　　PC-6 Neiguan　　/

Explanation:
- ST-40 Fenglong and LI-11 Quchi remove phlegm;
- RN-12 Zhongwan reinforces the middle-jiao to decrease production of phlegm;

- GB-20 Fengchi and PC-6 Neiguan relieve symptoms of the head and chest.

Secondary points according to conditions:
1 Nausea or vomiting—SP-9 Yinlingquan [- ^], ST-36 Zusanli [+ ^] and ST-8 Touwei [-];
2 Severe dizziness — DU-20 Baihui [-].

3. Over-Activity of Yang with Yin Deficiency

Manifestations: High blood pressure, headache, dizziness, tinnitus, irritability, insomnia, soreness and weakness of the lower back and knees, numbness or trembling of the limbs.

Tongue: Red body with little coating.

Pulse: Thready and wiry.

Treatment Principle: Nourish yin and restrain yang.

Point Prescription & Manipulation:
Primary points:
    BL-18 Ganshu   +
    BL-23 Shenshu   +
    LR-3 Taichong   -
    SP-6 Sanyinjiao   /
    GB-20 Fengchi   /
    PC-6 Neiguan   /

Explanation:
- BL-18 Ganshu and BL-23 Shenshu tonify the kidney and liver yin and nourish blood for the treatment of the root of this syndrome;
- LR-3 Taichong and GB-20 Fengchi pacify the liver to restrain yang from rising and calm wind;
- SP-6 Sanyinjiao and PC-6 Neiguan reinforce yin and calm the mind.

Secondary points according to conditions:
1 Insomnia and palpitations—HT-7 Shenmen is punctured to HT-6 Yinxi;
2 Dizziness — EX-HN-3 Yintang [-];
3 Severe numbness of the limbs —LI-11 Quchi [-] and GB-34 Yanglingquan [-].

4. Deficiency of Yin and Yang

Manifestations: High blood pressure, dizziness, blurred vision, palpitations, tinnitus, soreness and weakness of the lower back and knees, insomnia, frequent urination in the night.

Tongue: Red body with little coating.

Pulse: Deep and weak.

Treatment Principle: Nourish yin and reinforce yang.

Point Prescription & Manipulation:
Primary points:
    BL-23 Shenshu   +
    RN-4 Guanyuan   +
    RN-6 Qihai   +
    DU-20 Baihui   /
    GB-20 Fengchi   /
    SP-6 Sanyinjiao   +

Explanation:
- BL-23 Shenshu, RN-6 Qihai and RN-4 Guanyuan tonify kidney yin and yang;
- SP-6 Sanyinjiao reinforces kidney yin;
- DU-20 Baihui and GB-20 Fengchi soothe the liver and calm wind.

Secondary points according to conditions:
1 Insomnia and palpitations—HT-7 Shenmen [/];
2 Dizziness — EX-HN-1 Sishencong [/];
3 Dry throat and tongue — KI-3 Taixi [+];
4 Edema of the lower limbs—SP-9 Yinlingquan [+].

II. EXPERIENTIAL TREATMENT

1. Puncturing ST-9 Renying

Indication: Hypertension.

Point Prescription:
    ST-19 Renying

Manipulation: Insert a needle into the point perpendicularly 1 cun deep, place the needle body near to the artery but do not injure the artery, retain the needle for 5 minutes. The treatment is given once every other day, with five treatments as a course. Usually, after treatment, high blood pressure will be lowered immediately. Some cases can be cured by the treatment.

2. Warming Needling on RN-5 Shimen

Indication: Hypertension belonging to yang deficiency.

Point prescription:
RN-5 Shimen

Manipulation: Insert a needle into the point perpendicularly about 2.5 cun deep, rotate the needle to induce arrival of qi, and retain the needle for 30 minutes. During the retention, apply moxibustion by performing the warm needle manipulation. The treatment is given once daily or every other day, with 10 treatments as a course.

3. Puncturing EX-HN-18 Pressure-Lowering Point

Indication: Hypertension.

Point Prescription:
EX-HN-18 Pressure-lowering Point, located at the midpoint of the line connecting BL-1 Jingming and BL-2 Cuanzhu.

Manipulation: Insert a needle perpendicularly into the point 0.3-0.5 cun deep, rotate the needle at a small amplitude to induce the needling sensation and retain the needle for 30 minutes. The treatment is given once every other day, with five treatments as a course. Generally, after three treatments, high blood pressure will be lowered greatly.

4. Puncturing BL-65 Shugu

Indication: Intractable high diastolic blood pressure in old patients.

Point Prescription:
BL-65 Shugu

Manipulation: Insert a needle into the point obliquely 0.5 cun with its tip toward the tip of the small toe. Thrust, lift and rotate the needle to induce arrival of qi, retain it for 40 minutes and manipulate it every 10 minutes. The treatment is given once daily, with five treatments as a course. Usually, after three treatments the patient's condition will be obviously improved.

Comment:
Acupuncture is effective in lowering blood pressure, and some patients' hypertension can be cured by Zhenjiu treatment. Patients with hypertension are advised to keep a good emotional condition, give up smoking and drinking, and reduce intake of greasy food.

Notes:

5. Arrhythmic Disorder

Arrhythmic disorder refers to quick heart beating, slow heart beating or irregular heart beating. It may be caused by organic diseases of the heart and functional disorders of the nervous system. Arrhythmic disorder includes tachycardia, bradycardia and arrhythmia. Clinically, it is marked by palpitation, accompanied by dizziness, distressing sensation in the chest, or even nausea. According to TCM, arrhythmic disorder belongs to Xin Ji (palpitation), and is caused by emotional depression or improper diet. This leads to stagnation of qi and blood with internal generation of phlegm that interferes with the heart, or causes deficiency of qi and blood and lack of nourishment of the heart.

I. STANDARD TREATMENT

Arrhythmic disorder is generally divided into five types — heart qi deficiency, heart blood deficiency, heart yin deficiency with hyperactivity of fire, blood stasis, and attack of the heart by retained phlegm. Points of the Pericardium, Heart and Bladder Meridians are frequently selected in its treatment.

1. Heart Qi Deficiency

Manifestations: Palpitation, fear and fright, restlessness, insomnia, dream-disturbed sleep.

Tongue: Thin and white coating.

Pulse: Feeble.

Treatment Principle: Nourish heart qi, relieve timidity and calm the mind.

Point Prescription & Manipulation:
Primary points:
    HT-7 Shenmen /
    PC-6 Neiguan /
    KI-3 Taixi +
    ST-36 Zusanli +
    RN-6 Qihai +
    BL-15 Xinshu +

Explanation:
* ST-36 Zusanli and RN-6 Qihai reinforce the middle-jiao and tonify qi;
* HT-T Shenmen and BL-15 Xinshu nourish the heart and calm the mind to relieve timidity;
* KI-3 Taixi and PC-6 Neiguan communicate with the heart and kidney to calm the mind.

Secondary points according to conditions:
1▢ Severe palpitation — LU-9 Taiyuan [+] and HT-9 Shaochong [/];
2▢ Chest oppression or pain — RN-14 Juque [+].

2. Heart Blood Deficiency

Manifestations: Palpitation, dizziness, pale complexion, and lassitude.

Tongue: Pale body.

Pulse: Thready and weak.

Treatment Principle: Replenish blood, nourish heart and calm the mind.

Point Prescription & Manipulation:
Primary points:
    HT-7 Shenmen /
    ST-36 Zusanli +
    RN-6 Qihai +
    BL-15 Xinshu +
    SP-6 Sanyinjiao +
    BL-18 Ganshu +

Explanation:
* ST-36 Zusanli and RN-6 Qihai reinforce the middle-jiao and tonify qi to promote blood production;
* SP-6 Sanyinjiao and BL-18 Ganshu reinforce the liver and nourish blood;
* HT-7 Shenmen and BL-15 Xinshu nourish the heart and calm the mind.

Secondary points according to conditions:
1▢ Night sweating — HT-6 Yinxi [-];
2▢ Dizziness and blurred vision — KI-3 Taixi [+] and GB-20 Fengchi [-].

3. Heart Yin Deficiency with Hyperactivity of Fire

Manifestations: Palpitation, restlessness, insomnia, dizziness, hot sensation in the palms, soles and chest, tinnitus, soreness of the lower back and knees.

Tongue: Red body.

Pulse: Thready and rapid.

Treatment Principle: Replenish yin, clear heat, nourish heart and calm the mind.

Point Prescription & Manipulation:
Primary points:
    HT-7 Shenmen /
    PC-6 Neiguan /
    KI-3 Taixi +
    LR-3 Taichong -
    BL-15 Xinshu /
    BL-23 Shenshu +

Explanation:
- KI-3 Taixi, BL-15 Xinshu and BL-23 Shenshu replenish yin of the heart and kidney;
- LR-3 Taichong clears heat;
- HT-7 Shenmen and PC-6 Neiguan calm the mind.

Secondary points according to conditions:
1. Night sweating — HT-6 Yinxi [-];
2. Hot sensation — LU-9 Taiyuan [-] and SI-4 Wangu [-];
3. Dizziness and blurred vision—GB-20 Fengchi [-].

4. Blood Stasis of the Heart

Manifestations: Palpitation, pain in the chest, purplish lips.

Tongue: Purple body with ecchymotic spots.

Pulse: Unsmooth.

Treatment Principle: Promote circulation of qi and blood, activate the collaterals.

Point Prescription & Manipulation:
Primary points:
    HT-7 Shenmen /
    BL-17 Geshu - ^
    BL-18 Ganshu / ^
    BL-15 Xinshu / ^
    RN-17 Danzhong /
    LR-3 Taichong -

Explanation:
- HT-7 Shenmen calms the mind;
- BL-17 Geshu , BL-18 Ganshu and BL-18 Xinshu promote blood circulation and activate collaterals of the heart;
- RN-17 Danzhong and LR-3 Taichong promote qi circulation.

Secondary points according to conditions:
1. Severe pain in the chest — PC-5 Jianshi [-] and RN-14 Juque [/].

5. Attack of Heart by Retained Phlegm

Manifestations: Palpitation, fullness in the chest and epigastrium, edema of the lower limbs, nausea.

Tongue: White and slippery body.

Pulse: Wiry and smooth.

Treatment Principle: Invigorate heart yang, reinforce qi and transform phlegm.

Point Prescription & Manipulation:
Primary points:
    HT-7 Shenmen /
    RN-17 Danzhong / ^
    RN-4 Guanyuan + ^
    ST-40 Fenglong - ^
    SP-9 Yinlingquan / ^

Explanation:
- RN-17 Danzhong and RN-4 Guanyuan tonify qi and invigorate heart yang;

- ST-40 Fenglong and SP-9 Yinlingquan strengthen the middle-jiao and resolve phlegm;
- HT-7 Shenmen nourishes the heart and calms the mind.

Secondary points according to conditions:
1□ Nausea and severe palpitation— LI-4 Hegu [-], PC-6 Neiguan [-] and ST-36 Zusanli [+];
2□ Severe pain in chest — PC-4 Ximen [-];
3□ Edema — BL-15 Xinshu [+ ^] and BL-23 Shenshu[+^];
4□ Unbearable palpitation — The twelve Jing-Well Points are pricked to bleed.

II. EXPERIENTIAL TREATMENT

1. Puncturing BL-2 Cuanzhu

Indication: Supraventricular tachycardia.

Point Prescription:
    BL-2 Cuanzhu

Manipulation: Puncture 0.3-0.5 cun deep, manipulate the needles to induce arrival of qi, retain the needles for 15 minutes, and manipulate them every 5 minutes. The treatment is given once every other day with 10 treatments as a course. Usually several courses are needed.

2. Puncturing PC-6 Neiguan, etc.

Indication: Sinus bradycardia.

Point Prescription:
Primary points:
    PC-6 Neiguan
    LU-7 Lieque
    RN-17 Danzhong
    ST-36 Zusanli

Secondary points according to conditions:
1□ Dream-disturbed sleep and night sweating— HT-7 Shenmen and SP-6 Sanyinjiao;
2□ Distressing sensation and pain in the chest — BL-17 Geshu.

Manipulation: Puncture with even reinforcing-reducing manipulation by rotating the needles.

The treatment is given once every other day, with 10 treatments as a course. Usually, several courses are needed.

3. Puncturing EX-UE-14 Xiadu

Indication: Bradycardia.

Point Prescription:
    EX-UE-14 Xiadu located on the dorsum of the hand, 0.5 cm proximal to the web between the fourth and fifth fingers.

Manipulation: Ask the patient to make a fist with the left hand. Puncture the left point along the inter-space of the metacarpal bones 0.5-1 cun deep, rotate the needle about 10 turns to induce arrival of qi. Retain the needle for 20-60 minutes and manipulate every 10 minutes. Usually, within 15 minutes the effective result will come. If not, puncture the opposite point the same way additionally.

4. Puncturing PC-6 Neiguan

Indication: Various types of arrhythmia.

Point Prescription:
    PC-6 Neiguan

Manipulation: Puncture obliquely upward 1-1.2 cun. Thrust, lift and rotate the needles to induce soreness, numbness, heaviness and distention to the patient. Use mild stimulation on old or weak patients, but strong stimulation on patients with a hardy bodily constitution. Retain the needles for 15-30 minutes, and manipulate them every 5 minutes. The treatment is given once every other day, with 10 treatments as a course. Usually, arrhythmia will be relieved immediately after the treatment.

Comment:
Zhenjiu is effective in treating arrhythmia. For functional arrhythmia, Zhenjiu can bring about a radical result, but for arrhythmia due to an organic disorder of the heart, Zhenjiu is mainly used to relieve symptoms.

Notes:

6. Angina Pectoris

Angina pectoris, a type of coronary heart disease, it is caused by coronary spasm or coronary arteriosclerosis resulting in temporary or long-term myocardial ischemia and subsequent damage to the cardiac muscle. Its etiology is still not well known. Typical angina pectoris is marked by paroxysmal constrictive pain in the retrosternal region or left chest, radiating to the left arm and shoulder. It is induced by physical exertion, emotional disturbance, over-eating or attack by cold, and is usually relieved quickly by rest and treatment. According to TCM, angina pectoris belongs to Xiong Bi (chest blockage syndrome), Jue Xin Tong (precordial pain with cold limbs), and Zhen Xin Tong (real heart pain). It is caused by emotional injury resulting in stagnation of the liver qi and heart blood, or obstruction of the collaterals by turbid phlegm.

I. STANDARD TREATMENT

Angina pectoris is generally divided into five types — stagnation of qi and blood by turbid phlegm, obstruction of collaterals by stagnant blood, deficiency of heart and spleen, deficiency of heart and kidney yang and collapse of qi and yang. Points of the Bladder, Heart and Pericardium Meridians are frequently selected in its treatment.

1. Stagnation of Qi and Blood by Turbid Phlegm

Manifestations: Chest pain radiating to the shoulder and back, suffocation feeling of the chest, palpitation, shortness of breath, nausea, profuse sputum.

Tongue: Pale body with white, thick and sticky coating.

Pulse: Wiry and smooth or deep and wiry.

Treatment Principle: Invigorate yang, eliminate turbid phlegm and relieve stagnation.

Point Prescription & Manipulation:

Primary points:
    BL-15 Xinshu   + ^
    PC-6 Neiguan   /
    RN-14 Juque   +
    RN-17 Danzhong   -
    ST-40 Fenglong   -
    ST-36 Zusanli   + ^

Explanation:
During attack with cardiac pain, perform strong stimulation, manipulate the needle until the pain becomes mild and retain the needles until the pain disappears. During the remission stage, perform mild stimulation.

- BL-15 Xinshu and RN-14 Juque, the Back-Shu and Front-Mu Points of the Heart, invigorate heart yang, activate heart blood circulation and stop cardiac pain;
- RN-17 Danzhong, the Influential Point of qi, promotes qi circulation to relieve pain of the chest;
- PC-6 Neiguan promotes qi circulation and activates the collaterals to relieve cardiac pain;
- ST-40 Fenglong and ST-36 Zusanli reinforce the spleen and stomach and transform phlegm.

Secondary point:
1🗌 Severe chest pain — PC-4 Ximen [-].

2. Obstruction of Collaterals by Stagnant Blood

Manifestations: Fixed pain in the chest, suffocation feeling of the chest, shortness of breath.

Tongue: Dark purple body with ecchymosis.

Pulse: Thready and unsmooth or regularly or irregularly interrupted.

Treatment Principle: Promote blood circulation, remove blood stasis and activate collaterals.

Point Prescription & Manipulation:
Primary points:

BL-15 Xinshu   + ^
PC-6 Neiguan   /
RN-14 Juque   /
RN-17 Danzhong   -
BL-17 Geshu   - ^
PC-4 Ximen   -

Explanation:
Manipulation is the same as above.

* BL-15 Xinshu   and RN-14 Juque, the Back-Shu and Front-Mu Points of the heart, invigorate heart yang, activate heart blood circulation and stop cardiac pain;
* RN-17 Danzhong, the Influential Point of qi, promotes qi circulation to relieve pain of the chest;
* BL-17 Geshu promotes blood circulation and removes blood stasis;
* PC-6 Neiguan and PC-4 Ximen promote circulation of qi of the Heart Meridian and relieve pain.

Secondary points according to conditions:
1□ Severe chest pain — HT-6 Yinxi [-];
2□ Chest oppression and enlarged tongue body — ST-36 Zusanli [+ ^] and ST-40 Fenglong [+ ^].

3. Deficiency of Heart and Spleen

Manifestations: Dull cardiac pain, palpitation, shortness of breath, poor appetite, loose stools, fatigue, listlessness.

Tongue: Pale body.

Pulse: Deep and thready pulse or irregularly or regularly interrupted.

Treatment Principle: Tonify heart and spleen, reinforce qi and blood, and promote circulation of qi and blood.

Point Prescription & Manipulation:
Primary points:
BL-15 Xinshu   + ^
PC-6 Neiguan   /
RN-17 Danzhong   /

BL-20 Pishu   + ^
ST-36 Zusanli   + ^
BL-17 Geshu   / ^
BL-14 Jueyinshu + ^

Explanation:
* BL-15 Xinshu, BL-20 Pishu and BL-17 Geshu, the Back-Shu Points of the heart and spleen and the Influential Point of blood, tonify blood of the heart and spleen; Moxibustion is applied to strengthen the effect of warming yang qi, and promote blood circulation to relieve cardiac pain;
* BL-14 Jueyinshu, the Back-Shu Point of the pericardium, good for weakness of the chest yang, can be used to warm the heart yang and disperse cold evil;
* PC-6 Neiguan promotes qi circulation to relieve cardiac pain;
* ST-36 Zusanli tonifies the spleen and stomach to reinforce qi.

Secondary points according to conditions:
1□ Poor appetite — RN-12 Zhongwan [+ ^];
2□ Regularly or irregularly interrupted pulse — HT-7 Shenmen [/].

4. Deficiency of Heart and Kidney Yang

Manifestations: Suffocation sensation or dull pain of the chest, palpitation, shortness of breath, which are aggravated by exertion, aversion to cold, cold limbs, soreness, weakness and coldness of the lower back and knees, swelling of the lower limbs.

Tongue: Pale body.

Pulse: Thready and weak or interrupted.

Treatment Principle: Benefit heart, kidney and warm yang.

Point Prescription & Manipulation:
Primary points:
BL-15 Xinshu + ^
PC-6 Neiguan   -
RN-4 Guanyuan + ^
RN-6 Qihai   + ^

BL-23 Shenshu + ^
ST-36 Zusanli + ^

Explanation:
- BL-15 Xinshu and BL-23 Shenshu, the Back-Shu Points of the heart and kidney, tonify the heart and kidney;
- RN-4 Guanyuan and RN-6 Qihai invigorate yang;
- ST-36 Zusanli reinforces the middle-jiao to promote production of yang qi;
- PC-6 Neiguan promotes heart qi circulation to relieve cardiac pain.

Secondary point:
1 Swelling — SP-9 Yinlingquan [^].

5. Collapse of Qi and Yang

Manifestations: Acute, colic and stabbing pain in the chest, which radiates to the upper back and shoulder, dark complexion, cold limbs, profuse sweating, purple lips, or even coma

Tongue: Purple body.

Pulse: Deep and feeble or intermittent.

Treatment Principle: Restore yang and rescue the life from collapse.

Point Prescription & Manipulation:
Primary points:
    BL-14 Jueyinshu + ^
    PC-6 Neiguan   -
    RN-8 Shenque ^
    RN-6 Qihai   ^
    RN-4 Guanyuan ^
    DU-20 Baihui ^
    ST-36 Zusanli + ^

Explanation:
Rotate the needles in DU-25 Shuigou, DU-26 Suliao, and PC-6 Neiguan with strong stimulation until the patient recovers his consciousness. Apply moxibustion with moxa stick on RN-8 Shenque, RN-4 Guanyuan, RN-6 Qihai and DU-20 Baihui for 20-40 minutes.

- RN-8 Shenque, RN-6 Qihai, RN-4 Guanyuan and DU-20 Baihui warm primary yang, reinforce qi and rescue the life from collapse;
- ST-36 Zusanli stabilizes the body resistance;
- PC-6 Neiguan and BL-14 Jueyinshu promote qi and blood circulation to relieve cardiac pain.

Secondary points according to conditions:
1 Coma — DU-25 Shuigou [-];
2 Feeble breath — DU-26 Suliao [-].

II. EXPERIENTIAL TREATMENT

1. Puncturing PC-6 Neiguan

Indication: Angina pectoris.

Point Prescription:
    PC-6 Neiguan

Manipulation: Puncture perpendicularly 2 cun deep, quickly rotate the needle for 2 minutes to induce needling sensations of soreness, numbness, heaviness and distention which radiate to the elbow, armpit and chest. In case the needling sensation is limited in the PC-6 Neiguan region, repeat the manipulation and press the running course of the Pericardium Meridian from PC-6 Neiguan upward to the armpit to induce the radiation of the needling sensation. Then, retain the needle for 30 minutes, and manipulate it once during the retention. The treatment is given once daily, with 10 treatments as a course.

2. Pressing with Finger

Indication: Acute onset of angina pectoris.

Point Prescription:
    DU-9 Zhiyang

Manipulation: Hold the patient's shoulder with the left hand and press the point forcefully with the right thumb until the pain becomes greatly relieved, usually, for 1-6 minutes. Alternatively, hold a coin with the thumb and index finger of the right hand to press the point heavily in replace of pressing the point with the thumb.

3. Bleeding

Indication: Acute onset of angina pectoris.

Point Prescription:
    PC-9 Zhongchong
    The tip of the tongue

Manipulation: Prick the points with a thick needle to cause bleeding. The pain can be relieved immediately by this method.

Comment:

Zhenjiu is effective in treatment of angina pectoris. Pressing DU-9 Zhiyang with finger has proven to be effective in relieving cardiac pain due to angina pectoris, so it can be chosen for patients with attack of angina pectoris in case of lack of needle or medicine.

Notes:

7. Chronic Bronchitis

Chronic bronchitis refers to a chronic nonspecific inflammation of the mucosa and peripheral tissues of the trachea and bronchi. Always it comes from acute bronchitis. Clinically, it is marked by long-standing intermittent cough with sputum induced by or aggravated by cold or overstrain, usually accompanied by shortness of breath, and lasts for more than 3 months every year for 2 years or more. Chronic bronchitis is usually caused by infection of virus or/and bacteria, and related to smoking, air pollution, and sensitivity to some materials, such as bacteria, dusts and chemical air. According to TCM, chronic bronchitis belongs to the categories of Ke Sou (cough) and Chuan Zheng (asthma). It is caused by attack of the lung by exogenous pathogens, leading to the failure of the lung qi in descending; or attack of the lung by phlegm and dampness resulting from spleen deficiency; or failure of the kidney in receiving qi due to long-standing illness resulting in kidney deficiency.

I. STANDARD TREATMENT

Bronchitis is generally divided into three types — attack of the lung by damp-phlegm, deficiency of lung and kidney yin, and deficiency of spleen and kidney yang. Points of the Large Intestine, Kidney, Spleen and Stomach Meridians are frequently selected in its treatment.

1. Attack of Lung by Damp-Phlegm

Manifestations: Cough with profuse white and sticky sputum, distressing sensation in the chest and epigastrium, poor appetite.

Tongue: White and sticky coating.

Pulse: Wiry and smooth.

Treatment Principle: Invigorate spleen, remove dampness, resolve phlegm and check cough.

Point Prescription & Manipulation:

Primary points:
    BL-13 Feishu   / ^
    BL-20 Pishu   / ^
    ST-36 Zusanli   + ^
    ST-40 Fenglong   - ^
    LU-9 Taiyuan   -

Explanation:
Acupuncture and moxibustion are applied with reducing manipulation during the onset stage and even reinforcing-reducing manipulation during the remission stage.

- BL-20 Pishu, ST-36 Zusanli and ST-40 Fenglong reinforce spleen to transform phlegm and dampness;
- BL-13 Feishu, the Back-Shu Point of the lung, disperses lung qi and relieves cough;
- LU-9 Taiyuan assists BL-13 Feishu to disperse lung qi and relieve cough.

Secondary points according to conditions:
1 Shortness of breath or asthma—RN-22 Tiantu [/], RN-17 Danzhong [-] and RN-6 Qihai [+ ^].

2. Deficiency of Lung and Kidney Yin

Manifestations: Cough with a little sticky sputum, dizziness, soreness and weakness of the lower back and knees, heat sensation of the chest, palms and soles, dry mouth and throat.

Tongue: Red body with little coating.

Pulse: Thready and rapid.

Treatment Principle: Nourish kidney, moisten lung and arrest cough.

Point Prescription & Manipulation:
Primary points:
    BL-13 Feishu   +
    BL-43 Gaohuang   +
    BL-23 Shenshu   +
    KI-3 Taixi   +
    RN-22 Tiantu   +
    LU-5 Chize   +

Explanation:
- BL-13 Feishu, BL-43 Gaohuang and LU-5 Chize nourish lung yin;
- BL-23 Shenshu and KI-3 Taixi nourish kidney yin;
- RN-22 Tiantu disperses lung qi to arrest cough.

Secondary points according to conditions:
1 Severe cases — KI-6 Zhaohai [+] and LU-7 Lieque [+];
2 Night sweating — HT-6 Yinxi [+].

3. Deficiency of Spleen and Kidney Yang

Manifestations: Cough with shortness of breath or asthma, poor appetite, loose stool, soreness, weakness and coldness of the lower back and knees.

Tongue: Pale body with white coating.

Pulse: Deep and weak.

Treatment Principle: Warm yang and strengthen spleen, tonify lung and kidney and help absorbing qi.

Point Prescription & Manipulation:
Primary points:
    BL-20 Pishu   + ^
    BL-23 Shenshu   + ^
    BL-13 Feishu   + ^
    ST-36 Zusanli   + ^
    ST-40 Fenglong   + ^
    RN-22 Tiantu   +
    LU-10 Yuji   +

Explanation:
- BL-20 Pishu, BL-23 Shenshu and BL-13 Feishu, the Back-Shu Points of the spleen, kidney and lung, reinforce yang qi of these three organs. Cupping may be applied on them to strengthen their action of relieving cough;
- ST-36 Zusanli and ST-40 Fenglong reinforce the middle-jiao and transform phlegm;
- RN-22 Tiantu and LU-10 Yuji disperse lung qi to relieve cough.

Secondary points according to conditions:
1. Edema and dysuria—SP-9 Yinlingquan [-^];
2. Chest oppression and palpitation — BL-15 Xinshu [+ ^] and PC-6 [/].

II. EXPERIENTIAL TREATMENT

1. Puncturing and Cupping DU-14 Dazhui

Indication: Childhood chronic bronchitis.

Point Prescription:
   DU-14 Dazhui

Manipulation: Prick DU-14 Dazhui and the point 6 cm lateral to DU-14 Dazhui to bleed a little, and apply cupping on the punctured region for 20 minutes. The treatment is given once a week, with five treatments as a course.

2. Moxibustion

Indication: Chronic bronchitis.

Point Prescription:
   RN-22 Tiantu
   BL-13 Feishu
   BL-12 Fengmen
   DU-14 Dazhui
   BL-43 Gaohuang

Manipulation: Apply moxibustion with moxa stick on each point 5-10 minutes until the local skin becomes flushed. The treatment is given once daily, with 10 treatments as a course.

3. Puncturing and Cupping A Group of Points

Indication: Chronic bronchitis.

Point Prescription:
Primary points:
   DU-12 Shenzhu
   RN-17 Danzhong

Secondary points according to conditions:
1. Fever — LI-4 Hegu and DU-14 Dazhui;
2. Profuse sputum — ST-40 Fenglong;
3. Asthma — EX-B-1 Dingchuan and LU-10 Yuji;
4. Severe cough — RN-22 Tiantu and LU-7 Lieque.

Manipulation: Ask the patient to sit down upright. First, puncture DU-12 Shenzhu 0.8-1.2 cun deep, and rotate the needle. Then, puncture RN-17 Danzhong obliquely downward 0.5 deep, rotate the needle to induce distention sensation to the patient. Retain the needles for 20 minutes and manipulate them every 5 minutes. After removing the needles, apply cupping on the punctured region 10-15 minutes. For severe cases, prick the punctured points before applying cupping. Acupuncture is applied every day and cupping every other day. When puncturing the Secondary points according to conditions, use the ordinary manipulation.

4. Ear Acupuncture

Indication: Chronic bronchitis.

Ear Point Prescription:
   Bronchia, Lung, Chest, Spleen, Kidney, Large Intestine, Endocrine, Shenmen.

Manipulation: See page 255.

Comment:
Zhenjiu is effective in relieving symptoms of bronchitis and improving the patient's condition. As having an action of strengthening the body's resistance, moxibustion on ST-36 Zusanli can be frequently applied to prevent acute attack of chronic bronchitis.

Notes:

8. Bronchial Asthma

Bronchial asthma is an allergic condition of the bronchi. An asthma attack often occurs as an allergic response in the environment, but it can also be triggered by internal reactions to too much exercise or cold air, or even to emotional stress. Clinically, it is marked by paroxysmal dyspnea and wheezing in the throat, usually accompanied by a feeling of fullness in the chest, shortness of breath, productive cough, cyanosis and orthopnia. Its etiology is closely correlated to heredity, and its attack is mostly induced by the inhalation of, or contact with allergens, such as pollens, dusts, insects, germs, etc. According to TCM, bronchial asthma belongs to the category of Xiao Chuan (asthma), and is caused by exogenous factors, improper diet, emotional injury, or overstrain which stir the interior phlegm, causing it to rise and obstruct the bronchi.

I. STANDARD TREATMENT

Bronchial asthma is generally divided into four types — cold phlegm, heat phlegm, deficiency of lung and spleen, and deficiency of lung and kidney. Points of the Lung, Urinary Bladder and Kidney Meridians are frequently selected in its treatment.

1. Cold Phlegm

Manifestations: Asthma, shortness of breath, dyspnea, fullness and stuffiness in the chest, cough with white and sticky or thin and frothy sputum.

Tongue: White and sticky coating.

Pulse: Floating and tense.

Treatment Principle: Disperse wind and cold, transform phlegm, and stop asthma.

Point Prescription & Manipulation:
Primary points:
  BL-12 Fengmen   - ^

BL-13 Feishu   - ^
RN-22 Tiantu   -
RN-17 Danzhong   -
LU-5 Chize   -
LU-9 Taiyuan   -

Explanation:
- BL-12 Fengmen and BL-13 Feishu disperse the Taiyang Meridian and dispel wind-cold. Additionally, cupping may be applied on them to strengthen their action of relieving asthma;
- LU-5 Chize and LU-9 Taiyuan disperse the Taiyin Meridian and clear the lung for removing phlegm;
- RN-22 Tiantu subdues the adverse flow of the lung qi and relieves asthma;
- RN-17 Danzhong checks the adverse flow of lung qi for relieving asthma.

Secondary points according to conditions:
1⬚ Severe attack of asthma — LU-7 Lieque [-], DU-14 Dazhui [- ^], LI-4 Hegu [-] and EX-B-1 Dingchuan [- ^].

2. Heat Phlegm

Manifestations: Asthma, shortness of breath, paroxysmal choking cough with thick, sticky and yellow sputum that is difficulty to expectorate, stuffiness in the chest, irritability, sweating, thirst.

Tongue: Red body with yellow and sticky coating.

Pulse: Smooth and rapid.

Treatment Principle: Clear heat from the lung, transform phlegm and stop asthma.

Point Prescription & Manipulation:
Primary points:
  BL-13 Feishu   -
  LU-5 Chize   -
  LU-7 Lieque   -
  RN-22 Tiantu   -
  RN-17 Danzhong   -
  ST-40 Fenglong   -
  LI-4 Hegu   -

Explanation:
- LU-5 Chize and LU-7 Lieque clear heat from the lung;
- BL-12 Feishu disperses the lung to relieve asthma;
- ST-40 Fenglong transforms phlegm;
- LI-4 Hegu clears heat;
- RN-22 Tiantu subdues the adverse flow of the lung qi and relieves asthma;
- RN-17 Danzhong promotes circulation of the chest qi.

Secondary points according to conditions:
1〕 Severe attack of asthma—EX-B-1 Dingchuan [-].

3. Qi Deficiency of Lung and Spleen

Manifestations: Asthma, shortness of breath which is aggravated by exertion, cough with profuse dilute sputum, sweating, aversion to cold, poor appetite, loose stools.

Tongue: Pale body with white sticky coating.

Pulse: Soft and thready.

Treatment Principle: Reinforce lung and spleen, transform phlegm and stop asthma.

Point Prescription & Manipulation:
Primary points:
BL-13 Feishu   + ^
BL-20 Pishu   + ^
BL-43 Gaohuang   + ^
RN-17 Danzhong   +
RN-6 Qihai   + ^
ST-36 Zusanli   + ^
LU-9 Taiyuan +
SP-3 Taibai +

Explanation:
- LU-12 Feishu and BL-43 Gaohuang regulate the lung qi and tonify deficiency;
- BL-20 Pishu and RN-6 Qihai reinforce the spleen and tonify qi;
- ST-36 Zusanli reinforces the spleen and transforms phlegm;

- RN-17 Danzhong checks the adverse flow of lung qi for relieving asthma;
- LU-9 Taiyuan, the Yuan-Source and Primary Point of the Lung Meridian, reinforces the lung qi;
- SP-3 Taibai, the Yuan-Source Point of the Spleen Meridian, which pertains to earth, reinforces the lung because the lung belongs to metal and there is a mother-son relationship between the earth and metal.

Secondary points according to conditions:
1〕 Profuse sputum — ST-40 Fenglong [+ ^].

4. Yang Deficiency of Lung and Kidney

Manifestations: Asthma, shortness of breath which is aggravated by exertion, aversion to cold, cold limbs, scanty urine, edema, soreness, coldness and weakness of the lower back and knees.

Tongue: Pale and enlarged body with white and sticky coating.

Pulse: Deep and weak.

Treatment Principle: Tonify kidney and assist in its function of absorption of qi, reinforce lung, stop asthma.

Point Prescription & Manipulation:
Primary points:
BL-13 Feishu   + ^
BL-23 Shenshu   + ^
RN-4 Guanyuan   + ^
RN-6 Qihai 6 + ^
ST-36 Zusanli   +   ^
RN-22 Tiantu   /

Explanation:
- Bl-13 Feishu and BL-23 Shenshu tonify the lung and kidney;
- RN-4 Guanyuan and RN-6 Qihai warm yang and reinforce the kidney;
- RN-22 Tiantu subdues the adverse flow of the lung qi and relieves asthma;
- ST-36 Zusanli reinforces the spleen and transforms phlegm.

Secondary points according to conditions:
1□ Severe cases—RN-17 Danzhong [+], DU-12
Shenzhu [+ ^] and BL-43 Gaohuang [+ ^];
2□ Edema and dysuria—SP-9 Yinlingquan [+^].

II. EXPERIENTIAL TREATMENT

1. Puncturing LU-10 Yuji

Indication: Bronchial asthma in the attack period
or at the remission period.

Point Prescription:
LU-10 Yuji of one side and the other side are
used alternatively.

Manipulation: Puncture 0.5 cun with the needle
tip toward to the center of the palm, rotate the
needle to induce needling sensation, retain it for
20-30 minutes, and rotate it every 5 minutes
during the retention. The treatment is given once
daily, with 10 treatments as a course. Generally,
1-4 courses are needed.

2. Puncturing LU-6 Kongzui

Indication: Bronchial asthma in attack period.

Point Prescription:
LU-6 Kongzui

Manipulation: Puncture 1-2 cun, rotate the
needles at frequency of 120-180 times/minute to
induce a needling sensation that radiates
downward to the tips of the thumb and index
finger and upward to the chest. Retain the needles
for 30-60 minutes, and rotate them every 10
minutes during the retention.

3. Puncturing & Cupping

Indication: Bronchial asthma in attack or
remission period.

Point Prescription:
DU-14 Dazhui
BL-12 Fengmen
BL-13 Feishu
EX-B-1Dingchuan

Manipulation: Firstly, puncture the points,
manipulate the needles to induce arrival of qi, and
retain them for 30 minutes. Then, remove the
needles from BL-12 Fengmen and BL-13 Feishu
and leave the needles in DU-14 Dazhui and EX-
B-1 Dingchuan, and apply cupping on all of the
points for 10-15 minutes. The treatment is given
once daily, with 10 treatments as a course.
Generally, after three treatments, the patient's
condition will be greatly improved.

4. Ear Acupuncture

Indication: Bronchial asthma in attack or
remission period.

Ear Point Prescription:
Trachea, Lung, Chest, Spleen, Kidney, Large
Intestine, Sympathetic, Apex of Antitragus,
Adrenal Gland, Endocrine, Shenmen.

Manipulation: See page 255.

Comment:
Zhenjiu is effective in controlling the patients'
condition due to attack of asthma. However, in
the case of severe attacks, it is suggested not to
refuse other medical treatment methods, which
have also been proven effective. Generally,
allergic asthma can be cured by Zhenjiu
treatment, and radical treatment should be applied
in summer, the hottest period of a year, no matter
whether the patient has an attack of asthma or not
during that period.

Notes:

9. Vomiting

Vomiting is a common symptom of many diseases and disorders including acute gastroenteritis, cardiospasm, pylorospasm, hepatitis, pancreatitis, cholecystitis and cerebral problems. According to TCM, vomiting, called Ou Tu in Chinese, is due to adverse flow of the stomach qi caused by overeating, attack of the stomach by hyperactive liver qi, and deficiency of the spleen and stomach.

I. STANDARD TREATMENT

Vomiting is generally divided into three types — retention of food in the stomach due to overeating, attack of the stomach by hyperactive liver qi and deficiency of the spleen and stomach. Points of the Stomach, Spleen, Pericardium and Ren Meridians are frequently selected in its treatment.

1. Retention of Food in Stomach due to Overeating

Manifestations: Vomiting of acid-fermented contents of the stomach, fullness and distention in the epigastrium and abdomen, belching and anorexia, loose and foul stools.

Tongue: Thick and sticky coating.

Pulse: Slippery and forceful.

Treatment Principle: Improve digestion, relieve stagnation, regulate the stomach and conduct the adverse flow of qi.

Point Prescription & Manipulation:
Primary points:
    RN-12 Zhongwan -
    PC-6 Neiguan -
    ST-36 Zusanli +
    SP-4 Gongsun -
    RN-10 Xiawan -

Explanation:

- RN-12 Zhongwan, the Front-Mu Point of the stomach, ST-36 Zusanli, the He-Sea Point of the Stomach Meridian, and RN-10 Xiawan regulate the middle-jiao to promote digestion;
- PC-6 Neiguan, the Luo-Connecting Point of the Hand-Jueyin Meridian which connects downward the three jiaos, and the Crossing Point of the Yinwei Meridian which functions to control the interior of the body, regulates the qi activity of the upper- and middle-jiao and acts as the key point for relieving vomiting;
- SP-4 Gongsun, the Luo-Connecting and Yuan-Source Point of the Spleen Meridian, and one of the Eight Confluent Points that connects with the Chong Meridian, regulates the middle-jiao and causes rebellious qi to descend;
- PC-6 Neiguan and SP-4 Gongsun are combined, one of the pair-points of the Eight Confluent Points, to have very good effect to relieve fullness of the chest and abdomen.

Secondary points according to conditions:
1️⃣ Constipation— ST-25 Tianshu [-];
2️⃣ Severe vomiting— EX-HN-12 Jinjin and EX-HN-13 Yuye are pricked to bleed.

2. Attack of Stomach by Hyperactive Liver Qi

Manifestations: Vomiting, acid regurgitation, belching, fullness and pain in the costal and hypochondriac region, irritability.

Tongue: Red border and sticky coating.

Pulse: Wiry.

Treatment Principle: Soothe the liver and regulate the stomach.

Point Prescription & Manipulation:
Primary points:
    RN-12 Zhongwan -
    ST-36 Zusanli +
    PC-6 Neiguan -
    SP-4 Gongsun -
    LR-3 Taichong -

Explanation:
- LR-3 Taichong soothes liver qi;
- RN-12 Zhongwan, the Front-Mu Point of the stomach, and ST-36 Zusanli, the He-Sea Point of the Stomach Meridian, reinforce the middle-jiao and regulate stomach qi;
- PC-6 Neiguan, the Luo-Connecting Point of the Hand-Jueyin Meridian which connects downward the three jiaos, and one of the Eight Confluent Points which connects with the Yinwei Meridian which functions to control the interior of the body, soothes liver qi, regulates the qi activity of the upper- and middle-jiao and acts as the key point for relieving vomiting;
- SP-4 Gongsun, the Luo-Connecting Point of the Spleen Meridian, one of the Eight Confluent Points that connects with the Chong Meridian, regulates the middle-jiao and causes rebellious qi to descend.

Secondary points according to conditions:
1️⃣ Abdominal distention —BL-21 Weishu [-];
2️⃣ Acid regurgitation and frequent belching — GB-34 Yanglingquan [-];
3️⃣ Severe vomiting— EX-HN-12 Jinjin and EX-HN-13 Yuye are pricked to bleed.

3. Deficiency of the Spleen and Stomach

Manifestations: Vomiting after over eating, sallow complexion, poor appetite, abdominal distention, loose stools and fatigue.

Tongue: Pale body with thin and white coating.

Pulse: Thready and weak.

Treatment Principle: Reinforce the spleen and stomach, and check the adverse qi.

Point Prescription & Manipulation:
Primary points:
    RN-12 Zhongwan   + ^
    PC-6 Neiguan   /
    ST-36 Zusanli   + ^
    SP-4 Gongsun   + ^

Explanation:
- RN-12 Zhongwan, the Front-Mu Point of the stomach, and ST-36 Zusanli, the He-Sea Point of the Stomach Meridian, warm and reinforce the middle-jiao;
- PC-6 Neiguan, the Luo-Connecting Point of the Hand-Jueyin Meridian which connects downward the three jiaos, and one of the Eight Confluent Points which connects with the Yinwei Meridian which functions to control the interior of the body, regulates the qi activity of the upper- and middle-jiao and acts as the key point for relieving vomiting;
- SP-4 Gongsun, the Luo-Connecting Point of the Spleen Meridian, and one of the Eight Confluent Points that connects with the Chong Meridian, regulates the middle-jiao and causes rebellious qi to descend.

Secondary points according to conditions:
1️⃣ If vomiting lasts for a long period— BL-20 Pishu [+ ^] and BL-21 Weishu [+ ^];
2️⃣ Severe vomiting— EX-HN-12 Jinjin and EX-HN-13 Yuye are pricked to bleed.

II. EXPERIENTIAL TREATMENT

1. Blood Letting

Indication: Acute or intractable vomiting caused by acute gastritis.

Point Prescription:
    EX-HN-26 Neidicang, located on the mucus of the inside of the mouth, opposite to ST-4 Dicang.

Manipulation: Prick the point with the three-edged needle 0.2-0.5 cun deep to bleed a little. Generally, within 5 minutes of the pricking, vomiting will stop or become obviously relieved.

2. Puncturing EX-UE-19 Zitu

Indication: Vomiting caused by acute various factors.

Point Prescription:
EX-UE-19 Zitu, located on the medial aspect of the hand, 0.5 cun distal to the midpoint of the transverse crease of the wrist.

Manipulation: Insert a 1-1.5-cun needle through the point and push the needle horizontally at an angle of 15-30 degrees, with its tip towards the tip of the middle finger. Rotate the needle at large amplitude to induce strong stimulation, and retain the needle for 10 minutes. Generally, only one treatment is needed to stop vomiting. If not, repeat this treatment 5-6 hours later or the next day.

3. Puncturing GB-21 Jianjing

Indication: Vomiting caused by various factors.

Point Prescription:
GB-21 Jianjing

Manipulation: Acupuncture is applied with reinforcing manipulation for deficiency syndrome or reducing manipulation for excessive syndrome. This treatment can be given 1-3 times a day according to the patient's condition. Generally, vomiting will stop immediately. If not, this treatment can be repeated next day.

4. Puncturing KI-1 Yongquan

Indication: Vomiting caused by various factors.

Point Prescription:
KI-1 Yongquan of the left side for the male and the right side for the female.

Manipulation: Insert a 1-cun needle into the point, rotate the needle with even reinforcing and reducing manipulation to induce arrival of qi, and retain the needle for 20-40 minutes. Generally, only one treatment is needed to stop vomiting.

5. Puncturing EX-RN-10 Xiawan

Indication: Neurogenic vomiting.

Point Prescription:
EX-RN-10 Xiawan

Manipulation: Insert a 5-cun needle through the skin of the point, push the needle horizontally with its tip arriving at the region under the skin of RN-14 Juque. Rotate the needle to induce arrival of qi and pull the needle downward but do not withdraw it. Manipulate the needle 10 minutes before removing it. This treatment is given once daily with 10 treatments as a course.

6. Puncturing PC-6 Neiguan

Indication: Neurogenic vomiting, or vomiting during anesthesia for surgical operation.

Point Prescription:
PC-6 Neiguan

Manipulation: Insert a 2.5-cun needle perpendicularly 2 cun deep, rotate, lift and thrust the needle for 10 minutes or until vomiting is relieved. This treatment is given while the patient is vomiting, and two or three treatments can be given within one day.

Comment:
Zhenjiu is effective to relieve vomiting due to various factors. However, vomiting is only a symptom of many diseases. Usually, treatment of these diseases should be done simultaneously.

Notes:

10. Phrenospasm

Phrenospasm refers to spasm of the diaphragm. Its cause is uncertain. Clinically, it is marked by frequent and quick hiccup, which lasts for several minutes to hours. In severe cases, epigastric pain due to long-term onset of the spasm of the diaphragm may be present. According to TCM, phrenospasm belongs to the category of E Ni (hiccup), and is due to attack of stomach by cold pathogen or improper intake of food, or stagnation of qi resulting in adverse flow of the stomach qi.

I. STANDARD TREATMENT

Phrenospasm is generally divided into three types — cold in the stomach, accumulation of food, and qi stagnation. Points of the Stomach, Du and Ren Meridians are frequently selected in its treatment.

1. Cold in the Stomach

Manifestations: Hiccup that is alleviated by warmth and aggravated by cold.

Tongue: White and sticky coating.

Pulse: Slow.

Treatment Principle: Warm the stomach and check the adverse qi.

Point Prescription & Manipulation:
Primary points:
    RN-12 Zhongwan + ^
    PC-6 Neiguan /
    ST-36 Zusanli + ^
    BL-17 Geshu / ^
    RN-13 Shangwan + ^

Explanation:
- RN-12 Zhongwan, the Front-Mu Point of the stomach, and ST-36 Zusanli, the He-Sea Point of the Stomach Meridian, warm and reinforce the middle-jiao;

- PC-6 Neiguan, the Luo-Connecting Point of the Hand-Jueyin Meridian which connects downward the three jiaos, and one of the Eight Confluent Points which connects with the Yinwei Meridian which functions to control the interior of the body, regulates the qi activity of the upper- and middle-jiao and acts as the key point for causing rebellious stomach qi to descend;
- BL-17 Geshu and RN-13 Shangwan check the adverse flow of stomach qi and relieve spasm.

Secondary points according to conditions:
1〗 Severe cases — HT-7 Shenmen [+].

2. Retention of Food

Manifestations: Loud and clear hiccup, abdominal distention and pain, belching, foul smell in the mouth, anorexia.

Tongue: Thick and sticky coating.

Pulse: Slippery and forceful.

Treatment Principle: Promote digestion and regulate the stomach.

Point Prescription & Manipulation:
Primary points:
    PC-6 Neiguan -
    RN-12 Zhongwan -
    ST-44 Neiting -
    ST-36 Zusanli /
    BL-17 Geshu -

Explanation:
- RN-12 Zhongwan, the Front-Mu Point of the stomach, and ST-36 Zusanli, the He-Sea Point of the Stomach Meridian, regulate the middle-jiao to promote digestion;
- PC-6 Neiguan, the Luo-Connecting Point of the Hand-Jueyin Meridian which connects downward the three jiaos, and one of the Eight Confluent Points which connects with the Yinwei Meridian that functions to control the interior of the body, regulates the qi

activity of the upper- and middle-jiao and acts to relieve hiccup;
- BL-17 Geshu regulates the diaphragm and relieves its spasm;
- ST-44 Neiting clears the stomach to remove retained food.

Secondary points according to conditions:
1） Severe cases — RN-14 Juque [-];
2） Constipation and abdominal distention— ST-25 Tianshu [-].

3. Qi Stagnation

Manifestation: Continual hiccups, which are aggravated by bad emotional stimulation, distention and pain of the chest and hypochondrium.

Tongue: Thin coating.

Pulse: Wiry and forceful.

Treatment Principle: Soothe the liver and regulate the stomach.

Point Prescription & Manipulation:
Primary points:
LR-3 Taichong -
RN-17 Danzhong -
BL-17 Geshu /
RN-12 Zhongwan -
PC-6 Neiguan -
ST-36 Zusanli +

Explanation:
- LR-3 Taichong and PC-6 Neiguan soothe the liver and check adverse flow of stomach qi;
- RN-12 Zhongwan, the Front-Mu Point of the stomach, and ST-36 Zusanli, the He-Sea Point of the Stomach Meridian, regulate the middle-jiao to promote digestion;
- RN-17 Danzhong and BL-17 Geshu regulate the diaphragm and relieve its spasm.

Secondary points according to conditions:
1） Bitter taste in the mouth — GB-34 Yanglingquan [-];
2） Chronic cases — BL-20 Pishu[/] and BL-21

Weishu [/]

II. EXPERIENTIAL TREATMENT

1. Pressing with Finger

Indication: Phrenospasm.

Point Prescription:
BL-1 Jingming
KI-1 Yongquan
LU-11 Shaoshang

Manipulation: Firstly, press KI-1 Yongquan. Ask the patient to lie on the back, press KI-1 Yongquan of the one side for 1-2 minutes with enough force to induce strong but tolerable stimulation to the patient. Usually, the patient will stop hiccuping during this treatment. If not, then select BL-1 Jingming. Press BL-1 Jingming bilaterally with the thumbs, and increase pressure gradually until the patient cannot stand. Ask the patient to breathe in deeply and hold his/her breath as long as he/she can. Usually, about 30 seconds later, hiccuping will stop. If not, select LU-11 Shaoshang. Press LU-11 Shaoshang of the left side with the thumb tightly to induce soreness and distention for 30 seconds, within which, generally, hiccup will stop. The above procedure may be repeated if hiccuping will not stop.

2. Puncturing KI-1 Yongquan

Indication: Intractable phrenospasm.

Point Prescription:
KI-1 Yongquan

Manipulation: Insert a 1-cun needle into KI-1 Yongquan bilaterally, lift, thrust and rotate the needles with reducing manipulation to induce arrival of qi, and retain the needles for 20-40 minutes. This treatment may be given 1-2 times daily, and generally, hiccups will stop within two treatments. If hiccup relapses, apply this treatment again.

3. Ear Acupuncture

Indication: Phrenospasm.

Point Prescription:
Diaphragm, Stomach, Spleen, Liver, Sympathetic, Shenmen, Subcortex.

Manipulation: Insert needles into 3-5 points bilaterally, rotate them to induce strong stimulation which is tolerable to the patient and retain the needles for 20 minutes. Alternatively, press the points with match sticks or the needle handles to induce strong stimulation that is tolerable to the patient, until the hiccup stops. Generally, hiccup will stop within several minutes during this treatment.

Comment:
Zhenjiu is effective to relieve phrenospasm due to various factors. However, phrenospasm may be only a symptom of many diseases, and treatment of these diseases should be done simultaneously. The patient should be advised not to take cold or irritative food, not to drink alcohol or have emotional pressure during the treatment period.

Notes:

11. Gastritis

Gastritis is an inflammatory condition of the gastric mucosa. It is classified into acute and chronic types. Acute gastritis includes acute simple gastritis, acute corrosive gastritis, acute erosive gastritis and acute purulent gastritis. Chronic gastritis includes chronic superficial gastritis, chronic atrophic gastritis and chronic hypertrophic gastritis. Chronic gastritis and acute simple gastritis are indications for acupuncture treatment. Clinically, acute simple gastritis is marked by distention and pain in the epigastric region, poor appetite, nausea, vomiting, belching, and acid regurgitation; and chronic gastritis is marked by epigastric pain with burning sensation, abdominal distention and fullness, belching, acid regurgitation and poor appetite. The causes of acute gastritis may include overfilling the stomach with food and drinking too much alcohol. The etiology of chronic gastritis is not well understood, but is usually related to administration of irritating drugs and food, bile regurgitation, buccal inflammation or autoimmunity. According to TCM, gastritis belongs to Wei Wan Tong (epigastric pain) and Pi Zhong (fullness sensation in the epigastrium). It is due to attack of the stomach by exogenous pathogens, improper food intake, emotional depression leading to stagnation of liver qi, deficiency of the spleen and stomach due to poor body constitution, or due to long-term disease, which results in the stagnation of qi of the spleen and stomach.

I. STANDARD TREATMENT

Gastritis is generally divided into five types — qi stagnation due to cold, obstruction of damp-heat in the middle-jiao, stagnation of liver qi, deficient cold of the spleen and stomach, and stomach heat due to yin deficiency. Points of the Yangming Meridian, Spleen Meridian and Liver Meridian are frequently selected.

1. Qi Stagnation due to Cold

Manifestations: Abrupt attack of severe stomachache, which is aggravated by cold and alleviated by warmth.

Tongue: Thin and white coating.

Pulse: Wiry and tight.

Treatment Principle: Warm the middle-jiao, dispel cold, and regulate the stomach and arrest pain.

Point Prescription & Manipulation:
Primary points:
  RN-12 Zhongwan   - ^
  PC-6 Neiguan   -
  ST-36 Zusanli   + ^
  SP-4 Gongsun   -

Explanation:
Acupuncture, moxibustion and cupping are applied together. Acupuncture is performed with reducing manipulation and strong stimulation, and with the needles retained in the points for 20-40 minutes. Moxibustion by warming the needle is applied on RN-12 Zhongwan and ST-36 Zusanli during the retention of the needle. Cupping is applied only on RN-12 Zhongwan after removing the needle.

* RN-12 Zhongwan, the Front-Mu Point of the stomach, warms the middle-jiao to dispel cold;
* ST-36 Zusanli   regulates and strengthens the middle-jiao qi;
* PC-6 Neiguan and SP-4 Gongsun, one pair of the Eight Confluent Points, harmonize the stomach, warm the middle-jiao, promote qi circulation to relieve pain.

Secondary points according to conditions:
1□ Severe vomiting — BL-21 Weishu [+ ^]
2□ Severe epigastric pain — ST-34 Liangqiu [+ ^];
3□ Fever and aversion to cold —DU-14 Dazhui [+ ^] and LI-4 Hegu [-].

2. Obstruction of Damp-Heat in the Middle-Jiao

Manifestations: Epigastric distending pain with burning sensation which is aggravated by taking food, uncomfortable sensation in the abdomen, acid regurgitation, bitter taste and dry throat.

Tongue: Red body with yellow and sticky coating.

Pulse: Soft and rapid.

Treatment Principle: Clear heat and dry dampness.

Point Prescription & Manipulation:
Primary points:
  RN-12 Zhongwan   -
  PC-6 Neiguan   -
  SP-4 Gongsun -
  ST-36 Zusanli   /
  ST-44 Neiting   -
  SP-6 Sanyinjiao   -
  SP-9 Yinlingquan   -

Explanation:
* PC-6 Neiguan and SP-4 Gongsun, one pair of the Eight Confluent Points, harmonize the stomach, warm the middle-jiao, and promote qi circulation to relieve pain.
* RN-12 Zhongwan and ST-36 Zusanli regulate stomach qi and relieve pain;
* ST-44 Neiting clears heat from the stomach;
* SP-6 Sanyinjiao and SP-9 Yinlingquan drain dampness.

Secondary points according to conditions:
1□ Bitter taste in mouth and constipation — ST-45 Lidui [-] and ST-25 Tianshu [-].

3. Stagnation of Liver Qi

Manifestations: Distention and fullness sensation of the epigastrium, distending pain of the hypochondria, distressing sensation in the chest, and frequent belching, which are aggravated by anger or poor emotional condition.

Tongue: Thin and white coating.

Pulse: Wiry.

Treatment Principle: Relieve depressed liver qi, regulate the stomach, and arrest pain.

Point Prescription & Manipulation:
Primary points:
    RN-12 Zhongwan   +
    BL-18 Ganshu   -
    LR-13 Qimen   -
    PC-6 Neiguan   -
    ST-36 Zusanli   +
    GB-34 Yanglingquan   -

Explanation:
- BL-18 Ganshu and LR-14 Qimen, the Back-Shu and Front-Mu Points of the liver, soothe the liver to relieve the depression;
- PC-4 Neiguan and GB-34 Yanglingquan regulate the liver qi and cause the rebellious qi to descend;
- RN-12 Zhongwan and ST-36 Zusanli strengthen the stomach to prevent or treat attack from the stagnant liver qi, harmonize the stomach and stop pain.

Secondary points according to conditions:
1️⃣ Acute and severe epigastric pain—LR-3 Taichong [-];
2️⃣ Hematemesis and tarry stools—BL-17 Geshu [-] and SP-10 Xuehai [-].

4. Insufficiency-Cold of Spleen and Stomach

Manifestations: Persistent dull pain in the epigastrium which is alleviated by warmth and pressure and aggravated by coldness, poor appetite, epigastric distention, sallow complexion, aversion to cold and cold limbs, fatigue, loose stools.

Tongue: Pale and slippery with white coating.

Pulse: Thready and weak.

Treatment Principle: Warm the middle-jiao, dispel cold and regulate the stomach.

Point Prescription & Manipulation:
Primary points:
    BL-20 Pishu   + ^
    BL-21 Weishu   + ^
    RN-12 Zhongwan   + ^
    LR-13 Zhangmen + ^
    ST-36 Zusanli   + ^
    SP-9 Yinlingquan   + ^
    RN-4 Guanyuan   + ^

Explanation:
- BL-20 Pishu, the Back-Shu Point of the spleen, and SP-9 Yinlingquan, the He-Sea Point of the Spleen Meridian, warm the spleen;
- LR-13 Zhangmen, the Front-Mu Point of the spleen, expels cold and relieves pain;
- BL-21 Weishu, the Back-Shu Point of the stomach, RN-12 Zhongwan, the Front-Mu Point of the stomach, and ST-36 Zusanli, the He-Sea Point of the Stomach Meridian, warm the stomach;
- RN-4 Guanyuan reinforces yang, expels cold and stops pain.

Secondary points according to conditions:
1️⃣ Hematemesis or bloody stools—BL-17 Geshu [+].

5. Heat in Stomach due to Yin Deficiency

Manifestations: Epigastric dull pain with burning sensation and discomfort, hungry but without desire to take food, thirst, dry stools.

Tongue: Red body with little coating.

Pulse: Thready and rapid.

Treatment Principle: Tonify yin and clear heat from the stomach.

Point Prescription & Manipulation:
Primary points:
    BL-21 Weishu   +
    PC-6 Neiguan   -
    RN-12 Zhongwan   +
    SP-6 Sanyinjiao   +
    KI-3 Taixi   +

ST-44 Neiting   -

Explanation:
- BL-21 Weishu and RN-12 Zhongwan, the Back-Shu and Front-Mu Points of the stomach, nourish the stomach yin, regulate the stomach qi and relieve pain;
- SP-6 Sanyinjiao and PC-6 Neiguan nourish yin, reinforce the stomach and regulate qi;
- KI-3 Taixi nourishes yin and moistens dryness.

Secondary points according to conditions:
1□ Constipation and thirst — BL-57 Chengshan [-].

II. EXPERIENTIAL TREATMENT

1. Puncturing RN-15 Jiuwei

Indication: Acute simple gastritis.

Point Prescription:
RN-15 Jiuwei

Manipulation: Insert a 1-cun needle perpendicularly or obliquely downward 0.5 cun deep, and rotate, lift and thrust needle 5 minutes before taking out it. Generally, only one treatment is needed to cure this disease. In case it does not, another treatment may be given the next day.

2. Puncturing DU-7 Zhongshu

Indication: Acute simple gastritis or chronic gastritis with epigastric pain as its main symptom.

Point Prescription:
DU-7 Zhongshu

Manipulation: Ask the patient to sit down with the body a little bit bent forward. Insert two needles perpendicularly into the point 0.2-0.5 cun deep, lift the needles slightly and thrust them with their tips respectively toward the lateral sides and upward and downward 0.2-0.5 cun deep. After arrival of qi, retain the needles for 30 minutes. During needle retention, if the pain is not relieved noticeably, manipulate the needles with the same technique 1-2 times. Generally, the pain will be completely stopped in 1-3 treatments.

3. Puncturing EX-HN-3 Yintang

Indication: Superficial gastritis.

Point Prescription:
EX-HN-3 Yintang

Manipulation: Insert a 1-cun needle obliquely downward 0.3-0.5 cun deep, lift, thrust and rotate the needle until the patient feels soreness, distention and heaviness in the tip of the nose, retain the needle for 30 minutes, and manipulate it every 10 minutes. The treatment is given once daily, with 10 treatments as a course. Generally, 2-3 courses are needed in its treatment.

4. Ear Acupuncture

Indication: Various types of gastritis.

Ear Point Prescription:
Stomach, Spleen, Liver, Subcortex, Endocrine, Sanjiao, Abdomen.

Manipulation: See page 255.

Comment:
Presently, there is no satisfactory treatment of chronic atrophic gastritis in Western medicine. Zhenjiu has been proven effective in its treatment. Therefore, Zhenjiu can be taken as its main treatment. Additionally, Zhenjiu is effective in treatment of other types of gastritis. The patient should be advised not to take cold, greasy or irritative food, not to drink, not to have emotional stress during the treatment period.

Notes:

12. Volvulus of Stomach

Volvulus of the stomach refers to torsiversion malposition of the stomach. Its cause is uncertain. It is divided into acute and chronic types. Acute volvulus of the stomach is clinically marked by an abrupt attack of acute or colic epigastric pain, frequent dry vomiting, abdominal distention and palpable mass in the epigastrium. Intermittent epigastric pain and distention, vomiting, and tender epigastrium mark chronic type. X-ray examination is significant in its diagnosis. According to TCM, volvulus of the stomach belongs to the categories of Wei Wan Tong (epigastric pain) and Ou Tu (vomiting), and is due to disharmony between the liver and stomach or external injury, leading to stagnation of qi of the liver and stomach.

I. STANDARD TREATMENT

Volvulus of stomach is divided into two types — stagnation of qi of liver and stomach and stagnation of qi with blood stasis. Points of the Stomach, Liver and Ren Meridians are frequently selected in its treatment.

1. Stagnation of Qi of Liver and Stomach

Manifestations: Epigastric distending pain, belching, vomiting, distention and fullness of the chest and hypochondria.

Tongue: Thin and pale coating.

Pulse: Wiry and tight.

Treatment Principle: Promote circulation of qi and regulate stomach.

Point Prescription & Manipulation:
Primary points:
```
RN-13 Shangwan      -  ^
ST-36 Zusanli       / ^
LR-3 Taichong       -
GB-34 Yanglingquan  -
BL-21 Weishu        -  ^
PC-6 Neiguan        -
```

Explanation:
- RN-13 Shangwan, the local point of the stomach, BL-21 Weishu, Back-Shu Point of the stomach, and ST-36 Zusanli, Lower He-Sea Point of the Stomach Meridian, regulate the stomach;
- PC-6 Neiguan and LR-3 Taichong promote circulation of qi, cause the rebellious qi to descend, and relieve pain.

Secondary points according to conditions:
1⚬ Colic epigastric pain—ST-34 Lianqiu [-] and LR-6 Zhongdu [-].

2. Stagnation of Qi with Blood Stasis

Manifestations: Acute or colic epigastric pain, palpable mass in the epigastrium, frequent vomiting.

Tongue: Purple and dark body.

Pulse: Wiry and tight.

Treatment Principle: Promote circulation of qi, remove blood stasis and regulate stomach.

Point Prescription & Manipulation:
Primary points:
```
BL-17 Geshu      - ^
BL-21 Weishu     - ^
BL-18 Ganshu     - ^
RN-12 Zhongwan   +
LR-3 Taichong    -
PC-6 Neiguan     -
SP-4 Gongsun     - ^
```

Explanation:
- BL-21 Weishu, the Back-Shu Point of the stomach, and RN-12 Zhongwan, the Front-Mu Point of the stomach, regulate the stomach;
- PC-6 Neiguan and SP-4 Gongsun, one pair of the Eight Confluent Points which are indicated in stomach disorders, promote circulation of the middle-jiao qi;
- LR-3 Taichong, BL-18 Ganshu and BL-17 Geshu promote qi circulation and remove blood stasis.

Secondary points according to conditions:
1️⃣ Epigastric pain radiating to chest — RN-17 Danzhong [-].

II. EXPERIENTIAL TREATMENT

1. Puncturing Two Groups of Points

Indication: Chronic volvulus of stomach.

Point Prescription:
   Group 1: ST-36 Zusanli, LR-3 Taichong, RN-12 Zhongwan.

   Group 2: BL-20 Pishu, BL-21 Weishu, BL-17 Geshu.

These two groups are selected alternatively.

Manipulation: Rotate needles with even reinforcing and reducing manipulation to induce arrival of qi, retain the needles for 30 minutes and manipulate them once during the retention. The treatment is given once daily with 10 treatments as a course. Generally, 2 courses are needed.

2. Scalp Acupuncture

Indication: Acute and chronic volvulus of stomach.

Line Prescription:
   Line 2 Lateral to Forehead
   Middle 1/3 of Line of Forehead-Vertex

Manipulation: Insert a needle on Line 2 Lateral to Forehead from the above downward and on Middle 1/3 of Line of Forehead-Vertex from the posterior to the anterior, with lifting and thrusting manipulation at small amplitude. Ask the patient to hold his/her breathing, then do abdominal breathing, and turn the waist right during the manipulation, or to turn around the body in the direction of clock several times on the bed with the needles in the body. Then, tap on the back of the left side with the palm forcefully several times. Retain the needles for 30 minutes, and manipulate them 2-3 minutes every 10 minutes. The treatment is given once daily with 5 treatments as a course.

Comment:
Usually, volvulus of stomach is treated through surgical operation, and there is no satisfactory treatment for it with drugs in Western medicine. However, Zhenjiu can relieve the patient's condition of volvulus of stomach, or even to cure it. Therefore, Zhenjiu can be taken as the first or main treatment.

Notes:

13. Chronic Enteritis

Chronic enteritis refers to chronic inflammation of the intestines. It is usually due to infection by pathogenic microorganisms or intestinal hypersensitivity. Clinically, it is marked by repeated and prolonged attacks of abdominal pain and distention, diarrhea, borborygmus, loose stools, mucous stools, or bloody, purulent stools and tenesmus, or alternating attacks of diarrhea and constipation. According to TCM, chronic enteritis belongs to the categories of Xie Xie (diarrhea), and Xia Li (dysentery), and is caused mainly by retention of dampness in the intestines and deficiency of spleen and kidney.

I. STANDARD TREATMENT

Chronic enteritis is generally divided into four types — fluid retention in the intestines, attack of the spleen by liver qi, spleen deficiency, and kidney deficiency. Points of the Stomach, Spleen and Urinary Bladder Meridians are frequently selected in its treatment.

1. Fluid Retention in the Intestines

Manifestation: Diarrhea with clear watery or frothy stools, abdominal distention, and borborygmus.

Tongue: Pale body with white and slippery coating.

Pulse: Soft.

Treatment Principle: Invigorate spleen, eliminate dampness and stop diarrhea.

Point Prescription & Manipulation:
Primary points:
ST-36 Zusanli + ^
SP-9 Yinlingquan + ^
SP-4 Gongsun / ^
PC-6 Neiguan /
ST-25 Tianshu / ^
RN-12 Zhongwan / ^
Explanation:

- ST-36 Zusanli and RN-12 Zhongwan warm the middle-jiao and invigorate the spleen;
- SP-9 Yinlingquan reinforces the spleen and drain dampness;
- SP-4 Gongsun and PC-6 Neiguan, one pair of the Eight Confluent Points which are indicated in stomach disorders, regulate the middle-jiao and relieve pain;
- ST-25 Tianshu strengthens the large intestine to stop diarrhea.

Secondary points according to conditions:
1 Severe diarrhea — ST-37 Shangjuxu [+ ^], BL-25 Dachangshu [+^] and RN-4 Guanyuan [+ ^].

2. Attack of Spleen by Liver Qi

Manifestation: Diarrhea induced by emotional stress, abdominal pain and distention which are not alleviated by bowel movements, hypochondriac distention, belching, poor appetite.

Tongue: Slightly red body.

Pulse: Wiry pulse.

Treatment Principle: Restrain the liver, invigorate spleen and stop diarrhea.

Point Prescription & Manipulation:
Primary points:
ST-25 Tianshu +
ST-36 Zusanli +
SP-6 Sanyinjiao +
LR-3 Taichong -
LI-4 Hegu -
RN-12 Zhongwan /

Explanation:
- ST-36 Zusanli and RN-12 Zhongwan strengthen the middle-jiao and invigorate the spleen;
- LR-3 Taichong and LI-4 Hegu promote qi circulation and soothe the liver;
- ST-25 Tianshu strengthens the large intestine to stop diarrhea.

Secondary points according to conditions:
1️⃣ Irritability and hypochondriac pain—GB-34 Yanglingquan [-] and LR-14 Qimen [/];
2️⃣ Prolonged diarrhea — SP-9 Yinlingquan [+] and BL-20 Pishu [+].

3. Deficiency of Spleen

Manifestation: Diarrhea with undigested food, or loose stools, increase bowel movements after eating greasy food, poor appetite, abdominal distention, lassitude, sallow complexion.

Tongue: Pale body with white coating.

Pulse: Weak and thready.

Treatment Principle: Invigorate spleen, reinforce qi, transform dampness and stop diarrhea.

Point Prescription & Manipulation:
Primary points:
    BL-20 Pishu + ^
    BL-25 Dachangshu + ^
    ST-25 Tianshu + ^
    ST-36 Zusanli + ^
    SP-9 Yinlingquan + ^
    RN-6 Qihai + ^

Explanation:
* ST-36 Zusanli and SP-9 Yinlingquan, the He-Sea Points of the Stomach and Spleen Meridians, and BL-20 Pishu, the Back-Shu Point of the Spleen, reinforce the stomach and spleen and drain dampness;
* BL-25 Dachangshu and ST-25 Tianshu strengthen the large intestine to stop diarrhea;
* RN-6 Qihai reinforces qi and warms yang.

Secondary points according to conditions:
1️⃣ Prolonged diarrhea leading to prolapse of rectum — DU-20 Baihui [+ ^] and DU-1 Changqiang [+ ^];
2️⃣ Epigastric distention and fullness and acid regurgitation—LR-13 Zhangmen [/], BL-21 Weishu [/] and RN-12 Zhongwan [/].

4. Kidney Deficiency

Manifestation: Diarrhea at dawn following abdominal pain and borborygmus, both of which are relieved after bowel movements, cold limbs, soreness, coldness and weakness in the lower back and knees.

Tongue: Pale body with white coating.

Pulse: Deep and thready.

Treatment Principle: Warm the kidney, invigorate spleen, promote astringency and stop diarrhea.

Point Prescription & Manipulation:
Primary points:
    BL-20 Pishu + ^
    BL-23 Shenshu + ^
    DU-4 Mingmen + ^
    BL-25 Dachangshu + ^
    ST-25 Tianshu + ^
    RN-6 Qihai + ^
    RN-4 Guanyuan + ^
    ST-36 Zusanli + ^

Explanation:
* BL-20 Pishu and RN-6 Qihai warm the middle-jiao, reinforce the spleen and tonify qi;
* BL-23 Shenshu and DU-4 Mingmen warm the kidney and strengthen yang;
* BL-25 Dachangshu and ST-25 Tianshu, the combination of the Back-Shu and Front-Mu Points of the large intestine, strengthen the intestine and stop diarrhea;
* RN-4 Guanyuan, the Crossing Point of the three Foot-Yin Meridians with Ren Meridian and the Front-Mu Point of the small intestine, tonifies qi of the three Foot-Yin Meridians and improves the small intestine's function of separating the clear from the turbid and transforming the turbid.

Secondary points according to conditions:
1️⃣ Prolonged diarrhea — DU-20 Baihui [+ ^] and LR-13 Zhangmen [+];
2️⃣ Prolonged diarrhea leading to prolapse of

rectum — DU-20 Baihui [+ ^] and DU-1 Changqiang [+ ^].

II. EXPERIENTIAL TREATMENT

1. Puncturing RN-8 Shenque

Indication: Chronic enteritis with frequent diarrhea.

Point Prescription:
RN-8 Shenque

Manipulation: Puncture perpendicularly 0.3-0.8 cun deep, perform reinforcing manipulation to induce arrival of qi, and remove the needle without retention. Usually, only one treatment is needed for stopping diarrhea. If not, the treatment can be repeated next day.

2. Moxibustion on EX-LE-20 Fuxietexiaoxue

Indication: Chronic enteritis with frequent diarrhea.

Point Prescription:
EX-LE-20 Fuxietexiaoxue, located on the lateral aspect of the foot, directly below the tip of the external malleolus, at the junction of the red and white skin.

Manipulation: Apply moxibustion with moxa stick and keep the ignited end 1 cun from the point for about 10-15 minutes. The treatment is given 1-3 times a day, with 5 days as a course. Usually, within one course, diarrhea will be stopped.

3. Ear Acupuncture

Indication: Chronic enteritis with frequent diarrhea.

Point Prescription:
Large Intestine, Small Intestine, Rectum, Abdomen, Endocrine and Subcortex.

Manipulation: See page 255.

Comment:
Zhenjiu is effective in the treatment of acute and chronic enteritis. Compared to other treatments, Zhenjiu is a good therapy for chronic enteritis, but long-term treatment is needed. The patient should be advised not to take cold, greasy or irritative food and not to drink alcohol during the treatment period.

Notes:

14. Gastrointestinal Neurosis

Gastrointestinal neurosis is a functional disorder of the stomach and intestine caused by disturbance of gastrointestinal movement and secretion. Its cause is mainly related to emotional factors, but in some cases, it is a sequel of some gastrointestinal diseases. It includes intestinal neurosis and gastric neurosis. The former is clinically marked by abdominal pain, discomfort sensation of the abdomen, abdominal distention, borborygmus, and diarrhea or constipation; and the latter, by anorexia, belching, acid regurgitation, nausea, vomiting, burning sensation of the epigastrium, and abdominal distention or pain. According to TCM, gastrointestinal neurosis belongs to the categories of Yu Zheng (depression syndrome), Mei He Qi (globus hysterics), Wei Wan Tong (epigastric pain), Ou Tu (vomiting), Fu Xie (diarrhea), or Bian Bi (constipation), and it is due to stagnation of liver qi resulting from emotional depression and attacking the stomach and spleen.

I. STANDARD TREATMENT

Gastrointestinal neurosis is generally divided into three types — disharmony between the liver and stomach, disharmony between the liver and spleen, and deficiency of the heart and spleen. Points of the Spleen, Stomach and Liver Meridians are frequently selected in its treatment.

1. Disharmony Between Liver and Stomach

Manifestations: Epigastric fullness and distention, belching, poor appetite, emotional depression, distressing sensation in the chest, symptoms aggravated by emotional stress.

Tongue: White and thin coating.

Pulse: Wiry.

Treatment Principle: Relieve depressed liver qi and regulate the stomach.

Point Prescription & Manipulation:

Primary points:
    LR-3 Taichong   -
    PC-6 Neiguan   -
    RN-12 Zhongwan   -
    ST-36 Zusanli   +
    BL-18 Ganshu   -
    BL-21 Weishu   /

Explanation:
* BL-18 Ganshu and LR-3 Taichong soothe the liver and relieve the depression;
* RN-12 Zhongwan and BL-21 Weishu, the combination of Front-Mu and Back-Shu Points of the stomach, strengthen the stomach and regulate middle-jiao qi;
* PC-6 Neiguan and ST-36 Zusanli promote qi circulation, regulate the stomach and cause the rebellious qi to descend.

Secondary points according to conditions:
1〕 Hypochondriac pain—GB-34 Yanglingquan [-];
2〕 Hiccup — BL-17 Geshu [-].

2. Disharmony Between Liver and Spleen

Manifestations: Hypochondriac pain and distressing sensation of the chest, epigastric and abdominal distention and fullness, poor appetite, borborygmus, abdominal pain, loose stools or constipation, which are aggravated by emotional stimulation.

Tongue: Thin and white coating.

Pulse: Wiry.

Treatment Principle: Relieve depressed liver qi, and regulate spleen.

Point Prescription & Manipulation:
Primary points:
    LR-3 Taichong   -
    BL-18 Ganshu   -
    BL-20 Pishu   +
    BL-25 Dachangshu / ^
    ST-25 Tianshu   / ^
    ST-36 Zusanli   +
    RN-6 Qihai   + ^

SP-6 Sanyinjiao   +

Explanation:
- BL-18 Ganshu and LR-3 Taichong soothe the liver and relieve the depression;
- BL-20 Pishu, ST-36 Zusanli and SP-6 Sanyinjiao reinforce the spleen's function of transformation and transportation;
- BL-25 Dachangshu and ST-25 Tianshu, the combination of the Front-Mu and Back-Shu Points of the large intestine, regulate the gastrointestinal function;
- RN-6 Qihai reinforces qi and relieves abdominal pain.

Secondary points:
1 Constipation — SJ-6 Zhigou [-] and ST-37 Shangjuxu [-];
2 Hiccup — BL-17 Geshu [-].

3. Deficiency of Heart and Spleen

Manifestations: Poor appetite, abdominal distention, loose stools, sallow complexion, listlessness, fatigue, palpitation, shortness of breath, insomnia, poor memory.

Tongue: Pale body with white and thin coating.

Pulse: Thready and feeble.

Treatment Principle: Tonify the heart and spleen.

Point Prescription & Manipulation:
Primary points:
HT-7 Shenmen   +
ST-36 Zusanli   +
BL-15 Xinshu   + ^
BL-20 Pishu   + ^
RN-12 Zhongwan   + ^
RN-6 Qihai   + ^
ST-25 Tianshu   / ^
SP-6 Sanyinjiao   + ^

Explanation:
- BL-15 Xinshu and BL-20 Pishu, Back-Shu Points of the heart and spleen, tonify the heart and spleen;

- ST-36 Zusanli, Lower He-Sea Point of the Stomach Meridian, and RN-12 Zhongwan, Front-Mu Point of the stomach, tonify the stomach and spleen and reinforce qi;
- RN-6 Qihai, ST-25 Tianshu and SP-6 Sanyinjiao tonify qi and reinforce the spleen;
- HT-7 Shenmen nourishes the heart and calms the mind. Combining with each other, HT-7 and SP-6 have the action of regulating the heart and spleen, calming spirit, good for insomnia.

Secondary points:
1 Amenorrhea — RN-4 Guanyuan [+ ^] and SP-10 Pishu [+ ^].

II. EXPERIENTIAL TREATMENT

1. Puncturing through PC-6 Neiguan to SJ-5 Waiguan

Indication: Gastrointestinal neurosis with gastrointestinal spasm as main manifestation.

Point Prescription:
PC-6 Neiguan

Manipulation: Insert a 2-cun needle perpendicularly into the point and push the needle deep until the tip reaches the area under the skin of SJ-5 Waiguan. Then, lift and thrust the needle quickly with small amplitude. While manipulating the needle, touch and knead the abdomen gently 1-2 minutes, and ask the patient to do deep breath. Repeat this course every 5 minutes until the abdominal pain disappears. Take out the needle after retaining it in the point for 15 minutes. Generally, only one treatment is needed to arrest abdominal pain.

2. Puncturing PC-6 Neiguan

Indication: Gastrointestinal neurosis with vomiting as main manifestation.

Point Prescription:
PC-6 Neiguan

Manipulation: Give acupuncture treatment after eating but before vomiting. Insert the needle perpendicularly. Then, lift and thrust the needle with quick frequency and with small amplitude, and ask the patient to take deep breaths 2-3 times during the manipulation. Then, repeat this course every 10-15 minutes, and retain the needle for 30 minutes. The treatment is given once daily and generally, 3-9 treatments are needed.

3. Ear Acupuncture

Indication: Intestinal neurosis.

Ear Point Prescription:
Small Intestine, Large Intestine, Abdomen, Spleen, Liver, Subcortex, Endocrine and Sympathetic.

Manipulation: See page 255.

Comment:
Zhenjiu is a good therapy for gastrointestinal neurosis, usually bringing about satisfactory results. As emotional stress or improper diet habit play an important role in causing and aggravating this disease, the patient should be advised not to take cold, greasy or irritative food, not to drink, to try to avoid emotional stress during the treatment period.

Notes:

15. Constipation

Constipation refers to difficult and infrequent defecation. It is a common symptom of various diseases and disorders such as habitual constipation, gastrointestinal neurosis, fever, and problems in the rectum and anus. According to TCM, constipation, called Bian Bi in Chinese, is caused mainly by accumulation of heat in the intestines which consumes the intestinal fluids, or by deficiency of qi, blood, or bodily fluids causing lack of moisture in the intestines.

I. STANDARD TREATMENT

Constipation is generally divided into four types — constipation due to heat, constipation due to stagnation of qi, constipation due to blood deficiency, and constipation due to yang deficiency. Points of the Stomach and Urinary Bladder Meridians are frequently selected in its treatment.

1. Constipation due to Heat

Manifestations: Constipation with dry stools and difficulty in passing them at a frequency of every three to eight days, scanty urine, flushed face, irritability, abdominal distention and pain, foul breath.

Tongue: Red body with dry and yellow coating.

Pulse: Smooth and rapid.

Treatment Principle: Clear heat and moisten the intestines.

Point Prescription & Manipulation:
Primary points:
ST-25 Tianshu   -
BL-25 Dachangshu   -
SP-15 Daheng   -
ST-44 Neiting   -

Explanation:
- ST-25 Tianshu and BL-25 Dachangshu, combination of the Front-Mu and Back-Shu

Points of the large intestine, purge heat from the large intestine and move the stools;

- SP-15 Daheng, the Crossing Point of the Spleen and Yinwei Meridians, relieves abdominal pain and distention;
- ST-44 Neiting, the Ying-Spring Point of the Stomach Meridian, purges excessive heat from Yangming Meridian.

Secondary points according to conditions:
1️⃣ Fever — LI-4 Hegu [-] and LI-11Quchi [-];
2️⃣ Yin injury due to excessive heat— KI-6 Zhaohai [+].

2. Constipation due to Stagnation of Qi

Manifestations: Constipation with difficulty in passing stools although there is an urge to defecate, frequent belching, fullness in the costal and hypochondriac region or even abdominal distending pain, poor appetite.

Tongue: Thin and sticky coating.

Pulse: Wiry.

Treatment Principle: Circulate qi and relieve stagnation.

Point Prescription & Manipulation:
Primary points:
RN-6 Qihai /
ST-25 Tianshu -
BL-32 Ciliao -
SJ-6 Zhigou -
GB-34 Yanglingquan -
LR-3 Taichong -

Explanation:
- LR-3 Taichong soothes the liver and relieves the depression;
- RN-6 Qihai and ST-25 Tianshu promote qi movement of the large intestine and move stools;
- SJ-6 Zhigou, GB-34 Yanglingquan and BL-32 Ciliao regulate qi activities of the Sanjiao and move stools.

Secondary points according to conditions:
1️⃣ Frequent belching — RN-12 Zhongwan [/]

and ST-36 Zusanli [/].

3. Constipation due to Blood Deficiency

Manifestations: Constipation with dry stools, pale complexion, dizziness, palpitation, blurred vision, pale lips.

Tongue: Pale body.

Pulse: Thready and weak.

Treatment Principle: Nourish blood and moisten intestines.

Point Prescription & Manipulation:
Primary points:
BL-20 Pishu +
BL-17 Geshu +
SJ-6 Zhigou -
ST-25 Tianshu /
KI-6 Zhaohai +
ST-36 Zusanli +

Explanation:
- BL-20 Pishu, the Back-Shu Point of the spleen, ST-36 Zusanli, the He-Sea Point of the Stomach Meridian, and BL-17 Geshu, the Influential Point of blood, reinforce the spleen, tonify blood and moisten the intestine;
- KI-6 Zhaohai promotes production of body fluids and moistens the intestines;
- SJ-6 Zhigou and ST-25 Tianshu regulate the Sanjiao and move the stools.

Secondary points according to conditions:
1️⃣ Thirst, restlessness, and red tongue with little moisture due to heat generating from blood deficiency — PC-6 Neiguan [/] and SP-6 Sanyinjiao [+].

4. Constipation due to Yang Deficiency

Manifestations: Constipation, weakness and cold sensation in the lower back.

Tongue: Pale body with moist white coating.

Pulse: Deep and slow.

Treatment Principle: Warm yang and relieve constipation.

Point Prescription & Manipulation:
Primary points:
    BL-23 Shenshu + ^
    RN-4 Guanyuan + ^
    RN-6 Qihai + ^
    SP-15 Daheng + ^
    SP-6 Sanyinjiao + ^

Explanation:
- BL-23 Shenshu and RN-4 Guanyuan reinforce kidney yang and remove cold accumulation;
- RN-6 Qihai and SP-15 Daheng reinforce qi and promote qi circulation;
- SP-6 Sanyinjiao warms qi of the three Foot-Yin Meridians.

Secondary points according to conditions:
1️⃣ Prolonged cases— RN-8 Shenjue [^];
2️⃣ Old persons — DU-4 Mingmen [+ ^].

II. EXPERIENTIAL TREATMENT

1. Puncturing Five Points

Indication: Intractable constipation.

Point Prescription:
    ST-40 Fenglong
    ST-28 Shuidao of the left side
    ST-29 Guilai of the left side
    Point 2 cun lateral to the left ST-28 Shuidao
    Point 2 cun lateral to the left ST-29 Guilai

Manipulation: Puncture points on the abdomen 2.5-3 cun deep, and the points on the leg 1.5 cun deep, rotate the needles to induce the needling sensation, and retain the needles for 30 minutes. Usually, one hour after the treatment, the patient will have bowel movement.

2. Pressing ST-25 Tianshu with Finger

Indication: Habitual constipation.

Point Prescription:
    ST-25 Tianshu

Manipulation: Ask the patient to lie on the back with the knee joints bent. Firstly, press the left point with the thumb and knead it clockwise with strong force for 5 minutes. Then, repeat the manipulation on the right point. The treatment is given once daily, with 7 treatments as a course. Usually, the patient will have bowel movement next day after the first treatment, and will have bowel movement every day or every other day after one course of the treatment.

3. Puncturing BL-57 Chengshan

Indication: Habitual constipation.

Point Prescription:
    BL-57 Chengshan

Manipulation: Puncture perpendicularly 1.5-2.5 cun deep, rotate the needles to induce arrival of qi, retain the needles for 20-30 minutes, and rotate the needles every 10 minutes during the retention. The treatment is given once every other day, with 5 treatments as a course. Usually, 10 treatments are needed to cure this disorder.

4. Puncturing SJ-6 Zhigou

Indication: Constipation.

Point Prescription:
    SJ-6 Zhigou

Manipulation: Puncture perpendicularly 1-1.5 cun deep, perform even reinforcing and reducing manipulation to induce arrival of qi, retain the needles for 20-40 minutes, and manipulate the needles every 10 minutes during the retention. Usually, after one treatment, the patient will have bowel movement.

Comment:
Being effective but having no side effect, Zhenjiu is a good therapy for constipation, especially for chronic constipation, which usually needs a long term of treatment. Additionally, the custom of having a bowel movement everyday at a regular time is very important in the treatment of habitual constipation.

Notes:

16. Gastroptosis

Gastroptosis refers to an abnormally low position of the stomach (the lower region of the greater curvature of the stomach is often 5 or more cm below the level of the inter-iliac-crest line) accompanied with a decrease in gastric emptying function. Clinically, it is marked by abdominal distention characterized by aggravation after eating and relief by lying down, nausea, belching, irregular epigastric pain, and constipation or diarrhea occasionally. According to TCM, gastroptosis belongs to the categories of Wei Xia (low position of the stomach), Wei Huang (relaxed stomach), and Xu Zheng (deficiency syndrome), and it is due to deficiency of the spleen and stomach leading to sinking of the middle-jiao qi.

I. STANDARD TREATMENT

Gastroptosis is generally divided into three types — sinking of qi due to deficiency of the spleen, disharmony between the spleen and stomach, and deficiency of qi and yin. Points of the Ren, Stomach and Bladder Meridians are frequently selected in its treatment.

1. Sinking of Qi due to Deficiency of Spleen and Stomach

Manifestations: Abdominal distention, fullness, heaviness and sinking sensation in the abdomen which are aggravated by taking food and relieved by lying down, sallow complexion, emaciation, restlessness, fatigue, shortness of breath, loose stools.

Tongue: Pale body with thin white coating.

Pulse: Weak.

Treatment Principle: Tonify the middle-jiao, reinforce qi and raise the sunken qi.

Points Prescription & Manipulation:
Primary points:
    DU-20 Baihui   + ^

    BL-20 Pishu   + ^
    RN-12 Zhongwan   + ^
    ST-36 Zusanli   + ^
    RN-6 Qihai   ^
    RN-14 Juque   /

Explanation:
On DU-20 Baihui and RN-6 Qihai, apply moxibustion with the moxa stick for 15 minutes; on BL-20 Pishu, RN-12 Zhongwan and ST-36 Zusanli, insert needles into the points, manipulate to induce arrival of qi, retain the needles in the points for 30-40 minutes, and during the retention apply moxibustion by warming the needles. On RN-14 Juque, insert a 7-cun needle horizontally downward to reach the area of KI-16 Huangshu, rotate the needle to induce arrival of qi, rotate the needle in one direction until there is a sensation of tightness and unevenness around the needle tip felt by the operator, and retain the needle for 30-40 minutes; on RN-9 Shuifen, SP-9 Yinlingquan and PC-6 Neiguan, apply puncture with reducing manipulation, and retain the needles in the points for 30-40 minutes; and on ST-25 Tianshu, apply acupuncture with even reinforcing and reducing manipulation, and retain the needle for 30-40 minutes too. The treatment is given 3 hours after taking food, on RN-14 Juque once every other day, and on the other points once every day, and 15 days as a course.

- DU-20 Baihui, the Crossing Point of the Du Meridian with the three Hand- and Foot-Yang Meridians, tonifies qi and raises yang and raises the sunken qi;
- BL-20 Pishu and RN-12 Zhongwan reinforce the spleen and regulate the middle-jiao;
- ST-36 Zusanli and RN-6 Qihai reinforce the middle-jiao and tonify qi;
- RN-14 Juque raises the stomach.

Secondary points according to conditions:
1□ Sound due to water in the stomach — ST-40 Fenglong [-];
2□ Vomiting — PC-6 Neiguan [-];
3□ Abdominal distention and diarrhea—ST-25 Tianshu [/].

2. Disharmony Between Spleen and Stomach

Manifestations: Abdominal distention and fullness, and heaviness and sinking sensation in the abdomen, which are aggravated by taking food and relieved by lying down, intermittent and dull pain of the abdomen, poor appetite, belching, abdominal discomfort, constipation or diarrhea.

Tongue: Pale body.

Pulse: Wiry.

Treatment Principle: Reinforce qi, harmonize the middle-jiao and regulate the spleen and stomach.

Point Prescription & Manipulation:
Primary points:
    BL-20 Pishu   + ^
    BL-21 Weishu + ^
    RN-12 Zhongwan   + ^
    ST-36 Zusanli   + ^
    RN-6 Qihai   + ^
    SP-16 Fuai   + ^

Explanation:
On SP-16 Fuai, insert a needle horizontally and push it to reach the region near RN-8 Shenque with the same manipulation as on RN-14 Juque mentioned above; on BL-57 Chengshan perform reducing manipulation; and on the other points perform reinforcing manipulation. The retention of the needles and treatment course are the same as those in Sinking of Qi due to Deficiency of the Spleen and Stomach.

- BL-20 Pishu and BL-21 Weishu reinforce the spleen and stomach and harmonize the middle-jiao;
- RN-12 Zhongwan and ST-36 Zusanli reinforce the middle-jiao and tonify qi;
- RN-6 Qihai reinforces and raises qi;
- SP-16 Fuai raises the stomach.

Secondary points according to conditions:
1❏ Loose stools — ST-25 Tianshu [+ ^];
2❏ Constipation— BL-57 Chengshan [-].

3. Deficiency of Qi and Yin

Manifestations: Abdominal distention and fullness, and heaviness and sinking sensation in the abdomen, which are aggravated by taking food and relieved by lying down, thirst, belching, dull pain of the stomach, hungry but without desire to take food, emaciation, listlessness, fatigue, dry stools.

Tongue: Red body with little coating.

Pulse: Thready, rapid and weak.

Treatment Principle: Reinforce qi and nourish yin, and raise the sunken.

Point Prescription & Manipulation:
Primary points:
    RN-12 Zhongwan   + ^
    RN-6 Qihai   + ^
    PC-6 Neiguan   /
    SP-6 Sanyinjiao   +
    KI-3 Taixi   +
    BL-20 Pishu   +
    RN-14 Juque   +

Explanation:
On RN-14 Juque perform the same manipulation mentioned above; on SJ-6 Zhigou perform reducing manipulation with strong stimulation to induce arrival of qi, and retain the needle in the point for 20-30 minutes; and on the other points perform reinforcing manipulation to induce arrival of qi, and retain the needles in the points for 20-30 minutes. The treatment course is the same as that in Sinking of Qi due to Deficiency of the Spleen and Stomach.

- RN-12 Zhongwan reinforces the middle-jiao and tonifies qi;
- RN-6 Qihai reinforces and raises qi;
- PC-6 Neiguan and KI-3 Taixi nourish yin, clear heat, and promote qi circulation for regulating the stomach;
- SP-6 Sanyinjiao reinforces the three Foot-Yin Meridians and tonifies yin;
- BL-20 Pishu promotes the spleen's function and moistens the stomach.

Secondary points according to conditions:
1️⃣ Constipation — SJ-6 Zhigou [-].

II. EXPERIENTIAL TREATMENT

1. Puncturing RN-11 Jianli

Indication: Gastroptosis.

Point Prescription:
RN-11 Jianli

Manipulation: Insert 2 needles 3 cun into the point, push them downward under the skin 2-3 cun deep to induce the needling sensation. Lift and thrust the needles several times, and retain the needles for 20 minutes. After removing the needles, ask the patient to wrap his or her waist with a girdle, and remove it when sleeping. The treatment is given once daily with 10 treatments as a course. After an interval of 2-3 days the next course is given. Generally, the patient's condition will be greatly improved through three courses of the treatment. Ask the patient to receive the treatment when the stomach is empty and to have a rest after the treatment.

2. Puncturing ST-21 Liangmen

Indication: Gastroptosis.

Point Prescription:
ST-21 Liangmen

Manipulation: Insert a 4-cun needle through the point, push the needle horizontally downward under the skin 3 cun deep, rotate the needle to induce arrival of qi, withdraw the needle in both sides simultaneously so slowly that the needles will be taken out by 2-3 minutes. The treatment is given once daily, with 10 treatments as a course. After an interval of 2-3 days the next course of the treatment is given. Generally, 2-3 courses are needed.

3. Applying Ginger Moxibustion

Indication: Gastroptosis belonging to qi deficiency.

Point Prescription:
RN-13 Shangwan
RN-12 Zhongwan
RN-10 Xiawan
ST-21 Liangmen
RN-6 Qihai
ST-36 Zusanli

Manipulation: Apply moxibustion on three or four points with 5-7 moxa cones each. The treatment is given once daily and 20 treatments are needed.

4. Acupuncture and Moxibustion on Two Groups of Points in Cooperation with the Patient's Exercise

Indication: Gastroptosis.

Point Prescription:
Primary points:
Group 1: RN-12 Zhongwan, EX-CA-4 Weishang, located on the abdomen, 4 cun lateral to RN-10 Xiawan, ST-36 Zusanli.

Group 2: BL-21 Weishu, BL-20 Pishu, DU-20 Baihui.

These two groups are selected alternatively.

Secondary points according to conditions:
1️⃣ Severe cases—RN-6 Qihai   and RN-4 Guanyuan;
2️⃣ Duodenal ulcer — SP-4 Gongsun, ST-21 Liangmen and PC-6 Neiguan.

Manipulation: On RN-12 Zhongwan, insert a needle perpendicularly 1.5-2 cun or horizontally with the needle tip towards the umbilicus. Lift, thrust and rotate the needle until the patient feels contracture, distention and heaviness in the epigastrium. On EX-AC-4 Weishang, insert a needle through the skin of the point, push it horizontally 2-3 cun deep with its tip facing the umbilicus or ST-25 Tianshu, lift, thrust and rotate the needle until the patient feels abdominal distention, spasm of the umbilicus region, and contracture of the stomach. On ST-36 Zusanli, insert a needle perpendicularly 1.5-2 cun deep, and perform reinforcing manipulation by lifting, thrusting and rotating the needle to induce soreness and distention radiating downward to the dorsum of the foot and upward to the knee. On BL-21 Weishu and BL-20 Pishu, insert a needle obliquely 1-1.5 cun deep with its tip facing the center of the vertebra, perform reinforcing manipulation by lifting, thrusting and rotating the needle to induce sensations of local soreness, distention, numbness and spasm; and on DU-20 Baihui, insert a needle horizontally backward 0.5-1 cun deep, and rotate the needle until the patient feels local distention and pain. Retain the needle in each point for 15-30 minutes. Apply moxibustion on RN-12 Zhongwan and BL-21 Weishu during the retention. The treatment is given once daily with 10 treatments as a course. After an interval of 5-7 days, the next course can be given.

Advise the patient to perform the following exercises:

    a. Breathing with the abdomen: Lying on the back and breathing deeply with the abdomen 10-20 times; and

    b. Lying down and raising the upper body, and repeat this course as far as possible.

5. Acupuncture with A Long Needle

Indication: Gastroptosis.

Point Prescription:
    RN-14 Juque
    DU-20 Baihui
    RN-12 Zhongwan
    RN-6 Qihai

Manipulation: Ask the patient to lie down on the back, breathe naturally, and relax the abdomen. On RN-14 Juque, insert a 7-cun needle through the skin of the point, push the needle horizontally under the skin slowly to the umbilicus region, rotate the needle in one direction 3-5 turns to circle the needle body by muscular fibril. Spend 5-10 minutes to slowly withdraw the needle encircled by the fibulas and make the patient feel strong sensations of soreness, distention and contracture. Then, withdraw the needle, and repeat this course after 10 minutes. In one

treatment, repeating this procedure for 3 times is needed. The treatment is given once every other day, and 10-20 treatments are needed to cure this disease. During the treatment, apply moxibustion on the other points, each with moxa stick for 10-20 minutes, or with ginger moxibustion for 5-7 moxa cones.

Comment:

Presently there is no better way to treat gastroptosis than by Zhenjiu or herbal medicine. Zhenjiu is effective to restore the normal position of the stomach, and it can be taken as the first choice for gastroptosis. During the Zhenjiu treatment period and for three months after the treatment, the patient should be advised to rest a lot and avoid violent physical exertion. Additionally, it is advised to take food which is easily digested, increase eating frequency with reducing amount of food in each eating, lie on the back for 30 minutes or more after eating. It is strongly advised to do physical excise to improve the muscular tone of the abdomen.

Notes:

17. Peptic Ulcer

Peptic ulcer refers to circular or oval lesions on the wall of the stomach or duodenum, occurring primarily on the gastric pylorus or the duodenal bulb. The etiology of peptic ulcer, in spite of a variety of theories about it, has not been well understood. Peptic ulcer is clinically characterized by regularly occurring pain in the epigastric region, accompanied by belching, acid regurgitation, nausea, vomiting and poor appetite. Onset of pain is generally related to intake of food; in cases of gastric ulcer the pain usually occurs 30 minutes to 2 hours after eating and disappears sometimes before the next meal. In cases of duodenal ulcer, the pain usually starts three to four hours after eating and is relieved after eating the next meal. According to TCM, peptic ulcer is classified as Wei Wan Tong (epigastric pain), and is caused either by mental injury resulting in stagnation of the liver qi and subsequent attack on the stomach by hyperactive liver qi, or by improper eating habits such as irregularity of taking meals or overindulgence in raw, cold, or spicy food, resulting in injury to the stomach and spleen. The main pathogenesis of peptic ulcer is stagnation of qi and blood, which affects the stomach, spleen and liver.

I. STANDARD TREATMENT

Peptic ulcer is usually divided into four types—stagnation of qi of the liver and stomach, qi and blood stagnation, stagnant heat in the liver and stomach, and stomach yin deficiency. Points of the Stomach, Spleen Bladder and Liver Meridians are frequently selected in its treatment.

1. Stagnation of Qi of Liver and Stomach

Manifestations: Epigastric distending pain, discomfort and distention of the hypochondria, belching, acid regurgitation, poor appetite, which are induced or aggravated by emotional stress.

Tongue: Thin and white coating.

Pulse: Wiry.

Treatment Principle: Relieve depression of liver and regulate qi, harmonize stomach to stop pain.

Point Prescription & Manipulation:
Primary points:
    BL-17 Geshu   -
    BL-18 Ganshu   -
    BL-21 Weishu   /
    RN-12 Zhongwan   /
    LR-14 Qimen   -
    LR-3 Taichong   -
    ST-36 Zusanli   /

Explanation:
- BL-18 Ganshu and LR-14 Qimen, the combination of Front-Mu and Back-Shu Points of the liver, soothe the liver and relieve constrained qi;
- BL-17 Geshu promotes circulation of qi in the chest;
- BL-21 Weishu, Back-Shu Point of the stomach, RN-12 Zhongwan, Front-Mu Point of the stomach, and ST-36 Zusanli, He-Sea Point of the Stomach Meridian, regulate qi of the middle-jiao to relieve pain.

Secondary points according to conditions:
1️⃣ Nausea and vomiting — PC-6 Neiguan [/];
2️⃣ Severe epigastric pain — ST-21 Liangmen [/] and ST-34 Liangqiu [/];
3️⃣ Acid regurgitation and discomfort of the stomach — BL-20 Pishu [/].

2. Stagnation of Qi and Blood

Manifestations: Epigastric stabbing and fixed pain which is aggravated by pressing, or may be accompanied with vomiting blood, or bloody stool.

Tongue: Dark and purplish body with ecchymosis patch or spots.

Pulse: Uneven or wiry.

Treatment Principle: Promote qi circulation and activate blood, resolve blood stasis, arrest bleeding and stop pain.

Point Prescription & Manipulation:
Primary points:
    BL-17 Geshu   - ^
    BL-18 Ganshu - ^
    BL-20 Pishu - ^
    RN-12 Zhongwan   -
    ST-36 Zusanli   + ^

Explanation:
* BL-17 Geshu, the Influential Point of the blood, BL-18 Ganshu, the Back-Shu Point of the liver whose pertaining organ — liver is responsible to keep qi flowing freely and store blood, and BL-20 Pishu, the Back-Shu Point of the spleen whose pertaining organ — spleen has function to produce blood and keep the blood circulating in blood vessels, promote qi circulation, remove blood stasis and stop bleeding;
* RN-12 Zhongwan and ST-36 Zusanli reinforce the spleen and regulate the stomach.

Secondary points according to conditions:
1ⁿ Hemoptysis or bloody stools—PC-6 Neiguan [-], SP-6 Sanyinjiao [-] and SP-10 Xuehai [-].

3. Stagnant Heat in Liver and Stomach

Manifestations: Acute epigastric pain with burning sensation which is aggravated by eating, dry mouth and bitter taste, acid regurgitation and discomfort of the stomach, dry stool, dark-red urine.

Tongue: Red body with yellow coating.

Pulse: Wiry and rapid.

Treatment Principle: Relieve depression of the liver and clear heat, harmonize the stomach to relieve pain.

Point Prescription & Manipulation:
Primary points:
    BL-18 Ganshu   -
    BL-21 Weishu   -
    RN-12 Zhongwan   -
    ST-36 Zusanli   -
    ST-44 Neiting   -

    LR-2 Xingjian   -
Explanation:
* BL-18 Ganshu and LR-2 Xingjian clear fire from the liver;
* BL-21 Weishu and RN-12 Zhongwan, the combination of Front-Mu and Back-Shu Points of the stomach, harmonize the middle-jiao and relieve pain;
* ST-36 Zusanli and ST-44 Neiting regulate stomach qi, clear heat from the stomach and arrest pain.

Secondary points according to conditions:
1ⁿ Severe epigastric pain —ST-34 Liangqiu [-] and SP-6 Sanyinjiao [-];
2ⁿ Constipation— SJ-6 Zhigou [-] and BL-57 Chengshan [-].

4.   Stomach Yin Deficiency

Manifestations: Epigastric dull pain, discomfort of the stomach with hungry sensation but without desire to take food, epigastric distention and fullness after intake of food, restlessness, insomnia, thirst and dry mouth, constipation with dry stool.

Tongue: Red body with little coating.

Pulse: Thready and rapid.

Treatment   Principle: Nourish   yin   and harmonize the stomach.

Point Prescription & Manipulation:
Primary points:
    BL-20 Pishu   +
    BL-21 Weishu   +
    RN 12 Zhongwan   /
    PC-6 Neiguan   /
    ST-36 Zusanli   +
    SP-6 Sanyinjiao   +
    KI-3 Taixi   +

Explanation:
* BL-20 Pishu and SP-6 Sanyinjiao promote the spleen's function to nourish the middle-jiao and generate fluids;

- BL-21 Weishu and RN 12 Zhongwan nourish the stomach, generate fluids and clear heat from the stomach;
- PC-6 Neiguan and KI-3 Taixi clear heat, tonify yin and relieve pain;
- ST-36 Zusanli reinforces the stomach and stops pain.

Secondary points according to conditions:
1️⃣ Poor appetite and epigastric distention and fullness — ST-21 Liangmen [/] and ST-25 Tianshu [/];
2️⃣ Constipation with dry stool — SJ-6 Zhigou [/] and BL-57 Chengshan [/].

5. Deficient Cold of Spleen and Stomach

Manifestations: Dull epigastric pain which is aggravated by hunger and relieved by taking food, warmth and pressure, pale complexion, lassitude and weakness, loose stools.

Tongue: Pale body with white coating.

Pulse: Deep and thready.

Treatment Principle: Reinforce the spleen and tonify qi, warm the middle-jiao to harmonize the stomach.

Point Prescription & Manipulation:
Primary points:
    BL-20 Pishu + ^
    BL-21 Weishu + ^
    RN-12 Zhongwan + ^
    ST-25 Tianshu + ^
    ST-36 Zusanli + ^
    LR-13 Zhangmen /
    RN-6 Qihai + ^

Explanation:
BL-20 Pishu, BL-21 Weishu, RN-12 Zhongwan and LR-13 Zhangmen, the Front-Mu and Back-Shu Points of the spleen and stomach, warm the spleen and stomach and dispel cold;
RN-6 Qihai and ST-36 Zusanli warm yang and reinforce qi;
RN-12 Zhongwan, ST-25 Tianshu and RN-6 Qihai, a traditional classic combination and named the "Four Door Points", are effective to treat abominal distention, pain, and diarrhea.

Secondary points according to conditions:
1️⃣ Diarrhea — ST-25 Tianshu [+ ^];
2️⃣ Hemoptysis and bloody stools — BL-17 Geshu [+ ^].

II. EXPERIENTIAL TREATMENT

1. Puncturing with 5 Needles

Indications: Gastric or duodenal ulcer.

Point Prescription:
    PC-6 Neiguan
    ST-36 Zusanli
    RN-12 Zhongwan

Manipulation: Use 2-cun needles to insert into PC-6 Neiguan and ST-36 Zusanli as well as RN-12 Zhongwan. Rotate, lift and thrust the needles with even manipulation and middle-degree force stimulation. After arrival of qi, retain the needles in the points for 40 minutes, and manipulate them every 10 minutes. Give the treatment once daily with 10 treatments as a course. After an interval of 3-5 days, apply the next therapeutic course. Three courses are needed in total.

2. Ear Acupuncture

Indications: Gastric or duodenal ulcer.

Ear Point Prescription:
    Stomach, Duodenum, Abdomen, Spleen, Liver, Synthetic, Subcortex, Shenmen.
Manipulation: See page 255.

Comment:
As bad emotional stress and improper diet play an important role in causing and aggravating peptic ulcer, the patient should be advised not to take cold, greasy or irritative food, not to drink or smoke, and avoid emotional stresses during the treatment period. For patients with deficiency syndrome, moxibustion is recommended to use for a long period to get a good result.

Notes:

18. Cystitis

Cystitis is a bacterially caused inflammation of the internal wall of the urinary bladder. Acute cystitis is clinically marked by sudden onset of lower abdominal pain and frequent, dripping, and painful urination, accompanied by macroscopic blood in the urine and pyuria. The manifestations of chronic cystitis are similar to or milder than those of acute cystitis, and reoccur frequently. According to TCM cystitis belongs to the category of Lin Zhen (stranguria), and is caused by attack of exogenous damp-heat or internal production of damp-heat, leading to accumulation of damp-heat in the lower-jiao.

I. STANDARD TREATMENT

Cystitis is generally divided into two types — damp-heat in the lower-jiao and deficiency of the spleen and kidney. Points of the Bladder, Gallbladder, Ren and Spleen Meridians are frequently selected in its treatment.

1. Damp-Heat in the Lower-Jiao

Manifestations: Frequent, painful, and dripping urination with burning sensation, dark or turbid urine.

Tongue: Red body with yellow and sticky coating.

Pulse: Soft and rapid.

Treatment Principle: Clear heat, promote diuresis and relieve stranguria.

Point Prescription & Manipulation:
Primary points:
>   RN-3 Zhongji   -
>   BL-28 Pangguanshu   -
>   SP-6 Sanyinjiao   -
>   SP-9 Yinlingquan   -
>   BL-39 Weiyang   -
>   KI-2 Rangu   -
>   GB-34 Yanglingquan   -

Explanation:
- RN-3 Zhongji, KI-2 Rangu and BL-28 Pangguanshu clear damp-heat from the urinary bladder;
- SP-6 Sanyinjiao and SP-9 Yinlingquan promote the spleen's function of transportation of water to drain dampness;
- BL-39 Weiyang and GB-34 Yanglingquan clear damp-heat in the lower-jiao.

Secondary points according to conditions:
1． Difficulty in urination— BL-32 Ciliao [-] and BL-33 Zhongliao [-];
2． Hematuria— SP-10 Xuehai;
3． High fever — LI-11 Quchi [-];
4． Sandy urine—LI-4 Hegu [-], LR-4 Zhongfeng [-];
5． Turbid urine— KI-6 Zhaohai [-].

2. Deficiency of Spleen and Kidney

Manifestations: Intermittent dripping urination with dull pain, which is induced by exertion, fatigue, listlessness, soreness and weakness of the loins and knees, poor appetite, loose stools.

Tongue: Pale tongue.

Pulse: Weak or feeble.

Treatment Principle: Reinforce the spleen, invigorate the kidney and relieve stranguria.

Point Prescription & Manipulation:
Primary points:
>   BL-20 Pishu   + ^
>   BL-23 Shenshu   + ^
>   RN-3 Zhongji   + ^
>   RN-4 Guanyuan   + ^
>   ST-36 Zusanli   + ^
>   SP-6 Sanyinjiao   + ^
>   DU-4 Mingmen   + ^

Explanation:
- BL-20 Pishu, ST-36 Zusanli and SP-6 Sanyinjiao reinforce the spleen and tonify qi;
- BL-23 Shenshu, RN-4 Guanyuan and DU-4 Mingmen reinforce the kidney and tonify yang;

- RN-3 Zhongji regulates the urinary bladder to relieve stranguria.

Secondary points according to conditions:
1〕 Poor appetite and abdominal distention—RN-12 Zhongwan [/].

II. EXPERIENTIAL TREATMENT

1. Puncturing BL-54 Zhibian

Indications: Acute cystitis or acute urethritis.

Point Prescription:
BL-54 Zhibian

Manipulation: Insert a 3-cun needle through the skin at the point, push the needle with its tip toward the perineum 3 cun deep. Rotate the needle to induce needling sensation radiating to the perineum, retain the needle for 20 minutes, and rotate the needle once during the retention. The treatment is given once a day. Generally, one treatment will bring about effective results and three treatments are needed in total.

2. Acupuncture and Moxibustion on KI-6 Zhaohai

Indications: Chronic cystitis or urethritis.

Point Prescription:
KI-6 Zhaohai

Manipulation:
Insert a needle perpendicularly into the point, lift, thrust and rotate it to induce arrival of qi, retain the needle for 30-40 minutes, and manipulate it every 10 minutes. If the patient's condition belongs to category of yang deficiency, apply moxibustion on the point. Ignite a moxa stick, hold the stick and keep the ignited end 0.5-1 cun from the skin of the point until the patient feels slight burning pain. Usually, apply the moxibustion on each side for 5-7 minutes. The treatment with acupuncture or moxibustion is given once daily, with 10 treatments as a course. For mild cases, only 2-3 treatments are needed, and to severe cases, two or three courses may be given.

3. Ear Acupuncture

Indications: Acute or chronic cystitis or urethritis.

Ear Point Prescription:
Primary points:
Bladder, Abdomen, Pelvic Cavity.

Secondary points according to conditions:
1〕 Damp-heat syndrome—Sanyinjiao, Endocrine and Shenmen;
2〕 Yang deficiency syndrome with a long-term course — Kidney and Spleen.

Manipulation: See page 255.

Comment:
Zhenjiu is effective in relieving symptoms of cystitis, and is a good therapy for chronic cystitis. In some cases, chronic cystitis can be cured by Zhenjiu therapy.

Notes:

19. Seminal Emission

Seminal emission refers to ejaculation of the male without sexual intercourse. It is due to functional disorders of the cerebral cortex or the sexual active center in the spinal cord, usually resulting from over sexual life or a too strong sexual desire. Seminal emission that occurs while asleep and dreaming is called oneirogmus; spontaneous seminal emission that occurs while awake is called spermatorrhea. It is normal for healthy men to experience oneirogmus several times a month, but several times a week or every night is considered abnormal. Seminal emission is usually accompanied by weakness and soreness of the lower back and knees, dizziness, tinnitus, lassitude, and poor memory. According to TCM, oneirogmus, called Yi Jing in Chinese (seminal emission is also called Yi Jing in Chinese), is caused by mental injury or excessive masturbation leading to imbalance between the heart and kidney. Spermatorrhea, called Hua Jing in Chinese, is due to excessive sexual activity or weak constitution after protracted illness, leading to deficiency of the kidney essence.

I. STANDARD TREATMENT

Seminal emission is generally divided into three types — deficiency of yin with hyperactivity of fire, kidney deficiency with impaired storage function, and retained damp-heat. Points of the Ren, Du, Bladder, Heart, Kidney and Liver Meridians are frequently selected in its treatment.

1. Deficiency Yin with Hyperactivity of Fire

Manifestations: Nocturnal seminal emission, restlessness, insomnia, dizziness, blurred vision, tinnitus, soreness and weakness of the lower back and knees, hot sensation in the palms, soles and chest, scanty urine.

Tongue: Red body.

Pulse: Thready and rapid.

Treatment Principle: Nourish yin, reduce fire, calm the mind, and consolidate essence.

Point Prescription & Manipulation:
Primary points:
  HT-7 Shenmen /
  BL-15 Xinshu -
  KI-3 Taixi +
  BL-52 Zhishi +
  LR-3 Taichong -
  SP-6 Sanyinjiao -
  DU-20 Baihui -

Explanation:
- HT-7 Shenmen and BL-15 Xinshu clear fire from the heart;
- KI-3 Taixi and BL-52 Zhishi strengthen the kidney to restrain the essence;
- LR-3 Taichong clears heat from the lower-jiao;
- DU-20 Baihui calms spirit;
- SP-6 Sanyinjiao, the Crossing Point of the three Foot-Yin Meridians, reinforces yin to reduce fire.

Secondary points according to conditions:
1① Bitter taste in the mouth and painful urination — RN-3 Zhongji [/] and GB-43 Xiaxi [-];
2① Over susceptibility to erect penis—GB-34 Yanglingquan [-].

2. Kidney Deficiency with Impaired Storage Function

Manifestations: Frequent nocturnal emission or even spontaneous emission at day or night, particularly if there is a desire for sex, dizziness, pale complexion, lassitude, listlessness, soreness and weakness of the lower back and knees.

Tongue: Pale.

Pulse: Deep, thready and weak.

Treatment Principle: Replenish kidney yang, nourish essence, and consolidate the essence gate.

Point Prescription & Manipulation:
Primary points:

    BL-23 Shenshu + ^
    KI-12 Dahe + ^
    SP-6 Sanyinjiao + ^
    RN-4 Guanyuan + ^
    DU-4 Mingmen + ^
    DU-20 Baihui + ^

Explanation:
- BL-23 Shenshu and KI-12 Dahe reinforce kidney yang;
- DU-20 Baihui raises the sunken qi to consolidate the essence gate;
- SP-6 Sanyinjiao, the Crossing Point of the three Foot-Yin Meridians, nourishes yin and warms yang;
- RN-4 Guanyuan, the Crossing Point of the Ren and three Foot-Yin Meridians, and DU-4 Mingmen tonify kidney yang and restrain the essence.

Secondary points according to conditions:
1❑ Prolonged course —BL-42 Gaohuang [+ ^], BL-52 Zhishi [+ ^] and KI-3 Taixi [+];
2❑ Frequent urination— BL-28 Pangguanshu [+ ^].

3. Retained Damp-Heat

Manifestations: Seminal emission, restlessness, insomnia, bitter taste in the mouth, hot urination with scanty urine.

Tongue: Red body with sticky and yellow coating.

Pulse: Soft and rapid.

Treatment Principle: Clear damp-heat.

Point Prescription & Manipulation:
Primary points:

    LR-3 Taichong -
    RN-3 Zhongji -
    SP-6 Sanyinjiao -
    GB-34 Yanglingquan -
    PC-6 Neiguan -

Explanation:
- LR-3 Taichong and GB-34 Yanglingquan clear damp-heat from the lower-jiao;
- RN-3 Zhongji clears heat from the essence palace and restrains the essence;
- SP-6 Sanyinjiao drains dampness, clears heat from the three Foot-Yin Meridians and restrains the essence;
- PC-6 Neiguan calms the mind to help restrain the essence.

Secondary points according to conditions:
1❑ Turbid urination and dysuria—BL-32 Ciliao [-] and BL-28 Pangguanshu [-].

II. EXPERIENTIAL TREATMENT

1. Acupuncture and Moxibustion on RN-3 Zhongji

Indication: Intractable seminal emission.

Point Prescription:
    RN-3 Zhongji

Manipulation: Puncture perpendicularly 1.5 cun deep, constantly rotate, thrust and lift the needle to induce an electric shock sensation radiating to the tip of the penis. Retain the needle for 20 minutes. After removing the needle, apply warming moxibustion with moxa stick for 1 minute. The treatment is given once every other day, with 7 treatments as a course. Usually, 1-3 courses are needed.

2. Puncturing RN-1 Huiyin

Indication: Seminal emission.

Point Prescription:
    RN-1 Huiyin

Manipulation: Puncture perpendicularly 2 cun or more, rotate, thrust and lift the needle with medium stimulation until the patient cannot stand it, retain the needle for 20-30 minutes, and manipulate it every 5 minutes during the retention. The treatment is given once daily or every other day, with 7 treatments as a course. Usually, 1-2 courses are needed.

3. Puncturing Reaction Point on the Ear

Indication: Seminal emission.

Ear Point Prescription:
   Reaction point around the Endocrine and Testicle region.

Manipulation: Press the Endocrine and Testicle region on the ear to look for tender spot, puncture the tender spot about 0.2-0.3 cm deep, rotate the needle to induce strong pain to the patient, retain it for 20-30 minutes, and manipulate it twice with strong stimulation during the retention. The treatment is given once daily, with 7 treatments as a course. Usually, 1-2 courses are needed.

4. Puncturing and Taping Ear Points

Indication: Seminal emission.

Ear Point Prescription:
   Kidney, Liver, Spleen, Subcortex, Shenmen.

Manipulation: See page 255.

Comment:
Zhenjiu is effective for most cases of seminal emission. If it is applied in cooperation with avoiding emotional stress and giving up masturbation, the result will be better.

Notes:

20. Impotence

Impotence refers to a common male sexual dysfunction caused by functional disturbance of the central nervous system or organic disease. It is due to functional disorders of the cerebral cortex or the sexual center in the spinal cord, usually resulting from over sexual life or too much strong sexual desires, or psychic trauma which is related to sexuality. Impotence is clinically marked by inability to achieve or maintain an erection, making sexual intercourse problematic. According to TCM, impotence, Yang Wei called in Chinese, is caused by excessive masturbation or excessive sexual activity leading to decline of fire from the Gate of Life, or by mental injury which damages the heart and spleen or disturbs the kidney.

I. STANDARD TREATMENT

Impotence is generally divided into four types — decline of fire of the Gate of Life, damage to the heart and spleen, damage to kidney, and downward movement of damp-heat. Points of the Stomach, Du, Ren, and Bladder Meridians are frequently selected in its treatment.

1. Decline of Fire of the Gate of Life

Manifestations: Impotence, soreness and weakness of the lower back and knees, cold limbs, aversion to cold, lassitude, pale complexion, dizziness, blurred vision, poor appetite.

Tongue: Pale body with thin and sticky coating.

Pulse: Deep and weak.

Treatment Principle: Replenish the kidney essence and strengthen yang.

Point Prescription & Manipulation:
Primary points:
   BL-23 Shenshu   + ^
   DU-4 Mingmen   + ^
   RN-4 Guanyuan   + ^

RN-3 Zhongji   + ^
SP-6 Sanyinjiao +
BL-52 Zhishi   + ^
DU-20 Baihui   + ^

Explanation:
- BL-23 Shenshu, BL-52 Zhishi and DU-4 Mingmen warm and tonify primary yang of the kidney;
- RN-4 Guanyuan and RN-3 Zhongji, both being near to the penis and connecting with it through the Ren Meridian, directly warm and strengthen the penis;
- DU-20 Baihui raises the sunken yang;
- SP-6 Sanyinjiao nourishes yin to tonify yang.

Secondary points according to conditions:
1□ Poor appetite — ST-36 Zusanli [+].

2. Deficiency of Heart and Spleen

Manifestations: Impotence, palpitation, insomnia, lassitude, poor appetite, and loose stools, sallow complexion.

Tongue: Pale body with thin and sticky coating.

Pulse: Thready.

Treatment Principle: Invigorate heart and spleen, and replenish kidney.

Point Prescription & Manipulation:
Primary points:
    BL-15 Xinshu   +
    BL-20 Pishu   +
    BL-23 Shenshu   +
    RN-4 Guanyuan   +
    ST-36 Zusanli   + ^
    SP-6 Sanyinjiao + ^

Explanation:
- BL-15 Xinshu and BL-20 Pishu, the Back-Shu Points of the heart and spleen, tonify qi and blood of the heart and spleen;
- BL-23 Shenshu, the Back-Shu Point of the kidney, reinforces the kidney and strengthens its function;

- RN-4 Guanyuan, being near to the penis and connecting with it through the Ren Meridian, directly strengthens the penis;
- ST-36 Zusanli promotes production of qi and blood to nourish the heart and spleen;
- SP-6 Sanyinjiao nourishes yin to tonify yang.

Secondary points according to conditions:
1□ Insomnia — HT-7 Shenmen [-];
2□ Palpitation — PC-6 Neiguan [/].

3. Downward Movement of Damp-Heat

Manifestations: Impotence, scanty and dark urine, soreness of the lower limbs, bitter taste in the mouth.

Tongue: Red body with yellow sticky coating.

Pulse: Soft and rapid.

Treatment Principle: Clear heat and dampness.

Point Prescription & Manipulation:
Primary points:
    BL-28 Pangguanshu -
    BL-32 Ciliao   -
    RN-2 Qugu   -
    SP-6 Sanyinjiao -
    ST-40 Fenglong -
    LR-3 Taichong   -

Explanation:
- BL-28 Pangguanshu and BL-32 Ciliao clear damp-heat from the urinary bladder and essence palace;
- RN-2 Qugu clears damp-heat from the Ren Meridian and strengthens the penis;
- SP-6 Sanyinjiao drains dampness and clears heat from the three Foot-Yin Meridians and strengthens the penis;
- ST-40 Fenglong removes phlegm;
- LR-3 Taichong clears damp-heat from the Liver Meridian and benefits the penis.

Secondary points according to conditions:
1□ Moisture of the scrotum—GB-34 Yinlingquan [-].

Comment:
Zhenjiu can be effective to help most impotence patients eliminate this disorder. Impotence in most cases is a functional disorder, closely related to emotional pressure. Usually, mental stress, especially fear of sexual failure, can cause impotence or make it worse. It is suggested to talk with the patient and help him to feel confident in his sexual ability. If so, the Zhenjiu treatment result will be much better.

Notes:

21. Costal Chondritis

Costal chondritis is a chronic non-specific inflammation of the costal cartilage. It occurs primarily in young people and adults and is usually induced by chest trauma or infection of the respiratory tract. The costal cartilage of the second and third ribs are generally affected. It is clinically characterized by swelling and eminence of the affected costal cartilage and persistent dull pain aggravated by coughing, deep breathing, or movement of the chest or shoulders. The pain may spontaneously disappear after approximately one mouth, but recurs easily. According to TCM, costal chondritis is classified into Xie Tong (hypochondriac pain), and is caused by attack of the Shaoyang Meridian by pathogens or stagnation of liver qi, resulting in qi disorder of the Liver and Gallbladder Meridians, and obstruction of circulation of qi and blood.

I. STANDARD TREATMENT

Costal chondritis is generally divided into two types — qi stagnation with blood stasis and damp-heat in the liver and gallbladder. Points of the Liver and Gallbladder Meridians are frequently selected in its treatment.

1. Qi Stagnation and Blood Stasis

Manifestations: Hypochondriac pain with swelling of the local region, which is aggravated by pressing.

Tongue: Purplish body.

Pulse: Wiry.

Treatment Principle: Promote circulation of qi and activate blood to relieve pain.

Point Prescription & Manipulation:
Primary points:
    RN-17 Danzhong   -
    LR-3 Taichong   -
    GB-41 Zulinqi -
    PC-6 Neiguan -

Ashi Point -

Explanation:
- RN-17 Danzhong, the Influential Point of qi, and LR-3 Taichong, Shu-Stream and Yuan-Primary point of the Liver Meridian which runs through the hypochondrium, promote circulation of qi of the diseased region;
- GB-41 Zulinqi and PC-6 Neiguan promote qi circulation to relieve hypochondriac pain;
- Ashi Point activates the collaterals of the local region, removes blood stasis and relieves pain.

Secondary points according to conditions:
1〕 Stabbing pain — SP-21 Dabao [-], which can be pricked to bleed, BL-17 Geshu [-] and BL-18 Ganshu [-].

2. Damp-Heat in Liver and Gallbladder

Manifestations: Hypochondriac pain with swelling of the local region, bitter taste in the mouth, liable to lose temper.

Tongue: Yellow and sticky coating.

Pulse: Wiry and quick.

Treatment Principle: Clear heat and dampness from the liver and gallbladder, dissolve swelling to relieve pain.

Point Prescription & Manipulation:
Primary points:
    LR-3 Taichong -
    GB-34 Yanglingquan -
    LR-14 Qimen -
    GB-24 Riyue -
    Ashi Point -

Explanation:
- LR-3 Taichong and GB-34 Yanglingquan clear damp-heat from the Liver and Gallbladder Meridians;
- LR-14 Qimen and GB-24 Riyue, the Front-Mu Points of the liver and gallbladder and near the diseased region, clear damp-heat from the liver and gallbladder and relieve pain;

- Ashi Point activates the collaterals of the local region, removes blood stasis and relieves pain.

Secondary points according to conditions:
1〕 Dysuria — SP-9 Yinlingquan [-] ;
2〕 Prolonged course — LR-2 Xingjian [-] and ST-40 Fenglong [-];
3〕 High fever—LI-11 Quchi [-] and DU-14 Dazhui.

II. EXPERIENTIAL TREATMENT

1. Puncturing PC-6 Neiguan and the Tender Point

Indications: Costal chondritis.

Point Prescription:
    PC-6 Neiguan
    The border of the diseased region.

Manipulation: First, insert a needle into PC-6 Neiguan perpendicularly 0.5-0.8 cun deep, rotate, thrust and lift the needle to induce needling sensation to the patient. Then, insert a needle into 2 spots 1 cm away from the border of the diseased region obliquely or horizontally, with the needle tip directed at the most painful point. Gently manipulate the needle. Retain the needles in the points for 15-20 minutes. The treatment is given once every day and usually within 10 treatments the pain and swelling will disappear.

2. Hydro-Puncture on Tender Point

Indications: Prolonged costal chondritis.

Point Prescription:
    The most tender point of the diseased region.

Manipulation: Insert a syringe needle into the point 10-15 mm deep, withdraw the pistol to make sure there is no blood, inject 2-6 ml of 2% procaine slowly into the point. The treatment is given once every 4 days and 5 treatments are taken as a course.

3. Acupuncture with Cupping

Indications: Costal chondritis.

Point Prescription:

Primary points:
GB-21 Jianjing
PC-6 Neiguan
Ashi Points (located on the upper and lower borders of the diseased rib, 2 cun lateral to the midline of the chest, 4 points in total.)

Secondary points according to conditions:
1 Serious pain and suffocated sensation in the chest — LR-3 Taichong;
2 Prolonged course with obvious swelling of the diseased region — KI-3 Taixi;
3 Pain radiating to the back — BL-13 Feishu, and BL-42 Gaohuang.

Manipulation: Insert a needle into GB-21 Jianjing obliquely 0.5-0.6 cun deep, at an angle of 45 degree and with the needle tip toward the chest bone. Rotate the needle to induce sore and distending sensation that radiates to the chest wall and upper limbs. Insert a needle into PC-6 Neiguan 1 cun deep, with the needle tip toward the elbow, and rotate the needle to make the needling sensation radiate to the fingers, elbow, armpit and chest. Insert a needle into the Ashi Point horizontally 1 cun deep, at an angle of 15 degrees and with the needle tip toward the chest, and rotate the needle to induce the needling sensation. An assistant point is punctured with medium stimulation to induce needling sensation. Retain the needles in the points for about 20 minutes, and manipulate once during the retention. After withdrawing the needles, apply cupping on the chest and back of the diseased side. The treatment is given once every other day, with 10 treatments as a course.

4. Warming Needling

Indications: Prolonged costal chondritis.

Point Prescription:

Ashi Point (the center of the enlargement of the diseased region).
RN-17 Danzhong
SJ-5 Waiguan of the diseased side

Manipulation: Insert a 1-cun long needle into the Ashi Point perpendicularly about 0.5 cun deep, into SJ-5 Waiguan perpendicularly about 0.8 cun deep, and into RN-17 Danzhong obliquely downward about 0.8 cun deep. Rotate the needles to induce needling sensation, and retain the needles for about 20 minutes. During the retention, put a 20-mm long segment of moxa stick on each needle handle, and ignite them for moxibustion. When the moxa stick is extinguished, put on a new segment to continue moxibustion. 3 segments of moxa stick are needed on Ashi Points, and 2 segments needed on each of the other points. The treatment is given once every day with 7 treatments as a course.

Comment:
Zhenjiu is effective to relieve pain due to costal chondritis.

Notes:

22. Trigeminal Neuralgia

Trigeminal neuralgia refers to transient paroxysmal megalgia of the trigeminal nerve pathway. Its cause is uncertain, possibly related to compression of the trigeminal nerve root at its entry point into the brainstem. It is clinically marked by sudden onset of stabbing or burning pain along the pathway of the affected nerve, usually evoked by speaking, chewing, washing the face, brushing the teeth, catching cold, or touching "trigger points" on the face. According to TCM, trigeminal neuralgia belongs to the category of Mian Tong (facial pain), and is caused by attack of exogenous wind pathogen or by flaring-up of liver fire, obstructing the flow of qi and blood and resulting in pain in the teeth and face.

I. STANDARD TREATMENT

Trigeminal neuralgia is generally divided into four types — obstruction of the collaterals by wind-cold with phlegm, obstruction of the collaterals by wind-heat with phlegm, flaring up of liver fire, and blood stasis in the collaterals. Points of the Yangming and Shaoyang Meridians are frequently selected in its treatment.

1. Obstruction of the Collaterals by Wind-Cold with Phlegm

Manifestations: Sudden onset of paroxysmal severe stabbing pain in the face, which is aggravated by cold and relieved by warmth.

Tongue: Pale with white coating.

Pulse: Tight or wiry.

Treatment Principle: Disperse wind and cold, transform phlegm, dredge the collateral, stop pain.

Point Prescription & Manipulation:
Primary points:
    Ashi Points /
    GB-20 Fengchi   - ^

    SJ-5 Waiguan   - ^
    ST-40 Fenglong   - ^
    ST-36 Zusanli   / ^

Explanation:
The Ashi Points refer to the followings:
1□ BL-2 Cuanzhu, GB-14 Yangbai and EX-HN-4 Yuyao for pain in the first branch of the trigeminal nerve;
2□ ST-2 Sibai, SI-18 Quanliao and ST-3 Juliao for pain in the second branch of the trigeminal nerve;
3□ ST-6 Jiache, ST-7 Xiaguan and RN-24 Chengjiang for pain in the third branch of the trigeminal nerve.

- Ashi Points promote circulation of qi and blood in the diseased region to relieve pain;
- GB-20 Fengchi and SJ-5 Waiguan dispel external wind and cold pathogens;
- ST-40 Fenglong and ST-36 Zusanli reinforce the middle-jiao and transform phlegm.

Secondary points according to conditions:
1□ Severe pain — PC-6 Neiguan [-] and BL-17 Geshu [-].

2. Obstruction of Collaterals by Wind-Heat with Phlegm

Manifestations: Sudden onset of paroxysmal stabbing and burning pain in the face, which is aggravated by heat and relieved by cold, flushed face, red eyes, sweating, thirst, scanty and dark urine.

Tongue: Red body with yellow coating.

Pulse: Smooth or smooth and wiry.

Treatment Principle: Disperse wind and heat, transform phlegm, activate collaterals, and stop pain.

Point Prescription & Manipulation:
Primary points:
    Ashi Points (the same as above) -
    LI-1 Shangyang   -
    SJ-1 Guanchong   -

SI-1 Shaoze   -
LI-11 Quchi   -
ST-40 Fenglong -

Explanation:
Puncture LI-1 Shangyang, SJ-1 Guanchong and SI-1 Shaoze with the three-edged needle to bleed.

- Ashi Points   promote circulation of qi and blood in the diseased region to relieve pain;
- LI-1 Shangyang, SJ-1 Guanchong and SI-1 Shaoze, the Jing-Well Points of the three Hand-Yang Meridians, dispel wind-heat from the three Hand-Yang Meridians;
- LI-11 Quchi clears heat from Yangming Meridian;
- ST-40 Fenglong transforms phlegm.

Secondary points according to conditions:
1☐ Fever with headache — LI-4 Hegu [-] and GB-20 Fengchi [-].

3. Flaring-Up of Liver Fire

Manifestations: Sudden onset of paroxysmal stabbing and burning pain in the face, which is aggravated by heat and relieved by cold, flushed face, red eyes, irritability, distressed sensation in the chest and hypochondriac region, thirst, bitter taste in the mouth, dark urine, constipation.

Tongue: Red body with yellow coating.

Pulse: Wiry.

Treatment Principle: Clear liver fire.

Point Prescription & Manipulation:
Primary points:
Ashi Points (The same as above) -
SJ-2 Yemen   -
LR-2 Xingjian   -
GB-43 Xiaxi   -
LR-8 Ququan   -

Explanation:
- Ashi Points promote circulation of qi and blood in the diseased region to relieve pain;

- SJ-2 Yemen, LR-2 Xingjian and GB-43 Xiaxi clear fire from the liver;
- LR-8 Ququan nourishes the liver yin to reduce fire.

Secondary points according to conditions:
1☐ Distending fullness in chest and hypochondrium — SJ-6 Zhigou [-];
2☐ Dry stools — ST-44 Neiting [-];
3☐ Restlessness and over susceptibility to being angry — PC-7 Daling [-].

4. Blood Stasis in the Collaterals

Manifestations: Protracted course of repeated attack of paroxysmal pain in the face, which is stabbing and intolerable, dark complexion.

Tongue: Purplish body with ecchymotic spots.

Pulse: Unsmooth.

Treatment Principle: Remove blood stasis and activate collaterals.

Point Prescription & Manipulation:
Primary points:
Local tender points -
BL-17 Geshu   - ^
BL-18 Ganshu   - ^
SP-6 Sanyinjiao   / ^
ST-36 Zusanli   / ^

Explanation:
- Local tender points promote circulation of qi and blood in the diseased region to relieve pain;
- BL-17 Geshu, the Influential Point of blood, and BL-18 Ganshu, the Back-Shu Point of the liver, promote blood circulation and remove blood stasis;
- SP-6 Sanyinjiao and ST-36 Zusanli reinforce qi and blood and promote their circulation.

Secondary points according to conditions:
1☐ Severe pain with restlessness — HT-7 Shenmen [-] and PC-6 Neiguan [-].

II. EXPERIENTIAL TREATMENT

1. Puncturing EX-HN-4 Yuyao

Indication: Pain of the first branch of the trigeminal nerve.

Point Prescription:
EX-HN-4 Yuyao of the diseased side.

Manipulation: Insert a needle obliquely downwards 0.3-0.5 cun deep to induce an electric sensation to the patient, and gently lift and thrust the needle 20-50 times. The treatment is given once daily or every other day, with 10 treatments as a course.

2. Puncturing ST-2 Sibai

Indication: Pain of the second branch of the trigeminal nerve.

Point Prescription:
ST-2 Sibai of the diseased side.

Manipulation: Insert a needle obliquely upwards into the point at an angle of 45 degrees to induce an electric sensation radiating to the upper lip. Thrust and lift the needle 20-50 times. The treatment is given once daily or every other day, with 10 treatments as a course.

3. Puncturing ST-7 Xiaguan

Indication: Pain of the third or second branch of the trigeminal nerve.

Point Prescription:
ST-7 Xiaguan of the diseased side.

Manipulation: Puncture perpendicularly 1.5 cun to induce an electric sensation radiating to the bottom of the tongue or the mandible, thrust and lift the needle 20-50 times. The treatment is given once daily or every other day, with 10 treatments as a course.

4. Puncturing SI-18 Quanliao

Indication: Trigeminal neuralgia.

Point Prescription:
SI-18 Quanliao of the diseased side

Manipulation: Puncture perpendicularly about 2.5 cun to induce an electric sensation radiating over the whole face of the diseased side, retain the needle for 30 minutes, and manipulate it every 10 minutes. The treatment is given once daily or every other day. Usually, 1-3 courses are needed.

5. Puncturing SI-19 Tinggong

Indication: Trigeminal neuralgia.

Point prescription:
SI-19 Tinggong of the diseased side.

Manipulation: Puncture perpendicularly 0.6-0.8 cun deep, manipulate the needle gently to avoid inducing pain to the patient, retain the needle for 30-60 minutes, and manipulate it every 10 minutes. The treatment is given once daily or every other day, with 10 treatments as a course. Usually, after or during the treatment the patient's pain will be relieved.

Comment:
Trigeminal neuralgia is an obstinate disease, and no especially effective therapy has been discovered. As Zhenjiu is effective to relieve pain in most cases and does not have any side effect, it can be taken as the first choice for treatment of trigeminal neuralgia. In the Zhenjiu treatment, selection of the local points and selection of distal points should be combined, but the local points are chief. Generally, mild stimulation with long retention of the needles is applied on the local points, while strong stimulation with reducing manipulation is applied on the distal points. Usually, Zhenjiu will be more effective if massage is applied in cooperation.

Notes:

23. Facial Paralysis

Facial paralysis refers to facial palsy due to inflammation of a facial nerve. Its cause is uncertain. It is clinically marked by motor impairment of the facial muscles of the diseased side, and deviation of the mouth and eye. According to TCM, facial paralysis belongs to the categories of Kou Wai or Kou Pi (deviation of the mouth), Kou Yan Wai Xie (deviation of the mouth and eye), and is caused by deficiency of defending qi and empty collaterals, and attack of the meridians and collaterals by pathogenic wind, resulting in obstruction of the meridians and collaterals and failure of muscle to receive nourishment.

I. STANDARD TREATMENT

Facial paralysis is generally divided into two types — attack by exogenous wind and stirring of internal wind. Points of the Yangming Meridian and local points are frequently selected in its treatment.

1. Attack by Exogenous Wind

Manifestations: Sudden onset of deviation of the mouth and eye, numbness of the face on the diseased side, aversion to cold, fever.

Tongue: Thin and white coating.

Pulse: Floating.

Treatment Principle: Disperse wind and remove obstruction from the collaterals.

Point Prescription & Manipulation:
Primary points:
    GB-20 Fengchi -
    ST-4 Dicang of the diseased side /
    ST-6 Jiache of the diseased side /
    ST-2 Sibai of the diseased side /
    GB-14 Yangbai of the diseased side /
    LI-4 Hegu -

Explanation:

ST-4 Dicang of the diseased side, ST-6 Jiache of the diseased side, ST-2 Sibai of the diseased side and GB-14 Yangbai of the diseased side should be punctured very gently or even only moxibustion is applied on them. The other distal points should be punctured with strong stimulation.

- GB-20 Fengchi dispels wind and dredges the collaterals;
- ST-4 Dicang, ST-6 Jiache, ST-2 Sibai and GB-14 Yangbai activate the local collaterals;
- LI-4 Hegu, the key point of treatment of the head and face disorders, dispels wind, relieves exterior syndrome and regulates qi and blood of the face.

Secondary points according to conditions:
1⃞ Aversion to cold and fever — DU-14 Dazhui [-];
2⃞ Failure in closing the eye and lacrimation— BL-2 Cuanzhu [/] or EX-HN-4 Yuyao [/] of the diseased;
3⃞ Pain in the region posterior to the ear—SJ-17 Yifeng [-] of the diseased side;
4⃞ Hypogeusia—- RN-23 Lianquan [/].

2. Stirring-Up of Internal Wind

Manifestations: Prolonged course of deviation of the mouth and eye, numbness of the face and facial spasm of the diseased side, which are aggravated by emotional stimulation, difficulty in closing or opening the eye.

Tongue: Pale body with white and thin coating.

Pulse: Wiry and thin pulse.

Treatment Principle: Nourish blood and calm wind.

Point Prescription & Manipulation:
Primary points:
    ST-6 Jiache of the diseased side +
    ST-4 Dicang of the diseased side +
    LI-20 Yingxiang of the diseased side +
    ST-2 Sibai of the diseased side +
    SI-18 Quanliao of the diseased side +

GB-20 Fengchi   /
ST-36 Zusanli   +
LI-4 Hegu -
LR-3 Taichong -

Explanation:
Puncture the local points horizontally and gently. Puncture the other points perpendicularly. After acupuncture, apply moxibustion with moxa stick.

- ST-6 Jiache of the diseased side, ST-4 Dicang of the diseased side, LI-20 Yingxiang of the diseased side, ST-2 Sibai of the diseased side, and SI-18 Quanliao of the diseased side activate qi and blood circulation of the diseased region, nourish the local muscles and relieve spasm;
- GB-20 Fengchi calms wind and relieves spasm;
- ST-36 Zusanli reinforces the middle-jiao to generate blood;
- Combination of LR-3 Taichong and LI-4 Hegu, both belong to Four Gate Points, soothe the liver and calm spirit.

Secondary points according to conditions:
1) Distressed feeling in the chest and nausea—ST-40 Fenglong [-];
2) Difficulty in closing and opening the eye—BL-2 Cuanzhu [+] of the diseased side   and EX-HN-5 Taiyang [+] of the diseased side;
3) Intractable deviation of the mouth —DU-26 Shuigou [+] and RN-24 Chengjiang [+].

II. EXPERIENTIAL TREATMENT

1. Bleeding EX-HN-19 Neijiache

Indication: Facial paralysis.

Point Prescription:
  EX-HN-19 Neijiache of the diseased side, located on the mucosa of the mouth, opposite to ST-6 Jiache.

Manipulation: Prick the point with the three-edged needle 2-3 mm deep and squeeze the region to bleed. The treatment is given once daily or every other day. Usually, 10-20 treatments are needed to cure this disease.

2. Puncturing SJ-17 Yifeng

Indication: Facial paralysis.

Point Prescription:
  SJ-17 Yifeng of the diseased side

Manipulation: Puncture 1-1.5 cun deep with the needle tip towards the tip of the nose. Rotate, thrust and lift the needle to induce soreness and numbness radiating to the face, and retain the needle for 20-40 minutes. The treatment is given once daily or every other day. Usually, within 30 treatments, the disease will be cured.

3. Puncturing PC-6 Neiguan

Indication: Facial paralysis.

Point Prescription:
  PC-6 Neiguan of the diseased side.

Manipulation: Hold a needle handle with the thumb, index and middle fingers, insert the needle upwards quickly through the skin at an angle of 30 degrees. Push the needle horizontally along the subcutaneous layer 1.5 cun without rotating the needle, inducing no resistance felt by the operator and no needling sensation to the patient. In case there is soreness, numbness, distention and pain felt by the patient, withdraw the needle, change the insertion direction a little, and push the needle again with the same manipulation. Retain the needle for 30-40 minutes. The treatment is given once daily, with 10 treatments as a course. Usually, within 30 treatments, the disease will be cured.

Comment:
Zhenjiu is effective to treat facial paralysis. In cooperation with massage, Zhenjiu treatment will be more effective. Usually, at the early stage of facial paralysis, gentle manipulation of the needles in the diseased region is suggested, and electric acupuncture on the diseased region should be prohibited during the first 2 weeks of the disease.

Notes:

24. Intercostal Neuralgia

Intercostal neuralgia refers to pain in one or more of the intercostal spaces caused by inflammation of the intercostal nerves. Its cause may include pleuritis, pneumonia, costal chondritis, herpes zoster, or chest trauma resulting from inflammation of the intercostal nerves. It is marked by persistent or paroxysmal stabbing pain along the pathway of the affected intercostal nerves, radiating to the lumbar region of the affected side and aggravated by coughing or deep breathing, localized tenderness is also present. According to TCM, intercostal neuralgia is put in the category of Xie Tong (hypochondriac pain), and is caused by an attack of the Shaoyang Meridian by pathogens or stagnation of liver qi, resulting in qi disorder of the Liver and Gallbladder Meridians, and obstruction of the circulation of qi and blood.

I. STANDARD TREATMENT

Intercostal neuralgia is generally divided into three types — stagnation of liver qi, retention of phlegm, and deficiency of liver yin. Points from the Liver Meridian and Gallbladder Meridian are frequently selected.

1. Stagnation of Liver Qi

Manifestations: Hypochondriac distending pain which becomes worse with emotional change, distention in the chest and abdomen, poor appetite.

Tongue: Thin coating.

Pulse: Wiry pulse.

Treatment Principle: Soothe the liver, regulate qi and relieve pain.

Point Prescription & Manipulation:
Primary points:
    BL-18 Ganshu   /
    LR-14 Qimen   /
    LR-3 Taichong   -
    LI-4 Hegu -
    GB-40 Qiuxu   -

Explanation:
Cupping can be performed on BL-18 Ganshu and LR-14 Qimen.

- BL-18 Ganshu and LR-14 Qimen, the combination of Back-Shu and Front-Mu Points of the liver, soothe the liver, promote qi circulation and relieve pain;
- LR-3 Taichong and GB-40 Qiuxu, the Yuan-Primary Points of the Liver and Gallbladder Meridians, treat the interior and exterior simultaneously and relieve constrained liver qi.

Secondary points according to conditions:
1. Severe pain — PC-6 Neiguan [-], BL-17 Geshu [-] and SP-21 Dabao [-].

2. Retention of Phlegm

Manifestation: Distending pain in the hypochondriac region and chest, which is aggravated by breathing, cough with thin sputum, shortness of breath.

Tongue: White and sticky coating.

Pulse: Thready or wiry and smooth pulse.

Treatment Principle: Ventilate the lung, regulate qi, resolve phlegm, and relieve pain.

Point Prescription & Manipulation:
Primary points:
    LU-5 Chize   -
    LU-7 Lieque   -
    RN-17 Danzhong   -
    PC-6 Neiguan   -
    ST-36 Zusanli   /
    ST-40 Fenglong   /
    GB-41 Zulinqi   -
    SJ-5 Waiguan -

Explanation:
Apply reducing manipulation by rotating the needle on LU-5 Chize and LU-7 Lieque. Apply

even reinforcing and reducing manipulation on ST-36 Zusanli and ST-40 Fenglong. Remove the needle from RN-22 Tiantu after there is a needling sensation felt by the patient, and retain the needles on the other points for about 30 minutes.

- LU-5 Chize and LU-7 Lieque disperse lung qi to remove phlegm;
- RN-17 Danzhong and PC-6 Neiguan promote qi circulation to relieve cough and pain;
- ST-36 Zusanli and ST-40 Fenglong strengthen the middle-jiao and transform phlegm;
- GB-41 Zulinqi and SJ-5 Waiguan, one pair of Eight Confluent Points, regulate Sanjiao, promote water metabolism, move qi to relieve pain.

Secondary points according to conditions:
1▢ Mental depression — LR-3 Taichong [-].

3. Deficiency of Liver Yin

Manifestations: Constant and dull pain in the hypochondriac region, thirst, bitter taste in the mouth, restlessness, dizziness, blurred vision.

Tongue: Red body with little coating.

Pulse: Thready and rapid.

Treatment Principle: Nourish liver yin, activate the collaterals to relive pain.

Point Prescription & Manipulation:
Primary points:
　　BL-18 Ganshu ＋
　　LR-8 Ququan ＋
　　SP-6 Sanyinjiao ＋
　　KI-3 Taixi ＋

Explanation:
- BL-18 Ganshu, the Back-Shu Point of the Liver, and LR-8 Ququan, the He-Sea Point of the Liver Meridian, tonify the liver, nourish the collaterals, and relieve pain;
- SP-6 Sanyinjiao and KI-3 Taixi tonify yin

and generate fluids to nourish the collaterals.

Secondary points according to conditions:
1▢ Dizziness and blurred vision — GB-20 Fengchi [/].

II. EXPERIENTIAL TREATMENT

1. Puncturing EX-B-2 Jiaji

Indication: Intercostal neuralgia.

Point Prescription:
Primary points:
　　The corresponding EX-B-2 Jiaji Points
　　SJ-6 Zhigou
　　GB-34 Yanglingquan

Secondary points according to conditions:
1▢ Emotional distress— LR-2 Xingjian and LR-3 Taichong;
2▢ Stabbing and fixed pain in the hypochondrium—BL-17 Geshu, BL-18 Ganshu, and LR-14 Qimen;
3▢ Dull and persistent pain in the hypochondrium—BL-18 Ganshu, KI-3 Taixi, and SP-6 Sanyinjiao.

Manipulation: After insertion of needles, rotate, lift and thrust them with strong stimulation. After inducing the needling sensation to the patient, retain the needles for about 20 minutes, and rotate the needles for 2 minutes during the retention. The treatment is given once every day and 3-5 treatments are needed.

2. Puncturing from GB-40 Qiuxu to KI-6 Zhaohai

Indication: Severe intercostal neuralgia, any kind of hypochondriac pain.

Point Prescription:
Primary points:
　　GB-40 Qiuxu

Secondary points according to conditions:
1▢ Heat in the liver and gallbladder—SJ-6 Zhigou, GB-34 Yanglingquan and LR-2

Xingjian;
2⬚ Distressing feeling in the chest—PC-6
Neiguan and EX-B-2 Thoracic Jiaji 5-10.

Manipulation: Hold a 2-3-cun long filiform needle, insert it into GB-40 Qiuxu, mildly rotate and forcefully press the needle to insert it deeper. If it feels like that the needle tip meets some resistance, it means that the needle tip meets the bone. Withdraw the needle under skin, and change the direction to insert the needle again. Insert the needle until you can feel the needle tip under the skin of KI-6 Zhaohai with your other hand. Then rotate the needle until the pain is relieved greatly. Insert the needle obliquely into EX-B-2 thoracic Jiaji 5-10 0.5-1 cun (15-25 mm), with the tip toward the center of the spinal column, retain the needle for 15-20 minutes, and rotate it every 5 minutes. The other points are punctured with strong rotating, lifting and thrusting manipulation. After the needling sensation is induced, retain the needles in the points for about 30 minutes. The treatment is given once a day, and 3-5 treatments are needed if a curative result is to be achieved.

3. Puncturing GB-40 Qiuxu

Indication: Intercostal neuralgia.

Point Prescription:
GB-40 Qiuxu of the diseased side

Manipulation: Insert a needle perpendicularly 1-1.5 cun (25-40 mm), and constantly rotate it with large amplitude until the pain is relieved. Then, retain it for about 30 minutes, and rotate it once every 10 minutes. The treatment is given once every day and 5-7 treatments are needed.

4. Cutaneous Puncture with Cupping

Indication: Intractable Intercostal Neuralgia.

Point Prescription:
EX-B-2 Thoracic Jiaji 1-8
The running courses of the Urinary Bladder Meridian from BL-11 Dazhu to BL-26 Guanyuanshu on the back of the diseased side;

The intercostal space of the diseased region.

Manipulation: First, ask the patient to lie on the stomach, sterilize the local region of the selected points on the back, tap the skin from the top downwards 5 times with a blossom plum needle, and apply cupping to these places for about 5 minutes. Then, ask the patient to lie on the healthy side, tap the intercostal space of the diseased region from the back forward 5 times with a blossom plum needle. Namely, tap the intercostal space respectively above and below the diseased intercostal space twice and apply cupping on these spaces for about 5 minutes. The treatment is given once every day, with 5 treatments as one course. If the result is not satisfactory, the next course can be given after a 3-5 day interval.

5. Otopuncture (Ear Acupuncture)

Indication: Various type of intercostal neuralgia.

Ear Point Prescription:
Chest, Shenmen, Xiajiaoduan, Brain, Liver.
Each time 3-4 points are selected.

Manipulation: Insert a needle into the point, rotate it with strong stimulation, and retain the needles for 30-60 minutes. The treatment is given once a day, with 10 treatments as a course.

Comment:
Acupuncture is effective to relieve intercostal neuralgia, and some patients can be cured as a result of acupuncture treatment. In clinic, acupuncture can be chosen firstly.

Notes:

25. Sciatica

Sciatica refers to pain along the pathway of the sciatic nerve and the region distributed by the nerve. It is due to irritation or inflammation of the sciatic nerve, usually resulting from compression due to muscle strain or spasm, or a slipped disc. It is clinically marked by pain of the lumbar region, buttock, posterior aspect of the thigh, and lateral side of the leg. According to TCM, sciatica belongs to the category of Bi Zheng (Bi syndrome), and it is caused by an attack of exogenous wind-cold-dampness or trauma, resulting in stagnation of qi and blood in the meridians.

I. STANDARD TREATMENT

Sciatica is generally divided into three types — cold-dampness, qi and blood stasis and kidney deficiency. Points of the Gallbladder and Bladder Meridians are frequently selected in its treatment.

1. Cold-Dampness

Manifestations: Acute pain in the lumbar region and lower limb, difficulty in moving the hip and knee joints, numbness of the lateral side of the leg, which are aggravated by cold and relieved by warmth, heavy sensation of the body.

Tongue: White and sticky coating.

Pulse: Deep or tight.

Treatment Principle: Disperse cold and dampness, warm the meridians and activate the collaterals.

Point Prescription & Manipulation:
Primary points:
  EX-B-2 Jiaji from the 2nd to the 5th of the lumbar vertebrae / ^
  BL-54 Zhibian / ^
  GB-30 Huantiao   - ^
  GB-34 Yanglingquan / ^
  DU-3 Yaoyangguan + ^

Explanation:
- EX-B-2 Jiaji from the 2nd to the 5th of the lumbar vertebrae warms the meridians and dispels cold;
- BL-54 Zhibian and GB-30 Huantiao, located on the diseased region, activate the collaterals, promote blood circulation and relieve pain;
- GB-34 Yanglingquan, the Influential Point of the tendon, relieves spasm of the tendon and alleviates pain;
- DU-3 Yaoyangguan warms the meridian, dispels cold and dampness.

Secondary points according to conditions:
1□ Cold sensation in the lower back and poor appetite — DU-4 Mingmen [+ ^] and ST-36 Zusanli [+ ^].

2. Qi and Blood Stasis

Manifestations: History of external injury, stabbing pain in the lumbar region and lower limb, which is aggravated in the night, difficulty in moving lumber region and lower limbs.

Tongue: Purple body with ecchymotic spots.

Pulse: Unsmooth.

Treatment Principle: Promote qi and blood circulation, remove blood stasis, activate collateral, and stop pain.

Point Prescription & Manipulation:
Primary points:
  EX-B-2 Jiaji from the 2nd to the 5th of the lumbar vertebrae - ^
  BL-54 Zhibian   - ^
  GB-30 Huantiao   - ^
  GB-34 Yanglingquan   - ^
  BL-17 Geshu   - ^
  BL-40 Weizhong   - ^

Explanation:
- EX-B-2 Jiaji from the 2nd to the 5th of the lumbar vertebrae warms the meridians and activates the collaterals;

- BL-54 Zhibian and GB-30 Huantiao, located on the diseased region, activate the collaterals, promote blood circulation and relieve pain;
- GB-34 Yanglingquan, the Influential Point of the tendon, relieves spasm of the tendon and alleviates pain;
- BL-17 Geshu, the Influential Point of blood, and BL-40 Weizhong, one of the most important points of removing blood stasis, promote blood circulation and remove blood stasis.

Secondary points according to conditions:
1 Prolonged course — LR-3 Taichong [-] and GB-41 Zulinqi [-].

3. Kidney Deficiency

Manifestations: Prolonged course of pain in the lumber region and lower limbs with repeated attacks that are induced and aggravated by exertion, and relieved by rest, pressure and warmth; soreness and weakness of the lumber region and knees, pale complexion, listlessness.

Tongue: Purplish body.

Pulse: Deep and weak pulse.

Treatment Principle: Tonify kidney, strengthen the waist, remove obstruction from meridians, activate collaterals and relieve pain.

Point Prescription & Manipulation:
Primary points:
EX-B-2 Jiaji from the 2nd to the 5th of the lumbar vertebrae + ^
BL-54 Zhibian + ^
GB-30 Huantiao / ^
GB-34 Yanglingquan / +
BL-23 Shenshu + ^
ST-36 Zusanli + ^

Explanation:
- EX-B-2 Jiaji from the 2nd to the 5th of the lumbar vertebrae, located on the lumbar region, tonifies the kidney and warms the meridians;

- BL-54 Zhibian and GB-30 Huantiao, located on the diseased region, activate the collaterals, promote blood circulation and relieve pain;
- GB-34 Yanglingquan, the Influential Point of the tendon, relieves spasm of the tendon and alleviates pain;
- BL-23 Shenshu tonifies the kidney and strengthens the waist;
- ST-36 Zusanli tonifies qi and blood to nourish the kidney.

Secondary points according to conditions:
1 Chronic sciatica—LR-3 Taichong is punctured with the needle tip arriving the tissue near KI-1 Yongquan.

II. EXPERIENTIAL TREATMENT

1. Puncturing EX-LE-15 Huanzhongshang

Indication: Sciatica.

Point Prescription:
EX-LE-15 Huanzhongshang, located on the point 2 cun above and 0.5 cun lateral to the midpoint of the line connecting the end of the coccyx and the prominence of the great trochanter, of the diseased side.

Manipulation: Ask the patient to lie on the healthy side with the healthy leg extended and the diseased leg half bent. Puncture perpendicularly 3-4 cun deep, rotate, thrust and lift the needle to induce the needling sensation radiating to the foot. The treatment is given once daily with 7 treatments as a course. Usually within 4 courses, the pain will disappear.

2. Puncturing BL-24 Qihaishu

Indication: Sciatica.

Point Prescription:
BL-24 Qihaishu of the diseased side

Manipulation: Puncture perpendicularly 3-4 cun deep, rotate, thrust and lift the needle to induce the needling sensation radiating to the back of the thigh and lateral side of the leg. The treatment is given once daily, with 7 treatments as a course. Usually within 4 courses the pain will disappear.

3. Puncturing EX-B-11 Yaoer

Indication: Sciatica.

Point Prescription:
EX-B-11 Yao'er, located below the spinous process of the 2nd lumbar vertebra, and 1 cun lateral to the midline of the back, of the diseased side.

Manipulation: Puncture perpendicularly 3-4 cun deep, rotate and thrust and lift the needle to induce a needling sensation radiating to the foot. The treatment is given once daily with 7 treatments as a course. Usually, within 4 courses, the pain will disappear.

Comment:
Zhenjiu is effective to relieve sciatica pain, and in most cases, Zhenjiu can cure primary sciatica. When puncturing points on the back and buttock, it is required to induce the needling sensation radiating downwards to the diseased leg or even its extremity. But if an electric shock sensation is induced during manipulation, the needle should be withdrawn somewhat immediately in order to avoid injuring the nerve.

Notes:

26. Systremma

Systremma is a disorder caused by over strain of the lower limbs, cold stimulation, or lack of calcium. It is characterized by an abrupt attack of spastic pain and enlargement of the back of the leg, which is aggravated by extending the lower limb of the diseased side. It is called Tuiduzi Zhuangjing in Chinese.

I. STANDARD TREATMENT

Systremma is generally divided into two types — stagnation of qi and blood and yin deficiency of the kidney and liver. Points of the Bladder Meridian are frequently selected in its treatment.

1. Stagnation of Qi and Blood

Manifestations: Abrupt attack of spastic pain of the back of the leg during physical labor or exercise, limitation of movement of the leg.

Tongue and Pulse: Normal.

Treatment Principle: Promote circulation of qi and blood.

Point Prescription & Manipulation:
Primary points:
BL-57 Chengshan   - ^
BL-40 Weizhong   - ^
BL-60 Kunlun   - ^

Explanation:
* BL-57 Chengshan, located on the diseased region, activates qi and blood circulation, relieves spasms and alleviates pain;
* BL-40 Weizhong, one of the most important points to remove blood stasis, promotes blood circulation and removes blood stasis;
* BL-60 Kunlun, Jing-River Point of the Bladder Meridian, which runs through the diseased region, promotes circulation of qi of the Bladder Meridian and alleviates pain.

Secondary points according to conditions:
1〕 Severe pain — GB-34 Yanglingquan [-] and LR-3 Taichong [-];

2〕 Repeated attack ─ BL-17 Geshu [-].

2. Yin Deficiency of Kidney and Liver

Manifestations: Frequent attack of spastic pain of the back of the leg during rest, soreness and weakness of the knee and low back, lassitude.

Tongue: Red body with thin coating.

Pulse: Weak.

Treatment Principle: Reinforce kidney and liver yin to nourish the tendons and relieve pain.

Point Prescription & Manipulation:
Primary points:
    BL-23 Shenshu +
    BL-18 Ganshu +
    BL-57 Chengshan +
    KI-3 Taixi +

Explanation:
• BL-23 Shenshu and BL-18 Ganshu, the Back-Shu Points of the kidney and liver, tonify the kidney and liver and nourish yin;
• BL-57 Chengshan, located on the diseased region, activates qi and blood circulation, relieves spasms and alleviates pain;
• KI-3 Taixi nourishes kidney yin.

Secondary points according to conditions:
1〕 Restlessness and insomnia ─ PC-6 Neiguan [+] and SP-6 Sanyinjiao [+].

II. EXPERIENTIAL TREATMENT

1. Puncturing SI-3 Houxi

Indication: Attack of systremma.

Point Prescription:
    SI-3 Houxi

Manipulation: Insert needles bilaterally into SI-3 Houxi and rotate the needles with a large amplitude and strong stimulation until the spasmodic pain is relieved. Usually, after

manipulating the needles 2-10 minutes, the pain will be relieved.

2. Puncturing BL-57 Chengshan etc.

Indication: Acute attack of systremma, chronic systremma, prevention of attack of systremma.

Point Prescription:
    BL-57 Chengshan
    GB-34 Yanglingquan
    ST-36 Zusanli
    SP-6 Sanyinjiao

Manipulation: For an acute attack, insert needles into BL-57 Chengshan and GB-34 Yanglingquan of the diseased side to induce arrival of qi. Then, rotate, thrust and lift the needle with quick frequency and great amplitude to apply strong stimulation. Usually, the pain will be relieved within 10 minutes. For patients with a long history of frequent attacks of systremma, especially in the night, insert the needle into the same points mentioned above but rotate, thrust and lift the needle with slow frequency, small amplitude and mild or medium degree of stimulation. Additionally, insert needles into ST-36 Zusanli and SP-6 Sanyinjiao bilaterally. Retain the needles for 1-2 hours. If moxibustion on BL-57 Chengshan is applied in combination, the result will be better. The treatment is given once a day, with 5 treatments as one course. For patients who have attacks of systremma during physical exercise or labor, attack of systremma can be prevented by applying moxibustion on BL-57 Chengshan before physical exercise or labor.

3. Warm Needling on BL-57 Chengshan

Indication: Cases with attack or repeated attack of systremma.

Point Prescription:
    BL-57 Chengshan

Manipulation: Use a 2.5-cun long needle to insert into BL-57 Chengshan perpendicularly 1.5-2 cun deep; thrust and lift the needle to make the needling sensation radiate to the bottom of the

CHAPTER ONE: INTERNAL DISEASES 361

foot 3-4 times. Then, place a 1-cun long segment of moxa stick along the needle handle and ignite the moxa. After the moxa burns out, retain the needle for 15 minutes. The treatment is given once a day. Each time, BL-57 Chengshan is needled on one side only. Usually, within 5-7 treatments, the patient will no longer have attack of systremma.

4. Imbedding Needle in BL-57 Chengshan

Indication: Obstinate systremma.

Point Prescription:
BL-57 Chengshan of the diseased side

Manipulation: Insert a subcutaneous needle perpendicularly into the point, fix the needle with plaster, and remove the needle 5-7 days later. During the embedding period, if the patient feels pain in the local region, the needle should be taken out. This treatment is given only once.

5. Hydro-Puncture on BL-57 Chengshan

Indication: Repeated attack of systremma with atrophy of gastrocnemius muscle.

Point Prescription:
BL-57 Chengshan of the diseased side

Manipulation: Insert an injection needle into the point quickly, thrust and lift the syringe a little to induce needling sensation, withdraw the pistol to make sure no blood, and push the pistol down slowly to inject 10-20 ml of glucose into the point. After the treatment some patients may have mild fever and sweating which may last 1-7 days and disappear without need of treatment. The treatment is given once every other day with 10 treatments as a course.

Comment:
Zhenjiu is effective in the treatment and prevention of systremma. If massage is applied in combination, the treatment result will be better.

Notes:

27. Sequel of Cerebrovascular Accident

Cerebrovascular accident, including cerebral hemorrhage, cerebral thrombosis, cerebral embolism, and subarachnoid hemorrhage, is an acute encephalic disease caused by abnormal changes of the blood vessels of the brain or by a disorder of the systematic blood circulation. It is clinically characterized by sudden occurrence of disturbance of consciousness and paralysis of the limbs. According to TCM, Cerebrovascular accident belongs to the category of Zhong Feng (wind stroke), and is caused by bad emotional stimulation such as melancholy, anxiety and anger, bad diet customs such as over indulgence in drinking, eating sweet and greasy food, or bad life-style habits such as intemperance in sexual life, and excessive mental labor, causing deficiency of yin and hyperactivity of liver yang, disorder of qi and blood circulation, and internal generation of phlegm, blood stasis and fire, which go upwards to interfere with the mind and go horizontally to attack the meridians and collaterals. Generally, there are two types of wind stroke, attack on the zang-fu organs and attack on the meridians and collaterals. The first aid to wind stroke is seen in "105. Emergency Conditions" (Page 563).

The cerebrovascular accident sequel refers to hemiplegia, slurred speech, deviation of the mouth and eye, and other symptoms caused by acute cerebrovascular accident. According to TCM, these sequels are due to obstruction of the meridians and collaterals by blood stasis and phlegm and deficiency of qi and blood due to wind-stroke.

I. STANDARD TREATMENT

Generally, there are three types of Sequel of cerebrovascular accident — hemiplegia due to obstruction of the meridians by blood stasis, dysphasia due to obstruction of the collaterals by wind, phlegm and blood stasis and contortions of the facial muscles due to obstruction of the collaterals by wind, phlegm and blood stasis.

Points of the Yangming Meridians are frequently selected in the treatment.

1. Hemiplegia due to Blood Stasis

Manifestations: Motor impairment and numbness or total loss of sensation on one side of the body.

Tongue: Purplish body with ecchymotic spots.

Pulse: Wiry or unsmooth.

Treatment Principle: Promote circulation of qi and blood, remove blood stasis in the meridians.

Point Prescription & Manipulation:
a. For paralysis of the upper limbs:
> BL-11 Dazhu
> LI-15 Jianyu
> SJ-14 Jianliao
> LI-11 Quchi
> LI-10 Shousanli
> SJ-5 Waiguan
> LI-4 Hegu
> LI-3 Sanjian
> LU-5 Chize
> PC-3 Quze
> PC-6 Neiguan
> PC-7 Daling

b. For paralysis of the lower limbs:
> GB-30 Huantiao
> GB-31 Fengshi
> ST-31 Biguan
> ST-18 Futu
> GB-34 Yanglingquan
> ST-36 Zusanli
> GB-39 Xuanzhong
> BL-60 Kunlun
> GB-40 Qiuxu
> SP-6 Sanyinjiao
> BL-40 Weizhong
> LR-8 Ququan
> SP-9 Yinlingquan
> SP-5 Shangqiu

Explanation:
For patients with body resistance deficiency, perform reinforcing manipulation and puncture gently; for patients with stiff and hard limbs, apply reducing manipulation and puncture with strong stimulation; for patients with prolonged disease course, apply moxibustion in cooperation.

- BL-11 Dazhu, the Influential Point of bone, strengthens the bone;
- LI-15 Jianyu, LI-11 Quchi, LI-10 Shousanli, LI-4 Hegu and LI-3 Sanjian strengthen and remove obstruction from the Hand-Yangming Meridian;
- SJ-14 Jianliao and SJ-5 Waiguan strengthen and remove obstruction from the Hand-Shaoyang Meridian;
- LU-5 Chize strengthens and removes obstruction from the Hand-Taiyin Meridian;
- PC-3 Quze, PC-6 Neiguan and PC-7 Daling strengthen and remove obstruction from the Hand-Jueyin Meridian, and extinguish internal wind;
- ST-31 Biguan, ST-18 Futu, ST-36 Zusanli, and ST-40 Fenglong strengthen and remove obstruction from the Foot-Yangming Meridian, and generate qi and blood to nourish meridians, muscles and organs;
- GB-30 Huantiao, GB-31 Fengshi, GB-34 Yanglingquan, GB-39 Xuanzhong, and GB-40 Qiuxu strengthen and remove obstruction from the Foot-Shaoyang Meridian;
- BL-60 Kunlun and BL-40 Weizhong strengthen and remove obstruction from the Foot-Taiyang Meridian, and remove blood stasis;
- SP-6 Sanyinjiao, SP-9 Yinlingquan and SP-5 Shangqiu strengthen and remove obstruction from the Foot-Taiyin Meridian, and generate qi and blood to nourish meridians, muscles and organs;
- LR-8 Ququan remove obstruction from the Foot-Jueyin Meridian, and extinguish internal wind.

2. Dysphasia due to Wind, Phlegm and Blood Stasis

Manifestations: Dysphasia or aphasia, hypokinesia of the tongue, numbness of the limbs.

Tongue: Sticky coating.

Pulse: Wiry.

Treatment Principle: Eliminate wind and phlegm, remove blood stasis in the meridians.

Point Prescription & Manipulation:

Primary points:

RN-23 Lianquan -
LI-4 Hegu -
GB-20 Fengchi -
ST-40 Fenglong - ^
DU-15 Yamen -
HT-5 Tongli -
SP-6 Sanyinjiao - ^
KI-3 Taixi +

Explanation:

- RN-23 Lianquan and DU-15 Yamen, the experiential points for treatment of dysphasia;
- LI-4 Hegu and GB-20 Fengchi dispel wind, promote blood circulation and awake the mind;
- ST-40 Fenglong and SP-6 Sanyinjiao reinforce the middle-jiao and transform phlegm;
- HT-5 Tongli removes blood stasis from the Heart Meridian and improves the tongue's function;
- KI-3 Taixi nourishes kidney yin and communicates with the heart.

Secondary points according to conditions:

1️⃣ Stiffness of the tongue ─ EX-HN-12 Jinjin [-] and EX-HN-13 Yuye [-] are pricked to bleed.

3. Contortions of the Facial Muscles due to Wind, Phlegm and Blood Stasis

Manifestations: Deviation of the mouth and eye, numbness and weakness of the facial muscles on the affected side.

Tongue: Sticky coating.

Pulse: Wiry.

Treatment Principle: Eliminate wind, transform phlegm, activate blood circulation, and remove obstruction in the meridians.

Point Prescription and Manipulation:
See "Stirring-Up of Internal Wind" in "23. Facial Paralysis" (Page 352).

II. EXPERIENTIAL TREATMENT

1. Scalp Puncture

Indication: Paralysis of the limb due to cerebrovascular accident.

Scalp Line Prescription:
The line from DU-20 Baihui to GB-7 Qubin.

Manipulation: Insert a needle into DU-20 Baihui, push the needle under the scalp towards GB-7 Qubin about 1.5-2 cun; insert another needle into the point where the tip of the former needle reaches, and push the needle under the scalp towards GB-7 Qubin about 1.5-2 cun too. Insert another needle into the point where the tip of the second needle reaches, and push the needle under the scalp to GB-7 Qubin. Rotate these needles quickly at a frequency of 200 turns/minute for 5 minutes. Repeat the rotating manipulation after an interval of 5 minutes, 3 times in total, each time for 5 minutes. The treatment is given once daily with 15 treatments as a course. Usually, within the first five treatments, good results of the treatment will be noticeable.

2. Puncturing GB-20 Fengchi

Indication: Paralysis of the limb due to cerebral embolism.

Point Prescription:
GB-20 Fengchi

Manipulation: Puncture with a needle tip towards the opposite eyeball 0.5-1 cun deep, manipulate the needle to induce a soreness and distending sensation, retain the needles for 20 minutes, and manipulate them every 5 minutes during the retention. The treatment is given once daily with 10 treatments as a course.

3. Puncturing EX-HN-20 Yemen

Indication: Aphasia due to Cerebrovascular accident.

Point Prescription
EX-HN-20 Yemen, located on the surface of the tongue, 1 cm from the tongue tip.

Manipulation: Gently pull the tongue tip out of the mouth with one hand, insert the needle into the point, and push the needle along the direction of the running course of the vein and along the muscular layer of the tongue until the needle is near the root of the tongue. Remove the needle when the patient feels a hot sensation in the tongue or cannot stand it any longer. The treatment is given once every other day with 6 treatments as a course. Usually effective results will be present after 2-3 treatments.

Comment:
In treatment of sequel of cerebrovascular accident, Zhenjiu can be one of the most important treatments as it usually provides effective results. If Zhenjiu and massage are applied together, the result will be much better. Usually, Zhenjiu and massage can help patients recover from paralysis or aphasia due to cerebrovascular accident if the treatment is given within 6 months of the accident. Generally, the earlier the treatment is given, the less treatment times are needed and the better the treatment result will be. Additionally, Zhenjiu and massage may be effective to treat patients who have had paralysis or aphasia due to cerebrovascular accident for more than 5 years. According to our own experience, though a patient has had paralysis or aphasia for more then 5 years, Zhenjiu and massage are still effective to help the patient recover from the paralysis or aphasia.

Notes:

28. Traumatic Paraplegia

Traumatic paraplegia refers to paralysis of the limbs due to impairment of spinal cord or the cauda equina by fracture or dislocation of the vertebra from traumatic injury. According to TCM, it belongs to Shang Jin (impairment of tendon) or Wai Shang Wei Zheng (traumatic atrophy), and is caused by impairment of the tendons and vessels, leading to obstruction of the circulation of qi and blood which then fail to nourish the body. Generally, acupuncture is given to patients with traumatic paraplegia only after the patients have received the proper surgical operation or manipulation to rejoin the fractured bone or to reposition the displaced joint.

I. STANDARD TREATMENT

Traumatic paraplegia is generally divided into 2 types — obstruction of the meridians and vessels due to stagnation of qi and blood, and lack of nourishment of the tendons and bones due to deficiency of the liver and kidney. Points of the Du and Bladder Meridians are frequently selected in its treatment.

1. Obstruction of Meridians and Vessels due to Stagnation of Qi and Blood

Manifestations: Flaccid paralysis and atrophy of the lower limbs or the upper and lower limbs, retention of urine or unconscious urination, constipation or fecal incontinence.

Tongue: Yellow, sticky and thick coating.

Pulse: Wiry, thready and uneven.

Treatment Principle: Dredge the Du Meridian, regulate qi and blood.

Point Prescription & Manipulation:
Primary points:
The points of the interspaces of the vertebrae from the vertebra above the damaged vertebra down to the vertebra below the damaged vertebra - ^

EX-B-2 Jiaji of the same level - ^

Explanation:
Acupuncture and moxibustion are applied in cooperation on 10-20 points each treatment. Electric acupuncture should be applied additionally. When puncturing, reducing manipulation is performed on the points for constipation or retention of urine, and reinforcing manipulation is performed on the other points. A strong stimulation should be induced and the needles repeatedly manipulated. Retain the needles in the points for 20-40 minutes and during the retention apply moxibustion on the points punctured with reinforcing manipulation.

- The points of the interspaces of the vertebrae from the vertebra above the diseased vertebra down to the vertebra below the diseased vertebra strengthen the Du Meridian, promote circulation of qi of the Du Meridian and remove blood stasis from the meridian;
- EX-B-2 Jiaji of the same level promotes circulation of qi of the Du Meridian and removes blood stasis from the meridian.

Secondary points according to conditions:
1️⃣ For paralysis of the upper limbs: DU-14 Dazhui [- ^], LI-15 Jianyu [- ^], LI-11 Quchi [- ^], LI-1-0 Shousanli [- ^], SJ-5 Waiguan [- ^], LI-4 Hegu [-], and SI-3 Houxi [-];

2️⃣ For paralysis of the lower limbs: ST-31 Biguan [- ^], ST-32 Futu [- ^], ST-36 Zusanli [- ^], ST-41 Jiexi [-], GB-30 Huantiao [- ^], GB-31 Fengshi [- ^], GB-34 Yanglingquan [-], BL-37 Yinmen [-], BL-40 Weizhong [-], BL-57 Chengshan [- ^], BL-60 Kunlun [-], SP-10 Xuehai [- ^], LR-8 Ququan [-], SP-6 Sanyinjiao [- ^], and KI-3 Taixi [+];

3️⃣ For retention of urine or incontinence of urine: BL-23 Shenshu [+ ^], BL-32 Ciliao [+ ^], BL-28 Pangguanshu [+ ^], RN-3 Zhongji [- ^], and SP-9 Yinlingquan [+ ^];

4️⃣ For constipation: BL-25 Dachangshu [-], ST-25 Tianshu [-] and SJ-6 Zhigou [-];

5️⃣ For fecal incontinence: BL-25 Dachangshu [+ ^], RN-4 Guanyuan [+ ^], RN-6 Qihai [+ ^], and DU-1 Changqiang [+ ^].

2. Lack of Nourishment of the Tendons and Vessels due to Deficiency of Liver and Kidney

Manifestations: Paralysis and muscular stiffness, convulsion and atrophy of the limbs, dizziness, tinnitus, edema of the lower limbs, incontinence of urine and feces.

Tongue: Red body with little coating.

Pulse: Wiry and thready.

Treatment Principle: Tonify Liver and Kidney, nourish the tendons and bones.

Point Prescription & Manipulation:
Primary points:
The points of the interspaces of the vertebrae from the vertebra above the damaged vertebra down to the vertebra below the damaged vertebra + ^
EX-B-2 Jiaji of the same level + ^
BL-18 Ganshu + ^
BL-23 Shenshu + ^

Explanation:
Acupuncture and moxibustion are applied in cooperation on 10-15 points each treatment. Electric acupuncture should be applied additionally. On the points for incontinence of urine and feces reinforcing manipulation is performed, and on the points for persistent erection of the penis reducing manipulation performed. The other manipulations are the same as above.

- The points of the interspaces of the vertebrae from the vertebra above the diseased vertebra down to the vertebra below the diseased vertebra strengthen the Du Meridian, promote circulation of qi of the Du Meridian and remove blood stasis from the meridian;
- EX-B-2 Jiaji of the same level promotes circulation of qi of the Du Meridian and removes blood stasis from the meridian;

- BL-18 Ganshu and BL-23 Shenshu tonify the liver and kidney and nourish the tendons and bones.

Secondary points according to conditions:

1☐ For incontinence of urine: BL-28 Pangguanshu [+ ^], RN-4 Guanyuan [+ ^] and RN-3 Zhongji [- ^];

2☐ For fecal incontinence: BL-25 Dachangshu [+ ^], ST-25 Tianshu [+ ^], RN-6 Qihai [+ ^], and DU-1 Changqiang [+ ^];

3☐ For persistent erection of the penis: LR-2 Xingjian [-] and SI-5 Yanggu [-].

II. EXPERIENTIAL TREATMENT

1. Puncturing RN-5 Shimen

Indication: Retention of urine due to paraplegia.

Point Prescription:
RN-5 Shimen

Manipulation: Insert a needle obliquely downwards 2 cun deep, lift, thrust and rotate the needle with reducing manipulation, and press the patient's lower abdomen with two hands from the top downwards with gradually increasing force. Ask the patient to urine as forcefully as possible during the manipulation. Repeat the course until the bladder is completely empty. The treatment is given once or twice daily, and generally 10-30 treatments are needed.

2. Scalp Acupuncture

Indication: Traumatic Paraplegia.

Point Prescription:
The posterior 1/3 of the Line of Forehead-Vertex
The upper 1/3 of the Anterior Oblique Line of Vertex-Temporal
The upper 1/3 of the Posterior Oblique Line of Vertex-Temporal

Manipulation: On the posterior 1/3 of the Line of Forehead-Vertex, insert the needle from the anterior backwards; and on the Anterior and Posterior Lines of Vertex-Temporal, insert a 3-cun long needle. Manipulate the needles by lifting and thrusting them at small amplitude. Ask the patient to breathe deeply once, hold the breath, imagine the qi flowing to the diseased region, and do some active or non-active movement of the diseased limbs, such as extending and bending the legs. If the patient has incontinence of urine, ask the patient to press the lower abdomen with his/her hands and attempt urination. Repeat this course several times during puncturing on the posterior 1/3 of the Line of Forehead-Vertex. Retain the needles for 60 minutes and manipulate them 5 minutes every 20 minutes. The treatment is given once every other day with 10 treatments as a course.

Comment:

In treatment of traumatic paraplegia, Zhenjiu can be one of the most important treatments, and usually, it brings effective results. If Zhenjiu and massage are applied together, the result will be much better. Zhenjiu and massage can help some patients recover from paraplegia if the treatment is given soon after the accident. Generally, the earlier the treatment is given, the less treatment times are needed, and the better the treatment result will be. However, Zhenjiu and massage may also be effective to treat patients who have had traumatic paraplegia for more than 5 years. In our own experience, though a patient has had paraplegia for more then 5 years, Zhenjiu and massage are still effective to help the patient recover from the paraplegia.

Notes:

29. Epilepsy

Epilepsy refers to a disease caused by frequently recurring of abnormal neurogenic discharge leading to sudden and temporary dysfunction of the cerebrum. Its cause is mainly related to hereditary over susceptibility, infections like meningitis, and injuries to the brain during birth or from blows to the head. It is clinically marked by sudden seizure, falling down in a fit, loss of consciousness and spasm of the entire body which last from several seconds to fifteen minutes, or temporary disturbance of consciousness and mental confusion, which last from several minutes to half an hour. According to TCM, epilepsy belongs to the categories of Dian Ji (epilepsy) and Jiang Zheng (epilepsy), and is caused by deficiency of the liver and kidney leading to internal stirring of the liver-wind, or accumulation and obstruction of phlegm in the interior leading to failure of clean qi in ascending.

I. STANDARD TREATMENT

Epilepsy is generally divided into four types — liver-wind with accumulation of phlegm, blockage of orifice by phlegm-fire, Liver and kidney yin deficiency, and spleen and kidney deficiency. Points of the Du, Liver, Stomach and Bladder Meridians are frequently selected in its treatment. The first aid methods for severe attack of epilepsy are seen in "105. Emergency Conditions". (Page 563 for details)

1. Liver-Wind with Accumulation of Phlegm

Manifestations: Dizziness, headache, and distressed sensation in the chest before the seizure, falling down suddenly, loss of consciousness, convulsion, spitting foam, and clenched teeth during the seizure.

Tongue: White and sticky coating.

Pulse: Wiry and smooth.

Treatment Principle: Pacify the liver, calm wind, resolve phlegm and calm spirit.

Point Prescription & Manipulation:
Primary points:
   LR-3 Taichong   -
   ST-40 Fenglong   -
   DU-14 Dazhui   -
   PC-6 Neiguan   -
   DU-20 Baihui   /
   BL-18 Ganshu   -
   BL-15 Xinshu   -
   EX-HN-1 Sishencong -
   GB-13 Benshen -
   DU-24 Shenting -

Explanation:
During the onset, puncture DU-25 Shuigou, KI-1 Yongquan and PC-5 Jianshi with reducing manipulation by rotating, thrusting and lifting the needle, manipulate the needle until the patient becomes conscious, and retain the needle for 10 minutes. During the intermittent period, puncture the points with reinforcing manipulation, retain the needles for 20-40 minutes, and manipulate them every 10 minutes. The treatment is given once daily with 10 treatments as a course. When the attack frequency decreases greatly, puncture only 1-3 times a week for 3-6 months.

- LR-3 Taichong, BL-18 Ganshu and PC-6 Neiguan pacify the liver and extinguish internal wind;
- ST-40 Fenglong, the key point of transforming phlegm;
- DU-14 Dazhui, one of the most effective points of treatment of epilepsy;
- BL-15 Xinshu and DU-20 Baihui open the orifice, clear the brain and calm the mind;
- EX-HN-1 Sishencong, GB-13 Benshen and DU-24 Shenting, "three head spirit points" named by us and used very frequently for psychoses and mental disorders.

Secondary points according to conditions:
1️⃣ Loss of consciousness and convulsion—
   DU-25 Shuigou [-], KI-1 Yongquan [- ^] and PC-5 Jianshi [-];
2️⃣ Onset in the daytime—BL-62 Shenmai [-];

3〕 Onset in the night — KI-6 Zhaohai [+].

2. Blockage of Orifice by Phlegm-Fire

Manifestations: Falling down suddenly, loss of consciousness, convulsion, spitting foam during the attack, irritability, restlessness, insomnia, dizziness and headache, thirst, bitter taste in the mouth.

Tongue: Red body with yellow and sticky coating.

Pulse: Wiry, smooth and rapid.

Treatment Principle: Clear heat in the liver, resolve phlegm and restore consciousness.

Point Prescription & Manipulation:
Primary points:
    LR-2 Xingjian   -
    PC-6 Neiguan   -
    ST-40 Fenglong   -
    DU-14 Dazhui   -
    LI-11 Quchi   -
    BL-18 Ganshu   -
    BL-15 Xinshu   -
    EX-HN-1 Sishencong -
    GB-13 Benshen -
    DU-24 Shenting -

Explanation:
Manipulation is the same as above.

- LR-2 Xingjian, BL-18 Ganshu and PC-6 Neiguan pacify the liver, clear heat and extinguish internal wind;
- ST-40 Fenglong, the key point of transforming phlegm;
- DU-14 Dazhui one of the most effective points of treatment of epilepsy;
- BL-15 Xinshu, clears the heart and calms the mind;
- LI-11 Quchi clears heat;
- EX-HN-1 Sishencong, GB-13 Benshen and DU-24 Shenting, "three head spirit points" named by us and used very frequently for psychoses and mental disorders.

Secondary points according to conditions:
1〕 Restlessness and insomnia —HT-7 Shenmen [/];
2〕 Headache and dizziness — GB-20 Fengchi [-];
3〕 At the onset — DU-25 Shuigou [-], KI-1 Yongquan [-] and LU-11 Shaoshang [-].

3. Deficiency of Liver and Kidney Yin

Manifestations: Protracted course, dizziness, insomnia, poor memory, soreness and weakness of the lower back and knees.

Tongue: Red body with little coating.

Pulse: Thready and rapid.

Treatment Principle: Nourish the liver and kidney, calm the mind.

Point Prescription & Manipulation:
Primary points:
    DU-14 Dazhui   -
    BL-18 Ganshu   +
    BL-23 Shenshu   +
    KI-3 Taixi   +
    LR-3 Taichong   -
    HT-7 Shenmen   -
    SP-6 Sanyinjiao   +
    EX-HN-1 Sishencong +
    GB-13 Benshen +
    DU-24 Shenting +

Explanation:
- LR-3 Taichong, BL-18 Ganshu and SP-6 Sanyinjiao tonify liver yin, pacify liver yang and extinguish internal wind;
- DU-14 Dazhui one of the most effective points of treatment of epilepsy;
- BL-23 Shenshu and KI-3 Taixi tonify kidney yin;
- HT-7 Shenmen calms the mind;
- EX-HN-1 Sishencong, GB-13 Benshen and DU-24 Shenting, "three head spirit points" named by us and used very frequently for psychoses and mental disorders.

Secondary points according to conditions:
1️⃣ Dizziness and blurred vision—GB-20
   Fengchi [/].

4. Deficiency of Spleen and Kidney Qi

Manifestations: Protracted course, lassitude, dizziness, poor appetite, palpitation, pale complexion, weakness and soreness of the lower back and knees, pale tongue with white and sticky coating, thready and weak pulse.

Treatment Principle: Invigorate spleen and kidney, reinforce qi and resolve phlegm.

Point Prescription & Manipulation:
Primary points:
   RN-12 Zhongwan   + ^
   ST-40 Fenglong   - ^
   ST-25 Tianshu + ^
   ST-36 Zusanli   + ^
   PC-6 Neiguan   -
   RN-6 Qihai   + ^
   DU-14 Dazhui   - ^
   EX-HN-1 Sishencong +
   GB-13 Benshen +
   DU-24 Shenting +

Explanation:
- RN-12 Zhongwan, RN-6 Qihai and ST-25 Tianshu, the Four Door Points, strengthen the spleen and stomach and transform phlegm and dampness;
- ST-36 Zusanli reinforces the spleen, tonifies qi and transforms phlegm;
- ST-40 Fenglong transforms phlegm;
- PC-6 Neiguan calms the mind and extinguishes internal wind;
- DU-14 Dazhui, one of the most effective points of treatment of epilepsy;
- EX-HN-1 Sishencong, GB-13 Benshen and DU-24 Shenting, "three head spirit points" named by us and used very frequently for psychoses and mental disorders.

Secondary points according to conditions:
1️⃣ Prolonged course — BL-23 Shenshu [+ ^]
   and BL-20 Pishu [+ ^];
2️⃣ Impotence — DU-4 Mingmen [+ ^].

II. EXPERIENTIAL TREATMENT

1. Puncturing DU-14 Dazhui

Indication: Epilepsy.

Point Prescription:
   DU-14 Dazhui

Manipulation: Puncture upwards obliquely at an angle of 30 degree 1.5 cun deep. Thrust and lift the needle to induce an electric shock sensation in the patient and remove the needle immediately. The treatment is given once every other day with 10 treatments as a course. After an interval of 7 days, begin the next course. Generally, 3-4 courses are needed.

2. Puncturing EX-B-9 Yaoqi

Indication: Epilepsy.

Point Prescription:
   EX-B-9 Yaoqi

Manipulation: Ask the patient to lie on the stomach with the buttocks raised, insert a 3-cun needle into the point, rotate and push the needle along the spinal column upwards 2-2.5 cun deep. Rotate the needle to induce arrival of qi, retain the needle for 20-40 minutes, and manipulate it every 10 minutes. The treatment is given once daily until the patient's condition improves. Then the treatment is given 2-3 times a week for 3-6 months.

3. Puncturing DU-25 Shuigou

Indication: Epilepsy.

Point Prescription:
   DU-25 Shuigou

Manipulation: Hold the upper lip with the thumb and index finger to make it prominent, and puncture upwards at an angle of 45 degrees 0.3-0.5 cun deep. Rotate the needle to induce soreness, distention and an electric shock sensation, which radiates to the head and face. For severe cases with strong constitution, use a thicker needle to puncture, apply strong stimulation, and retain the needle for 1-2 hours. For mild cases or weak patients, use thinner needle, apply medium stimulation, and retain the needle for 20 minutes. The treatment is given once every other day with 10 treatments as a course.

Comment:
Emergency treatment should be given immediately if the patient has a severe seizure with loss of consciousness. Zhenjiu can be used for treatment of epilepsy either in seizure period or remission period. But in this chapter, treatment for epilepsy at its remission period is discussed mainly. Emergency treatment for epilepsy at its severe seizure period should be referred to "105. Emergency Conditions" (Page 563). Epilepsy is an obstinate disease. Zhenjiu can provide positive results in its treatment or even is effective to cure it in some patients, but a long-term treatment course is always needed. Usually, epilepsy patients take some Western medicines to control or prevent its attack. Upon beginning Zhenjiu treatment they should not stop taking their medication without advice from the doctor who wrote the prescription. Otherwise, it is very possible to induce a severe attack of epilepsy. However, after some treatments with Zhenjiu, if the patient's condition, including electroencephalogram condition, has been improved, the dosage of the medicines may be reduced gradually.

Notes:

30. Migraine

Migraine refers to a functional disorder of the cranial nerves, which is mainly manifested by headache. Its cause is uncertain, but evidence suggests a generally transmitted functional disturbance of intra- and extracranial circulation. According to TCM, migraine belongs to the categories of Tou Feng (wind in the head) and Pian Tou Tong (pain of the half head), and is caused mainly by internal injury by abnormal seven emotional factors leading to overactivity of liver yang.

I. STANDARD TREATMENT

Migraine is generally divided into two types — hyperactivity of liver yang and kidney yin deficiency. Points of the Shaoyang and Jueyin Meridians are frequently selected in its treatment.

1. Hyperactivity of Liver Yang

Manifestations: Headache blurred vision, restlessness, irritability, insomnia, a flushed face and red eyes, a bitter taste in the mouth.

Tongue: Red body with thin yellow coating.

Pulse: Taut and strong.

Treatment Principle: Pacify the liver and suppress yang.

Point Prescription & Manipulation:
Primary points:
    DU-20 Baihui -
    GB-20 Fengchi -
    GB-5 Xuanlu -
    LR-3 Taichong -
    GB-8 Shuaigu -
    Ashi Points -

Explanation:
Ashi Points can be tapped with the seven-star needle to bleed in severe case.

- Ashi Points unobstruct the meridians and collaterals and remove blood stasis for relieving pain;
- DU-20 Baihui, at the vertex where the Liver Meridian runs through, pacifies liver and restrains yang from rising;
- GB-20 Fengchi and GB-5 Xuanlu clear heat from Shaoyang Meridian which is due to hyperactivity of liver yang;
- LR-3 Taichong pacifies liver and restrains yang from rising.

Secondary points according to conditions:
1️⃣ Severe insomnia—HT-7 Shenmen [-] and PC-6 Neiguan [-];
2️⃣ Distending sensation of the head — LI-11 Quchi [-] and ST-40 Fenglong [-].

2. Kidney Yin Deficiency

Manipulations: Headache with an empty sensation in the head, dizziness, tinnitus, soreness and weakness in the lumbar region and knees, nocturnal emission.

Tongue: Red body.

Pulse: Deep, thready and weak.

Treatment Principle: Replenish yin and nourish the kidney.

Point Prescription & Manipulation:
Primary points:
    Ashi Points -
    GB-20 Fengchi   -
    DU-20 Baihui   /
    BL-23 Shenshu   +
    KI-3 Taixi   +
    GB-39 Xuanzhong +

Explanation:
- Ashi Points unobstruct the meridians and collaterals and remove blood stasis for relieving pain;
- GB-20 Fengchi and DU-20 Baihui, at the diseased region, activate the collaterals and alleviate pain;

- GB-39 Xuanzhong, the Influential Point of marrow, reinforces the kidney and strengthens the brain;
- BL-23 Shenshu and KI-3 Taixi tonify the kidney and nourish yin.

Secondary points according to conditions:
1️⃣ Insomnia— PC-6 Neiguan [-] and HT-7 Shenmen [/].

II. EXPERIENTIAL TREATMENT

1. Puncturing A Group of Points

Indication: Any type of migraine.

Point Prescription:
    GB-8 Shuaigu
    EX-HN-5 Taiyang
    GB-43 Xiaxi
    Ashi Point (the most painful or tender point).
    They are selected alternately and 2-4 points selected each time.

Manipulation: Puncture the points shallowly; rotate, lift and thrust the needles with strong stimulation until the patient has soreness, numbness and distention sensation. Then retain the needles for 20-30 minutes and manipulate them every 5 minutes during the retention. The treatment is given once a day with 10 treatments as a course.

2. Puncturing Through SJ-23 Sizhukong to GB-8 Shuaigu

Indication: Various type of migraine.

Point Prescription:
Primary points:
    SJ-23 Sizhukong of the diseased side

Secondary points according to conditions:
1️⃣ LI-4 Hegu, LU-7 Lieque, and GB-41 Zulinqi of the diseased side

Manipulation: Puncture SJ-23 Sizhukong with the 2.5-cun needle. After the needle passes through the skin, push it further along the skin towards GB-8 Shuaigu direction while rotating it and massaging the local skin from SJ-23 Sizhukong to GB-8 Shuaigu until the needle tip arrives at the subcutaneous tissue of GB-8 Shuaigu. Then, puncture LI-4 Hegu, LU-7 Lieque and GB-41 Zulinqi with the 1.2-cun needle and rotate, thrust and lift the needles with large amplitude. Retain the needles for 20 minutes. The treatment is given once every day, and within 5-7 treatments the migraine attacks will disappear.

3. Puncturing EX-B-2 Jiaji

Indication: Various migraines.

Point Prescription:
   EX-B-2 Jiaji 5, 7, 9, and 14
   GB-20 Fengchi

Manipulation: Insert a needle into EX-B-2 Jiaji points 1 cun deep, obliquely toward the vertebral body at an angle of 70 degrees, and rotate the needle gently and with small amplitude to make the needling sensation transmit along the spinal column or the rib. On GB-20 Fengchi, after inserting the needle towards the opposite eye about 25 mm deep, rotate the needle with a large amplitude. Retain the needles for 20-30 minutes, and manipulate them once during the retention. The treatment is given once every other day, with 10 treatments as a therapeutic course.

4. Ear Acupuncture by Taping

Indication: Obstinate Migraine.

Ear Point Prescription:
Primary points:
   Shenmen, Subcortex, Heart, Liver, Occiput.

Secondary points according to conditions:
   Endocrine, Upper Ear Root, Apex.

Manipulation: Prepare several pieces of 0.7x0.7 mm-sized plasters with a vaccaria seed in the center. Use the ear-point-probing instrument to find the sensitive points on the main ear point region, tape the plaster on each point with the seed directly over the sensitive spot. Press gently on the point to induce distention, heat sensation

or mild pain to the patient. Retain the plasters on the points for 3-5 days, and tell the patient to press the points 3-5 times daily during the retention to induce the same sensation. Then, use a filiform needle to prick Endocrine and Upper Ear Root, and bleed at Ear Apex. The treatment is given once every 5-7 days, and 5 treatments are taken as a therapeutic course.

5. Ear Acupuncture by Bleeding

Indications: Obstinate Migraine.

Point Prescription:
   The middle of 3 veins obviously seen on the upper 1/3 of the ear back and near the ear root on the diseased side.

Manipulation: Ask the patient to sit down. Gently knead and press the local region of the ear to cause local congestion so the vein becomes obvious, and apply regular local sterilization. Then, hold the ear with the left hand and the needle with the right hand, insert the needle into the vein quickly to cause about 5 ml of blood. If there is not enough blood, press and knead the local region to increase the bleeding. In case there is too much bleeding, press the local region with sterilized cotton ball until bleeding stops. Then, cover the wound with a sterilized cotton ball and fix it with a piece of plaster to prevent infection.

Comment:
Acupuncture is effective in relieving migraines. Migraine, in some patients, can be cured with acupuncture treatment. Bleeding by tapping Ashi Points with the seven-star needle is very effective to relieve severe migraine. If massage is applied in cooperation, the treatment result is much better.

Notes:

31. Post-Concussional Syndrome

Concussion of the brain is caused by cephalic trauma resulting in temporary loss of consciousness. Post-concussional syndrome refers to headache, dizziness, tinnitus, poor memory, and insomnia, which exist three months after concussion and are not accompanied by any corresponding organ impairment. According to TCM, post-concussional syndrome belongs to categories of Tou Tong (headache) and Xuan Yun (dizziness), and is caused by injury of the head, leading to obstruction of the qi and blood and disharmony of yin and yang.

I. STANDARD TREATMENT

Post-concussional syndrome is usually divided into two types — obstruction of qi and blood, and deficiency of the kidney and liver, and the local points and points of the Du, Bladder and Liver Meridians are frequently selected in its treatment.

1. Obstruction of Qi and Blood

Manifestations: Headache, dizziness, insomnia, poor memory and history of head injury.

Tongue: Dark red body.

Pulse: Wiry or uneven.

Treatment Principle: Tonify qi, activate blood and dredge the collaterals.

Point Prescription & Manipulation:
Primary points:
   Ashi Point /
   DU-20 Baihui   +
   EX-HN-1 Sishencong   +
   LR-3 Taichong   -
   BL-40 Weizhong   -
   DU-14 Dazhui   +
   GB-20 Fengchi   -
   PC-6 Neiguan   /
   LI-4 Hegu   /

Explanation:
These points are usually divided into two groups, and they are used alternatively.

- Ashi Point activates the collaterals, removes blood stasis and alleviates pain;
- DU-20 Baihui, DU-14 Dazhui and EX-HN-1 Sishencong reinforce the marrow, tonify the brain, dredge the collaterals, and clear the mind;
- LR-3 Taichong, PC-6 Neiguan and LI-4 Hegu promote qi circulation;
- BL-40 Weizhong removes blood stasis and alleviates pain.
- GB-20 Fengchi dredges the meridians, activates collaterals and alleviates pain;

Secondary points according to conditions:
1） Stabbing pain—BL-17 Geshu [-] and BL-18 Ganshu [-].

2. Deficiency of Liver and Kidney

Manifestation: Dull headache, dizziness, insomnia, poor memory, soreness and weakness of the lumber and knees, and history of head injury.

Tongue: Thin coating.

Pulse: Weak and deep.

Treatment Principle: Tonify kidney and liver, promote circulation of qi and blood.

Point Prescription & Manipulation:
Primary points:
   Ashi Point -
   DU-20 Baihui   /
   EX-HN-1 Sishencong   /
   LR-3 Taichong   -
   BL-40 Weizhong   -
   DU-14 Dazhui   -
   GB-20 Fengchi   -
   KI-3 Taixi   +
   BL-18 Ganshu   +
   BL-23 Shenshu   +

Explanation:
These points are usually divided into two groups, and they are used alternatively.

- Ashi Point activates the collaterals, removes blood stasis and alleviates pain;
- DU-20 Baihui and EX-HN-1 Sishencong tonify qi, dredge the collaterals, and clear the mind;
- LR-3 Taichong and DU-14 Dazhui promote qi circulation;
- BL-40 Weizhong removes blood stasis and alleviates pain;
- GB-20 Fengchi dredges the meridians, activates collaterals and alleviates pain;
- KI-3 Taixi, BL-18 Ganshu and BL-23 Shenshu tonify the kidney and liver and nourish yin.

Secondary points according to conditions:
1☐ Poor memory and insomnia—DU-24 Shenting [+] and GB-13 Benshen [+];
2☐ Lassitude and poor appetite—ST-36 Zusanli [+] and RN-4 Guanyuan [+].

II. EXPERIENTIAL TREATMENT

1. Pricking Weizhong BL-40 to Make Bleeding

Indication: Post-concussion with headache as its main symptom.

Point Prescription:
    BL-40 Weizhong

Manipulation: Insert the three-edged needle into the enlarged vein on the point region to cause bleeding of 3-4 drops. The treatment is given once every 4 days, and generally 3-4 treatments are needed.

2. Ear Acupuncture

Indication: Post-concussion at the early stage.

Ear Point Prescription:
    Kidney, Liver, Subcortex, Shenmen.

Manipulation: See page 255.

3. Scalp Puncture

Indication: Post-concussion.

Scalp Line Prescription:
Primary lines:
    Middle Line of Forehead
    Posterior 1/3 of Line of Forehead-Vertex

Secondary line:
    Lower 1/3 of Posterior Oblique Line of Vertex-Temporal

Manipulation: Puncture Middle Line of Forehead from the top downwards, and the posterior 1/3 of Line of Forehead-Vertex from the anterior backwards, and rotate the needles to induce arrival of qi. Ask the patient to relax himself/herself, be quiet, concentrate on Dantian (a region 4-finger breadth below the umbilicus), and take deep breaths with the abdomen during the manipulation of the needle. When puncturing and manipulating the needle in Posterior-Oblique Line of Vertex-Temporal, ask the patient to breathe in and hold breath, squeeze the nose, and send air to the ears. Repeat this course many times during the manipulation. Retain the needles for 60 minutes and manipulate them every 15 minutes. The treatment is given once daily and 5-7 treatments as a course.

Comment:
Zhenjiu is effective to relieve symptoms of post-concussional syndrome. In some cases it has a curative result. If massage is applied in cooperation the treatment result will be much better.

Notes:

32. Hysteria

Hysteria refers to a functional disorder caused by mental injury, occurring primarily in young people and more often in females than in males. Its manifestations are various, including: psychonosema, dyskinesia, sensory disturbance, vegetative nervous function disturbance and internal organ function disturbance, such as irrational laughing or crying, hysterical syncope, or mutism, hysterical paralysis, aphonia, spasm, blindness, deafness, globus hysterics, nervous vomiting, anorexia, hiccups, and frequent urination. According to TCM, hysteria belongs to the categories of Zang Zao (visceral irritation), Yu Zheng (melancholia), Bai He Bing (lily disease), and Jue Zheng (syncope syndrome), and is caused by mental injury which results in accumulation of phlegm in the interior or stagnation of the liver qi, leading to disorder of the mind.

I. STANDARD TREATMENT

Hysteria is generally divided into three types — stagnation of liver qi with wind-phlegm, depressed liver qi, and stagnation of liver qi and blood deficiency. Points of the Liver Meridian are frequently selected in its treatment.

1. Stagnation of Liver Qi and Wind-Phlegm

Manifestations: Falling down suddenly, loss of consciousness, possibly accompanied by spitting foam, convulsion, clenching fists, shaking the head and blinking, facial muscular trembling, or sudden paralysis or paraplegia.

Tongue: Sticky coating.

Pulse: Smooth and wiry.

Treatment Principle: Soothe the liver, tranquilize wind, remove phlegm and open the closed orifice.

Point Prescription & Manipulation:
Primary points:

LR-3 Taichong -
PC-6 Neiguan -
DU-20 Baihui - ^
DU-25 Shuigou -
LI-4 Hegu -
ST-40 Fenglong - ^

Explanation:
First, puncture DU-25 Shuigou and PC-6 Neiguan to restore consciousness with frequent rotating manipulation. Then, puncture the other points with thrusting, lifting and rotating manipulation to induce arrival of qi, retain the needles for 20-40 minutes, and manipulate once during the retention.

- LR-3 Taichong and LI-4 Hegu open the "Four Gates", activate the collaterals, promote blood circulation, extinguish wind and calm the mind;
- PC-6 Neiguan clams the mind and extinguishes wind;
- DU-20 Baihui and DU-25 Shuigou open the closed orifice and transform the turbid;
- ST-40 Fenglong transforms phlegm.

Secondary points according to conditions:
1□ Headache, irritability and insomnia —GB-20 Fengchi [-] and EX-HN-3 Yintang [-];
2□ If the patient has paralysis of lower limb— KI-1 Yongquan [-].

2. Depressed Liver Qi

Manifestations: Emotional depression, acid regurgitation, sighing, distressed sensation in the chest and hypochondria, or sensation of a foreign body in the throat which can't be swallowed down or spit out, or sudden aphasia, blindness, or deafness.

Tongue: Purplish body.

Pulse: Wiry.

Treatment Principle: Soothe the liver and relieve depression.

Point Prescription & Manipulation:

Primary points:
   RN-22 Tiantu   -
   RN-17 Danzhong   -
   LR-3 Taichong   -
   PC-6 Neiguan   -
   LI-4 Hegu   -

Explanation:
- RN-22 Tiantu and RN-17 Danzhong disperse qi stagnation in the diseased region and relieve depression;
- LR-3 Taichong and LI-4 Hegu open the "Four Gates", soothe the liver, relieve depression, extinguish wind and calm the mind;
- PC-6 Neiguan clams the mind and extinguishes wind.

Secondary points according to conditions:
1ᵒ Severe depression —GB-34 Yanglingquan [-] and LR-14 Qimen [-];
2ᵒ If the patient has dysphonia—DU-20 Baihui [-].

3. Stagnation of Liver Qi and Deficiency of Blood

Manifestations: Emotional depression, doubting mania, anxiety, blurred vision, dizziness, or onset of singing to replace speaking.

Tongue: Pale body with little coating.

Pulse: Thready and rapid.

Treatment Principle: Soothe the liver, nourish blood, and calm the mind.

Point Prescription & Manipulation:
Primary points:
   · DU-25 Shuigou   -
   SP-6 Sanyinjiao   +
   BL-18 Ganshu   +
   PC-6 Neiguan   -
   HT-7 Shenmen   +
   LI-3 Taichong   -

Explanation:

- DU-25 Shuigou tranquilizes the heart and calms the mind;
- SP-6 Sanyinjiao and BL-18 Ganshu nourish the liver and tonify blood;
- PC-6 Neiguan and LI-3 Taichong soothe the liver and relieve depressed qi;
- HT-7 Shenmen nourishes the heart and calms the mind.

Secondary points according to conditions:
1ᵒ Poor appetite and fatigue—ST-36 Zusanli [+], RN-12 Zhongwan [/] and RN-6 Qihai [+];
2ᵒ Paralysis — KI-1 Yongquan [-].

II. EXPERIENTIAL TREATMENT

1. Puncturing KI-1 Yongquan

Indication: Mental disorders or aphasia during the onset of hysteria, or hysterical mutism.

Point Prescription:
   KI-1 Yongquan

Manipulation:
a. For psychosis during hysterical attack
Puncture KI-1 Yongquan of one side. Thrust, lift and rotate the needle for 3 minutes, while speaking to the patient to give some verbal suggestions. Generally the patient's condition will be improved greatly. If not, puncture the opposite point additionally with the same method and manipulate the needles bilaterally alternatively until normal psychological condition of the patient is restored. Usually, one treatment is effective to restore the normal psychological condition.

b. For hysterical aphasia
Puncture bilateral KI-1 Yongquan. Perform thrusting, lifting and rotating manipulation with strong stimulation, connect the electric acupuncture instrument to give electric stimulation until the patient can speak.

c. For hysterical mutism
Puncture KI-1 Yongquan with a thick needle 0.6 cun deep. Rotate the needle with big amplitude to give strong stimulation for 1 minute, within which

most patients will be able to pronounce single sound, and continue manipulation until the patient can speak fluently, usually for 5-20 minutes. In case the disorder is not cured in one treatment, repeat the treatment the next day or the day after next.

2. Puncturing PC-6 Neiguan

Indication: Mental disorders during the onset of hysteria, or hysterical aphasia.

Point Prescription:
PC-6 Neiguan

Manipulation: Puncture the point with reducing manipulation by thrusting, lifting and rotating the needles for 2-5 minutes, and retain the needles for 20-30 minutes. Generally only one treatment is needed.

3. Puncturing HT-5 Tongli

Indication: Hysterical aphasia.

Point Prescription:
HT-5 Tongli

Manipulation: Insert a needle into the point 0.8 cun deep and perform reinforcing manipulation by lifting and thrusting the needle to induce arrival of qi. Then, gently rotate the needle with thumb moving forwards and the index finger moving backwards about one turn, press the needle handle downwards to the direction of the fingers to make the needle tip towards the upper arm and induce the needling sensation radiating to the elbow or upper limb, and keep this condition for 2 minutes. Finally, retain the needle for 15-20 minutes. Generally, only one treatment is needed to cure this problem.

4. Puncturing GB-30 Huantiao

Indication: Hysterical paralysis.

Point Prescription:
GB-30 Huantiao

Manipulation: Puncture 3 cun deep with the needle tip towards the genitalia, perform reducing manipulation by thrusting and lifting the needle to induce numbness or electric shock sensation radiating to the lower limbs, manipulate the needles 2-3 minutes, and remove the needle without retention. Generally, only one treatment is needed to cure this problem.

5. Puncturing RN-12 Zhongwan

Indication: Hysterical spasm.

Point Prescription:
RN-12 Zhongwan

Manipulation: Puncture the point 1.5 cun deep, perform reducing manipulation with strong stimulation, and manipulate the needle until the spasm stops. Generally, only one treatment is needed to stop spasm.

Comment:
Zhenjiu is effective to treat or even cure hysteria. As hysteria is very closely related to psychogenic factors, proper mental suggestion is important in the treatment of hysteria with Zhenjiu.

Notes:

33. Insomnia

Insomnia refers to the inability to have a normal sleep. It may be due to worries, excitement, nervous tension, and pain or noise sensitivity. It is clinically marked by difficulty in falling asleep, shallow sleep, difficulty to resume sleep once waking up in mild cases, and by inability to fall asleep for the whole night in severe cases. According to TCM, insomnia, called Shi Mian in Chinese, is caused by disorders of the heart, spleen, liver, kidney, and yin deficiency, leading to disharmony between hyperactive yang and insufficient yin.

I. STANDARD TREATMENT

Insomnia is generally divided into six types — hyperactivity of liver fire, internal disturbance of phlegm-heat, hyperactivity of fire due to yin deficiency, deficiency of heart and spleen, disharmony of the heart and kidney, and qi deficiency of heart and gallbladder. Points of the Heart, Pericardium, Kidney and Liver Meridians are frequently selected in its treatment.

1. Hyperactivity of Liver Fire

Manifestations: Insomnia, irritability, poor appetite, thirst, red eyes, bitter taste in the mouth, dark urine, constipation.

Tongue: Red body with yellow coating.

Pulse: Wiry and rapid.

Treatment Principle: Clear fire from the liver and calm the mind.

Point Prescription & Manipulation:
Primary points:
    LR-2 Xingjian   -
    PC-6 Neiguan   -
    HT-7 Shenmen   -
    ST-44 Neiting   -
    SP-6 Sanyinjiao   +

Explanation:

- LR-2 Xingjian and PC-6 Neiguan clear fire from the Jueyin Meridians;
- HT-7 Shenmen calms the min;
- ST-44 Neiting clears fire;
- SP-6 Sanyinjiao nourishes yin to restrain yang.

Secondary points according to conditions:
1□ Headache, dizziness and blurred vision— GB-20 Fengchi [-];
2□ Constipation — SJ-6 Zhigou [-].

2. Internal Disturbance of Phlegm-Heat

Manifestations: Insomnia, heavy sensation in the head, profuse sputum, stuffiness in the chest, poor appetite, belching, acid regurgitation, nausea, bitter taste in the mouth.

Tongue: Sticky and yellow coating.

Pulse: Smooth and rapid.

Treatment Principle: Transform phlegm, clear heat, harmonize the middle-jiao, calm the mind.

Point Prescription & Manipulation:
Primary points:
    HT-7 Shenmen   /
    GB-34 Yanglingquan -
    SP-6 Sanyinjiao   /
    ST-40 Fenglong   -
    LI-11 Quchi   -
    RN-12 Zhongwan /
    EX-HN-1 Sishencong -

Explanation:

- HT-7 Shenmen clears the heart and calms the mind;
- GB-34 Yanglingquan clears phlegm and heat;
- SP-6 Sanyinjiao, RN-12 Zhongwan and ST-40 Fenglong reinforce the middle-jiao and transform phlegm;
- LI-11 Quchi clears heat;
- EX-HN-1 calms the spirit.

Secondary points according to conditions:
1□ Chest oppression — PC-6 Neiguan [-].

3. Hyperactivity of Fire due to Yin Deficiency

Manifestations: Insomnia, restlessness, palpitation, dizziness, tinnitus, poor memory, soreness of the lower back and knees, nocturnal emission, hot sensation in the palms, soles and chest.

Tongue: Red body.

Pulse: Thready and rapid.

Treatment Principle: Replenish yin, clear heat, nourish the heart and calm the mind.

Point Prescription & Manipulation:
Primary points:
KI-6 Zhaohai +
BL-15 Xinshu +
BL-23 Shenshu +
HT-7 Shenmen +
LR-3 Taichong -

Explanation:
- KI-6 Zhaohai and BL-23 Shenshu tonify the kidney and nourish yin to restrain heart-fire;
- BL-15 Xinshu and HT-7 Shenmen nourish the heart, clear heat and calm the mind;
- LR-3 Taichong soothes the liver and clears heat.

Secondary points according to conditions:
1️⃣ Dizziness and tinnitus—GB-20 Fengchi [-].

4. Deficiency of Heart and Spleen

Manifestations: Insomnia, dream-disturbed sleep, shallow sleep, palpitation, poor memory, dizziness, blurred vision, lassitude, poor appetite, pale complexion.

Tongue: Pale body with thin coating.

Pulse: Thready and weak.

Treatment Principle: Tonify heart and spleen, reinforce qi and blood, and nourish the mind.

Point Prescription & Manipulation:

Primary points:
HT-7 Shenmen +
ST-36 Zusanli + ^
SP-6 Sanyinjiao +
RN-6 Qihai + ^
BL-20 Pishu + ^
BL-15 Xinshu + ^
SP-9 Yinlingquan +

Explanation:
- HT-7 Shenmen and BL-15 Xinshu nourish the heart and calm the mind;
- RN-6 Qihai, ST-36 Zusanli and SP-6 Sanyinjiao reinforce the middle-jiao to generate qi and blood;
- BL-20 Pishu and SP-9 Yinlingquan, the Back-Shu Point of spleen and He-Sea Point of the Spleen Meridian, reinforce the spleen's function to generate qi and blood.

Secondary points according to conditions:
1️⃣ Severe cases—DU-24 Shenting [+], EX-HN-1 Sishencong [+] and GB-13 Benshen [+], the three points of the head related to spirit which are effective in treatment of mental disorders;
2️⃣ Poor memory, dizziness, blurred vision— DU-20 Baihui [+ ^] BL-18 Ganshu [+ ^].

5. Qi Deficiency of Heart and Gallbladder

Manifestations: Insomnia, dream-disturbed sleep, shallow sleep, timidity, palpitation, liability to being frightened, shortness of breath, lassitude.

Tongue: Pale body.

Pulse: Thready.

Treatment Principle: Reinforce qi, nourish heart, and calm the mind.

Point Prescription & Manipulation:
Primary points:
RN-6 Qihai + ^
RN-17 Danzhong -
HT-7 Shenmen +
BL-15 Xinshu +
EX-HN-1 Sishencong +

ST-36 Zusanli   + ^

Explanation:
- RN-6 Qihai and ST-36 Zusanli reinforce qi;
- RN-17 Danzhong, the Influential Point of qi, regulates qi activity;
- HT-7 Shenmen and BL-15 Xinshu nourish the heart and calm the mind;
- EX-HN-1 Sishencong reinforces the brain and calms the mind.

Secondary points according to conditions:
1️⃣ Timidity — BL-19 Danshu [+ ^].

6. Disharmony of Heart and Kidney

Manifestations: Insomnia or even inability in fall asleep the whole night, dizziness, tinnitus, tidal fever, hot sensation in the palms, soles and chest, poor memory, soreness and weakness of the lower back and knees, nocturnal emission.

Tongue: Red body with little coating.

Pulse: Thready and rapid.

Treatment Principle: Reinforce kidney, clear heart, harmonize the heart and kidney, and calm spirit.

Point Prescription:
Primary points:
    DU-24 Shenting   +
    GB--13 Benshen   +
    EX-HN-1 Sishencong   /
    HT-7 Shenmen +
    KI-6 Zhaohai   +
    BL-15 Xinshu   +
    BL-23 Shenshu   +

Explanation:
- DU-24 Shenting, GB-13 Benshen and EX-HN-1 Sishencong, the three points on the head which are closely related to the spirit, calm the mind;
- HT-7 Shenmen and KI-6 Zhaohai reinforce kidney and calm the mind, harmonizing the heart and kidney;

- BL-15 Xinshu and BL-23 Shenshu, the Back-Shu Points of the heart and kidney, reinforce the heart and kidney.

Secondary points according to conditions:
1️⃣ Headache — GB-20 Fengchi [-].

II. EXPERIENTIAL TREATMENT

1. Puncturing EX-HN-16 Anmian

Indication: Insomnia.

Point Prescription:
    EX-HN-16 Anmian, located on the nape, at the midpoint of the line connecting GB-20 Fengchi and SJ-17 Yifeng.

Manipulation: Puncture perpendicularly 1.5 cun deep, rotate the needles to induce arrival of qi, and retain them for 30 minutes. The treatment is given once every day, with 10 treatments as a course. Usually after the first treatment the patient's sleep will be improved.

2. Acupuncture & Moxibustion on HT-7 Shenmen

Indication: Insomnia.

Point Prescription:
    HT-7 Shenmen

Manipulation: Puncture HT-7 Shenmen with reinforcing or reducing manipulation according to the patient's condition. Manipulate the needles to induce arrival of qi and retain them for 20-40 minutes. Ask the patient to apply moxibustion with moxa stick on HT-7 Shenmen for 20 minutes before going to bed. The treatment is given once daily with 12-15 treatments as a course. Usually, about 2-3 courses are needed to cure this disorder.

3. Puncturing BL-62 Shenmai

Indication: Insomnia.

Point Prescription:
    BL-62 Shenmai

Manipulation: Puncture with reinforcing or reducing manipulation according to the patient's condition. Manipulate the needles to induce arrival of qi and retain them for 15-30 minutes. The treatment is given once daily with 7 treatments as a course. Usually, within 4 courses, the disorder will be cured.

4. Puncturing EX-LE-21 Shimian

Indication: Insomnia.

Point Prescription:
EX-LE-21 Shimian, located on the bottom of the foot, at the Crossing Point of the perpendicular line from the tip of the external malleolus and the midline of the foot bottom.

Manipulation: Puncture shallowly about 0.1-0.2 cun deep, manipulate the needles gently, and retain them for 2-4 minutes. The treatment is given once daily, with 6 treatments as a course. Usually, within 4 courses of the treatment, the patient's sleep will be greatly improved.

5. Puncturing EX-HN-21 Tousanjiao

Indication: Insomnia with headache.

Point Prescription:
EX-HN-21 Tousanjiao, three points in total, located on the forehead, respectively at the Crossing Points of the perpendicular line from the inner canthus and the front hairline, and DU-23 Shangxing.

Manipulation: Puncture upwards along the scalp 1 cm, rotate the needles gently, retain them for 60 minutes. The treatment is given once daily with 10 treatments as a course. Usually, within 2 courses, the patient's condition will be improved greatly.

Comment:
Zhenjiu is effective to relieve insomnia.

Notes:

34. Cardiac Neurosis

Cardiac neurosis refers to a functional disorder of the cardiovascular system caused by disturbance of the central nervous system. It occurs mainly in adults, and more often in females than in males. It is clinically marked by pericardial dull pain lasting several hours or days, or stabbing pain in the apical region of the heart lasting one to five seconds. It is induced or aggravated primarily by exertion or mental injury. Other symptoms include lassitude, palpitation, shortness of breath, anxiety, restlessness, mild fever, perspiration, or trembling and numbness of the hands. According to TCM, cardiac neurosis belongs to the categories of Xin Ji (palpitation), Xin Tong (cardiac pain), or Yu Zhong (melancholia), and it is due to impairment of the heart and spleen due to over-thinking, leading to deficiency of the heart blood, or impairment of the kidney due to fright or fear, leading to disharmony of the heart and kidney.

I. STANDARD TREATMENT

Cardiac neurosis is generally divided into four types — qi deficiency of the heart and gallbladder, deficiency of the heart and spleen, disharmony of the heart and kidney, and stagnant liver qi and accumulation of phlegm. Back-Shu Points and points of the Heart and Pericardium Meridians are frequently selected in its treatment.

1. Qi Deficiency of Heart and Gallbladder

Manifestations: Palpitation, fear and fright, restlessness, insomnia, dream-disturbed sleep.

Tongue: Pale body with thin and white coating.

Pulse: Thready and weak.

Treatment Principle: Reinforce qi, nourish the heart, calm the mind, and relieve timidity.

Point Prescription & Manipulation:
Primary points:
BL-15 Xinshu   +

BL-19 Danshu +
PC-6 Neiguan /
HT-7 Shenmen /
ST-36 Zusanli + ^
RN-4 Guanyuan + ^
GB-34 Yanglingquan /
RN-17 Danzhong /

Explanation:
These points are usually divided into two groups, and they are used alternatively.

- BL-15 Xinshu and BL-19 Danshu, the Back-Shu Points of the heart and gallbladder, reinforce qi of the heart and gallbladder;
- PC-6 Neiguan and HT-7 Shenmen nourish the heart and calm the mind;
- ST-36 Zusanli and RN-4 Guanyuan tonify qi;
- GB-34 Yanglingquan promotes qi circulation and regulates the gallbladder;
- RN-17 Danzhong promotes qi circulation.

Secondary points according to conditions:
1☐ Spontaneous sweating — HT-6 Yinxi [+].

2. Deficiency of the Heart and Spleen

Manifestations: Palpitation, poor memory, insomnia, dream-disturbed sleep, fatigue and weakness, sallow complexion, poor appetite, abdominal distention.

Tongue: Pale body with thin and white coating.

Pulse: Thready and weak.

Treatment Principle: Tonify the heart and spleen, nourish blood and calm the mind.

Point Prescription & Manipulation:
Primary points:
BL-15 Xinshu +
BL-20 Pishu +
BL-17 Geshu +
PC-6 Neiguan /
ST-36 Zusanli +
RN-4 Guanyuan +
RN-17 Danzhong -

Explanation:
These points are usually divided into two groups, and they are used alternatively.

- BL-15 Xinshu and BL-17 Geshu, the Back-Shu Point of the heart and the Influential Point of blood, tonify the heart and nourish blood;
- BL-20 Pishu and ST-36 Zusanli tonify the spleen and generate qi;
- PC-6 Neiguan and RN-17 Danzhong promote qi circulation, regulate the heart and calm the mind;
- RN-4 Guanyuan tonifies Yuan-primary qi to strengthen the body constitution.

Secondary points according to conditions:
1☐ Abdominal distention and loose stools—ST-25 Tianshu [+];
2☐ Intractable insomnia — HT-7 Shenmen [+] and EX-HN-3 Yintang [/].

3. Disharmony of Heart and Kidney

Manifestations: Palpitation, restlessness, insomnia, dream-disturbed sleep, dizziness, tinnitus, heat sensation in the chest, palms and soles, dryness of the mouth and throat, night sweating, nocturnal emission, soreness and weakness of the loins and knees.

Tongue: Red body with little coating.

Pulse: Thready and rapid.

Treatment Principle: Tonify the heart and kidney, and calm the mind.

Point Prescription & Manipulation:
Primary points:
BL-23 Shenshu +
BL-15 Xinshu -
PC-6 Neiguan -
KI-3 Taixi +
SP-6 Sanyinjiao +
HT-7 Shenmen -
KI-7 Fuliu +

Explanation:
These points are usually divided into two groups, and they are used alternatively.

- BL-23 Shenshu and BL-15 Xinshu, the Back-Shu Points of the kidney and heart, tonify kidney yin, reduce deficient fire and harmonize the kidney and heart;
- PC-6 Neiguan, KI-3 Taixi and HT-7 Shenmen help BL-23 Shenshu and BL-15 Xinshu to reinforce the heart and kidney, and calm the mind;
- SP-6 Sanyinjiao and KI-7 Fuliu tonify the kidney, nourish yin and calm the mind.

Secondary points according to conditions:
1 Nocturnal emission—RN-4 Guanyuan [+].
2 Dizziness and tinnitus—GB-20 Fengchi [/]

4. Stagnation of Liver qi and Accumulation of Phlegm

Manifestations: Emotional depression or irritability and liability to lose temper, palpitation, distressed sensation in the chest, hypochondriac distending pain, poor appetite.

Tongue: White and sticky coating.

Pulse: Wiry and slippery.

Treatment Principle: Disperse depressed liver qi, resolve phlegm and accumulation.

Point Prescription & Manipulation:
Primary points:
BL-15 Xinshu -
BL-18 Ganshu -
PC-6 Neiguan -
LR-3 Taichong -
ST-40 Fenglong -
RN-17 Danzhong -
RN-12 Zhongwan -
EX-HN-1 Sishencong -

Explanation:
These points are usually divided into two groups, and they are used alternatively.

- BL-15 Xinshu and EX-HN-1 Sishencong calm the mind;
- BL-18 Ganshu, PC-6 Neiguan, LR-3 Taichong and RN-17 Danzhong soothe the liver, promote qi circulation, and relieve constrained qi;
- ST-40 Fenglong, the key point of transforming phlegm, and RN-12 Zhongwan, the Front-Mu Point of the stomach, regulate the middle-jiao and transform phlegm.

Secondary points according to conditions:
1 Feeling of obstruction in the throat by a foreign body — LI-17 Tianding [-];
2 Insomnia — HT-7 Shenmen [-].

II. EXPERIENTIAL TREATMENT

1. Puncturing HT-7 Shenmen

Indication: Cardiac neurosis with palpitation as its main symptom.

Point Prescription:
HT-7 Shenmen

Manipulation: Insert a 1-cun long needle perpendicularly into the point 0.5 cun deep, rotate the needle with medium stimulation to induce arrival of qi, retain the needle for 20-40 minutes and manipulate it every 10 minutes. The treatment is given once daily, and generally palpitation will be relieved greatly in 3-5 treatments.

2. Scalp Acupuncture

Indication: Cardiac neurosis.

Scalp Line Prescription:
Line 1 Lateral to Forehead of the right side
Middle Line of Forehead, the posterior 1/3 of the Middle Line of Vertex

Manipulation: On Line 1 Lateral to Forehead and Middle Line of Forehead, insert the needle from the top downwards; and on the 1/3 of the Middle Line of Vertex, insert the needle from the posterior to the anterior. After insertion of the needles, lift and thrust them at small amplitude to induce distention for 3 minutes, and repeat this course after an interval of 15 minutes. Ask the patient to keep quiet, relax himself/herself in the mind, breathe in and hold the breath, press the left chest and release the pressure to breathe deep with the chest during the manipulation of the needles. Retain the needles for 30 minutes in total.   The treatment is given once daily, with 10 treatments as a course.

3. Ear Acupuncture

Indication: Cardiac neurosis.

Ear Point Prescription:
   Heart, Chest, Liver, Small Intestine, Subcortex, Sympathetic.

Manipulation: See page 255.

Comment:
Zhenjiu is effective to treat cardiac neurosis, especially, to relieve palpitation and pain in the left chest due to cardiac neurosis.

Notes:

35   Hyperthyroidism

Hyperthyroidism refers to thyroid enlargement and hyper-secretion of thyroxin caused by auto-immunity or psychic trauma. It usually results from Graves' disease, toxic multinodular goiter, toxic adenoma, thyrotoxicosis factitia, subacute thyroiditis and silent thyroiditis. It is clinically marked by manifestations of hyperexcitation of the sympathetic nervous system and hypermetabolism, such as irritability, trembling of the fingers and tongue, lassitude, polyphagia, emaciation, frequent defecation, aversion to heat, profuse perspiration, mild or moderate diffuse thyroid enlargement, tremor and vascular murmur, premature heartbeat, paroxysmal tachycardia, and exophthalmus. According to TCM, hyperthyroidism belongs to the categories of Qi Ying (thyroid enlargement due to qi stagnation) and Zhong Xiao (emaciation with over drinking due to middle-jiao disorder), and it is caused by mental injury or improper diet leading to stagnation of the liver qi and accumulation of phlegm in the interior.

I. STANDARD TREATMENT

Hyperthyroidism is generally divided into three types — stagnation of qi and accumulation of phlegm, attack of the stomach by liver fire and yin deficiency with over-activity of fire. Points of the Liver, Stomach, Urinary Bladder and Heart Meridians are frequently selected in its treatment.

1. Qi Stagnation and Phlegm Accumulation

Manifestations: Thyroid enlargement, emotional depression or irritability, insomnia, sticky tongue coating, distressed sensation of the chest and epigastrium.

Tongue: Enlarged body.

Pulse: Wiry and smooth.

Treatment Principle: Dredge the liver, regulate qi and resolve phlegm.

Point Prescription & Manipulation:
Primary points:
   GB-20 Fengchi   -

ST-10 Shuitu /   SP-6 Sanyinjiao /
PC-6 Neiguan -   GB-20 Fengchi -
LR-3 Taichong -   BL-1 Jingming /
BL-18 Ganshu /   EX-HN-4 Yuyao -
ST-40 Fenglong -   GB-1 Tongziliao -

Explanation:

Puncture 1 or 2 local spots with the needle inserted through the border of the thyroid enlargement to the center of its bottom. Thrust, lift and rotate the needle at small amplitude, perform mild stimulation, and retain the needles for 30 minutes. Puncture the other points with reducing manipulation, retain the needles for 30 minutes after arrival of qi, and manipulate them every 10 minutes.

- GB-20 Fengchi and ST-10 Shuitu, local points, act at the diseased region to promote qi circulation and remove phlegm accumulation;
- PC-6 Neiguan, BL-18 Ganshu and LR-3 Taichong soothe the liver and relieve constrained qi;
- ST-40 Fenglong transforms phlegm and resolves the mass.

Secondary points according to conditions:

1□ The local spots [-] around the obvious thyroid enlargement.

2. Attack of Stomach by Liver Fire

Manifestations: Thyroid enlargement, exophthalmos, irritability, aversion to heat, profuse sweating, thirst with desire to drink, polyphagia, hunger.

Tongue: Red body with thin yellow coating.

Pulse: Wiry and rapid.

Treatment Principle: Clear heat from liver and stomach.

Point Prescription & Manipulation:
Primary points:
    LR-2 Xingjian -
    ST-44 Neiting -

Explanation:

Puncture the local spots with the same method mentioned above. Puncture BL-1 Jingming with a thin needle, push the eyeball outwards gently, and insert the needle perpendicularly 1 cun deep with no manipulation. Puncture the other points with reducing manipulation. Retain the needles for 20-40 minutes after arrival of qi.

- LR-2 Xingjian soothes the depressed liver and clears heat;
- ST-44 Neiting clears stomach fire;
- SP-6 Sanyinjiao strengthens the spleen and stomach to avoid attack by stagnant liver qi;
- GB-20 Fengchi, BL-1 Jingming, EX-HN-4 Yuyao and GB-1 Tongziliao clear fire from the liver and gallbladder, regulate qi and blood of the eye region to relieve exophthalmos.

Secondary points according to conditions:

1□ The local spots [/] around the obvious thyroid enlargement.

3. Yin Deficiency with Hyperactivity of Fire

Manifestations: Thyroid enlargement, exophthalmos, irritability, heat sensation in the chest, palms and soles, profuse sweating, hunger, trembling of the hands.

Tongue: Red body with little coating.

Pulse: Wiry, thready and rapid.

Treatment Principle: Nourish yin, descend fire, clear heart and nourish liver.

Point Prescription & Manipulation:
Primary points:
    BL-15 Xinshu +
    BL-23 Shenshu +

BL-18 Ganshu +
LR-3 Taichong -
KI-3 Taixi +
GB-34 Yanglingquan -
HT-7 Shenmen /

Explanation:
Puncture the local spots around the thyroid enlargement and orbital region with the same manipulation mentioned above, puncture the other points with even reinforcing-reducing manipulation, and retain the needles for 20-40 minutes after arrival of qi.

- BL-15 Xinshu and HT-7 Shenmen nourish the heart and clear heat;
- BL-23 Shenshu and KI-3 Taixi nourish the kidney and generate fluids to reduce deficient heat;
- BL-18 Ganshu nourishes yin and tonifies the liver;
- LR-3 Taichong and GB-34 Yanglingquan clear fire from the liver and gallbladder.

Secondary points according to conditions:
1□ The local points around the obvious thyroid enlargement [-]
2□ Obvious exophthalmos [-]—The points around the orbital region.

II. EXPERIENTIAL TREATMENT

1. Hydro-Puncture on LR-3 Taichong

Indication: Hyperthyroidism.

Point Prescription:
LR-3 Taichong.

Manipulation: Inject 2.5 ml of sterile water for injection into the point bilaterally. Give the treatment once every 3 days, with 4 treatments as a course. Generally, within 4 treatments the patient's condition will be improved and within 12 treatments, improved greatly possibly with the disappearance of all symptoms.

2. Puncturing EX-HN-22 Shangtianzhu and GB-20 Fengchi

Indication: Exophthalmus due to hyperthyroidism.

Point Prescription:
Primary points:
EX-HN-22 Shangtianzhu, 0.5 cun directly above BL-10 Tianzhu
GB-20 Fengchi

Secondary points according to conditions:
1□ Deficiency of qi and yin — PC-6 Neiguan, ST-36 Zusanli, SP-6 Sanyinjiao, KI-7 Fuliu, GB-14 Yangbai and SJ-23 Sizhukong;
2□ Yin deficiency with hyperactivity of fire— PC-5 Jianshi, LR-3 Taichong, KI-3 Taixi, EX-HN-5 Taiyang and BL-2 Cuanzhu.

Manipulation: Acupuncture is applied. Puncture EX-HN-22 Shangtianzhu, GB-20 Fengchi and points around the eye orbital region to induce the needling sensation radiating to the eyes, and puncture the other points with even reinforcing-reducing manipulation. Retain the needles for 20 minutes after arrival of qi, and manipulate them every 10 minutes. The treatment is given once daily with 10 treatments as a course.

3. Ear Acupuncture

Indication: Hyperthyroidism.

Ear Point Prescription:
Primary points:
Neck, Liver, Spleen, Kidney, Endocrine, Subcortex, and Yuanzhong
Secondary points according to conditions:
1□ Lower sexual function or irregular menstruation — Inner genitalia;
2□ Exophthalmus — Eye.

Manipulation: See page 255.

Comment:
Hyperthyroidism is an obstinate disease. Zhenjiu can provide positive results in its treatment. Additionally, if the patient takes the anti-hyperthyroidism medicine, Zhenjiu has a function to reduce their side effect and improve the patient's condition.

Notes:

36. Rheumatic Arthritis

Rheumatic arthritis refers to a frequently recurring collagen disorder of the joints caused by the Streptococcus rheumatosis bacteria. It is clinically marked by multiple, shifting, and symmetrical inflammation of the major joints, including the knees, ankles, shoulders, elbows, wrists, and hips. The affected area is usually red, swollen, hot, and painful. The joints may recover normal function with no residual deformity when the inflammation is relieved. According to TCM, rheumatic arthritis belongs to the category of Bi Zheng (Bi syndrome), and is due to attack of the meridians and collaterals by wind, cold and dampness, leading to obstruction of circulation of qi and blood.

I. STANDARD TREATMENT

Rheumatic arthritis is a result of three pathogenic factor wind, cold and dampness combining to attack the body. According to predominance of a certain pathogenic factor it is usually divided into four types — Wandering Bi, Painful Bi, Fixed Bi and Heat Bi (which is due to wind-cold-damp pathogens retained in the body for a long time to turning into heat). The local points are frequently selected in its treatment.

1. Wandering Bi

Manifestations: Wandering pain in the joints, especially the wrists, knees and ankles, limitation of movement, chills and fever.

Tongue: White and thin coating.

Pulse: Superficial or tight.

Treatment Principle: Dispel wind and cold, remove dampness, activate the collaterals to relieve pain.

Point Prescription & Manipulation:
Primary points:
  GB-20 Fengchi -
  SP-10 Xuehai -
  BL-17 Geshu _
  LR-3 Taichong -
  Ashi Points -

Explanation:
• GB-20 Fengchi dispels wind and expels superficial evils;
• SP-10 Xuehai and BL-17 Geshu, the Influential Point of blood, activate blood circulation and relieve pain;
• LR-3 Taichong regulates and promotes flow of qi and blood;
• Ashi Points activate collaterals and relieve pain.

Secondary points according to the diseased region:
1 *Shoulder joint*— SJ-14 Jianliao [- ^], LI-15 Jianyu [- ^], LI-16 Jugu [- ^], LI-11 Quchi [- ^], SI-10 Naoshu [- ^].

2 *Elbow joint* — LI-11 Quchi [- ^], LU-5 Chize [- ^], HT-3 Shaohai [- ^], LI-10 Shousanli [- ^].

3 *Wrist joint* — SJ-4 Yangchi [- ^], LI-5 Yangxi [- ^], PC-7 Daling [-], LI-4 Hegu [-], SJ-5 Waiguan [- ^].

4 *Metacarpophalangeal joint* — EX-UE-9 Baxie [- ^], LI-4 Hegu [-], LI-3 Sanjian [- ^].

5 *Phalangeal joint* —EX-UE-10 Sifeng [- ^].

6 *Hip joint* — GB-30 Huantiao [- ^], GB-29 Juliao [- ^], GB-34 Yanglingquan [- ^].

7 *Knee joint* — EX-LE-5 Xiyang [- ^], ST-34 Liangqiu [- ^], BL-40 Weizhong [-], GB-34 Yanglingquan [- ^], LR-8 Ququan [- ^], GB-33 Xiyangguan [- ^], EX-LE-2 Heding [- ^].

8 *Ankle joint* — BL-60 Kunlun [- ^], KI-3 Taixi [- ^], ST-41 Jiexi [- ^], GB-40 Qiuxu [- ^], KI-2 Rangu [- ^].

9 *Vertebral joint* — DU-14 Dazhui [+ ^],

DU-12 Shenzhu [+ ^], DU-3 Yaoyangguan [+ ^].

2. Painful Bi

Manifestations: Severe stabbing and fixed pain in the joints, alleviated by warmth and aggravated by cold, limitation of movement of the joints, cold limbs, aversion to cold, but no local redness and hotness.

Tongue: White and thin coating.

Pulse: Wiry or tight.

Treatment Principle: Dispel cold and wind, remove dampness, activate the collaterals and relieve pain.

Point Prescription & Manipulation:
Primary points:
BL-23 Shenshu   + ^
RN-4 Guanyuan   + ^
RN-8 Shenque ^

Explanation:
• BL-23 Shenshu, RN-8 Shenque and RN-4 Guanyuan are used in combination to tonify the kidney and activate yang qi so as to dispel cold and relieve pain.

Secondary points according to diseased region:
1 The same as above.

3. Fixed Bi

Manifestations: Numbness and heavy sensation of the limbs, fixed pain and soreness of the joints, aggravated on cloudy and rainy days.

Tongue: White sticky coating.

Pulse: Soft moderate.

Treatment Principle: Remove dampness, dispel cold and wind, activate the collaterals, and relieve pain.

Point Prescription & Manipulation:
Primary points:
ST-36 Zusanli   +
SP-9 Yinlingquan   +

Explanation:
• ST-36 Zusanli and SP-9 Yinlingquan strengthen the function of the spleen and stomach and resolve dampness.

Secondary points according to diseased region:
1 The same as above.

4. Heat Bi

Manifestations: Redness, swelling, pain and difficult movement of the joint, which are aggravated by heat and alleviated by cold.

Tongue: Red body with yellow and sticky coating.

Pulse: Wiry and rapid.

Treatment Principle: Dispel wind, clear away heat, remove dampness, and activate collaterals.

Point Prescription & Manipulation:
Primary points:
DU-14 Dazhui   -
DU-12 Shenzhu   -
LI-11 Quchi   -
LI-4 Hegu   -
LR-3 Taichong   -

Explanation:
• DU-14 Dazhui, DU-12 Shenzhu and LI-11 Quchi clear heat, dispel wind and remove dampness, and promote blood flow;
• LI-4 Hegu and LR-3 Taichong, the Four Gate Points, clear heat, promote qi flow, activate blood and relieve pain.

Secondary points according to diseased region:
1 The point prescription is the same as above, but only acupuncture with reducing manipulation is performed.

II. EXPERIENTIAL TREATMENT

1. Hydro-Puncture

Indication: Rheumatic arthritis with wind-heat-damp syndrome.

Point Prescription:
    BL-40 Weizhong

Manipulation: Mix 100mg of Vit. B1 and 100 mg Vit. B12 with injection water, and inject them into bilateral BL-40 Weizhong to induce soreness, distention and pain to the local region. The treatment is given once daily with 10 treatments as a course. After an interval of 5 days, next course may be given if the disease is not cured.

2. Puncturing ST-9 Renying

Indication: Rheumatic arthritis with wind-heat-damp syndrome.

Point Prescription:
    ST-9 Renying

Manipulation: Slowly insert a 1-cun needle perpendicularly into the point. If the needle handle trembles with the beating pulse, retain the needle for 1-3 minutes or remove the needle without retention. Strong stimulation is prohibited. The treatment is given once daily, with 5 treatments as a course.

3. Puncturing EX-LE-5 Xiyang

Indication: Rheumatic arthritis of the knee joint.

Point prescription:
    EX-LE-5 Xiyang

Manipulation: Insert the needle into the point 0.6 cun deep with the tip towards the center of the joint. Rotate the needle to induce arrival of qi, retain the needle in the point for 30-40 minutes, and manipulate it every 10 minutes. The treatment is given once daily, with 10 treatments as a course.

4. Ear Acupuncture

Indication: Rheumatic arthritis.

Ear Point Prescription:
    Endocrine, Adrenal Gland, Shenmen, Liver Spleen, Kidney, the point corresponding to the diseased joint.
Manipulation: See page 255.

Comment:
Zhenjiu is effective to relieve the pain of rheumatic arthritis. For severe cases, other treatments are needed in addition to Zhenjiu. Generally, the patients should pay attention to not catching wind, cold and dampness from climatic changes, avoid improper dwelling conditions and lack of physical excise, and do their best to get treatment at the early stage of the disease so as to avoid impairment of the joint function.

Notes:

37. Rheumatoid Arthritis

Rheumatoid arthritis is a non-suppurative inflammation of the small joints primarily due to auto-immunity. Its cause is uncertain. It is clinically characterized by chronic, multiple, and symmetrical inflammation of the small joints. The paracentral interphalangeal joints of the hands are most commonly affected, followed by the joints of the toes, ankles, and wrist. In the initial stage, there are pain, rigidity, swelling, and tenderness of the affected joints, most severe in the morning and gradually lessening with mild movement. In the intermediate stage, symptoms worsen, with the joints becoming swollen and deformed. In the advanced stage, stiffness and deformity of the affected joints may be accompanied by atrophy of the surrounding muscles. General symptoms may include lassitude, emaciation, mild fever, poor appetite, and mild anemia. According to TCM, rheumatoid arthritis is classified as a Bi Zheng (Bi syndrome), and is caused by internal deficiency of qi and blood and external invasion by wind-cold or damp-heat. The combination of internal and external factors results in obstruction of qi and blood and insufficient nourishment of the tendons, muscles, and bones.

I. STANDARD TREATMENT

Rheumatoid arthritis is generally divided into attack by wind-dampness, obstruction by phlegm and blood stasis, and retention of pathogen with body deficiency. The local points are selected frequently.

1. Attack by Wind-Cold-Dampness

Manifestations: Pain, stiffness, swelling and tenderness of the joint, aggravated by cold and relieved by warmth, aversion to cold.

Tongue: Pale body with white and sticky coating.

Pulse: Soft.

Treatment Principle: Dispel cold and remove dampness, dispel wind and dredge the collaterals.

Point Prescription & Manipulation:
General selection:
    DU-14 Dazhui   - ^
    RN-6 Qihai   + ^
    RN-4 Guanyuan   + ^
    LI-4 Hegu -
    LR-3 Taichong /

Explanation:
Four to eight points (including the secondary points) are punctured or punctured in combination with moxibustion each treatment session. After insertion of the needles, uniform reinforcing-reducing manipulation is applied to induce arrival of qi. Then, the needles are retained in the points for 20-40 minutes. During the retention, moxibustion can be applied. But RN-4 Guanyuan, RN-6 Qihai and RN-8 Shenque are applied with moxibustion only. The moxibustion can be applied until the local skin become flushed. The treatment is given once a day, with 10 treatments as a course. The next course begins after a 5-10 days interval.

- DU-14 Dazhui, the confluence place of all of the yang meridians, regulates qi, activities all of the yang meridians and dispels external wind-cold-damp pathogens;
- LI-4 Hegu and LR-3 Taichong, the Four Gate Points, regulate qi and blood, calm spirit and relieve pain;
- RN-6 Qihai and RN-4 Guanyuan strengthen primary yang and tonify primary qi to consolidate the exterior.

Selection according to diseased part:
1￻ *Shoulder joint*: LI-15 Jianyu [- ^], SJ-14 Jianliao [- ^], LI-16 Jugu [- ^], LI-11 Quchi [- ^].

2￻ *Elbow joint*: LI-11 Quchi [- ^], LU-5 Chize [- ^], HT-3 Shaohai [- ^], PC-3 Quze [- ^], LI-10 Shousanli [- ^].

3￻ *Wrist Joint*: SJ-4 Yangchi [- ^], LI-5 Yangxi [- ^], PC-7 Daling [-], LI-4 Hegu [-], SJ-5 Waiguan [- ^].

4￻ *Interphalangeal joints of the hand*: EX-UE-9

Baxie   [- ^], LI-4 Hegu [-], LI-3 Sanjian [- ^], SI-3 Houxi [-].

5□ *Interphalangeal joints of the foot*: EX-LE-10 Bafeng [- ^].

6□ *Hip joint*: GB-30 Huantiao [- ^], GB-29 Juliao [- ^], GB-34 Yanglingquan [- ^].

7□ *Sacral-iliac joint*: BL-26 Guanyuanshu [+ ^],   BL-30 Baihuanshu [+^], BL-27 Xiaochangshu [+ ^].

8□ *Knee joint*: ST-35 Dubi [- ^], EX-LE-4 Xiyan [- ^], GB-33 Xiyangguan   [-^], ST-34 Liangqiu [- ^], BL-40 Weizhong [-], LR-8 Ququan [- ^], GB-34 Yanglingquan [- ^], SP-9 Yinlingquan [- ^], BL-55 Heyang [- ^], EX-LE-2 Heding [- ^].

9□ *Ankle joint*: BL-60 Kunlun [- ^], KI-3 Taixi [- ^], ST-41 Jiexi [- ^], GB-40 Qiuxu [- ^], KI-2 Rangu [- ^], SP-5 Shangqiu [- ^], BL-62 Shenmai [-], KI-6 Zhaohai [- ^].

10□ *Wrist joint*: EX-LE-10 Bafeng [- ^], ST-44 Neiting [- ^], LR-3 Taichong [-], ST-41 Jiexi [- ^], SP-3 Gongsun [- ^], GB-41 Zulinqi [-].

11□ *Cervical vertebral joints*: GB-20 Fengchi [-], BL-10 Tianzhu [-], DU-14 Dazhui[+ ^].

12□ *Thoracic and lumbar vertebral joints*: DU-14 Dazhui [+ ^], DU-12 Shenzhu [+], DU-3 Yaoyangguan [+ ^], EX-B-2 Huatuo Jiaji [+ ^] of the diseased region.

13□ *Lumbar-sacral vertebral joints*: DU-3 Yaoyangguan [+ ^], EX-B-8 Shiqizhuixia [+ ^], BL-26 Guanyuanshu [+ ^].

2. Obstruction by Phlegm and Blood Stasis

Manifestations: Acute pain, deformity and swelling of the joint, difficulty in movement of the joint.

Tongue: Dark body with ecchymotic patches or spots.

Pulse: Thready and uneven.

Treatment Principle: Dispel phlegm and resolve blood stasis, activate blood and dredge collateral.

Point Prescription & Manipulation:
General selection:
    RN-6 Qihai   + ^
    RN-4 Guanyuan   + ^
    LI-4 Hegu -
    LR-3 Taichong /
    SP-10 Xuehai -
    ST-36 Zusanli   +

Explanation:
Four to eight points are punctured with filiform needles each time. After insertion of the needles, lift, thrust and rotate them to induce arrival of qi. Then, they are retained for 20-40 minutes with manipulation of them every 10 minutes. The treatment is given once daily with 10 treatments as a course. The next course can be given after a 5-10 days interval.

- SP-10 Xuehai and ST-36 Zusanli reinforce the spleen and stomach, transform dampness and phlegm and promote blood flow;
- LI-4 Hegu and LR-3 Taichong, the Four Gate Points, regulate qi and blood, calm spirit and relieve pain;
- RN-6 Qihai and RN-4 Guanyuan strengthen primary yang and tonify primary qi to consolidate the exterior.

Selection according to diseased part:
1□ The same as above.

3. Retention of Pathogen with Body Resistance Deficiency

Manifestations: Malformation,   pain   and swelling of the joint with difficulty in movement, muscular atrophy, fatigue, listlessness.

Tongue: Red body with little coating.

Pulse: Thready and quick.

Treatment Principle: Reinforce yin and nourish blood, activate blood and dredge collateral.

Point Prescription & Manipulation:
General selection:
    BL-18 Ganshu +
    BL-23 Shenshu +
    ST-36 Zusanli +
    RN-4 Guanyuan +

Explanation:
Four to eight points are punctured with the filiform needles each time. After insertion of the needles, lift, thrust and rotate them with uniform reinforcing-reducing manipulation in the local points and with reinforcing manipulation in the other points. The retention and therapeutic course are similar to those in the above syndromes. Moxibustion can be applied to patients with yang deficiency.

- BL-18 Ganshu and BL-23 Shenshu tonify the liver and kidney and strengthen the tendons and bones;
- ST-36 Zusanli and RN-4 Guanyuan tonify primary qi and strengthen the body constitute.

Selection according to the diseased location:
1☐ The point prescription is the same as those in "Attack by Wind-Cold-Dampness", but only acupuncture with reinforcing manipulation is performed.

II. EXPERIENTIAL TREATMENT

1. Puncturing the Tender Point on the Ear

Indication: Rheumatoid arthritis at any stage.

Ear Point Prescription:
    The tender point or nodule on the corresponding region of the diseased joint on the ear.

Manipulation: Use a probing needle to press the corresponding region of the joint on the ear to find the tender point or nodule first. Then, strictly and carefully sterilize the local region, and insert a needle into the spot or nodule about 0.2-0.3 cun deep. Rotate the needle to induce strong stimulation, and retain it for 20-40 minutes with manipulation every 10 minutes. The treatment is given once daily with 10 treatments as a course. The next course can be given after a 5-10 day interval.

2. Moxibustion on the Ashi Point

Indication: Rheumatoid arthritis at the early or middle stage.

Point Prescription:
    The painful or tender point at the diseased joint.

Manipulation: Ignite a grain-size moxa cone. When it is burning strongly, press it on the point until it is extinguished. Repeat this course 5 times. Each treatment session 3-5 points are selected. The treatment is given once every other day, with 10 treatments as a course.

Comment:
Acupuncture and moxibustion are effective in relieving pain and improving the general condition in rheumatoid arthritis.

Notes:

38. Sunstroke

Sunstroke refers to a disorder of the peripheral circulation due to over accumulation of heat in the body and of thermotactic dysfunction caused by exposure of the body to a high temperature environment. It is clinically marked by dizziness, headache, fever, thirst, nausea, suffocating sensation in the chest, palpitation, lassitude; or even pale face, vomiting, lowering of blood pressure, coma and convulsion. According to TCM, sunstroke belongs to the categories of Shang Shu (summer-heat injury), Shu Feng (summer-heat convulsion), Shu Jue (summer-heat exhaustion), and Fa Sha (exanthema), and it is caused by an attack of turbid qi of summer heat or summer damp-heat, leading to over accumulation of pathogenic heat which obstructs the clear orifice.

I. STANDARD TREATMENT

Sunstroke is usually divided into two types — injury of qi and nutritive phases by summer-heat and collapse of qi and yin, and points of the Ren and Du Meridians are frequently selected in its treatment.

1. Injury of Qi and Yin (Mild Type)

Manifestation: Fever, over-sweating, thirst, restlessness, dizziness, headache, distressed sensation of the chest, nausea, listlessness, red tongue with little moisture.

Tongue: Yellow coating.

Pulse: Full, rapid and hollow.

Treatment Principle: Clear summer heat, reinforce qi and nourish yin.

Point Prescription & Manipulation:
Primary points:
　EX-HN-5 Taiyang -
　PC-6 Neiguan -
　LI-11 Quchi -
　DU-14 Dazhui -

　LI-4 Hegu -

Explanation:
Prick EX-HN-5 Taiyang first to bleed several drops, then puncture the other points with reducing manipulation. Retain the needles until the symptoms are greatly relieved.

- DU-14 Dazhui, LI-11 Quchi and LI-4 Hegu clear summer-heat, purge Yangming Meridians to reduce fire;
- PC-6 Neiguan, opening to the Yinwei Meridian which runs into the abdominal region, and having the action of not only protecting the heart by tranquilizing the mind, but also regulating the stomach by lowering the adverse flow of qi, opens the closing of the pericardium, clears heat from the three jiaos, getting rid of irritability and arresting vomiting;
- EX-HN-5 Taiyang reduces heat and clears the mind.

Secondary points according to conditions:
1〇 Restlessness — HT-7 Shenmen [/].

2. Collapse of Qi and Yin (Severe Type)

Manifestation: Sudden onset of coma, hot trunk with cold limbs, convulsion.

Pulse: Thready, rapid and weak pulse.

Treatment Principle: Open the closed orifice and rescue the collapsed qi and yin.

Point Prescription & Manipulation:
Primary points:
　DU-25 Shuigou -
　PC-6 Neiguan -
　KI-1 Yongquan - ^
　EX-UE-11 Shixuan -
　RN-4 Guanyuan + ^
　DU-20 Baihui ^
　BL-40 Weizhong -

Explanation:
Acupuncture and moxibustion are applied. First, prick EX-UE-11 Shixuan and BL-40 Weizhong

with the three-edged needle to bleed. Then, puncture DU-25 Shuigou, PC-6 Neiguan and KI-1 Yongquan with reducing manipulation by thrusting, lifting and rotating the needle with a big amplitude until the patient recovers consciousness. Apply moxibustion on RN-6 Qihai, RN-4 Guanyuan and DU-20 Baihui. Puncture LI-11 Quchi and GB-34 Yanglingquan with even reinforcing and reducing manipulation.

- DU-20 Baihui and RN-4 Guanyuan recuperate depleted yang;
- BL-40 Weizhong, the He-Sea Point of the Bladder Meridian, removes heat from blood by bleeding;
- DU-25 Shuigou, KI-1 Yongquan and PC-6 Neiguan reduce heat, open the orifice, and awake the mind;
- EX-UE-11 Shixuan, the Connecting Points of the Yin and Yang Meridians, communicate yin and yang, induce resuscitation and restore consciousness.

Secondary points according to conditions:
1〕 Convulsion ── LI-11 Quchi [-] and GB-34 Yanglingquan [-].

II. EXPERIENTIAL TREATMENT

1. Holding with Fingers & Scraping

Indication: Mild sunstroke or severe sunstroke after recovery of consciousness.

Point Prescription:
EX-HN-3 Yintang
LI-18 Futu
DU-15 Yamen
LU-5 Chize
BL-40 Weizhong
The lines of the Bladder Meridian on the upper back

Manipulation: Dip fingers into water or alcohol, flex the fingers, hold the points up with the second finger joints of the index finger and middle finger and stop the holding movement immediately to make a sound "Pa". Repeat the holding and releasing action until the local skin

becomes purple-red due to congestion of blood. Then, dip a smooth spoon into water or vegetable oil, scrape the Bladder Meridian lines with the spoon until purplish red color appears at these regions. When scraping, be careful not to break the skin.

Comment:
1).   Although Zhenjiu is quite effective in treating sunstroke, other emergency methods should be applied in severe cases.

2). After the onset of sunstroke, first move the patient to a room where fresh air ventilates, give cool drink to the patient.

3). If the patient appears to be in circulation failure with dehydration and coma, the emergent therapy in combination with Chinese and Modern Medicines should be given.

Notes:

CHAPTER TWO
EXTERNAL DISEASES

39. Cystic Hyperplasia of the Breast

Cystic hyperplasia of the breast refers to cystogenesis of the mammary tissues caused by hyperplasia of acinar epithelia. It occurs primarily in women above forty years old who have a history of irregular menstruation, infertility, or miscarriage. It is marked clinically by periodic distending pain in the breast, aggravated by mental injury or before menstruation and alleviated after menstruation. Multiple masses in the breast occur and may be circular, oval, or lobulated, with an indistinct border and adhesion to peripheral tissues. The masses may vary with the menstrual cycle and state of mind. According to TCM, cystic hyperplasia of the breast is classified into Ru Pi (breast tumor), and it is due to internal emotional injury leading to stagnation of liver qi, disharmony of the Chong and Ren Meridians, and accumulation of internal phlegm.

I. STANDARD TREATMENT

Cystic hyperplasia of the breast is usually divided into two types — accumulation of phlegm and stagnation of liver qi, and disharmony of the Chong and Ren Meridians. The local points and points of the Stomach Meridian and Liver Meridian are frequently selected in its treatment.

1. Accumulation of Phlegm and Stagnation of Liver Qi

Manifestations: Distending pain or stabbing pain of the breast which is aggravated before menstruation and relieved after menstruation, masses in the breast which change in size according to emotional changes. This syndrome is usually seen in younger women who are at bad temperament, easy to loose temper, or have poor emotional condition.

Tongue: White and thin coating.

Pulse: Wiry and smooth.

Treatment Principle: Soothe liver and regulate circulation of qi, reinforce spleen and resolve phlegm.

Point Prescription & Manipulation:
Primary points:
    ST-18 Rugen   -
    GB-21 Jianjing -
    LR-3 Taichong -
    PC-6 Neiguan -
    ST-40 Fenglong -
    RN-17 Danzhong -

Explanation:
- LR-3 Taichong and PC-6 Neiguan promote circulation of qi of the Jueyin Meridians and soothe the liver;
- ST-40 Fenglong, the key point of transforming phlegm;
- RN-17 Danzhong, the Influential Point of qi, disperses qi stagnation;
- ST-18 Rugen, a local point and effective point for treatment of breast disorders, has function of promoting circulation of qi of the breast;
- GB-21 Jianjing, an experiential point for treatment of breast disorders.

Secondary points according to conditions:
1〕 Distention in chest and hypochondriac region —SI-1 Shaoze [-] and GB-34 Yanglingquan [-];
2〕 Stabbing pain in chest — BL-17 Geshu [-] and BL-18 Ganshu [-].

2.　Disharmony of Chong and Ren Meridians

Manifestations:　Masses and distending pain of the breast, irregular menstruation or amenorrhea, restlessness, and liability to being angry, headache, and dizziness. This type is usually seen in woman over 35 years old.

Tongue: White coating.

Pulse: Deep and thready.

Treatment Principle: Harmonize the Chong and Ren Meridians, relieve depression and resolve phlegm.

Point Prescription & Manipulation:
Primary points:
    SP-6 Sanyinjiao /
    LR-3 Taichong -
    PC-6 Neiguan -
    KI-3 Taixi +
    BL-18 Ganshu +
    BL-23 Shenshu +
    RN-17 Danzhong /
    ST-40 Fenglong /
    ST-18 Rugen /
    ST-36 Zusanli +
    GB-21 Jianjing /

Explanation:
The points mentioned above might be divided into two groups, and they are selected alternatively.

- LR-3 Taichong and PC-6 Neiguan relieve liver depression;
- KI-3 Taixi and BL-23 Shenshu tonify the kidney to regulate the Ren Meridian;
- BL-18 Ganshu tonifies the liver to regulate the Chong Meridian;
- SP-6 Sanyinjiao, the Crossing Point of the three Foot-Yin Meridians, reinforces yin and assists BL-18 Ganshu and BL-23 Shenshu to reinforce the liver and kidney and to regulate the Chong and Ren Meridians;
- RN-17 Danzhong, the Influential Point of qi, disperses qi stagnation;
- ST-40 Fenglong and ST-36 Zusanli strengthen the stomach and transform phlegm;
- ST-18 Rugen, a local point and effective point for treatment of breast disorders, has the function of promoting circulation of qi of the breast;
- GB-21 Jianjing, an experiential point for treatment of breast disorders.

Secondary points according to conditions:
1〕 Distention in chest — SI-1 Shaoze [-].
2〕 Stabbing pin in chest— BL-17 Geshu [-] and

BL-18 Ganshu [-].

II. EXPERIENTIAL TREATMENT

1. Circling Puncture on the Mass

Indication: Cystic hyperplasia of the breast with obvious mass.

Point Prescription:
The border of the mass.

Manipulation: Insert 4 needles respectively into the upper, lower, left and right points of the mass border. After insertion of the needles through the skin, push the needles deep with the tips toward the center of the bottom of the mass while slowly rotating the needles. After the needle tips reach the center, rotate, lift and thrust the needles with small amplitude to induce arrival of qi. Then, retain the needles in the points for 30-50 minutes and manipulate them every 10 minutes. When inserting and manipulating the needles, attention should be paid to the depth to avoid injury of the pleura. The treatment is given once daily with 10 treatments as a course. The next course begins after an interval of 3-5 days. Generally, 2-5 courses are needed depending on the size of the mass.

2. Ear Acupuncture

Indication: Cystic hyperplasia of the breast with masses of small size.

Ear Point Prescription:
Chest, Thoracic Vertebra, Liver, Spleen, Stomach, Endocrine.

Manipulation: See page 255-256.

Comment:
Zhenjiu is effective in treating hyperplasia of the breast, and in some cases, it is effective to cure this disease.

Notes:

40. Cholecystitis

Cholecystitis is an acute or chronic inflammation of the gallbladder. Its cause is mainly related to cholelithiasis or improper diet. The acute type is marked by sudden persistent pain in the right upper abdomen with paroxysmal exacerbation and radiation to the right shoulder and back, usually accompanied by nausea, vomiting, and fever. It occurs primarily in middle-aged women and is usually induced by overindulgence in greasy food. There is usually a history of acute cholecystitis in cases of chronic cholecystitis. The manifestations of an acute attack of chronic cholecystitis are similar to those of acute cholecystitis. The remission stage of chronic cholecystitis is marked by distention and discomfort in the upper abdomen after eating, belching, and aversion to greasy food, usually accompanied by dull pain in the right shoulder and back which is aggravated by standing, movement, or cold showers. According to TCM, cholecystitis is classified into the category of Xie Tong (hypochondriac pain), and caused by exogenous or endogenous damp-heat leading to dampness and heat in the gallbladder and liver and subsequent disharmony between the stomach and spleen.

I. STANDARD TREATMENT

Cholecystitis is generally divided into two types — damp-heat in the liver and gallbladder and stagnation of the liver and gallbladder qi. Points of the Liver and Gallbladder Meridians are frequently selected in its treatment.

1. Damp-Heat in Liver and Gallbladder

Manifestations: Abrupt attack, constant distending pain in the right upper abdomen, poor appetite, bitter taste in the mouth or even nausea or vomiting, constipation, yellow urination, fever.

Tongue: Red body with yellow and sticky coating.

Pulse: Wiry and quick.

Treatment Principle: Clear heat and remove dampness, relieve depressed liver qi and normalize function of the gallbladder.

Point Prescription & Manipulation:
Primary points:
    GB-24 Riyue   -
    BL-19 Danshu   -
    LR-14 Qimen   -
    GB-34 Yanglingquan   -
    LI-11 Quchi   -
    LR-2 Xingjian   -
    EX-LE-6 Dannang   -
    SP-9 Yinlingquan   -

Explanation:
- GB-24 Riyue and BL-19 Danshu, the Front-Mu and Back-Shu Points of the gallbladder, and LR-14 Qimen, the Front-Mu Point of the liver, all of them located at the diseased region, clear damp-heat from the gallbladder and liver, and promote flow of qi and blood for relieving hypochondriac pain;
- LI-11 Quchi clears heat;
- LR-2 Xingjian clears damp-heat from the Liver Meridian and promotes circulation of liver qi;
- EX-LE-6 Dannang and GB-34 Yanglingquan clear damp-heat from the Gallbladder and relieve pain.

Secondary points according to conditions:
1□ Fever — DU-14 Dazhui [-] and LI-4 Hegu [-];
2□ Constipation — SJ-6 Zhigou [-];
3□ Abdominal distention, nausea and vomiting — RN-12 Zhongwan [-] and ST-36 Zusanli [+];
4□ Jaundice — DU-9 Zhiyang [-].

2. Stagnation of Liver and Gallbladder Qi

Manifestations: Distending pain of the right hypochondriac region, which may radiate to the right shoulder, discomfort and distention of the stomach, poor appetite, acid regurgitation, nausea which are aggravated by anger and taking greasy food.

Tongue: Red body with yellow coating.

Pulse: Wiry.

Treatment Principle: Relieve depressed live qi and normalize the function of the gallbladder.

Point Prescription & Manipulation:
Primary points:
    LR-14 Qimen   /
    GB-24 Riyue   /
    LR-3 Taichong   -
    ST-36 Zusanli   +
    BL-18 Ganshu   /
    BL-19 Danshu   /
    GB-34 Yanglingquan   -
    RN-12 Zhongwan   /

Explanation:
The points mentioned above might be divided into two groups, and they are selected alternatively.

- LR-14 Qimen, GB-24 Riyue, BL-18 Ganshu, and BL-19 Danshu, the Front-Mu and Back-Shu Points of the liver and gallbladder, soothe the liver and gallbladder and relieve stagnation of liver and gallbladder qi;
- LR-3 Taichong and GB-34 Yanglingquan help the Front-Mu and Back-Shu Points to regulate the liver and gallbladder and relieve hypochondriac pain;
- ST-36 Zusanli and RN-12 Zhongwan strengthen the middle-jiao to prevent and treat attack of the spleen and stomach by abnormal liver qi.

Secondary points according to conditions:
1□ Hypochondriac pain radiating to chest and shoulder — GB-20 Jianjing [-] and PC-6 Neiguan [-].

II. EXPERIENTIAL TREATMENT

1. Puncturing Point Through Point

Indication: Acute or chronic cholecystitis.

Point Prescription:

GB-40 Qiuxu
LI-11 Quchi

Manipulation: First, insert a 2-cun long needle into LI-11 Quchi of both sides, manipulate the needle to induce arrival of qi, and retain the needle. Then, insert a 2-cun-long needle into GB-40 Qiuxu of both sides, rotate and push the needle deep until the needle tip reaches under the skin of the KI-6 Zhaohai, and retain the needle for 30-50 minutes. If the patient has severe hypochondriac pain, rotate the needle in GB-40 Qiuxu constantly with medium stimulation. Generally, during or after one treatment, the pain will be obviously relieved. The treatment is given once every day, with 10 treatments as a course. The next course can be given after an interval of 5-7 days.

2. Moxibustion on RN-8 Shenque

Indication: Acute attack of chronic cholecystitis marked by right hypochondriac pain.

Point Prescription:
    RN-8 Shenque

Manipulation: Ask the patient to lie on the healthy side. Ignite a moxa stick, hold the moxa stick 1-2 cun over RN-8 Shenque for moxibustion, and constantly rotate the stick. Apply moxibustion for about 15 minutes so the patient feels a heat sensation on the local region but can withstand it. Usually, during and after the moxibustion, the pain will be obviously relieved.

3. Ear Acupuncture

Indication: Acute and chronic cholecystitis.

Ear Point Prescription:
    Pancreas, Gallbladder, Liver, Abdomen, Thoracic Vertex, Spleen, Stomach, Sanjiao, Ermen, Endocrine.

Manipulation: See page 255-256.

Comment:
Zhenjiu is effective to relieve the symptoms of cholecystitis, especially hypochondriac pain. However, it is advisable to use other treatments in cooperation with Zhenjiu in order to cure this disease.

Notes:

41. Biliary Ascariasis

Biliary ascariasis is an acute abdominal condition caused by roundworm in the biliary tract. It is clinically marked by acute paroxysmal colic pain in the right upper abdomen, accompanied by nausea, vomiting, or even pale complexion and cold limbs. According to TCM, biliary ascariasis belongs to the category of You Jue (colic caused by ascaris).

I. STANDARD TREATMENT

Biliary ascariasis is usually diagnosed in differentiation as qi obstruction in its attack stage. Points of the Stomach, Gallbladder and Liver Meridians are frequently selected.

Qi Obstruction

Manifestations: Acute paroxysmal colic pain in the right upper abdomen, accompanied by nausea, vomiting, or even pale complexion and cold limbs.

Tongue: Purplish body.

Pulse: Tight or wiry.

Treatment Principle: Calm the ascaris, promote function of the gallbladder, relieve spasm and arrest pain.

Point Prescription & Manipulation:
Primary points:
    ST-19 Burong -
    LR-14 Qimen /
    GB-34 Yanglingquan -
    RN-13 Shangwan -
    LR-3 Taichong -
    PC-6 Neiguan -

Explanation:
Acupuncture is applied with repeated lifting, thrusting and rotating manipulation until the pain is relieved. This treatment can be given twice or more a day according to the patient's condition.

- ST-19 Burong, located at the diseased place, and LR-14 Qimen, located at the diseased place and being the Front-Mu Point of the liver, promote circulation of qi of the liver and gallbladder, relieve pain;
- GB-34 Yanglingquan promotes gallbladder qi movement and arrests pain;
- RN-13 Shangwan and PC-6 Neiguan regulate the stomach to stop vomiting;
- LR-3 Taichong and PC-6 Neiguan promote qi circulation to relieve pain.

Secondary points according to conditions:
1 Constipation and abdominal distention—ST-25 Tianshu [-] and SJ-6 Zhigou [-].

II. EXPERIENTIAL TREATMENT

1. Puncturing Through LI-20 Yingxiang to ST-2 Sibai

Indication: Biliary ascariasis.

Point Prescription:
    LI-20 Yingxiang
    ST-2 Sibai

Manipulation: Insert a 1.5-cun needle into LI-20 Yingxiang perpendicularly about 0.5 cm deep to induce needling sensation, then push the needle horizontally with its tip towards ST-2 Sibai until the needle tip reaches the region of ST-2 Sibai. Manipulate the needle to induce local numbness and distention to the patient, retain the needle until the pain is relieved. During the retention of the needle manipulate the needle every 5-10 minutes.

2. Puncturing EX-UE-12 Jinling

Indication: Biliary ascariasis.

Point Prescription:
    EX-UE-12 Jinling located on the dorsum of the hand, at the proximal border of the inter-space of the 4th and 5th metacarpal bones, in the depression at the midpoint between the transverse crease of the wrist and the small head of the metacarpal bone.

Manipulation: Insert a 1-cun needle into the point of the right side 0.3-0.5 cun deep. Lift, thrust, and rotate the needle with medium stimulation to induce soreness, numbness and distention that radiate to the tip of the finger. If the pain is not relieved, retain the needle for 10 minutes and manipulate the needle several times to strengthen the stimulation. Generally, the pain will be obviously relieved within 10 minutes after arrival of qi.

3. Puncturing with Finger

Indication: Biliary ascariasis.

Point Prescription:
EX-LE-6 Dannang

Manipulation: Press EX-LE-6 Dannang bilaterally with thumbs forcefully for 3 minutes, and knead the point until the pain is relieved.

Comment:
Zhenjiu is very effective to relieve pain due to an attack of biliary ascariasis and causes no side effects. Generally, Zhenjiu can be taken as the first choice when treating patients with an attack of biliary ascariasis. However, after the pain is relieved, root treatment with some other therapeutic methods for this disease should be given.

Notes:

42.   Prostatitis

Prostatitis is an acute or chronic inflammation of the prostate gland. Acute prostatitis occurs mainly in young people and adults and is clinically marked by frequent, painful, or dripping urination, sudden high fever, chills, and distending or severe pain in the lumbosacral region and perineum.   It is usually caused by overindulgence in alcohol, excessive sexual activity or suppression of ejaculation, injury of the perineum, acute urethritis, or the common cold.   Chronic prostatitis is marked by increased frequency of urination, burning sensation during urination, turbid terminal urine, and sinking pain in the lumbosacral region, perineum, and scrotum.   It may be accompanied by sexual dysfunction including pain during ejaculation or impotence, and neurosis.   There is usually a history of acute prostatitis.   According to TCM, prostatitis is classified into Lin Zheng or Lin Syndrome (stranguria syndrome), and it is caused primarily by accumulation of damp-heat in the lower-jiao leading to stagnation of qi.

I. STANDARD TREATMENT

Prostatitis is usually divided into two types— down flow of damp-heat and deficiency of kidney qi. Points of the Liver, Kidney, Urinary Bladder and Ren Meridians are selected in its treatment.

1. Down-Flow of Damp-Heat

Manifestations: Frequent, urgent and painful urination with burning sensation, white or turbid secretion dripping from the urethra following urination or bowel movement, pain in the perineum, testicle, and lumbosacral region.

Tongue: Red body with yellow sticky coating.

Pulse: Soft and rapid.

Treatment Principle: Clear heat and promote diuresis, separate the clear from the turbid and resolve the turbid-dampness.

Point Prescription & Manipulation:
Primary points:

    RN-2 Qugu   -

    SP-9 Yinlingquan   /

    LR-5 Ligou   -

    LR-1 Dadun   -

    ST-28 Shuidao   -

    BL-33 Zhongliao   /

Explanation:

Three to four points are punctured with filiform needles each treatment session. After inserting the needle, rotate, lift and thrust the needles at great amplitude to make the needling sensation of the points on the lower abdomen and lumbosacral region radiate to the external genitalia.

- RN-2 Qugu and BL-33 Zhongliao clear damp-heat in the lower-jiao;
- SP-9 Yinlingquan promotes diuresis and removes dampness;
- LR-1 Dadun and LR-5 Ligou, the Jing-Well and Luo-Connecting Points of the Liver Meridian which runs through the lower anterior yin region (the external genitalia region), clear damp-heat from the Liver Meridian and relieve pain;
- ST-28 Shuidao promotes diuresis.

Secondary points according to conditions:

1️⃣ Hematuria — SP-10 Xuehai [-];

2️⃣ High fever — DU-14 Dazhui [-] and LI-11 Quchi [-];

3️⃣ Repeated attack — ST-40 Fenglong [-], BL-32 Ciliao [/] and BL-54 Zhibian [/].

2. Deficiency of Kidney Qi

Manifestations: Frequent and urgent urination, turbid terminal urine, soreness of the lumbar region, impotence.

Tongue: Pale body with white coating.

Pulse: Deep and thready.

Treatment Principle: Reinforce the kidney and resolve the turbid-dampness.

Point Prescription & Manipulation:
Primary points:

    BL-23 Shenshu   + ^

    ST-36 Zusanli   + ^

    RN-3 Zhongji   /

    RN-4 Guanyuan   + ^

    DU-4 Mingmen   + ^

    BL-54 Zhibian   + ^

Explanation:

Three to four points are selected and acupuncture and moxibustion are applied in combination. After insertion, lift, thrust and rotate the needle with reinforcing manipulation to induce arrival of qi and make the needling sensation of RN-3 Zhongji and RN-4 Guanyuan radiate to the external genitalia. Then, retain the needles in the points for 20-40 minutes and warm the needles with burning moxa until the local skin becomes flushed.

- ST-36 Zusanli reinforces the middle-jiao and tonifies qi;
- BL-23 Shenshu, RN-4 Guanyuan and DU-4 Mingmen warm yang, tonify qi and consolidate the kidney;
- RN-3 Zhongji and BL-54 Zhibian regulate the urinary bladder for promoting diuresis, and promote flow of qi and blood for relieving local distention and pain.

Secondary points according to conditions:

1️⃣ Spontaneous emission — ST-29 Guilai [+ ^] and RN-2 Qugu [+ ^];

2️⃣ Edema — SP-9 Yinlingquan [+ ^];

3️⃣ Lower abdominal pain radiating to testis— LR-1 Dadun [^] and LR-8 Ququan [-];

4️⃣ Kidney yin deficiency manifested by hot sensation in palms and soles, night sweating, nocturnal emission, and burning sensation when urining — SP-6 Sanyinjiao [+] and KI-3 Taixi [+] are added, and moxibustion and DU-4 Mingmen are deleted.

II.   EXPERIENTIAL TREATMENT

1. Puncturing EX-CA-2 Huiyinhou

Indication: Chronic prostatitis.

Point Prescription:

EX-CA-2 Huiyinhou — located on the midpoint of the line connecting the perineum and anus.

Manipulation: Ask the patient to lie on one side. Insert a 3-cun long needle into the point to a depth of 1.5-2 cun, rotate, lift and thrust the needle with small amplitude to induce arrival of qi. Then, retain the needle in the point for 20-30 minutes, and manipulate it every 10 minutes. The treatment is given once daily with 10 treatments as a course. The next course can be given after an interval of 5-10 days.

2. Ear Acupuncture

Indications: Acute or chronic prostatitis.

Ear Point Prescription:
Angle of Superior Concha, Urethra, Kidney, Sanjiao, Liver, Endocrine, Subcortex, Shenmen, Internal Genitalia.

Manipulation: See page 255-256.

Comment:
Zhenjiu provides some beneficial effects in the treatment of prostatitis; However, it is not usually the main method of treatment chosen for this disease. In most cases, herbs may be more effective than Zhenjiu in the treatment of prostatitis.

Notes:

43. Hyperplasia of the Prostate

Hyperplasia of the prostate is a common problem of older men, and is also a common cause of such disorders as retention of urine, urinary tract infection, and uremia. Its cause is mainly related to repeated infection of the prostate, especially due to sexually transmitted disease, and hormonal changes that occur as men get older, similar to the menopausal changes that occur in women. It is clinically characterized in the initial stage by frequent urination, more severe at night and worsening over time. As the condition develops, difficulty in urination, weak urinary stream, urinary stuttering, or interrupted urination may occur. In the advanced stage, there may be acute urinary retention or incontinence. According to TCM, hyperplasia of the prostate is classified into Lin Zheng or Lin Syndrome (stranguria), and it is caused by deficiency of the kidney qi and accumulation of damp-heat in the lower-jiao. The combination of deficient antipathogenic qi and excessive pathogens results in the protracted course of the disease.

I. STANDARD TREATMENT

Hyperplasia of the prostate is usually divided into two types — damp-heat and deficient cold. Points of the Urinary Bladder, Spleen, Liver, and Ren Meridians are frequently selected in its treatment.

1. Damp-Heat

Manifestations: Frequent urination with burning sensation, difficulty and pain on urination, hematuria, or even retention of urine.

Tongue: Red tongue with yellow and sticky coating.

Pulse: Soft and rapid.

Treatment Principle: Clear heat and promote diuresis.

Point Prescription & Manipulation:
Primary points:
    RN-3 Zhongji   -
    SP-9 Yinlingquan -
    SP-6 Sanyinjiao   -
    RN-1 Huiyin   -
    LR-2 Xingjian   -
    BL-54 Zhibian - (punctured with the needle
    tip to ST-28 Shuidao)

Explanation:
* BL-54 Zhibian, RN-3 Zhongji and RN-1
  Huiyin clear damp-heat in the lower-jiao,
  resolve accumulation and promote diuresis;
* SP-9 Yinlingquan and SP-6 Sanyinjiao
  promote diuresis and remove dampness;
* LR-2 Xingjian clears damp-heat from the
  Liver Meridian, which runs through the
  anterior yin (the external genitalia region).

Secondary points according to conditions:
1⦿ Difficult urination and pain in lumbosacral
   region— BL-33 Zhongliao [-] and ST-28
   Shuidao [-];
2⦿ High fever— LI-11 Quchi [-] and DU-14 [-].

2.   Kidney Deficiency

Manifestations: Difficulty in urination or even
retention of urine, pale complexion, soreness and
coldness of the lumbar region.

Tongue: Pale body.

Pulse: Weak.

Treatment Principle: Warm the kidney and
activate yang.

Point Prescription & Manipulation:
Primary points:
    DU-4 Mingmen   + ^
    BL-23 Shenshu   + ^
    RN-4 Guanyuan   + ^
    KI-3 Taixi   + ^
    BL-54 Zhibian   + ^
    SP-6 Sanyinjiao + ^

Explanation:

* DU-4 Mingmen and BL-23 Shenshu warm
  and tonify kidney yang and dispel deficient
  cold;
* RN-4 Guanyuan   warms and tonifies
  primary yang and consolidates the essence;
* KI-3 Taixi tonifies the kidney and promotes
  diuresis;
* BL-54 Zhibian warms the urinary bladder
  and promotes diuresis;
* SP-6 Sanyinjiao promotes diuresis.

Secondary points according to conditions:
1⦿ Spontaneous emission— ST-29 Guilai [+ ^]
2⦿ Lower abdominal pain radiating to testis—
   and RN-2 Qugu [+ ^]; LR-1 Dadun [^] and
   LR-8 Ququan [-];
3⦿ Kidney yin deficiency manifested by hot
   sensation in palms and soles, night sweating,
   nocturnal emission, and burning sensation in
   urination—DU-4 Mingmen and Moxibustion
   are deleted.

II. EXPERIENTIAL TREATMENT

1. Puncturing to Relieve Retention of Urine

Indication: Hyperplasia of prostate with
retention of urine.

Point Prescription:
    PC-6 Neiguan
    DU-26 Renzhong
    BL-54 Zhibian
    RN-3 Zhongji
    SP-29 Guilai

Manipulation: When puncturing at PC-6
Neiguan, insert the needle perpendicularly and
apply reducing manipulation for about 1 minutes.
When puncturing at DU-26 Renzhong, insert the
needle obliquely with the needle tip toward the
nasal septum, lift and thrust the needle quickly
until the eyes are filled with tears; when
puncturing at BL-54 Zhibian, ask the patient to
lie on the side with knees flexed, insert a 6 cun-
long needle into the point with its tip reaching
under the skin of ST-28 Shuidao, and lift and
thrust the needle to induce the needling sensation
radiating to the external genitalia. If the patient is

diagnosed with deficiency of the kidney, the warming needle method is applied on BL-23 Shenshu, DU-4 Mingmen, RN-4 Guanyuan, ST-36 Zusanli and SP-6 Sanyinjiao. If the patient's condition belongs to damp-heat, puncture SP-6 Sanyinjiao, SP-9 Yinlingquan, KI-7 Fuliu and BL-26 Pangguanshu with reducing manipulation by lifting and thrusting the needles.

2. Ear Acupuncture

Indication: Hyperplasia of the prostate.

Ear Point Prescription:
Angle of Superior Concha, Urethra, Kidney, Sanjiao, Liver, Endocrine, and Subcortex.

Manipulation: See page 255-256.

Comment:
Zhenjiu can provide good results in the treatment of hyperplasia of the prostate. For some cases with retention of urine, acupuncture with massage can be taken as the first choice to induce urination and relieve an urgent condition, but it is not usually the main method to cure this disease. In most cases, a comprehensive treatment including herbs and Zhenjiu may be needed.

Notes:

44. Proctoptosis

Proctoptosis, commonly known as "prolapse of rectum", refers to a pathological condition of displacement and prolapse of the rectum and anal canal or even a part of the sigmoid colon, most commonly seen in children, old people, multiparae and weak youngsters and the middle aged. It is mainly caused by long-term diarrhea or constipation, or weak constitution. According to TCM, proctoptosis, called Tuo Gan in Chinese, is caused by deficiency of the middle-jiao qi, or by downward flow of damp-heat, resulting in failure to keeping the normal position of the rectum.

I. STANDARD TREATMENT

Proctoptosis is generally divided into two types — sinking of middle-jiao qi and downward flow of damp-heat. Points of the Stomach, Du and Bladder Meridians are frequently selected in its treatment.

1. Sinking of Middle-Jiao Qi

Manifestations: Prolapse of rectum induced by defecation, cough, walking, or long term standing, accompanied by fatigue, weakness, shortness of breath, dizziness, palpitation, poor appetite, loose stools.

Tongue: Pale and slippery body.

Pulse: Weak.

Treatment Principle: Replenish middle-jiao qi, raise the sunken qi.

Point Prescription & Manipulation:
Primary points:
DU-20 Baihui   + ^
BL-32 Ciliao   + ^
ST-36 Zusanli   + ^
RN-6 Qihai   + ^
BL-20 Pishu   + ^

Explanation:
- DU-20 Baihui, located on the highest place of the body and a point of the Du Meridian which governs all of yang meridians, raises the sunken;
- BL-32 Ciliao promotes circulation of qi and blood and raises the sunken;
- ST-36 Zusanli and BL-20 Pishu reinforce the spleen and stomach and tonify qi;
- RN-6 Qihai tonifies qi and consolidates the intestines.

Secondary points according to conditions:
1️⃣ Cough—BL-13 Feishu [+ ^] and LU-9 Taiyuan [-];
2️⃣ With kidney yang deficiency —DU-4 Mingmen [+ ^] and BL-23 Shenshu [+ ^].

2. Down-Flow of Damp-Heat

Manifestations: Prolapse of the rectum with burning sensation, swelling and pain, flushed face, thirst, distressed sensation in the chest and epigastric region, abdominal distention, constipation, scanty and dark urine.

Tongue: Red tongue with yellow and sticky coating.

Pulse: Soft and rapid.

Treatment Principle: Clear heat and dampness.

Point Prescription & Manipulation:
Primary points:
　　BL-32 Ciliao   -
　　BL-57 Chengshan   -
　　SP-9 Yinlingquan   -
　　BL-25 Dachangshu   -
　　ST-44 Neiting   -

Explanation:
- BL-32 Ciliao and BL-25 Dachangshu clear damp-heat from the intestines and promote bowel movement;
- BL-57 Chengshan, an experiential point for promoting bowel movement;
- SP-9 Yinlingquan removes dampness;

- ST-44 Neiting clears heat from the Yangming Meridians.

Secondary points according to conditions:
1️⃣ Constipation — ST-25 Tianshu [-].

II. EXPERIENTIAL TREATMENT

1. Puncturing DU-20 Baihui

Indication: Prolapse of the rectum.

Point Prescription:
　　DU-20 Baihui

Manipulation: Puncture horizontally backwards at an angle of 15 degrees, push the needle into the point 1.5 cun, and manipulate the needle to induce a heavy and distending sensation. Retain it for 20 minutes, and manipulate once during the retention. The treatment is given once daily, with 3 treatments as a course. Usually, only 1-3 treatments are needed to cure this disease.

2. Moxibustion on DU-1 Changqiang

Indication: Prolapse of the rectum due to qi deficiency.

Point Prescription:
　　DU-1 Changqiang

Manipulation: Apply moxibustion with moxa stick on DU-1 Changqiang for about 10-20 minutes, until the patient cannot tolerate it. The treatment is given once daily with 5 treatments as a course.   Usually one course is needed.

3. Puncturing DU-1 Changqiang

Indication: Prolapse of the rectum.

Point Prescription:
　　DU-1 Changqiang

Manipulation: Ask the patient to lie down on the knees and chest. Puncture 2-3 cun along the medial (anterior) border of the coccyx, perform reinforcing manipulation to induce numbness sensation around the anus, and withdraw the needle without retention. Usually, only 1-3 treatments are needed to cure this disease.

4. Moxibustion on RN-8 Shenque

Indication: Prolapse of the rectum.

Point Prescription:
RN-8 Shenque
BL-25 Dachangshu

Manipulation: On RN-8 Shenque, to manipulation see "Moxibustion" in Part One. On ST-25 Dachangshu, puncture perpendicularly 1.2 cun and warm the needle with moxa wool until the local region becomes flushed and the patient cannot bear it. Usually, only 1-5 treatments are needed to cure this disease.

Comment:
Zhenjiu can be effective to cure proctoptosis.

Notes:

45. Hemorrhoids

Hemorrhoids refers to venous masses caused by backflow obstruction of the hemorrhoidal veins resulting in dilation and varicosity of the submucosal venous plexus of the blind end of the rectum and the submucosal venous plexus of the anal canal. It is mainly caused by constipation, but obesity, pregnancy, a sedentary lifestyle and lack of exercise, or standing or sitting for long periods of time also may result in hemorrhoids. It is classified into three types according to the location of the venous masses. Internal hemorrhoids are marked by bleeding during defecation, prolapse of the hemorrhoids, or severe pain when complicated by infection. External hemorrhoids are marked by sensation of a foreign body in the anus, and severe pain aggravated by defecation, walking, or sitting, any of which may cause thrombosis or splitting of the hemorrhoidal veins to occur. Mixed hemorrhoids have characteristics of both internal and external hemorrhoids, but the condition is more severe than either alone. Hemorrhoids are called Zhi or Zhi Chuan in Chinese. According to TCM, hemorrhoids are caused primarily by over indulgence in spicy or greasy food, or by protracted diarrhea or constipation, resulting in stagnation of qi and blood and subsequently injury of the collaterals of the anus.

I. STANDARD TREATMENT

Hemorrhoids are generally divided into two types — down flow of damp-heat and deficiency of qi and blood. Points of the Stomach, Spleen, Bladder and Du Meridians are frequently selected in its treatment.

1. Down-Flow of Damp-Heat

Manifestations: Stool with red blood, itching and pain of the anus which is aggravated by touching, dry stool, scanty and dark urine, thirst.

Tongue: Red tongue with yellow and sticky coating.

Pulse: Slippery and rapid.

Treatment Principle: Clear heat and remove dampness, cool blood to stop bleeding.

Point Prescription & Manipulation:
Primary points:

    EX-UE-2 Erbai   -
    DU-1 Changqiang   -
    SP-9 Yinlingquan   -
    ST-37 Shangjuxu   -
    SP-6 Sanyinjiao   /
    BL-57 Chengshan   -

Explanation:
- EX-UE-2 Erbai, an experiential point for hemorrhoids;
- DU-1 Changqiang, at the anal region, removes the stagnation of qi and blood of the anal region;
- SP-9 Yinlingquan and SP-6 Sanyinjiao clear damp-heat, and cool blood and stop bleeding;
- BL-57 Chengshan, an experiential point for hemorrhoids;
- ST-37 Shangjuxu, the Lower He-Sea Point of the large intestine, purges heat from the large intestine.

Secondary points according to conditions:
1️⃣ Swelling and pain of the anus—BL-54 Zhibian [/];
2️⃣ Bleeding from the anus— SP-10 Xuehai [/] and BL-24 Qihaishu [/];
3️⃣ Severe pain — LI-7 Wenliu [-], the Xi-Cleft Point of the Large Intestine Meridian;
4️⃣ Constipation — ST-25 Tianshu [-] and BL-25 Dachangshu [-].

2. Deficiency of Qi and Blood

Manifestations: Prolapse of the internal hemorrhoids which are difficult to return to the normal position, sinking sensation of the anus, sallow complexion, palpitation, shortness of breath, fatigue.

Tongue: Pale body with thin white coating.

Pulse: Thready and weak.

Treatment Principle: Tonify qi and blood, raise qi.

Point Prescription & Manipulation:
Primary points:

    DU-20 Baihui   + ^
    RN-8 Shenque   ^
    SP-6 Sanyinjiao   + ^
    BL-35 Huiyang   + ^
    BL-58 Feiyang   + ^

Explanation:
Acupuncture is not applied on RN-8 Shenque, only moxibustion with salt or ginger moxibustion can be applied. Usually 5-7 cones of moxa are needed.

- DU-20 Baihui, located on the highest place of the body and a point of the Du Meridian which governs all yang meridians, raises the sunken;
- RN-8 Shenque and SP-6 Sanyinjiao tonify qi and blood;
- BL-35 Huiyang promotes circulation of qi and blood of the anal region;
- BL-58 Feiyang, an experiential point for hemorrhoids.

Secondary points according to conditions:
1️⃣ Poor appetite — ST-36 [+ ^] and BL-20 Pishu [+ ^];
2️⃣ Frequent urination— RN-4 Guanyuan [+ ^].

II. EXPERIENTIAL TREATMENT

1. Puncturing DU-1 Changqiang

Indications: Internal hemorrhoids, external hemorrhoids, mixed hemorrhoids.

Point Prescription:
    DU-1 Changqiang

Manipulation: Ask the patient to lie on the stomach with buttocks raised and the legs separated at 35 degrees. Insert a 3-cun filiform needle into the point, gradually push while rotating the needle until 2 cun deep to induce heat, numbness and distention sensations to the patient. Then, retain the needle in the point for 20 minutes and manipulate it every 5 minutes. Give the treatment once daily in the first two days and then once every other day. Five treatments are taken as a course, and 2-4 courses are needed.

2. Puncturing BL-57 Chengshan

Indications: Attack of pain due to hemorrhoids.

Point Prescription:
   BL-57 Chengshan

Manipulation: Ask the patient to lie on the stomach. Insert a filiform needle into the point 1.5 cun deep, rotate the needle at a frequency of about 350 times per minute, and with strong manipulation to cause soreness, numbness and distention radiating to the popliteal fossa, lower leg, and bottom of the foot, or induce local distention and pain only. Then, retain the needle for 30 minutes in the point and manipulate it every 5 minutes. Generally, a few hours later the pain will be relieved.

3. Breaking

Indications: Internal hemorrhoids, external hemorrhoids, mixed hemorrhoids.

Point Prescription:
   Positive spots on the back and lumbar sacral region or BL-25 Dachangshu

Manipulation: Look for positive circle-shaped spots about 0.5 cm long, which are slightly raised above the skin, grayish white, dark brown, or dark red, and do not fade in color under pressure. Use a three-edged needle to break a 1-cm long section of superficial skin on the positive spot, and break several fibroid materials. In one treatment session two spots are broken, and one week later the next treatment is given, with 3 treatments as a therapeutic course. If no positive spots are found, break the BL-25 Dachangshu with the same method. This treatment is only done under strict sterilization.

Comment:
Having a bowel movement every day at a regular time is very important in treating and preventing hemorrhoids. This viewpoint should be stressed to the patients very well. Zhenjiu is effective in the treatment of hemorrhoids. In some cases it can be cured by Zhenjiu treatment.

Notes:

46.   Thromboangitis Obliterans

Thromboangitis obliterans, also called Buerger's Disease, refers to chronic and progressive inflammation of the peripheral arteries and veins of the body. It occurs predominantly in men aged 20 to 40 who smoke cigarettes. Only about 5% of cases occur in women. This suggests that cigarette smoking is its primary etiologic factor. It is clinically marked in the initial stage by numbness and coldness of the extremities, fixed pain, and intermittent claudication.   In the intermediate and advanced stages, there is persistent severe pain worsening at night, myoatrophy, and black pigmentation or dry or moist necrosis of the affected region.   According to TCM, thromboangitis obliterans is classified into Bi Zheng   (blockage syndrome), Tuo Ju (gangrene of finger or toe), and it is caused by exogenous cold or dampness, trauma, or mental injury, which leads to stagnation of qi and blood and subsequent insufficient nourishment of the muscles and skin.

I. STANDARD TREATMENT

Usually, thromboangitis obliterans is divided into two types — cold-damp syndrome and blood stasis syndrome. Points on the Yang Meridians are frequently selected in its treatment.

1. Cold-Dampness

Manifestations: Coldness and numbness of the diseased limb, pale color of the local skin, weak or even disappearing of the artery pulse beating of the dorsum of the foot or leg, intermittent claudication.

Tongue: Pale body with white sticky coating.

Pulse: Deep, thready and slow.

Treatment Principle: Warm the meridian, dispel cold, activate blood circulation and dredge the collateral.

Point Prescription & Manipulation:

According to the diseased region:
On the lower limb:
   ST-36 Zusanli
   ST-41 Jiexi
   SP-9 Yinlingquan
   LR-2 Xingjian
   DU-4 Mingmen
   KI-3 Taixi

On the upper limb:
   LI-11 Quchi
   SJ-5 Waiguan
   LI-4 Hegu
   SJ-3 Zhongzhu
   DU-14 Dazhui
   PC-7 Daling

Explanation:
Acupuncture is taken as the main the treatment, and moxibustion as the assistant. At first, only 1-2 points are needed to induce obvious good results. After 5-15 treatments, it is needed to increase the number of acupoints gradually and to select the points alternately in order to sustain the result. Additionally, the needling manipulation should increase from mild to heavy, and the retention of the needles from short to long periods of time. During the retention moxibustion can be applied in cooperation.

- ST-36 Zusanli and ST-41 Jiexi dredge the Foot-Yangming Meridian, promote generation of qi and blood, and dispel coldness;
- SP-9 Yinlingquan reinforces the spleen and removes dampness;
- LR-2 Xingjian and ST-41 Jiexi promote flow of the meridian qi in the lower limbs;
- DU-4 Mingmen and KI-3 Taixi warm kidney yang to dispel cold and dampness;
- LI-11 Quchi and LI-4 Hegu dredge the Hand-Yangming Meridian, promote generation of qi and blood, and dispel coldness;
- DU-14 Dazhui warms yang to dispel cold;
- PC-7 Daling, SJ-5 Waiguan and SJ-3 Zhongzhu promote flow of the meridian qi of the upper limbs.

2. Blood Stasis

Manifestations: Constant pain of the diseased limb, which is aggravated in the night, purple-yellow, dark-red or purple color of the diseased limb with atrophy of the skin.

Tongue: Purple-dark body.

Pulse: Deep, thready and uneven.

Treatment Principle: Activate blood, remove blood stasis, and dredge the collaterals.

Point Prescription & Manipulation:
According to the diseased region:
On the lower limb:
  BL-40 Weizhong
  BL-60 Kunlun
  KI-3 Taixi
  ST-41 Jiexi
  ST-43 Xiangu
  EX-LE-10 Bafeng

On the upper limb:
  LI-11 Quchi
  SJ-5 Waiguan
  LI-4 Hegu
  SJ-3 Zhongzhu
  EX-UE-9 Baxie
  PC-3 Quze

Explanation:
BL-40 Weizhong is pricked to cause bleeding. Manipulation on the other points is the same as above.

- BL-40 Weizhong removes blood stasis;
- BL-60 Kunlun, KI-3 Taixi, ST-41 Jiexi, and ST-43 Xiangu promote flow of the meridian qi in the lower limbs;
- EX-LE-10 Bafeng relieves foot pain.
- LI-11 Quchi, SJ-5 Waiguan, LI-4 Hegu and SJ-3 Zhongzhu promote flow of the meridian qi in the upper limbs;
- PC-3 Quze and EX-UE-9 Baxie promote flow of qi and blood and relieve hand pain.

II. EXPERIENTIAL TREATMENT

1. Puncturing EX-LE-16 Tongmai

Indication: Thromboangitis obliterans at the early stage or middle stage.

Point Prescription:
  EX-LE-16 Tongmai of the diseased side, located at the supero-bacterior aspect of the buttock, at the Crossing Point of the line starting from BL-30 Baihuanshu and going down perpendicularly and the line starting from EX-LE-13 Huanzhong and going horizontally.

Manipulation: Ask the patient to lie on the stomach with the lower limbs extended, insert a 4-cun long needle perpendicularly into the point 3 cun deep, and constantly lift, thrust and rotate the needle for about 5 minutes to make the needling sensation radiate to the bottom of the foot. Retain the needle in the point for 20-40 minutes and manipulate it every 10 minutes.

2. Puncturing the Reaction Points

Indication: Thromboangitis obliterans at the early or middle stage.

Point Prescription:
According to the diseased region:
1） *On the lower limb*—EX-B-12 Maigen, located on the lower back, 0.5 cun below the level of the second spinal process of the sacrum and 3 cun lateral to the spinal column; EX-LE-22 Shangququan, located on the posterior border of the thigh and 3 cun directly above LR-8 Ququan. If the toe is diseased, SP-9 Yinlingquan and SP-8 Diji are added; if the dorsum of the foot and the second and third toes are diseased, Zusanli ST 36 and ST-40 Fenglong added; and if the fourth toe and lateral side of the leg are diseased, GB-34 Yanglingquan is added.

2） *On the upper limb*—LI-11 Quchi, HT-3 Qingling, EX-UE-20 Shouni, located on the midline of the medial aspect of the arm, at the midpoint of the line connecting the transverse crease of the wrist and elbow. If the diseased site is the thumb, LI-10 Shousanli is added; the ring finger, SJ-5 Waiguan added; and the small finger, HT-5 Tongli is added.

Manipulation: After insertion of the needles, lift, thrust and rotate them with medium stimulation to induce arrival of qi. Then retain the needles for 20-40 minutes.

3. Ear Acupuncture

Indication: Thromboangitis obliterans at the early or middle stage.

Ear Point Prescription:
The corresponding region, Heart, Lung, Kidney, Liver, Spleen, Sympathetic, Subcortex, Ear Apex.

Manipulation: See page 255-256.

Comment:
As thromboangitis obliterans is usually aggravated by coldness, emotional depression, and smoking, the patient should be advised to keep warm, avoid bad emotional stimulation and give up smoking. Zhenjiu may be one of the best treatment methods for thromboangitis obliterans. It can act to effectively relieve the patient's condition and prevent his/her condition from becoming worse. However, this disease is obstinate, and long-term treatment in cooperation with some other therapeutic methods, such as herbs, is generally needed.

Notes:

47. Scapulohumeral Periarthritis

Scapulohumeral periarthritis refers to a chronic retrograde inflammation of the soft tissues, including muscles, tendons, and joint capsule, peripheral to the shoulder joint. It occurs primarily in people above fifty years old, and more often in females than in males. Its cause is uncertain, though it is closely related to retrograde affection, and may be caused by trauma, chronic overuse, inflammation arthritis, and acute or chronic infection. It is clinically marked by pain and limited abduction, outward rotation, backward extension, and raising of the shoulder joint. According to TCM, scapulohumeral periarthritis belongs to the categories of Jian Ning (restricted movement of shoulder), Lou Jian Feng (omalgia), or Dong Jie Jian (congealed shoulder), and is caused by trauma or by the pathogenic factors of wind, coldness or dampness, resulting in obstruction of qi and blood in the meridians and insufficient nourishment of the tendons and muscles.

I. STANDARD TREATMENT

Scapulohumeral periarthritis is generally divided into three types — wind-cold-dampness, blood stasis and deficiency of liver and kidney and the local points and points of the three yang meridians are frequently selected in its treatment.

1. Wind-Cold-Dampness

Manifestations: Aching pain or stabbing pain in the shoulder, rigidity and tension of the arm, numbness of the fingers, which are related to weather changes and fatigue.

Tongue: White coating.

Pulse: Tight or wiry.

Treatment Principle: Disperse wind, dispel cold and dampness, warm the meridians, remove obstruction in the meridians, and stop pain.

Point Prescription & Manipulation:
Primary points:
    GB-21 Jianjing -
    ST-15 Jianyu - ^
    SJ-14 Jianliao - ^
    LI-11 Quchi - ^
    SJ-5 Waiguan - ^
    SI-3 Houxi -
    Ashi Points -

Explanation:
- Ashi Points, GB-21 Jianjing, ST-15 Jianyu and SJ-14 Jianliao, located at the diseased region, warm the meridians, dispel wind-cold-damp pathogens, activate the collaterals and arrest pain;
- LI-11 Quchi, SJ-5 Waiguan and SI-3 Houxi, the points of the three Hand-Yang Meridians, and located far from the diseased region, dredge the qi of the three meridians.

Secondary points according to conditions:
1️⃣ Stiffness of neck — DU-14 Dazhui [+ ^];
2️⃣ According to the diseased meridian—LI-4 Hegu [-], SJ-3 Zhongzhu [-], or SI-3 Houxi [-] is added.

2. Blood Stasis

Manifestations: Stabbing pain or aching in the shoulder joint, and limitation of the shoulder joint movement, which last for a period of time.

Tongue: Purplish body with ecchymotic spots.

Pulse: Wiry or unsmooth.

Treatment Principle: Relieve rigidity of muscles, activate the collaterals, remove blood stasis, and relieve pain.

Point Prescription & Manipulation:
Primary points:
    GB-21 Jianjing - ^
    ST-15 Jianyu - ^
    ST-14 Jianliao - ^
    Ashi Points -
    SJ-5 Waiguan -
    LI-11 Quchi -

    SI-3 Houxi -
    BL-17 Geshu -
    BL-40 Weizhong -

Explanation:
- Ashi Points, GB-21 Jianjing, ST-15 Jianyu and ST-14 Jianliao, located at the diseased region, warm the meridians, promote blood and qi movement, activate the collaterals, remove blood stasis, and arrest pain;
- LI-11 Quchi, SJ-5 Waiguan and SI-3 Houxi, the points of the three Hand-Yang Meridians, and located far from the diseased region, dredge the qi of the three meridians;
- BL-17 Geshu, the Influential Point of blood, and BL-40 Weizhong, an experiential point of removing blood stasis.

Secondary points according to conditions:
1️⃣ Prolonged cases — LR-3 Taichong [-] and KI-6 Zhaohai [+];
2️⃣ Stiffness of neck — DU-14 Dazhui [+ ^].

3. Deficiency of Liver and Kidney

Manifestations: Dull pain in the shoulder joint, atrophy of the local muscles, and limited movement of the shoulder joint, which last for a long time, dizziness, blurred vision, insomnia, soreness of the lower back and knees.

Tongue: Red body with little coating.

Pulse: Deep and weak.

Treatment Principle: Tonify liver and kidney, relieve rigidity of the muscles and activate collaterals, and stop pain.

Point Prescription & Manipulation:
Primary points:
    Ashi Points / ^
    GB-21 Jianjing / ^
    ST-15 Jianyu / ^
    SJ-14 Jianliao / ^
    SJ-5 Waiguan -
    BL-23 Shenshu + ^
    BL-18 Ganshu + ^

Explanation:

- Ashi Points, GB-21 Jianjing, ST-15 Jianyu and ST-14 Jianliao, located at the diseased region, warm the meridians, promote blood and qi movement, activate the collaterals and arrest pain;
- SJ-5 Waiguan dredges the Hand-Shaoyang Meridian;
- BL-23 Shenshu and BL-18 Ganshu, the Back-Shu Points of the kidney and liver, tonify the kidney and liver and strengthen the tendons and bones.

Secondary points according to conditions:

1️⃣ According to the diseased meridian — LI-4 Hegu [-], SJ-3 Zhongzhu [-], or SI-3 Houxi [-] is added;

2️⃣ Prolonged cases — LR-3 Taichong [-] and KI-6 Zhaohai [+].

II. EXPERIENTIAL TREATMENT

1. Puncturing ST-38 Tiaokou Toward BL-57 Chengshan

Indication: Scapulohumeral periarthritis.

Point Prescription:
     ST-38 Tiaokou of the diseased side.

Manipulation: Puncture with a needle tip toward BL-57 Chengshan and insert the needle deep until its tip reaches the area under the skin of BL-57 Chengshan. Then, rotate the needle with strong stimulation and ask the patient to move the shoulder joint during the manipulation until the pain and limitation become greatly relieved. Retain the needle for 20 minutes and rotate it during the retention 2-3 times. The treatment is given once daily or every other day. Usually immediately after the treatment the pain will be greatly relieved.

2. Puncturing GB-34 Yanglingquan

Indication: Scapulohumeral periarthritis.

Point Prescription:

GB-34 Yanglingquan of the diseased side or both sides.

Manipulation: Ask the patient to sit down. Puncture to induce arrival of qi and then partially withdraw the needle until it is just under the skin. Then, ask the patient to breathe in deeply once and raise the hand as far as the patient can. Push the needle perpendicularly about 3 cun deep while rotating it. Then, withdraw the needle until it is just under the skin, and at the time ask the patient to lower his hand and breathe out slowly during the withdrawal. Repeat this course 2-3 times before removing the needle. The treatment is given once daily. Usually within 15 treatments the disease will be cured.

3. Puncturing EX-LE-17 Zhongping

Indication: Scapulohumeral periarthritis.

Point Prescription:
     EX-LE-17 Zhongping of the healthy side, located on the leg, 1 cun directly below ST-36 Zusanli.

Manipulation: Puncture perpendicularly about 3 cun deep, rotate, thrust and lift the needle for 1 minutes, and ask the patient to perform movements of the shoulder joint. Then retain the needle 30 minutes, and manipulate it every 5 minutes. The treatment is given once daily with 7 treatments as a course. Usually, for patients with short-term disease course, only one or two treatments are needed to cure this disease. For the others, one or two courses are needed.

4. Puncturing EX-LE-18 Taijian

Indication: Scapulohumeral periarthritis.

Point Prescription:
     EX-LE-18 Taijian of the diseased side, located on the leg, 0.8 cun directly below SP-9 Yinlingquan.

Manipulation: Puncture perpendicularly 1.5-3 cun, rotate the needle in cooperation with some thrusting and lifting manipulation to induce arrival of qi. During the manipulation, ask the patient to move the shoulder joint. The treatment is given once daily with 7 treatments as a course. Usually within 2-3 courses the pain will disappear.

5. Pressing LI-10 Shousanli with Finger

Indication: Scapulohumeral periarthritis.

Point Prescription:
LI-10 Shousanli of the diseased side.

Manipulation: Ask the patient to sit down. Stand at the diseased side of the patient. If the patient has pain in the left shoulder joint, hold his left arm with your right hand, press the point with your right thumb forcefully, knead the point clock-wise to induce soreness, numbness, pain or electric shock sensation which radiate to the shoulder. Then, help the patent to move the shoulder joint. The treatment is given once daily with 10 treatments as a course. Usually 5-30 treatments are needed to cure this disease.

Comment:
Zhenjiu is effective in the treatment of scapulohumeral periarthritis. In most cases, it can be cured by Zhenjiu treatment. In clinic Zhenjiu can be taken as the first choice in its treatment.

Notes:

48. External Humeral Epicondylitis

External humeral epicondylitis, commonly called tennis elbow, refers to laceration, bleeding, adhesion or aseptic inflammatory change in the general tendon of the extensor muscle at the origin of the external epicondyle of the humerus. Its cause is uncertain, though it may be caused by repetitive strenuous supination of the wrist against resistance, as in manual use of a screwdriver, or by violent extension of the wrist with the hand pronated, as in tennis. It is clinically marked by pain on the lateral side of the elbow joint, usually radiating to the lateral side of the forearm or shoulder and aggravated when making a fist or wringing a towel. There is extreme tenderness on the external humeral epicondyle, but no swelling or impairment of joint movement. According to TCM, external humeral epicondylitis is classified into Shang Jin (injury of the tendon) or Zhou Tong (pain of the elbow), and is caused by strain of the elbow leading to localized obstruction of qi and blood.

I. STANDARD TREATMENT

External humeral epicondylitis is divided into two types—stagnation of qi and blood and deficiency of kidney yang. Points in the local area and the Kidney Meridian are frequently used.

1. Stagnation of Qi and Blood

Manifestations: Pain and heaviness or swelling and distending sensation of the elbow, which are aggravated by movement and relieved by rest.

Pulse and Tongue: Normal.

Treatment Principle: Promote circulation of qi, activate blood and relieve pain.

Point Prescription & Manipulation:
Primary points:
LI-12 Zhouliao - ^
LI-11 Quchi - ^

LI-10 Shousanli   - ^
SJ-10 Tianjing   - ^
Ashi Point - ^

Explanation:
On Ashi Points, puncture each spot with the needle tip toward several directions (point toward point puncturing), or puncture each spot with two or more needles.

• LI-12 Zhouliao, LI-11 Quchi, LI-10 Shousanli, SJ-10 Tianjing and Ashi Point, located at the diseased region, warm the meridians, activate the collaterals, promote qi and blood circulation, and arrest pain;

Secondary points according to conditions:
1▢ Severe and stabbing pain — BL-17 Geshu [-] and PC-6 Neiguan [-].

2. Deficiency of Kidney Yang

Manifestations: Soreness, swelling and discomfort of the elbow joint, which is aggravated by wind and cold, weakness and fatigue of the elbow joint.

Tongue: Pale body with white coating.

Pulse: Weak.

Treatment Principle: Warm the kidney, activate the collateral, and relieve pain.

Point Prescription & Manipulation:
Primary points:
    RN-4 Guanyuan   + ^
    BL-23 Shenshu   + ^
    LI-12 Zhouliao   + ^
    SJ-10 Tianjing   + ^
    Ashi Point   + ^

Explanation:
Ashi Points are punctured with the same manipulation mentioned above.

• RN-4 Guanyuan and BL-23 Shenshu warm and tonify kidney yang;

• LI-12 Zhouliao, SJ-10 Tianjing and Ashi Point, located at the diseased region, warm the meridians, activate the collaterals, promote qi and blood circulation, and arrest pain.

Secondary points according to conditions:
1▢ Dizziness, soreness of waist and knees and tinnitus — BL-18 Ganshu [+] and SP-6 Sanyinjiao [+].

II. EXPERIENTIAL TREATMENT

1. Puncturing LU-5 Chize

Indication: External humeral epicondylitis.

Point Prescription:
    LU-5 Chize of the diseased side.

Manipulation: Acupuncture is taken as the main the treatment and moxibustion as the assistant. Ask the patient to sit down with the diseased elbow bent at an angle of 90 degrees. First look for the obvious tender point around the external humeral epicondyle. Then, insert a 2-cun long needle into LU-5 Chize with its tip toward the tender point as deep as possible. Lift, thrust and rotate the needle to induce a painful and distending sensation in the elbow joint. Finally, retain the needle for 20 minutes and apply moxibustion on the diseased place during the retention.   The treatment is given once daily or every other day, with 10 treatments as a course.

2. Acupuncture and Moxibustion on the Tender Point

Indication: External humeral epicondylitis.

Point Prescription:
    The tender point on the area of the epicondyle.

Manipulation: Ask the patient to sit down with the elbow bent at an angle of 90 degrees and place the arms on a desk.   Look for the most obvious tender point on the area of the epicondyle, insert a filiform needle into the point, and rapidly rotate the needle with strong stimulation for 5 minutes. Then, remove the needle and apply moxibustion on the punctured region for 5-10 minutes until the patient cannot stand it. The treatment is given once daily, with 8 treatments as a course.

3. Puncturing ST-42 Chongyang

Indication:
External humeral epicondylitis at the acute stage.

Point Prescription:
ST-42 Chongyang

Manipulation: After insertion of needles, rotate them with even reinforcing and reducing manipulation until arrival of qi. Then, retain the needles for 20 minutes, and manipulate them every 5 minutes to strengthen the needling sensation. The treatment is given once daily and usually 5 times are needed.

4. Ear Acupuncture

Indication: External humeral epicondylitis, which lasts for a long time.

Ear Point Prescription:
Elbow, Sanjiao, Liver, and Shenmen.

Manipulation: See page 255-256. Generally, after 2-3 treatments, symptoms will be relieved greatly.

Comment:
1). Zhenjiu is effective in the treatment of external humeral epicondylitis. In most cases, it can be cured by Zhenjiu treatment. In clinics, Zhenjiu can be taken as the first choice in the treatment.

2). The earlier the treatment is given, the better the result will be. Among Zhenjiu treatment methods, puncture with warming needle often induce obvious effect result, therefore it may be selected firstly.

3). During the treatment period, the patient should decrease activities of the diseased elbow joint movement. As the disease very easily

reoccurs, after the treatment, he/she should avoid over usage of the diseased elbow joint so as to prevent reoccurrence.

4). If combined with massage or some other treatment, the Zhenjiu treatment result may be improved.

Notes:

49.   Myofascitis of Neck and Shoulder

Myofascitis of neck and shoulder refers to myofascitis taking place in the neck and shoulder. It may be induced or intensified by physical or mental stress, poor sleep, trauma, exposure to dampness or cold. It is clinically marked by pain and limitation of movement of the neck and shoulder. According to TCM, myofascitis of neck and shoulder is classified into Jing Xiang Tong (neck pain), Bei Tong (back pain), and Jian Bei Tong (pain of the shoulder and back), and it is caused by attack by wind-cold-damp, resulting in stagnation and obstruction of the collaterals.

I. STANDARD TREATMENT

Myofascitis of neck and shoulder is usually divided into two types—attack by wind-cold-damp and stagnation of qi and blood. Points of the three yang meridians are frequently selected in its treatment.

1. Attack by Wind-Cold--Damp

Manifestations: Stiffness, heaviness, soreness and pain of the neck and shoulder.

Tongue: Pale body with white and sticky coating.

Pulse: Slow or soft.

Treatment Principle: Dispel wind and cold, remove dampness and dredge the collaterals.

Point Prescription & Manipulation:
Primary points:
    GB-20 Fengchi   -
    BL-12 Fengmen   + ^
    SI-12 Bingfeng   / ^
    SI-11 Tianzong   + ^
    SI-14 Jianwaishu   + ^
    SI-3 Houxi   -
    Ashi Point + ^

Explanation:

- GB-20 Fengchi and BL-12 Fengmen dispel pathogenic wind-cold-dampness;
- SI-12 Bingfeng, SI-11 Tianzong, SI-14 Jianwaishu, and Ashi Point, located at the diseased region, warm the meridians, dispel pathogenic wind-cold-dampness, promote blood and qi movement, activate the collaterals, and arrest pain;
- SI-3 Houxi promotes qi and blood flow, activates the meridian and relieves pain.

Secondary points according to conditions:
1 Difficulty in moving the head forward and backward—BL-60 Kunlun [-] and LU-7 Lieque [-];
2 Difficulty in turning the head left and right — SI-7 Zhizheng [-].

2. Stagnation of Qi and Blood

Manifestations: Stabbing and fixed pain in the neck and shoulder.

Tongue: Purplish body with ecchymosis or petechiae.

Pulse: Uneven or wiry.

Treatment Principle: Promote circulation of qi and activate blood, dredge the collateral and relieve pain.

Point Prescription & Manipulation:
Primary points:
    BL-10 Tianzhu   /
    BL-17 Geshu   -
    SI-13 Quyuan   -
    SI-12 Bingfeng   -
    SI-11 Tianzong   -
    Ashi Point   -

Explanation:
Acupuncture is taken as the main and cupping as the assistant. Three to five points are selected each time. After insertion of the needles, lift, thrust and rotate them with reducing manipulation to induce arrival of qi. Retain the needles for 20-40 minutes, and enlarge the needle holes by shaking the needles before withdrawing them.

Then, apply cupping immediately on the punctured region to make a little bleeding.

- BL-10 Tianzhu promotes flow of the Bladder Meridian qi;
- BL-17 Geshu, the Influential Point of blood, removes blood stasis;
- SI-13 Quyuan, SI-12 Bingfeng, SI-11 Tianzong, and Ashi Point, located at the diseased region, warm the meridians, promote blood and qi movement, activate the collaterals, remove blood stasis, and arrest pain.

Secondary points according to conditions:
1□ Severe neck pain —DU-14 Dazhui [- ^], GB-39 Xuanzhong [+] and SL-3 Houxi [-].

II. EXPERIENTIAL TREATMENT

1. Puncturing SI-12 Bingfeng

Indication: Myofascitis of neck and shoulder.

Point Prescription:
SI-12 Bingfeng of the diseased side.

Manipulation: Ask the patient to sit down with the head slightly bent and the arm of the diseased side raised. After insertion of the needle, press the needle deep to 0.3-0.5 cun perpendicularly to induce arrival of qi, constantly lift, thrust and rotate the needle with strong stimulation to make the needling sensation radiating along the Hand-Taiyang Meridian to the neck. Then, withdraw the needle. If the patient has difficulty in holding material with the hand of the diseased side, LI-15 Jianyu is punctured additionally; if the patient has difficulty in bending the head, BL-11 Dazhu is punctured additionally. When puncturing LI-15 Jianyu, insert the needle perpendicularly 1.2 cun deep, rotate the needle with reinforcing manipulation, and retain the needle for 20 minutes; when puncturing BL-11 Dazhu, insert the needle perpendicularly 0.5 cun deep, rotate the needle with reducing manipulation, and retain the needle for 20 minutes too. The treatment is given once every other day, with 10 treatments as a course.

2. Puncturing SI-3 Houxi

Indication: Acute Myositis of neck and shoulder.

Point Prescription:
SI-3 Houxi of the diseased side.

Manipulation:
Insert a 1-cun long needle into the point perpendicularly 0.5-0.8 cun deep, repeatedly rotate the needle with strong stimulation while the patient is being asked to move the neck and shoulder until there is a little sweating on the these regions. Usually, within 3 treatments, the disease will be cured.

Comment:
Zhenjiu is effective in the treatment of Myositis of neck and shoulder. In most cases, it can be cured by Zhenjiu treatment. In clinics, usually, Zhenjiu can be taken as the first choice in the treatment.

Notes:

50.   Acute Soft Tissue Injury

Acute soft tissue injury refers to sprain or contusion of the soft tissues, including the muscles, tendons, ligaments, or joint capsules. It usually occurs on the neck, shoulder, elbow, wrist, fingers, limbs, hip, knee, or ankle, clinically marked by swelling, pain, and limitation of the joint movement. According to TCM, acute soft tissue injury is classified into Shang Jing (impairment of the tendon).

Among acute soft tissue injury, lumbar sprain, wrist sprain, and ankle sprain are introduced respectively in   "52. Acute Lumbar Sprain", "53. Acute Wrist Sprain", and   "54. Acute Ankle Sprain" because they are commonly seen in clinics and there is a necessity to discuss them separately.

I. STANDARD TREATMENT

Acute soft injury is generally diagnosed in differentiation as syndrome of stagnation of qi and blood.

Stagnation of Qi and Blood

Manifestations: Abrupt attack of pain, swelling and impaired joint movement of the local region after external injury.

Tongue: Normal.

Pulse: Wiry and tight or normal.

Treatment Principle: Activate blood and resolve blood stasis, dredge the meridian and activate the collateral, promote circulation of qi and relieve pain.

Point Prescription & Manipulation:
According to the different injured place, points are selected as the following:
Neck:
    BL-10 Tianzhu
    BL-11 Dazhu
    SI-3 Houxi

GB-20 Fengchi
GB-39 Xuanzhong

Shoulder:
    LI-15 Jianyu
    SJ-14 Jianliao
    SI-19 Jianzhen

Elbow:
    LI-11 Quchi
    SI-8 Xiaohai
    SJ-10 Tianjing
    LI-10 Shousanli
    SJ-9 Sidu

Hip:
    GB-30 Huantiao
    BL-54 Zhibian
    BL-36 Chengfu
    GB-39 Xuanzhong
    LR-3 Taichong

Explanation:
Three to four points are selected at each treatment session. Firstly, insert the filiform needle into the point, lift, thrust and rotate it to induce arrival of qi, and retain it in the points for 20-40 minutes. Then, apply moxibustion on the painful spot of the injured region for 10-15 minutes, or tap the spot with seven-star needle and apply cupping on it to make bleeding. Generally speaking, after withdrawing the needles in the diseased area, the needles in the distal points should be twisted greatly to induce strong stimulation, while the patient is asked to move the diseased part in a gradual increasing amplitude. If it is done, the pain will be milder immediately in most cases. The treatment is given once daily, and about 5 treatments are needed.

Neck:
- BL-10 Tianzhu, BL-11 Dazhu, and GB-20 Fengchi, located at the diseased region, warm the meridians, promote blood and qi movement, activate the collaterals, remove blood stasis, and arrest pain;
- SI-3 Houxi, at the diseased meridian, promotes qi and blood circulation of the meridian;

- GB-39 Xuanzhong, the Influential Point of Marrow, strengthens the bone.

Shoulder:
- LI-15 Jianyu, SJ-14 Jianliao and SI-19 Jianzhen, located at the diseased region, warm the meridians, promote blood and qi movement, activate the collaterals, remove blood stasis, and arrest pain.

Elbow:
- LI-11 Quchi, SI-8 Xiaohai, and SJ-10 Tianjing, located at the diseased region, warm the meridians, promote blood and qi movement, activate the collaterals, remove blood stasis, and arrest pain;
- LI-10 Shousanli and SJ-9 Sidu, at the diseased meridians, promote qi and blood circulation of the meridians.

Hip:
- GB-30 Huantiao, BL-54 Zhibian, and BL-36 Chengfu, located at the diseased region, warm the meridians, promote blood and qi movement, activate the collaterals, remove blood stasis, and arrest pain;
- GB-39 Xuanzhong, the Influential Point of Marrow, and at the diseased meridian, promotes qi and blood circulation of the meridian.

II. EXPERIENTIAL TREATMENT

1. Puncturing with Shallow Insertion and Gentle and Slow Manipulation

Indication: Acute soft tissue injury at early or medium stage.

Point Prescription:
Local points or Ashi Points.

Manipulation: One or two points are selected each treatment session. After insertion of the needle, push the needle deep with slow rotation until arrival of qi. Then, rotate the needle with small amplitude to strengthen the needling sensation, retain the needle for about 30 minutes, and manipulate it 3 minutes every 10 minutes. If the patient has aversion to cold and prefers

warmth in the local region, warming needling method should be applied as well. The treatment is given once daily, and usually within 3 treatments pain will disappear.

2. Puncturing the Corresponding Point

Indication: Acute sprain of limbs.

Point Prescription:
The point on the healthy limb but at the diseased side corresponds to the most painful spot of the injured region. Namely, if the injury is on the lower limb, the point on the upper limb of the same side corresponding to the most painful spot is selected and vice verso.

Manipulation: Insert a 1-cun long needle into the Corresponding Point horizontally at 15 degrees to 0.8 cun, rotate the needle for 15 seconds gently, inducing no needling sensation or little to the patient. Then, retain the needle in the point for 20 minutes. Ask the patient to move the diseased part during the retention. The treatment is given once daily, and usually within 3 treatments the pain will disappear.

3. Puncturing EX-UE-14 Xiadu

Indication: Acute neck sprain.

Point Prescription:
EX-UE-14 Xiadu of the diseased side, extraordinary point, located on the dorsum of the hand, between the 4th and 5th metacarpal bones, and proximal to the metacarpophalangeal joint.

Manipulation: Insert a filiform needle obliquely 1-1.2 cun deep to induce arrival of qi. Then, lift, thrust and rotate the needle with large amplitude 1-2 minutes, and ask the patient to move the neck at the same time. Retain the needle in the point for 10-15 minutes, and manipulate it twice during the retention. Usually, only 1 or 2 treatments are needed to cure this disease.

4. Puncturing ST-38 Tiaokou Toward BL-57 Chengshan

Indication: Acute or chronic shoulder sprain.

Point Prescription:
ST-38 Tiaokou of the diseased side.

Manipulation: Insert a 3-cun or 4-cun long needle into ST-38 Tiaokou of the diseased side, rotate and push the needle deeply with the needle tip towards BL-57 Chengshan until the tip reaches the area under the skin of the BL-57 Chengshan. Then, rotate, lift and thrust the needle with large amplitude for about 5 minutes, and ask the patient to move the shoulder joint in the same time. The treatment is given once daily, and usually within 3 treatments the pain will be relieved.

5. Ear Acupuncture

Indication: Acute soft tissue injury.

Ear Point Prescription:
The tender point, Shenmen, Liver, Spleen, Heart.

Manipulation: See page 255-256.

Comment:
Zhenjiu is effective in the treatment of acute soft tissue injury. In most cases, it can be cured by Zhenjiu treatment. In clinics, usually, Zhenjiu can be taken as the first choice of treatment. It is always important in the treatment that one has the patient's cooperation by moving the diseased part when the needle in the distal point is twisted, thrust and lifted.

Notes:

51. Stiff Neck

Stiff neck refers to rigidity, pain and limited movement of the neck. It is usually caused by improper posture when sleeping or exposure to dampness or cold during sleeping. It is clinically marked by rigidity of the neck and pain which usually radiates to one or both shoulders and upper arms, accompanied by muscular tension of the neck, extreme tenderness on the medial angle of the scapula, and impairment of movement of the neck. According to TCM, stiff neck, called Luo Zhen in Chinese, is caused by improper sleeping position, strain, sprain, or attack by wind-cold, resulting in obstruction of qi and blood in the meridians.

I. STANDARD TREATMENT

Stiff neck is always manifested as the syndrome of obstruction of the meridians by attack of wind-cold. Points of the Small Intestine, Gallbladder and Urinary Bladder Meridians are frequently selected in its treatment.

Obstruction of Meridian due to Attack of Wind-Cold

Manifestations: Sudden onset of spasm, rigidity, soreness and pain in one side of the neck, limitation of neck movement, accompanied with pain and tenderness in the shoulder, upper back and arm.

Tongue: Normal or white coating.

Pulse: Wiry and floating or normal.

Treatment Principle: Disperse wind and cold, dredge the meridians, and relieve pain.

Point Prescription & Manipulation:
Primary points:
Ashi Point - ^
BL-10 Tianzhu - ^
SI-14 Jianwaishu - ^
SI-3 Houxi -
GB-39 Xuanzhong - ^

Explanation:
Generally speaking, after withdrawing the needles in the diseased area, the needles in SI-3 Houxi and GB-39 Xuanzhong should be twisted greatly to induce strong stimulation, while the patient is asked to move the diseased part in a gradually increasing amplitude. If it is done, the pain will become milder immediately in most cases.

- Ashi Point, BL-10 Tianzhu and SI-14 Jianwaishu, located at the diseased region, warm the meridians, promote blood and qi movement, activate the collaterals, remove blood stasis, and arrest pain;
- SI-3 Houxi, Shu-Stream Point of the Small Intestine Meridian and one of the Eight Confluent Points communicating with the Du Meridian, promotes qi and blood circulation of the meridian, activates the collaterals, and relieves pain and stiffness of the neck;
- GB-39 Xuanzhong, the Influential Point of marrow, strengthens the bones.

Secondary points according to conditions:
1□ Headache — GB-20 Fengchi [-].

II. EXPERIENTIAL TREATMENT

1. Puncturing LI-4 Hegu, SJ-5 Waiguan, SI-3 Houxi, or GB-41 Zulinqi

Indication: Stiff neck.

Point Prescription:
LI-4 Hegu, SJ-5 Waiguan, SI-3 Houxi, or GB-41 Zulinqi of the diseased side. Only one of them is punctured, which is at the meridian where the most painful or tender spot locates.

Manipulation: Puncture perpendicularly 1-1.5 cun deep, rotate the needle quickly at a frequency of 200 turns per minute, retain the needle for 30 minutes, and manipulate it 2 times during the retention. Ask the patient to move the neck as much as possible during the manipulation and retention. Usually, one treatment is effective to cure this disorder. If not, repeat this course next day.

2. Puncturing PC-6 Neiguan

Indication: Stiff neck.

Point Prescription:
PC-6 Neiguan of the diseased side.

Manipulation: Puncture perpendicularly 1.2 cun deep to induce arrival of qi, rotate, thrust and lift the needle for 5 minutes, and remove the needle. Ask the patient to move the neck during the manipulation. Usually, only one treatment is effective to stop pain. If not, repeat this course next day.

3. Moxibustion on Ashi Point and SI-11 Tianzong

Indication: Stiff neck.

Point Prescription:
Ashi Point and SI-11 Tianzong of the diseased side.

Manipulation: Apply moxibustion with moxa stick on each point for about 10 minutes. The treatment can be given twice a day. Usually after one or two days of treatment, the disorder will be cured.

Comment:
Zhenjiu is very effective in the treatment of stiff neck. In most cases, it can be cured by Zhenjiu treatment. It is always important in the treatment that one has the patient's cooperation in moving the diseased part when the needle in the distal point is twisted, thrust and lifted. In clinics, usually, Zhenjiu can be taken as the first choice of treatment.

Notes:

52. Acute Lumbar Sprain

Acute lumbar sprain refers to acute sprain of lumbar muscle and fasciae. It is marked by an apparent traumatic history, followed by sharp pain in the lumbus on one or both sides, limitation of movement in the area, spasm and tenderness in the sacrospinal muscle and pain which can radiate to the buttock and posterior side of the thigh. It is called Ji Xing Yao Niu Shang or Shang Yao in Chinese.

I. STANDARD TREATMENT

Acute lumbar sprain is generally diagnosed in differentiation as syndrome of stagnation of qi and blood.

Stagnation of Qi and Blood

Manifestations: Abrupt attack of sharp pain in the lambar area on one or both sides, which can radiate to the buttock and posterior side of the thigh, limitation of lumbar movement, and spasm and tenderness in the sacrospinal muscle following external injury of the lumbus.

Tongue: Normal.

Pulse: Wiry and tight or normal.

Treatment Principle: Activate blood and resolve blood stasis, dredge the meridian and activate the collateral, promote circulation of qi and relieve pain.

Point Prescription & Manipulation:
Primary points:
> The tender points in the lumbus - ^
> BL-23 Shenshu + ^
> BL-52 Zhishi + ^
> DU-3 Yaoyangguan + ^
> BL-40 Weizhong - (pricked to bleed)
> BL-57 Chengshan -

Explanation:
- The Tender points in the lumbus, BL-23 Shenshu, BL-52 Zhishi BL and DU-3

Yaoyangguan, located in the diseased region, warm the meridians, promote blood and qi movement, activate the collaterals, remove blood stasis, and arrest pain;
- BL-40 Weizhong and BL-57 Chengshan promote flow of the Bladder Meridian qi and remove blood stasis.

Secondary points according to conditions:
1. Stabbing pain—DU-28 Yinjiao [-] (pricked to bleed), BL-17 Geshu [-] and SP-10 Xuehai [-];
2. Stiffness of spinal column—EX-B-2 Jiaji [-] and BL-25 Dachangshu [-].

II. EXPERIENTIAL TREATMENT

1. Puncturing EX-UE-13 Shangdu

Indication: Acute lumbar sprain.

Point Prescription:
> EX-UE-13 Shangdu of the diseased side, located on the dorsum of the hand, between the second and third metacarpophalangeal joints.

Manipulation: Ask the patient to sit or stand, and make a loose fist with its center facing downward. Insert a 2-cun long needle into the point with tip toward the palm center to 1-1.5 cun, and rotate the needle with reducing manipulation with stimulation tolerable to the patient. After arrival of qi, retain the needle in the point for 20 minutes, and ask the patient to turn at the waist until there is sweating in the diseased lumbar region. The treatment is given once daily and usually, 1-3 treatments are needed to cure the disease.

2. Ear Acupuncture

Indication: Acute lumbar sprain.

Ear Point Prescription:
> Shenmen

Manipulation: Use the handle of the needle to press the region of Shenmen to find out the most painful spot, insert a 0.5-cun long needle into the spot, manipulate the needle 3-5 minutes with strong stimulation to induce soreness, numbness and distention to the patient. Then, retain the needles in the points for 10 minutes, and manipulate them during the retention to strengthen the needling sensation. Usually, 1 treatment is enough to relieve the pain.

3. Pressing EX-B-9 Yaoqi with Finger

Indication: Acute sprain of the waist.

Point Prescription:
> EX-B-9 Yaoqi, located on the dorsum of the foot, between LR-2 Xingjian and LR-3 Taichong.

Manipulation: Ask the patient to sit or stand with the feet 15-20 cm apart. Press bilateral EX-B-9 Yaoqi with the tip of the index fingers simultaneously and forcefully and release. Repeat for 2-3 minutes, ask the patient to turn at the waist in conjunction. The treatment is given once daily and within 3 days, generally, acute lumbar sprain will be cured. If there is an obvious tender point near EX-B-9 Yaoqi, press the tender point to replace EX-B 9 Yaoqi. The result will be better than pressing on EX-B-9 Yaoqi.

4. Puncturing SI-3 Houxi

Indication: Acute lumbar sprain.

Point Prescription:
> SI-3 Houxi

Manipulation: Puncture perpendicularly 1 cun deep, perform reducing manipulation to induce soreness, heaviness, numbness, and distention which radiate to the elbow or even the shoulder, retain the needles for 30 minutes, and manipulate them during the retention. Ask the patient to turn at his/her lumbus after arrival of qi. In most cases the disorder will be cured with only one treatment. If not cured, the treatment can be repeated next day.

5. Puncturing EX-UE -15 Shanyao

Indication: Acute lumbar sprain.

Point Prescription:
> EX-UE-13 Shanyao, three points in total, located on the arm, at the three points of an equilateral triangle. LI-11 Quchi is its upper point, point 1 cun radial to the midpoint of the line connecting LI-11 Quchi and LI-10 Shousanli is one of the bottom point, and point on the line from the olecranon to LI-11 Quchi and 1 cun lateral to LI-11 Quchi is the other bottom point.

Manipulation: Puncture perpendicularly 1-1.5 cun deep, manipulate the needles to induce arrival of qi, retain them for 20-30 minutes, and manipulate them every 5 minutes. Ask the patient to move his lumbus during the manipulation and retention. Usually, only one treatment is effective to cure this disease. If not, the treatment can be given next day.

6. Puncturing RN-17 Danzhong

Indication: Acute lumbar sprain.

Point Prescription:
> RN-17 Danzhong

Manipulation: Puncture 0.5-0.8 cun horizontally at an angle of 10 degrees, with the needle tip toward RN-15 Jiuwei if the most painful spot is in the spinal column, toward the region left lateral to RN-15 Jiuwei if the most painful spot is at the left lumbus, or towards the region right lateral to RN-15 Jiuwei if the most painful spot is at the right lumbus, manipulate the needle forcefully to induce strong stimulation for 20 seconds, and retain the needle for 30 minutes. Ask the patient to move the lumbus during the retention. Usually, within 3 treatments, the disease will be cured.

7. Pressing BL-59 Fuyang with Finger

Indication: Acute lumbar sprain.

Point Prescription:
> BL-59 Fuyang

Manipulation: Ask the patient to lie on the stomach with the hands extended forwards and legs backwards. Firstly massage the lumbus several minutes to relax the muscular spasms. Then, press the BL-59 Fuyang with the tip of the thumb and increase the pressure gradually. Ask the patient to cough several times to know whether the pain becomes relieved or not. After the pain is relieved, ask the patient to support the body with hands, kneel on the bed, and move the buttock to touch the lower leg, and to repeat this course several times. Usually, one or two treatments are effective to cure this disease.

Comment:

Zhenjiu is very effective in the treatment of acute lumbar sprain. In most cases, it can be cured by Zhenjiu treatment. In clinics, usually, Zhenjiu can be the first choice of treatment. It is always important in the treatment that one has the patient's cooperation by moving the diseased part when the needle in the distal point is twisted, thrust and lifted.

Notes:

53. Acute Wrist Sprain

Acute wrist sprain refers to acute sprain of the wrist muscle and fasciae. It is marked by an apparent trauma history, followed by sharp pain, tenderness, and swelling in the wrist on one or both sides, limitation of the wrist joint movement. It is called Wan Niu Shang in Chinese.

I. STANDARD TREATMENT

Acute wrist sprain is generally diagnosed in differentiation as a syndrome of stagnation of qi and blood.

Stagnation of Qi and Blood

Manifestations: Abrupt onset of sharp pain, tenderness and swelling in the wrist region on one or both sides, and limitation of the wrist joint movement following external injury of the wrist joint.

Tongue: Normal.

Pulse: Wiry and tight or normal.

Treatment Principle: Activate blood and resolve blood stasis, dredge the meridian and activate the collateral, promote circulation of qi and relieve pain.

Point Prescription & Manipulation:
Primary points:
    The tender points in the wrist region - ^
    SJ-4 Yangchi   - ^
    SI-5 Yanggu - ^
    LI-5 Yangxi - ^
    SJ-5 Waiguan - ^

Explanation:
* The Tender points in the wrist region, SJ-4 Yangchi, SI-5 Yanggu, LI-5 Yangxi, located at the diseased region, warm the meridians, promote blood and qi movement, activate the collaterals, remove blood stasis, and arrest pain;

- SJ-5 Waiguan promotes flow of the Shaoyang Meridian qi.

Secondary points according to conditions:
1□ Stabbing pain — BL-17 Geshu [-].

II. EXPERIENTIAL TREATMENT

1. Puncturing the Corresponding Point on the Ankle

Indication: Acute wrist sprain.

Point Prescription:
The Corresponding Point, which is on the ankle of the healthy side, and corresponds to the most painful spot of the injured region in location. Namely, if the injury is on the left wrist joint, the Corresponding Point is the spot on the right ankle, which corresponds to the most painful spot on the diseased wrist.

Manipulation:
Method 1: Insert a 1-cun long needle into the Corresponding Point on the ankle, lift, thrust and rotate the needle repeatedly to induce and keep the needling sensation. Constantly manipulate the needle for 15-20 minutes, and ask the patient to move the diseased joint simultaneously during the manipulation. Usually, pain will be milder immediately. If not, the same spots but on the diseased side is also punctured in the same way. The treatment is given once daily. Generally, the pain will be relieved greatly after one treatment.

Method 2: Insert a 1-cun long needle into the Corresponding Point horizontally at 15 degrees to 0.8 cun, rotate the needle for 15 seconds gently, inducing no needling sensation or little to the patient. Then, retain the needle in the point for 20 minutes. Ask the patient to move the diseased region during the retention. Usually, pain will be milder immediately. If not, the same spot but on the diseased side is also punctured with the same way. The treatment is given once daily, and usually within 3 treatments the pain will disappear.

2. Puncturing the Corresponding Point on the Wrist

Indication: Acute wrist sprain.

Point Prescription:
The Corresponding Point, which is on the wrist of the healthy side, and corresponds to the most painful spot on the injured region. Namely, if the injury on the left wrist joint, the Corresponding Point is the spot on the right wrist which corresponds to the most painful spot on the left wrist.

Manipulation: The same as above.

3. Ear Acupuncture

Indication: Acute wrist sprain.

Ear Point Prescription:
The tender point, Shenmen, Liver, Spleen, Heart.

Manipulation: See page 255-256.

Comment:
Zhenjiu is very effective in the treatment of acute wrist sprain. In most cases, it can be cured by Zhenjiu treatment. In clinics, usually, Zhenjiu can be taken as the first choice in its treatment. It is always important in the treatment that one has the patient's cooperation by moving the diseased part when the needle in the distal point is twisted, thrust and lifted.

Notes:

54. Acute Ankle Sprain

Acute ankle sprain refers to acute sprain of the ankle muscles and fasciae. It is clinically marked by an apparent history of trauma, followed by sharp pain, tenderness, and swelling in the ankle on one or both sides, and limitation of the joint movement. It is called Huai Niu Shang in Chinese.

I. STANDARD TREATMENT

Acute ankle sprain is generally diagnosed in differentiation as syndrome of stagnation of qi and blood.

Stagnation of Qi and Blood

Manifestations: Abrupt onset of sharp pain, tenderness and swelling in the ankle region on one or both sides, and limitation of the ankle joint movement following an external injury of the ankle joint.

Tongue: Normal.

Pulse: Wiry and tight or normal.

Treatment Principle: Activate blood and resolve blood stasis, dredge the meridian and activate the collateral, promote circulation of qi and relieve pain.

Point Prescription & Manipulation:
Primary points:
> The tender points in the ankle region ^
> ST-41 Jiexi   - ^
> BL-60 Kunlun   - ^
> GB-40 Qiuxu   - ^
> GB-39 Xuanzhong   - ^

Explanation:
• The tender points in the ankle region, ST-41 Jiexi, BL-60 Kunlun, and GB-40 Qiuxu, located at the diseased region, warm the meridians, promote blood and qi movement, activate the collaterals, remove blood stasis, and arrest pain;

• GB-39 Xuanzhong, the Influential Point of Marrow, strengthens the bones.

Secondary points according to conditions:
1□   Stabbing pain—BL-17 Geshu [-].

II. EXPERIENTIAL TREATMENT

1. Puncturing SJ-5 Waiguan

Indication: Acute and chronic ankle joint sprain.

Point Prescription:
> SJ-5 Waiguan of the diseased side.

Manipulation: Insert a 1.5-cun long needle perpendicularly into SJ-5 Waiguan 1-1.2 cun while rotating it. After arrival of qi, rotate, lift and thrust the needle repeatedly while asking the patient to move the diseased joint simultaneously during the manipulation.   When the pain becomes milder, retain the needle for about 20-40 minutes.   For a patient with recent sprain and obvious redness, swelling and pain of the diseased region, manipulate the needle with strong stimulation, and retain the needle for 10-15 minutes with manipulation every 5 minutes. For a patient with a chronic sprain and no obvious redness, swelling and pain of the diseased region, manipulate the needle with gentle stimulation, retain the needle for 30-40 minutes, and manipulate it every 10 minutes. The treatment is given once daily, and generally within 1-4 treatments the disease will be cured or greatly relieved.

2. Puncturing GB-34 Yanglingquan

Indication: Acute ankle joint sprain.

Point Prescription:
> GB-34 Yanglingquan of the diseased side.

Manipulation: Insert a 1.5-cun long needle perpendicularly into GB-34 Yanglingquan 1 cun, manipulate the needle with strong stimulation to induce arrival of qi. Then, retain the needle for 20 minutes, manipulating the needle 3-4 times during the retention to induce the needling sensation radiating to the ankle.   The treatment is given once daily. Generally, the pain will be relieved after one treatment, and cured within 3-5 treatments.

3. Puncture SJ-4 Yangchi

Indication: Acute ankle joint sprain.

Point Prescription:
SJ-4 Yangchi of the diseased side or of the healthy side.

Manipulation: If selecting SJ-4 Yangchi of the diseased side, puncture perpendicularly 0.3-0.5 cun, manipulate the needle to induce arrival of qi, retain the needle for 30 minutes, and ask the patient to massage the ankle region during the retention. If selecting the point on the healthy side, puncture perpendicularly 0.5-0.8 cun, perform strong stimulation, and ask the patient to move the ankle joint during the manipulation, and remove the needle when the pain becomes milder. Usually, after treatment, the pain will be immediately relieved or even disappear.

4. Puncturing the Corresponding Point on the Ankle

Indication: Acute wrist sprain.

Point Prescription:
The Corresponding Point, which is on the ankle of the healthy side, and corresponds to the most painful spot of the injured region. Namely, if the left ankle joint is injured, the Corresponding Point is the spot on the right ankle, which corresponds to the most painful spot on the left ankle.

Manipulation:
Method 1: Insert a 1-cun long needle in to the Corresponding Point on the ankle, lift, thrust and rotate the needle repeatedly to induce and keep the needling sensation. Constantly manipulate the needle for 15-20 minutes, and ask the patient to move the diseased joint simultaneously during the manipulation. Usually, pain will be milder immediately. The treatment is given once daily. Generally, the pain will be relieved greatly after one treatment.

Method 2: Insert a 1-cun long needle into the Corresponding Point horizontally at 15 degrees 0.8 cun, rotate the needle for 15 seconds gently, inducing no needling sensation or little to the patient. Then, retain the needle in the point for 20 minutes. Ask the patient to move the diseased part during the retention. Usually, pain will be milder immediately. The treatment is given once daily, and usually within 3 treatments the pain will disappear.

5. Ear Acupuncture

Indication: Acute ankle sprain.

Ear Point Prescription:
The tender point, Shenmen, Liver, Spleen, Heart.

Manipulation: See page 255-256.

Comment:
Zhenjiu is very effective in the treatment of acute ankle sprain. In most cases, it can be cured by Zhenjiu treatment. In clinics, usually, Zhenjiu can be taken as the first choice in treatment. It is always important in the treatment that one has the patient's cooperation in moving the diseased part when the needle in the distal point is twisted, thrust and lifted.

Notes:

55. Chronic Lumbar Muscle Strain

Chronic lumbar muscle strain refers to chronic lower back pain. It is usually caused by poor posture, overuse of the waist, and exposure to cold and dampness. It is clinically characterized by intermittent or persistent soreness, pain, and heaviness in the lumbar region, alleviated after appropriate movement and aggravated by extended sitting or standing or cold and rainy weather. There is usually a history of acute lumbar sprain. According to TCM, chronic lumbar muscle strain is classified into Yao Tong (lumbago), Shen Zhuo (chronic lumbago), and it is due to external trauma, or internal deficiency of body resistance and incision of wind-cold or cold-damp, resulting in obstruction of qi and blood in the meridians.

I. STANDARD TREATMENT

Chronic lumbar muscle strain is usually divided into three types—obstruction due to wind-cold and dampness, retention of blood stasis and deficiency of kidney yang. Points of the Urinary Bladder and Du Meridians are selected for its treatment.

1. Obstruction of the Meridian due to Wind-Cold-Damp

Manifestations: Repeated attack of alternatively mild or severe pain in the lumbar region, which is accompanied with soreness, distention, heaviness and stiffness, is relieved when warmth is given and aggravated when cold is given.

Tongue: Pale body with white and sticky coating.

Pulse: Soft and slow.

Treatment Principle: Dispel wind and cold, remove dampness, and dredge the collateral.

Point Prescription & Manipulation:
Primary points:
    Ashi Points
    DU-16 Fengfu   /

BL-25 Dachangshu + ^
BL-40 Weizhong - or /
SP-9 Yinlingquan - or /
ST-36 Zusanli + ^
BL-26 Guanyuanshu + ^
DU-3 Yaoyangguan + ^

Explanation:
Ashi Points are punctured by inserting the needle in several directions at each point.

- DU-16 Fengfu strengthens the Du Meridian and dispels wind and cold;
- Ashi Points, BL-26 Guanyuanshu, DU-3 Yaoyangguan, and BL-25 Dachangshu, located at the diseased region, warm the meridians, dispel wind-cold-dampness, promote blood and qi movement, activate the collaterals, remove blood stasis, and arrest pain.;
- BL-40 Weizhong removes blood stasis;
- SP-9 Yinlingquan and ST-36 Zusanli reinforce the spleen and stomach and remove dampness.

Secondary points according to conditions:
1️⃣ Lower back pain radiating to the leg — BL-60 Kunlun [-].

2. Internal Retention of Blood Stasis

Manifestations: Long-term repeated attacks of stabbing and fixed pain in the lumbar region, which is relieved when moving the lumbar region gently.

Tongue: Dark-red tongue with ecchymoses.

Pulse: Wiry and uneven.

Treatment Principle: Promote circulation of qi, activate blood, and dredge the collateral.

Point Prescription & Manipulation:
Primary points:
    Ashi Points
    BL-40 Weizhong
    BL-17 Geshu
    LR-3 Taichong

BL-25 Dachangshu
DU-3 Yaoyangguan
BL-23 Shenshu

Explanation:
Acupuncture is taken as the main, and cupping as the assistant. Three to five points are applied at each treatment. After insertion of the needles into the points, lift, thrust and rotate the needles with reducing manipulation to induce arrival of qi. Then, retain the needles for 20-40 minutes, and manipulate the needles every 10 minutes. Ashi Points are punctured by inserting the needle to several directions in each point. BL-40 Weizhong and the painful area may be pricked by the three-edged needle and cupping applied to cause bleeding 2-10 ml. The treatment with the filiform needle is given once daily and with three-edged needle and cupping once every 3-5 days.

- BL-40 Weizhong and BL-17 Geshu activate blood and remove blood stasis;
- LR-3 Taichong promotes qi flow to assist circulation of blood;
- BL-25 Dachangshu, DU-3 Yaoyangguan, BL-23 Shenshu, and Ashi Points, located in the diseased area, warm the meridians, promote blood and qi movement, activate the collaterals, remove blood stasis, and arrest pain.

Secondary points according to conditions:
1□ Lower back pain radiating to the leg — BL-60 Kunlun [-].

3. Deficiency of Kidney Yang

Manifestations: Dull pain with soreness and weakness in the lumbar region, which is aggravated by long-term standing or physical labor, pale expression, lassitude, listlessness, nocturnal emission, impotence.

Tongue: Pale body with white coating.

Pulse: Deep and weak.

Treatment Principle: Warm the kidney, strengthen yang and activate the collateral.

Point Prescription & Manipulation:
Primary points:
BL-23 Shenshu   + ^
BL-26 Guanyuanshu   + ^
KI-3 Taixi   + ^
BL-25 Dachangshu   + ^
DU-3 Yaoyangguan   + ^
ST-36 Zusanli   + ^

- BL-23 Shenshu, BL-26 Guanyuanshu, BL-25 Dachangshu, and DU-3 Yaoyangguan, located at the diseased region, warm the meridians, promote blood and qi movement, activate the collaterals, and arrest pain;
- KI-3 Taixi, BL-23 Shenshu and BL-26 Guanyuanshu tonify and warm the kidney yang;
- ST-36 Zusanli reinforces the spleen and stomach to promote generation of qi and blood.

Secondary points according to conditions:
1□ Impotence — DU-4 Mingmen [+ ^];
2□ Frequent urination — BL-28 Pangguanshu [+ ^].

II. EXPERIENTIAL TREATMENT

1. Puncturing BL-10 Tianzhu

Indication: Chronic Lumbar Strain.

Point Prescription:
BL-10 Tianzhu

Manipulation: Ask the patient to sit down with the head slightly bent. Press bilateral BL-10 Tianzhu with the thumbs and knead it a moment. Then, insert a 1.5-cun long needle into the point quickly and push the needle to 0.8 cun with its tip toward the corresponding intervertebral foramen. About 3-5 minutes after the insertion, usually the pain will be milder. Then, retain the needle for 20-30 minutes, and ask the patient to move the lumbar region until there is a little sweating on the lumbar region during the retention. The treatment is given once daily, with 10 treatments as a course.

2. Acupuncture & Moxibustion on Three Points

Indication: Chronic lumbar strain with syndrome of attack by wind-cold-damp.

Point Prescription:
  SI-6 Yanglao of the diseased side
  BL-52 Zhishi
  BL-23 Shenshu

Manipulation: Acupuncture and moxibustion are applied simultaneously. Firstly, ask the patient to raise the hand with the center of the palm facing inwards, insert a 2-cun long needle into SI-6 Yanglao at an angle of 45 degrees with its tip towards the elbow to 1.7 cun, frequently rotate the needle with even reinforcing and reducing manipulation to induce the needling sensation radiating to the elbow, back and lumbar region, and ask the patient to move the lumbar region until there is a little sweating there during the manipulation.   Then, Insert the needle perpendicularly into BL-23 Shenshu and BL-52 Zhishi 1.2 cun deep, and rotate the needles with reinforcing manipulation to induce the needling sensation.   Finally, retain the needles and apply warming needling method on the points until the local skin becomes flushed.   The treatment is given once daily, with 10 treatments as a course.

3. Ear Acupuncture

Indication: Chronic lumbar strain.

Ear Point Prescription:
  Waist, Sacral Vertebrae, Kidney, Urinary Bladder, Liver, Spleen, Shenmen.

Manipulation: See page 255-256.

Comment:
Zhenjiu is effective in the treatment of chronic lumbar sprain. But as this disease is obstinate, generally, in most cases, a long term of Zhenjiu treatment is needed, and some other treatment methods should be employed in addition.

Notes:

56. Thecal Cyst

Thecal cyst, called ganglion also, is a common benign tumor in the hand. It often occurs on the dorsum of the wrist. Its cause is uncertain. It is clinically marked by a cyst which is shaped as a ball, with smooth border and without adhesion with the surrounding tissue, and soft and plastic. Usually, it does not have symptoms.   According to TCM, thecal cyst belongs to the categories of Jin Liu (tumor of the tendon) or Rou Liu   (tumor of the muscle), and it is due to accumulation of qi and phlegm in the local region.

I. STANDARD TREATMENT

As thecal cyst does not have symptoms, no treatment based on differentiation of syndromes is given.

II. EXPERIENTIAL TREATMENT

1. Circling Puncture

Indication: Thecal cyst.

Point Prescription:
  The center point of the cyst as well as four points on the border of the cyst which are respectively above, below, left and right.

Manipulation: Insert a needle perpendicularly into the center point, and obliquely into the points on the border with the needle tip towards the center of the bottom of the cyst, lift, thrust and rotate the needles to induce the needling sensation, and retain the needles for 20 minutes. Then, take out the needles and squeeze or press the cyst. Generally, only one treatment is needed to cure this disease. In case it does not so, repeat the same treatment on the day after the next day.

2. Prick with Three-Edged Needle

Indication: Thecal cyst.

Point Prescription:
  The center of the cyst.

Manipulation: After sterilization, prick the center point of the cyst with three-edged needle to break the cyst, squeeze the cyst to let out all of the liquid of the cyst, place a coin which is the same size as the cyst, and bind the area with pressure for 3-5 days. Generally, only one treatment is needed to cure this disease. In case the thecal cyst relapses, use the same manipulation for its treatment.

Comment:

Zhenjiu is effective in the treatment of thecal cyst. In most cases, it can be cured by Zhenjiu treatment. In clinics, usually, Zhenjiu can be taken as the first choice in its treatment.

Notes:

57. Calcaneodynia

Calcaneodynia is a common symptom of various diseases of the heel, including calcaneal spur, epiphysitis of calcaneum, calcanitis and calcaneal bursitis. It is clinically marked by pain in the calcaneal region, aggravated by walking or standing. There is usually a tender point on the tuberosity of the calcaneus, but no redness or swelling. According to TCM, calcaneodynia belongs to Gen Tong (painful heels), and it is due to deficiency of kidney, leading to poor nourishment of the bone, or attack by cold-damp pathogen, leading to obstruction of the collaterals and vessels.

I. STANDARD TREATMENT

Calcaneodynia is generally divided into two types — excess and deficiency, and the local points are frequently selected in its treatment.

1. Excess

Manifestations: Abrupt attack of pain of the heel, which is usually induced by attack of cold and dampness, and marked by fixed pain, aggravated by cold and alleviated by warmth.

Tongue: White and thin coating.

Pulse: Wiry.

Treatment Principle: Warm the meridian, dispel cold, and arrest pain.

Point Prescription & Manipulation:
  BL-60 Kunlun   + ^
  KI-6 Zhaohai   + ^
  KI-3 Taixi   + ^

Explanation:
- BL-60 Kunlun, KI-6 Zhaohai and KI-3 Taixi, located at the diseased region, warm the meridians, dispel cold and dampness, promote blood and qi movement, activate the collaterals, remove blood stasis, and arrest pain.

2. Deficiency

Manifestations: Dull pain of the heel, which is gradually progressive, alleviated by warmth and pressure, and soreness and weakness of the low back and knees.

Tongue: Pale body.

Pulse: Wiry and thready.

Treatment Principle: Warm the kidney, strengthen the bone, and arrest pain.

Point Prescription & Manipulation:
    BL-60 Kunlun + ^
    KI-6 Zhaohai + ^
    KI-3 Taixi + ^
    BL-23 Shenshu + ^
    BL-18 Ganshu + ^

Explanation:
- BL-60 Kunlun, KI-6 Zhaohai and KI-3 Taixi, located at the diseased region, warm the meridians, promote blood and qi movement, activate the collaterals, and arrest pain;
- BL-23 Shenshu and BL-18 Ganshu, the Back-Shu Points of the kidney and liver, tonify the kidney and liver and strengthen the tendons and bones.

II. EXPERIENTIAL TREATMENT

1. Puncturing Heel Point of the Hand Acupuncture

Indication: Calcaneal spur.

Point Prescription:
    Heel Point of the Hand Acupuncture of the healthy side, located on the depression 0.8 cun directly distal to PC-7 Daling.

Manipulation: Insert a 1-cun needle through the skin of the point, push the needle obliquely upwards 0.3-0.5 cun deep, and manipulate the needle gently until the patient feels heat sensation of the palms, lumber and back, and obvious relief of pain in the heel. Then, rotate the needle at large amplitude, and ask the patient to stand with the painful heel on a hard material, pressing the material with the force gradually from mild to heavy. Repeat this course several times. The treatment is given once daily and 15 treatments are taken as a course.

2. Applying Bleeding & Moxibustion

Indication: Severe pain of the heel aggravated by walking.

Point Prescription:
    BL-57 Chengshan on the diseased side
    The tender point of the diseased heel

Manipulation: Look for the most painful point of the heel of the diseased side, prick the point and BL-57 Chengshan of the same side to make blood out 3-4 drops each, press the needle holes with sterilized cotton ball to stop bleeding. Then ignite a moxa stick and apply moxibustion on the heel for 10-15 minutes to make the local skin flushed and induce slight burning pain to the patient. Generally, only one treatment is needed for arrest the pain. In case not effective, repeat this course 5 days later.

3. Puncturing Scalp Lines

Indication: Calcaneodynia.

Line Prescription:
    Foot-Kinesthetic Sensory Area of the healthy side.

Manipulation: Insert a needle horizontally, rotate the needle at frequency of 150-200 times per minute for 2-3 minutes, and rotate the needle again after an interval of 10 minutes. Repeat this course 3 times. The treatment is given once every other day and 10 treatments taken as a course. Usually, 2-3 courses are needed to cure this disorder.

Comment:
Zhenjiu is effective in the treatment of calcaneodynia. In most cases, it can be cured by Zhenjiu treatment. In clinic, usually, Zhenjiu can be taken as the first choice in treatment.

Notes:

CHAPTER THREE
GYNECOLOGICAL
DISEASES

58. Dysmenorrhea

Dysmenorrhea is a common gynecological disorder, marked by pain in the lower abdomen or lower back before, during, or after menstruation. It is often accompanied by nausea, vomiting, headache, and dizziness. It may be divided into two types—primary or functional dysmenorrhea referring to the one which is not caused by organic diseases, and secondary dysmenorrhea referring to the one caused by organic diseases in reproductive system. Primary dysmenorrhea may be caused by lack of exercise, anxiety about menses, a narrow cervical os, and malposition of the uterus. Secondary dysmenorrhea may result from endometriosis, adenomyosis, and pelvic inflammatory diseases. According to TCM, dysmenorrhea, called Tong Jing in Chinese, is caused by attack of cold during the menstruation or stagnation of liver qi, resulting in blood stagnation, or by deficiency of blood, resulting in depriving the Chong and Ren Meridians of nourishment.

I. STANDARD TREATMENT

Dysmenorrhea is generally divided into four types — stagnation of qi and blood, accumulation of cold-dampness, qi and blood deficiency, and deficiency of liver and kidney. Points of the Ren, Liver, Spleen and Kidney meridians are frequently selected in its treatment.

1. Stagnation of Qi and Blood

Manifestations: Distending or colic pain in the lower abdomen, usually starting before menstruation or during menstruation, radiating to the lower back, and alleviated by passing out the clots, retarded and scanty and dark purple menses with clots, distending pain in the lower abdomen, distention in the hypochondriac region and breast.

Tongue: Purplish body with purple spots on its edge.

Pulse: Deep and wiry.

Treatment Principle: Promote circulation of qi and blood and stop pain.

Point Prescription & Manipulation:
Primary points:
    RN-6 Qihai /
    SP-8 Diji -
    LI-4 Hegu   -
    LR-3 Taichong -

Explanation:
- RN-6 Qihai regulates qi activities of the lower-jiao and arrests lower abdominal pain;
- SP-8 Diji, the Xi-Cleft Point of the Spleen Meridian, having a very good effect on dysmenorrhea, arrests pain;
- LR-3 Taichong and LI-4 Hegu, the Four Gate Points, soothe the liver, promote flow of qi and blood, and restore menstrual flow.

Secondary points according to conditions:
1⥎   Menses with clots — SP-10 Xuehai [-] and SP-6 Sanyinjiao [-].

2. Accumulation of Cold-Dampness

Manifestations: Colic pain and coldness in the lower abdomen, which are relieved by warmth, retarded and scanty purple menses with clots, cold limbs, and aversion to clod.

Tongue: White and sticky coating.

Pulse: Deep and tight.

Treatment Principle: Warm the meridians, disperse cold, remove dampness, and stop pain.

Point Prescription & Manipulation:
Primary points:
    RN-4 Guanyuan + ^
    SP-6 Sanyinjiao - ^
    BL-23 Shenshu + ^
    BL-32 Ciliao - ^

KI-12 Dahe   - ^

Explanation:
- RN-4 Guanyuan and BL-23 Shenshu warm the lower-jiao, and dispel cold-dampness from the uterus;
- SP-6 Sanyinjiao promotes flow of qi and blood and regulates menstruation;
- BL-32 Ciliao and KI-12 Dahe warm the Kidney and Bladder Meridians and dispel cold.

Secondary points according to conditions:
1⥎   Severe pain — SP-8 Diji [- ^] and DU-4 Mingmen [+ ^].

3. Deficiency of Qi and Blood

Manifestations: Dull pain in the lower abdomen, usually appearing during and after menstruation, accompanied with empty sensation in the lower abdomen, and alleviated by pressure, pink, scanty and thin menses, sallow complexion, lassitude, dizziness, blurred vision, palpitation.

Tongue: Pale body with thin coating.

Pulse: Thready and weak.

Treatment Principle: Tonify qi and blood and stop pain.

Point Prescription & Manipulation:
Primary points:
    RN-6 Qihai + ^
    ST-36 Zusanli + ^
    BL-20 Pishu + ^
    BL-21 Weishu + ^
    SP-6 Sanyinjiao + ^

Explanation:
- RN-6 Qihai tonifies qi and warms and nourishes the uterus;
- ST-36 Zusanli, BL-20 Pishu and BL-21 Weishu reinforce the spleen and stomach, and promote generation of qi and blood;

- SP-6 Sanyinjiao promotes flow of qi and blood, and regulates menstruation.

Secondary points according to conditions:
1꠱ Dizziness and blurred vision — BL-18 Ganshu [+ ^];
2꠱ Palpitation and insomnia —BL-15 Xinshu [+ ^].

4. Deficiency of Liver and Kidney

Manifestations: Dull pain in the lower abdomen, irregular menstruation, pink and scanty menses, soreness and weakness of the lower back and knees, dizziness, tinnitus, blurred vision.

Tongue: Red and thin body.

Pulse: Thready pulse.

Treatment Principle: Tonify liver and kidney.

Point Prescription & Manipulation:
Primary points:
  BL-18 Ganshu +
  BL-23 Shenshu +
  KI-6 Zhaohai +
  RN-4 Guanyuan +
  SP-6 Sanyinjiao +
  SP-10 Xuehai +

Explanation:
- BL-18 Ganshu and BL-23 Shenshu, the Back-Shu Points of the liver and kidney, tonify the liver and kidney, and regulate the Chong and Ren Meridians;
- KI-6 Zhaohai reinforces the kidney and nourishes the Ren Meridian;
- RN-4 Guanyuan tonifies essence and blood, reinforces the Liver, Kidney, Chong and Ren Meridians, and nourishes the uterus;
- SP-6 Sanyinjiao and SP-10 Xuehai reinforce qi of the three Foot-Yin Meridians, activate blood and promote menstrual flow.

Secondary points according to conditions:

1꠱ Insomnia — EX-HN-16 Anmian [+].

II. EXPERIENTIAL TREATMENT

1. Puncturing EX-B-8 Shiqizhui

Indication: Dysmenorrhea.

Point Prescription:
  EX-B-8 Shiqizhui

Manipulation: Puncture perpendicularly 1-1.5 cun to induce arrival of qi, rotate the needle quickly with strong stimulation to make the needling sensation radiating to the lower abdomen until the pain becomes mild of disappears, retain the needle for 10 minutes. Usually 1-3 treatments are needed to cure this disease.

2. Acupuncture & Moxibustion on BL-55 Heyang

Indication: Dysmenorrhea.

Point Prescription:
  BL-55 Heyang

Manipulation: Puncture perpendicularly 1-1.5 cun, perform even reinforcing and reducing manipulation to induce the needling sensation radiating to the bottom of the foot. Then, put a 0.5- or 1-cun long segment of moxa stick on the needle handle, and make moxibustion for about 15 minutes. The treatment is given once daily before or during the menstruation, with 5 treatments as a course. Usually, 2-3 courses of the treatment are needed to cure this disease.

3. Puncturing BL-32 Ciliao

Indication: Dysmenorrhea.

Point Prescription:
  BL-32 Ciliao

Manipulation: Puncture perpendicularly 2-3 cun to induce heaviness, distention or soreness and numbness in the lower abdomen, perform reducing manipulation by rotating the needles, retain the needles for 20-30 minutes, and manipulate them 1 or 2 times. Usually, only one treatment is effective to cure this disease.

4. Moxibustion on BL-67 Zhiyin

Indication: Dysmenorrhea belonging to cold syndrome.

Point Prescription:
BL-67 Zhiyin

Manipulation: Keep the ignited end of the moxa stick 1 cun away from the point for about 15-30 minutes until the local skin becomes flushed and the patient can not stand. The treatment is given once daily, from 3 days before the menstruation to the end of the menstruation. Usually, within 2 menstrual cycles of the treatment, the disease will be cured.

5. Puncturing BL-57 Chengshan

Indication: Dysmenorrhea due to blood stasis.

Point Prescription:
BL-57 Chengshan

Manipulation: Puncture perpendicularly 1.5 cun to induce arrival of qi, perform reducing manipulation for 2 minutes, retain the needles for 30 minutes, and manipulate every 10 minutes. The treatment is given before or during menstruation, once daily, with 3-7 times as a course. Usually, only one course of the treatment is needed to cure this disease.

Comment:
Zhenjiu is very effective in the treatment of dysmenorrhea. In most cases, it is effective to cure this disease. Generally, Zhenjiu treatment should be given 7-10 days before menstruation and until the menses comes, and another 1-2 courses of the treatment should be given after dysmenorrhea disappears in order to consolidate the result.

Notes:

59. Irregular Menstruation

Irregular menstruation refers to any abnormal change in menstrual cycle, in quantity and color of flow, and other accompanying symptoms. Its cause may include emotional, physical or mental hardships, improper diet, malnutrition, sexually transmitted diseases, pelvic infection diseases, endometriosis and ovarian cysts. Common cases are antedated and post-dated menstruation, irregular menstrual cycle. Menstruation earlier than due time by seven to eight days, or even twice a month, is regarded as antedated menstruation, while menses later than due time by eight to nine days or even once every forty to fifty days is considered as post-dated menstruation. According to TCM, irregular menstruation, called Yue Jing Bu Tiao in Chinese, is caused by many factors, such as exogenous pathogenic cold, heat, and dampness, emotional disturbances — worries, depressed rage, indulgence in sexual life, grand multiparity, etc., leading to the disharmony between qi and blood and the injury of the Chong and Ren Meridians.

I. STANDARD TREATMENT

Irregular menstruation is generally divided into three types — antedated menstruation, post-dated menstruation, and irregular menstrual cycles, and its treatment is always based on distinguishing deficiency and excess, cold and heat. Points of the Ren, Spleen, Bladder Meridians are frequently selected its treatment.

1. Antedated Menstruation

A. Blood Heat

Manifestations: Shortened cycle, menses coming 7 days or more earlier than the normal cycle, dark red and thick blood flow in large quantities, restlessness, fullness in the chest, brown urine.

Tongue: Red body with yellow coating.

Pulse: Rapid and forceful.

Treatment Principle: Clear heat from blood, regulate Chong and Ren Meridians.

Point Prescription & Manipulation:
Primary points:
    RN-3 Zhongji -
    SP-6 Xuehai -
    LR-3 Taichong -

Explanation:
- RN-3 Zhongji, the Crossing Point of the Ren Meridian and three Foot-Yin Meridians, clears heat from the uterus and regulates the Ren Meridian;
- SP-6 Xuehai cools blood;
- LR-3 Taichong clears heat from the Liver Meridian and regulates the Chong Meridian.

Secondary points according to conditions:
1☐ Blood heat of excess type — LI-11 Quchi [-];
2☐ Blood heat of deficiency type — SP-6 Sanyinjiao [+] and KI-2 Rangu [+];
3☐ Heat with phlegm — LR-2 Xingjian [-] and SP-8 Diji [-];
4☐ Headache — GB-20 Fengchi [-].

B. Qi Deficiency

Manifestations: Profuse, thin and light red menses in shortened cycles (menses coming 7 days or more earlier than the normal cycle), lassitude, palpitation, shortness of breath, empty and heavy sensation in the lower abdomen.

Tongue: Pale body with thin coating.

Pulse: Weak.

Treatment Principle: Reinforce spleen and replenish qi to restore its function in controlling blood.

Point Prescription & Manipulation:
Primary points:

    RN-6 Qihai + ^
    DU-20 Baihui + ^
    ST-36 Zusanli + ^
    SP-6 Sanyinjiao + ^
    BL-20 Pishu + ^
    BL-23 Shenshu + ^

Explanation:
- RN-6 Qihai reinforces qi, consolidates the Ren and Chong Meridians, and nourishes the uterus;
- DU-20 Baihui, a point of the Du Meridian which governs yang qi and located at the highest region of the body, raises the sunken and consolidates the uterus;
- ST-36 Zusanli, SP-6 Sanyinjiao and BL-20 Pishu reinforce the spleen's function of controlling blood;
- BL-23 Shenshu reinforces the kidney to strengthen the Ren Meridian.

Secondary points according to conditions:
1☐ Severe cases — RN-12 [+ ^] and SP-10 Xuehai [+];
2☐ Spontaneous sweating — BL-13 Feishu [+ ^] and LI-4 Hegu [/].

2. Post-Dated Menstruation

A. Blood Deficiency

Manifestations: Scanty and light red menses in delayed cycle (7 days later or 40-50 days in delayed menstrual cycle), empty and painful feeling in the lower abdomen, emaciation, sallow complexion, lusterless skin, dizziness and blurred vision, palpitation, insomnia.

Tongue: Pink body with little coating.

Pulse: Weak and thready.

Treatment Principle: Replenish qi, nourish blood, and regulate the Chong and Ren Meridians.

Point Prescription & Manipulation:
Primary points:

RN-4 Guanyuan + ^
RN-6 Qihai + ^
ST-36 Zusanli + ^
SP-6 Sanyinjiao + ^
BL-20 Pishu + ^
KI-13 Qixue + ^

Explanation:
- RN-4 Guanyuan and RN-6 Qihai reinforce qi, regulate the Ren and Chong Meridians, and nourish the uterus;
- ST-36 Zusanli and BL-20 Pishu reinforce the spleen and stomach and promote generation of qi and blood;
- KI-13 Qixue, the Crossing Point of the Kidney and Chong Meridians, regulates the Chong and Ren Meridians;
- SP-6 Sanyinjiao, the Crossing Point of three Foot-Yin Meridians, reinforces the spleen and promotes menstrual flow.

Secondary points according to conditions:
1☐ Severe cases — BL-17 Geshu [+ ^];
2☐ Dizziness and blurred vision — BL-18 Ganshu [+ ^];
3☐ Palpitation and insomnia —BL-15 Xinshu [+ ^].

B. Cold in Blood

Manifestations: Scanty and dark-colored menses in delayed cycle (7 days later or 40-50 days in delayed menstrual cycle), colic pain in the lower abdomen, slightly alleviated by warmth, cold limbs.

Tongue: Thin and white body.

Pulse: Deep and slow.

Treatment Principle: Disperse cold, warm the uterus, and promote circulation of blood.

Point Prescription & Manipulation:
Primary points:
RN-4 Guanyuan + ^
RN-6 Qihai + ^

ST-36 Zusanli + ^
SP-6 Sanyinjiao + ^

Explanation:
- RN-4 Guanyuan and RN-6 Qihai warm the lower-jiao and dispel cold from the uterus;
- ST-36 Zusanli and SP-6 Sanyinjiao strengthen the spleen and promote menstrual flow.

Secondary points according to conditions:
1☐ Pain during menses—SP-8 Diji [+ ^];
2☐ Cold excess syndrome—ST-29 Guilai [+ ^] and ST-25 Tianshu [+ ^}.

C. Qi Stagnation

Manifestations: Scanty menses in delayed cycle (7 days later or 40-50 days in delayed menstrual cycle), distending pain in the lower abdomen, mental depression, stuffy sensation in the chest and hypochondriac region, belching.

Tongue: Thin and white coating.

Pulse: Wiry.

Treatment Principle: Promote circulation of qi and regulate the Chong and Ren Meridians.

Point Prescription & Manipulation:
Primary points:
LR-3 Taichong -
SP-8 Diji -
SP-9 Sanyinjiao /
RN-6 Qihai /
RN-17 Danzhong -

Explanation:
- LR-3 Taichong soothes the liver and promotes qi flow;
- SP-8 Diji and SP-9 Sanyinjiao promote menstrual flow;
- RN-6 Qihai promotes qi flow and regulates the Chong and Ren Meridians;
- RN-17 Danzhong relieves qi stagnation.

Secondary points according to conditions:
1☐ Severe cases — LR-5 Ligou [-] and GB-34 Yanglingquan [-];
2☐ Headache — LI-4 Hegu [-] and GB-20 Fengchi [-].

3. Irregular Menstruation

A. Liver Qi Stagnation

Manifestations: Alteration of menstrual cycles and quantity of blood flow, thick, sticky, and purple colored menses difficult to flow, distention in the hypochondriac region and breast, distending pain in the lower abdomen, mental depression, frequent sighing.

Tongue: Thin and white coating.

Pulse: Wiry.

Treatment Principle: Relieve depressed qi in the liver, and regulate the Chong and Ren Meridians.

Point Prescription & Manipulation:
Primary points:
LR-3 Taichong -
PC-6 Neiguan -
RN-17 Danzhong -
SP-8 Diji -
KI-14 Siman -

Explanation:
• LR-3 Taichong and PC-6 Neiguan soothe the liver and promote qi flow;
• RN-17 Danzhong relieves qi stagnation;
• SP-8 Diji, an effective point to regulate menstruation, and KI-14 Siman, the Crossing Point of the Kidney Meridian with the Chong Meridian, regulate the Chong and Ren Meridians and regulate menstruation.

Secondary points according to conditions:
1☐ Chronic case — LI-4 Hegu [-] and LR-14 Qimen [-];

2☐ Headache — LI-4 Hegu [-] and GB-20 Fengchi [-].

B. Kidney Deficiency

Manifestations: Early or late menstrual cycle, scanty, light red blood flow in altering cycles, dizziness, tinnitus, soreness and weakness of the lower back and knees, frequent night urination, loose stools.

Tongue: Pale body with thin coating.

Pulse: Deep and weak.

Treatment Principle: Replenish the kidney qi and regulate the Chong and Ren Meridians.

Point Prescription & Manipulation:
Primary points:
RN-4 Guanyuan + ^
BL-23 Shenshu + ^
SP-6 Sanyinjiao + ^
KI-8 Jiaoxin + ^
BL-18 Ganshu + ^

Explanation:
• RN-4 Guanyuan strengthens the primary qi and nourishes the uterus;
• BL-23 Shenshu and BL-18 Ganshu, the Back-Shu Points of the kidney and liver, strengthen the kidney and liver and reinforce the Chong and Ren Meridians;
• SP-6 Sanyinjiao, the Crossing Point of the three Foot-Yin Meridians, and KI-8 Jiaoxin, having a good effect in treatment of irregular menstruation, nourish the kidney and liver, and regulate menstruation.

Secondary points according to conditions:
1☐ Chronic case — KI-3 Taixi [+] and KI-5 Shuiquan [+];
2☐ Pain during menses — SP-8 Diji [+ ^].

II. EXPERIENTIAL TREATMENT

1. Puncturing RN-4 Guanyuan, RN-6 Qihai and SP-6 Sanyinjiao

Indication: Post-dated menstruation due to deficiency.

Point Prescription:
Primary points:
  RN-4 Guanyuan
  RN-6 Qihai
  SP-6 Sanyinjiao

Secondary points according to conditions:
1. Poor appetite, borborygmus and diarrhea—RN-12 Zhongwan, ST-25 Tianshu and LR-13 Zhangmen;
2. Soreness and weakness of the loins and knees, cold limbs and fatigue — BL-18 Ganshu, BL-23 Shenshu and BL-26 Guanyuanshu;
3. Emotional depression, irritability, distressed feeling in the chest—BL-17 Geshu and BL-18 Ganshu.

Manipulation: Acupuncture is applied with reinforcing manipulation. The needle in RN-4 Guanyuan, RN-6 Qihai and SP-6 Sanyinjiao should be manipulated to induce a warm sensation radiating to the pubic region. After arrival of qi, the needles are retained for 20-40 minutes. The treatment is given once daily, with 10 treatments as a course.

2. Moxibustion on SP-1 Yinbai

Indication: Antedated menstruation due to qi deficiency.

Point Prescription:
  SP-1 Yinbai

Manipulation: Apply moxibustion with moxa stick 10 cm over the point for about 15-20 minutes to make the local skin flushed and burning sensation induced. The treatment can be given 3-5 times a day when there is a need to

arrest bleeding, and usually, the bleeding will be arrested on that day, and about 5 days of treatment are needed to prevent abnormal uterine bleeding in the next menstrual cycle.

Comment:
Zhenjiu is effective in the treatment of irregular menstruation. In some cases, it is effective to cure this disease. Generally, Zhenjiu treatment should be given 7-10 days before menstruation and until the menses comes, and another 1-2 courses of the treatment is needed after the menstrual cycle becomes normal in order to consolidate the result.

Notes:

60. Amenorrhea

Amenorrhea is classified into primary and secondary types. Primary amenorrhea refers to lack of onset of menstruation, even after eighteen years of age; secondary amenorrhea refers to cessation of previously normal menstruation for more than three months. Amenorrhea may be caused by malnutrition, over emotional stress, environmental change, and some reproductive organ diseases. According to TCM, amenorrhea belongs to Jing Bi (closing of menstruation), and it is caused by kidney deficiency, blood deficiency, phlegm and dampness, and attack of cold, leading to deficiency or obstruction of the Chong and Ren Meridians, resulting in disappearance of menstrual bleeding.

I. STANDARD TREATMENT

Amenorrhea is divided into five types—liver and kidney yin deficiency, spleen and kidney yang deficiency, deficiency of qi and blood, stagnation of qi and blood, and obstruction by phlegm and dampness. Points of the Ren, Kidney and Spleen Meridians are frequently selected in its treatment.

1. Liver and Kidney Yin Deficiency

Manifestations: Primary amenorrhea of a girl over 18 years old, or delayed menstruation cycle with scanty menstruation leading gradually to amenorrhea, constitutional debility, weakness and soreness of the loins and legs, dizziness, tinnitus, tide fever, night sweating.

Tongue: Reddish body with little coating.

Pulse: Deep and thready.

Treatment Principle: Tonify kidney and restore menstrual flow.

Point Prescription & Manipulation:

Primary points:
    BL-23 Shenshu +
    BL-52 Zhishi +
    RN-4 Guanyuan +
    SP-6 Sanyinjiao +
    KI-3 Taixi +

Explanation:
- BL-23 Shenshu, BL-52 Zhishi, and KI-3 Taixi tonify kidney yin;
- RN-4 Guanyuan, the Crossing Point of the Ren Meridian and three Foot-Yin Meridians, tonifies primary qi, nourishes the Chong and Ren Meridians, and promotes menstrual flow;
- SP-6 Sanyinjiao, the Crossing Point of the three Foot-Yin Meridians, tonifies yin and promotes menstrual flow.

Secondary points according to conditions:
1❑ Chronic cases — LR-3 Taichong [/] and SP-10 Xuehai [+];
2❑ Dizziness and blurred vision — BL-18 Ganshu [+];
3❑ Palpitation and insomnia —BL-15 Xinshu [+].

2. Spleen and Kidney Yang Deficiency

Manifestations: Primary amenorrhea of a girl over 18 years old, or delayed menstruation cycle with scanty menstruation leading gradually to amenorrhea, weakness and soreness of the loins, profuse night urination, poor appetite, loose stools or even diarrhea, cold limbs, aversion to cold, pale complexion.

Tongue: Pale body with white coating.

Pulse: Weak and deep.

Treatment Principle: Warm kidney, activate yang, and restore menstrual flow.

Point Prescription & Manipulation:
Primary points:
    BL-23 Shenshu + ^

DU-4 Minmen + ^
RN-4 Guanyuan + ^
RN-6 Qihai + ^
ST-29 Guilai + ^

Explanation:
- BL-23 Shenshu and DU-4 Minmen warm the kidney and strengthen yang;
- RN-4 Guanyuan and RN-6 Qihai reinforce primary qi, warm the Chong and Ren Meridians, and promote menstrual flow.
- ST-29 Guilai promotes qi movement and activates blood, and promotes menstrual flow.

Secondary points according to conditions:
1꘡ Edema — SP-9 Yinlingquan [+ ^] and KI-3 Taixi [+ ^]
2꘡ Poor appetite and loose stools — ST-25 Tianshu [+ ^], ST-36 Zusanli [+ ^] and SP-6 Yinlingquan [+ ^].

3. Deficiency of Qi and Blood

Manifestations: Gradual delay of menstruation with scanty blood which is thin and reddish, then leading to amenorrhea, pale complexion, dizziness, blurred vision, palpitation, lassitude.

Tongue: Pale body.

Pulse: Thready and weak.

Treatment Principle: Tonify qi and blood, restore menstrual flow.

Point Prescription & Manipulation:
Primary points:
ST-36 Zusanli + ^
SP-6 Sanyinjiao + ^
RN-6 Qihai + ^
ST-29 Guilai + ^
BL-20 Pishu + ^
BL-21 Weishu + ^

Explanation:

- ST-36 Zusanli, RN-6 Qihai, BL-20 Pishu and BL-21 Weishu reinforce the spleen and stomach, and promote generation of qi and blood;
- SP-6 Sanyinjiao and ST-29 Guilai promote qi circulation, activate blood movement and promote menstrual flow.

Secondary points according to conditions:
1꘡ Chronic cases — BL-18 Ganshu [+], BL-17 Geshu [+] and BL-23 Shenshu [+];
2꘡ Palpitation and dizziness—BL-15 Xinshu [+ ^] and BL-18 Ganshu [+ ^].

4. Qi Stagnation and Blood Stasis

Manifestations: Amenorrhea for several months, lower abdominal distending pain which is aggravated by pressure, mental distress, fidgets and liability to anger, distention and fullness in the chest and hypochondria.

Tongue: Purplish body with ecchymoses on the edges.

Pulse: Deep and uneven pulse.

Treatment Principle: Promote circulation of qi, remove blood stasis, and restore menstrual flow.

Points Prescription & Manipulation:
Primary points:
LI-4 Hegu -
LR-3 Taichong -
SP-6 Sanyinjiao -
SP-8 Diji -
SP-10 Xuehai -
ST-30 Qichong -

Explanation:
- LI-4 Hegu and LR-3 Taichong, the Four Gate Points, soothe liver, regulate qi and blood;
- SP-6 Sanyinjiao promotes qi movement, activates blood circulation, removes blood stasis, and promotes menstrual flow;

- SP-8 Diji and SP-10 Xuehai break blood stasis and promote menstrual flow;
- ST-30 Qichong, the point where the Chong Meridian qi is infused at the body surface, regulates the Chong Meridian and promotes menstrual flow.

Secondary points according to conditions:
1⦿ Chronic cases — RN-3 Zhongji [-] and BL-17 Geshu [/];
2⦿ Fixed and stabbing pain in lower abdomen — BL-17 Geshu [-] and SP-21 [-] are pricked to bleed.

5. Obstruction by Phlegm and Dampness

Manifestations: Gradual delay of menstruation leading to amenorrhea, excessive thin clear leukorrhea, obesity, distention and distressed feeling of the chest and abdomen, nausea, vomiting, sticky sensation of the mouth, spitting profuse sputum.

Tongue: Flattery body with sticky coating.

Pulse: Slippery.

Treatment Principle: Dry dampness, remove phlegm, and restore menstrual flow.

Point Prescription & Manipulation:
Primary points:
BL-20 Pishu + ^
BL-22 Sanjiaoshu + ^
BL-32 Ciliao + ^
RN-12 Zhongwan + ^
RN-3 Zhongji- ^
SP-6 Sanyinjiao/ ^
ST-40 Fenglong -

Explanation:
The points mentioned above might be divided into two groups and the two groups are used alternatively.

- BL-22 Sanjiaoshu regulates qi activities of the three jiaos and transforms phlegm;

- BL-32 Ciliao and RN-3 Zhongji, located at the lower abdomen and lower back, regulate the Chong and Ren Meridians and promote menstrual flow;
- SP-6 Sanyinjiao regulates the Chong and Ren Meridians and promotes menstrual flow;
- ST-40 Fenglong, the key point of transforming phlegm.

Secondary points according to conditions:
1⦿ Chronic cases — SP-8 Diji [-];
2⦿ Dizziness — GB-20 Fengchi [-];
3⦿ Oppressive feeling in the chest — PC-6 Neiguan [-].

II. EXPERIENTIAL TREATMENT

1. Puncturing DU-1 Changqiang

Indication: Amenorrhea.

Point Prescription:
DU-1 Changqiang

Manipulation: Ask the patient to lie down on the stomach, insert a 2-cun long needle into the point, manipulate the needle to induce strong stimulation, retain the needle for 20-40 minutes, and manipulate it every 5 minutes during the retention. The treatment is given once daily. Usually, within 3-5 treatments, menstruation will come. If 7 treatments have been given but the patient still does not have menstruation, it indicates the treatment is not effective to the patent and more time of the treatment is not advisable.

2. Puncturing EX-B-8 Shiqizhui

Indication: Amenorrhea.

Point Prescription:
EX-B-8 Shiqizhui

Manipulation: Ask the patient to lie down on the stomach, insert a 3-cun long needle into the point 2-2.5 cun while rotating the needle. Then, apply reinforcing or reducing manipulation according to the patient's condition. Retain the needle in the point for 20-40 minutes. The treatment is given once daily, with 10 days as a course.

3. Puncturing RN-4 Guanyuan, RN-6 Qihai and SP-6 Sanyinjiao

Indication: Amenorrhea due to deficiency.

Point Prescription:
Primary points:
    RN-4 Guanyuan
    RN-6 Qihai
    SP-6 Sanyinjiao

Secondary points according to conditions:
1️⃣ Poor appetite, borborygmus and diarrhea—RN-12 Zhongwan, ST-25 Tianshu and LR-13 Zhangmen;
2️⃣ Soreness and weakness of the loins and knees, cold limbs and fatigue — BL-18 Ganshu, BL-23 Shenshu and BL-26 Guanyuanshu;
3️⃣ Emotional depression, irritability, distressed feeling in the chest—BL-17 Geshu and BL-18 Ganshu.

Manipulation: Acupuncture is applied with reinforcing manipulation. The needle in RN-4 Guanyuan, RN-6 Qihai and SP-6 Sanyinjiao should be manipulated to induce the warm sensation radiating to the pubic region. After arrival of qi, the needles are retained for 20-40 minutes. The treatment is given once daily, with 10 treatments as a course.

4. Ear Acupuncture

Indication: Amenorrhea.

Ear Point Prescription:
    Inner Genitalia, Pelvic Cavity, Abdomen, Subcortex, Yuanzhong, Endocrine, Kidney, Spleen, Liver.

Manipulation: See page 255-256.

Comment:
Zhenjiu is effective in the treatment of secondary amenorrhea. In some cases, it can act to cure this disease. Generally, Zhenjiu treatment should be given 7-10 days before menstruation and until the menses comes, and another 1-2 courses of the treatment is needed after the menstrual cycle becomes normal in order to consolidate the result. To primary amenorrhea, Zhenjiu treatment is not always effective. Therefore, the primary causes should be treated in combination of Zhenjiu with some other therapies such as herb treatment. Secondary amenorrhea should be carefully distinguished from pregnancy.

Notes:

61. Dysfunctional Uterine Bleeding

Dysfunctional uterine bleeding refers to abnormal uterine bleeding caused by ovarian dysfunction, but with no accompanying organic or genital problems. It is mainly caused by disorder of endocrine function, but also may be induced by environmental change, over emotional stress, and over fatigue. Clinically, it is marked by disorders of menstrual cycle, prolonged and heavy bleeding. According to TCM, dysfunctional uterine bleeding belongs to Beng (metrorrhagia) or Lou (metrostaxis), and it is caused by disorder of qi and blood and debility of the Chong and Ren Meridians.

I. STANDARD TREATMENT

It is usually divided into three types—heat in blood, blood stasis and insufficiency of spleen. Points of the Spleen Meridian are frequently selected in its treatment.

1. Heat in Blood

Manifestations: Sudden and abnormal bursts of profuse menstrual bleeding or uterine bleeding prolonged and sustained for many days, with the blood being bright red, thick and sticky, accompanied with tidal fever.

Tongue: Thin and yellow coating.

Pulse: Thready and rapid.

Treatment Principle: Clear heat, and regulate menstruation to arrest bleeding.

Point Prescription & Manipulation:
Primary points:
    LR-1 Dadun -
    SP-1 Yinbai -
    SP-10 Xuehai -
    RN-3 Zhongji -
    SP-6 Sanyinjiao /

Explanation:
- LR-1 Dadun, the Jing-Well Point of the Liver Meridian, clears heat from the Liver Meridian and cools blood;
- SP-1 Yinbai, an effective point to arrest uterus bleeding;
- SP-10 Xuehai clears heat from blood;
- RN-3 Zhongji regulates the Chong and Ren Meridians and arrests bleeding from the uterus;
- SP-6 Sanyinjiao nourishes yin and regulates menstruation.

Secondary points according to conditions:
1ᴗ Excess heat — LI-11 Quchi [-] and DU-14 Dazhui [-];
2ᴗ Deficiency heat — KI-2 Rangu [+] and KI-10 Yingu [+];
3ᴗ Damp-heat — RN-3 Zhongji [-] and SP-9 Yinlingquan [-].

2. Blood Stasis

Manifestations: Abnormal and frequent bursts of menstrual bleeding, manifested as metrorrhagia or metrostaxis, marked by dark-colored blood with clots, accompanied with distending pain in the lower abdomen.

Tongue: Dull-purple body with white and thin coating.

Pulse: Chop.

Treatment Principle: Activate blood circulation, resolve blood stasis, arrest bleeding, and regulate menstruation.

Point Prescription & Manipulation:
Primary points:
    LR-3 Taichong -
    SP-6 Sanyinjiao /
    RN-4 Guanyuan -
    ST-30 Qichong/
    SP-8 Diji -

Explanation:
- LR-3 Taichong promotes qi flow and activates blood circulation;
- SP-6 Sanyinjiao and SP-8 Diji remove blood stasis and regulate menstruation;
- RN-4 Guanyuan regulates qi activities of the Chong and Ren Meridians and removes blood stasis from the uterus;
- ST-30 Qichong, the point where the qi of the Chong Meridian is infused at the body surface, regulates the Chong Meridian and removes blood stasis.

Secondary points according to conditions:
1⃞ Clots in bleeding and acute pain in lower abdomen — SP-21 Dabao [-] and BL-17 Geshu [-] are pricked to bleed;
2⃞ Severe bleeding — SP-12 Chongmen [-] and SP-1 Yinbai [-].

3. Insufficiency of Spleen

Manifestations: Irregular menstrual cycle, manifested as metrorrhagia or metrostaxis, prolonged menstruation, light-colored and thin menstrual blood, accompanied with shortness of breath, lack of spirit, pale complexion.

Tongue: Pale body with thin coating.

Pulse: Weak.

Treatment Principle: Tonify qi to keep the blood in the vessel, nourish blood to regulate menstruation.

Point Prescription & Manipulation:
Primary points:
SP-1 Yinbai ^
ST-36 Zusanli + ^
RN-6 Qihai + ^
DU-20 Baihui ^
SP-6 Sanyinjiao + ^
BL-20 Pishu + ^

Explanation:

- SP-1 Yinbai, an effective point to arrest abnormal bleeding from the uterus;
- ST-36 Zusanli and BL-20 Pishu reinforce the spleen, tonify qi and arrest bleeding;
- RN-6 Qihai and DU-20 Baihui strengthen qi and arrest bleeding;
- SP-6 Sanyinjiao regulates menstruation and arrests bleeding.

Secondary points according to conditions:
1⃞ Prolonged or chronic cases — BL-20 Pishu [+ ^] and BL-18 Ganshu [+ ^];
2⃞ Yang deficiency — DU-4 Mingmen [+ ^] and KI-8 Jiaoxin [-].

II. EXPERIENTIAL TREATMENT

1. Acupuncture & Moxibustion on EX-UE-16 Duanhong (Stopping the red)

Indication: Dysfunctional uterine bleeding belonging to qi deficiency in differentiation.

Point Prescription:
EX-UE-16 Duanhong, located on the dorsum of the palm, at the junction of the red and white skin, between the second and third phalangeal-carpal joints, namely, one of the EX-UE-9 Baxie.

Manipulation: Insert a 2-cun long needle through the skin of the point, push the needle horizontally along the inter-space of the carpal bones 1.5-1.8 cun while rotating it with gentle force, and retain the needle for 20 minutes. After withdrawing the needle, apply bird-pecking moxibustion on the point for 10-15 minutes. The treatment is given once a day when there is a need to arrest bleeding, and usually, within 2-3 treatments, bleeding will be arrested.

2. Moxibustion on SP-1 Yinbai

Indication: Dysfunctional uterine bleeding belonging to qi deficiency in differentiation.

Point Prescription:
SP-1 Yinbai

Manipulation: Apply moxibustion with moxa stick 10 cm over the point for about 15-20 minutes to make the local skin flushed and burning sensation induced. The treatment can be given 3-5 times a day when there is a need to arrest bleeding, and usually, bleeding will be arrested on that day and about 3 days of treatment are needed to treat or prevent uterine bleeding in the next menstrual cycle.

3. Puncturing SP-8 Diji

Indication: Dysfunctional uterine bleeding.

Point Prescription:
SP-8 Diji of the right side.

Manipulation: Insert a 1.5-cun long needle into the point 1.3 cun, lift, thrust and rotate it to induce a needling sensation radiating to the region posterior to the internal malleolus, and retain the needle for 10 minutes. Then, lift the needle to the region below the skin, insert it horizontally downwards along the running course of the Spleen Meridian 1 cun, and rotate it to induce a needling sensation, and retain it for 40 minutes. The treatment is given once daily, with 10 treatments as a course.

4. Ear Acupuncture

Indication: Dysfunctional uterine bleeding.

Ear Point Prescription:
Primary points:
Kidney, Uteri, Appendix, Pelvic, Endocrine, Subcortex, Adrenal Gland.

Secondary points according to conditions:
Diaphragm, Liver, Spleen, Heart.

Manipulation: See page 255-256

Comment:
Zhenjiu is effective in the treatment of dysfunctional uterine bleeding. In some cases, it can be used to cure this disease. It has been proved that SP-1 Yinbai and SP-6 Sanyinjiao are quite effective to arrest bleeding from the uterus, no matter whether acupuncture or moxibustion is applied. Generally, Zhenjiu treatment should be given 7-10 days before menstruation and until the menses comes, and another 1-2 courses of the treatment is needed after the menstrual cycle becomes normal in order to consolidate the result. The patient should be advised to take moor food rich in nutrition, give up smoking or drinking, have a good rest, and keep a good emotional state.

Notes:

62. Pre-Menstrual Syndrome

Pre-menstrual syndrome refers to a series of symptoms occurring in some women for several days before each menstrual period. It is caused by dysfunction of the cerebral subcortex and the autonomic nervous system and disturbance of the sex hormones. It is clinically characterized by nervousness, depression, anxiety, irritability, insomnia, headache, swelling of the hands, face, or feet, nausea, vomiting, diarrhea, cramps or sinking pain in the lower abdomen, lower back pain, and pain, swelling, redness or fever of the breasts. According to TCM, pre-menstrual syndrome is classified into Yu Zheng (depression syndrome), and is caused by emotional injury leading to depression of the liver qi.

I. STANDARD TREATMENT

It is divided into three types — stagnation of liver qi and deficiency of the spleen and heart. Points on the Liver Meridian are frequently selected in its treatment.

1. Stagnation of Liver Qi

Manifestations: Breast distention with dizziness, headache, abdominal distending pain radiating to the chest and hypochondriac region, and irritability before menstruation.

Tongue: Purplish body with thin coating.

Pulse: Wiry.

Treatment Principle: Soothe the liver and regulate qi.

Point Prescription & Manipulation:
Primary points:
    LR-3 Taichong -
    PC-6 Neiguan -
    LR-14 Qimen -
    HT-7 Shenmen /
    KI-3 Taixi +

    ST-36 Zusanli +
    SP-6 Sanyinjiao -

Explanation:
- LR-3 Taichong and PC-6 Neiguan soothe the liver and relieve qi stagnation;
- LR-14 Qimen, the Front-Mu Point of the liver, relieves stagnation of liver qi, and alleviates pain;
- HT-7 Shenmen and KI-3 Taixi regulate the heart and kidney, and calm the mind;
- ST-36 Zusanli and SP-6 Sanyinjiao strengthen the spleen and stomach and prevent or treat attack of the spleen and stomach by abnormal liver qi;
- SP-6 Sanyinjiao regulates menstruation and relieves pain.

Secondary points according to conditions:
1. Chronic cases — DU-20 Baihui [/] and GB-34 Yanglingquan [-];
2. Nausea—LI-4 Hegu [-] and SP-4 Gongsun [-];
3. Diarrhea and abdominal pain — RN-12 Zhongwan [/] and SP-4 Gongsun [/].

2. Deficiency of Heart and Spleen

Manifestations: Breast distention with dizziness, headache and abdominal pain or lower back pain before menstruation, insomnia, listlessness, fatigue, cold limbs.

Tongue: Pale body with white coating.

Pulse: Deep and thready.

Treatment Principle: Nourish the heart and reinforce the spleen.

Point Prescription & Manipulation:
Primary points:
    ST-36 Zusanli + ^
    SP-6 Sanyinjiao + ^
    RN-4 Guanyuan + ^
    PC-6 Neiguan /
    HT-7 Shenmen +

Explanation:
- ST-36 Zusanli and SP-6 Sanyinjiao strengthen the spleen, reinforce qi and tonify blood to nourish the heart and spleen;
- RN-4 Guanyuan tonifies primary qi and regulates the Chong and Ren Meridians;
- PC-6 Neiguan and HT-7 Shenmen nourish the heart and calm the mind.

Secondary points according to conditions:
1□ Chronic cases—BL-15 Xinshu [+], BL-20 Pishu [+] and EX-HN-3 Yintang [/];
2□ Dizziness and lower back pain—BL-18 Ganshu [+] and BL-23 Shenshu [+].

3. Fire due to Yin Deficiency

Manifestations: Headache, dizziness, irritability, insomnia, tinnitus, bitter taste in the mouth, sore mouth, epistaxis, hot sensation in the chest, palms and soles, and night sweating, which occur before menstruation or are aggregated before menstruation.

Tongue: Red body with little coating.

Pulse: Thread and rapid.

Treatment Principle: Nourish yin, clear fire and calm mind.

Point Prescription & Manipulation:
Primary points:
  BL-15 Xinshu +
  BL-23 Shenshu +
  EX-AC-1 Zigong +
  KI-3 Taixi +
  GB-43 Xiaxi -
  EX-HN-1 Sishencong /
  EX-HN-5 Taiyang -

Explanation:
- BL-15 Xinshu and BL-23 Shenshu, the Back-Shu Points of the heart and kidney, tonify yin and reinforce the heart and kidney;

- EX-AC-1 Zigong, an experiential point to treat menstrual disorders, and KI-3 Taixi reinforce the kidney and regulate menstruation;
- GB-43 Xiaxi clears fire;
- EX-HN-1 Sishencong and EX-HN-5 Taiyang check overactivity of yang, clear fire and calm mind.

Secondary points according to conditions:
1□ Poor appetite and abdominal distention— SP-6 Sanyinjiao[+] and RN-12 Zhongwan [+];
2□ Chronic cases — KI-6 Zhaohai [+] and SP-6 Sanyinjiao [+].

II. EXPERIENTIAL TREATMENT

Ear Acupuncture

Indication: Pre-menstrual syndrome.

Ear Point Prescription:
Primary points:
  Internal genitalia, Endocrine, Yuanzhong, Shenmen, Subcortex, Liver.

Secondary points according to conditions:
1□ Mental disorder — Heart;
2□ Gastrointestinal symptoms —Stomach and Abdomen;
3□ Low abdominal pain—Abdomen and Pelvic Cavity;
4□ Breast distending pain — Chest.

Manipulation: See page 255-256.

The treatment is given from 10 days before menstruation to the arrival of menstruation, and for 3 menstruation cycles.

Comment:
Zhenjiu is effective in the treatment of pre-menstrual syndrome. In most cases, it is effective to relieve their symptoms or even cure this disease. Generally, Zhenjiu treatment should

be given 7-10 days before menstruation and until the menses comes, and another 1-2 courses of the treatment are needed after the premenstrual syndrome disappears in order to consolidate the result.

Notes:

63. Menopausal Syndrome

Menopausal syndrome refers to a series of symptoms occurring in some women during the climacteric period. It is caused by gradual decline of ovarian function leading to disturbance of the endocrine and autonomic nervous systems. Women with anovarism due to trauma, surgery, or pelvic radiotherapy may also experience this condition before their climacteric period. Its main clinical manifestations include the following three aspects: firstly, symptoms of cardiovascular system such as intermittent flushing and sensations of heat on the face, neck and chest, accompanied by profuse perspiration, palpitation, discomfort or pain in the pericardial region, and numbness or pain of the limbs; secondly, mental symptoms such as restlessness, irritability, anxiety, insomnia, and poor memory; and thirdly, symptoms of metabolic dysfunction such as obesity and edema. According to TCM, menopausal syndrome is classified into Yu Zheng (depression syndrome) and Zan Zao (hysteria), and it is caused by gradual decline of the kidney yin or yang due to age, leading to dysfunction of the zang-fu organs.

I. STANDARD TREATMENT

Menopausal syndrome is usually divided into three types — over-activity of liver yang, deficiency of heart blood and stagnation of qi and phlegm. Points of the Liver, Kidney and Spleen Meridians are frequently selected in its treatment.

1. Over-Activity of Liver Yang

Manifestations: Headache, dizziness, flushed face, sweating, irritability, liability to loose temper, preceded menstrual cycle or irregular menstrual cycle, profuse or little bright red menstruation blood.

Tongue: Red body with little coating,

Pulse: Wiry and rapid.

Treatment Principle: Tonify yin to nourish kidney, soothe liver to restrain yang.

Point Prescription & Manipulation:
Primary points:
    LR-3 Taichong -
    KI-3 Taixi +
    DU-20 Baihui /
    EX-HN-1 Sishencong /
    DU-24 Shentin /
    GB-20 Fengchi -

Explanation:
- LR-3 Taichong and GB-20 Fengchi pacify overactivity of liver yang;
- KI-3 Taixi nourishes yin to restrain yang;
- DU-20 Baihui, EX-HN-1 Sishencong and DU-24 Shentin calm spirit and restrain floating yang.

Secondary points according to conditions:
1▢ Chronic cases — PC-6 Neiguan [/] and EX-HN-5 Taiyang [/];
2▢ Irritability — PC-7 Daling [-];
3▢ Flashed face and heat sensation of the upper of the body — KI-1 Yongquan [+] and KI-6 Zhaohai [+].

2. Deficiency of Heart Blood

Manifestations: Palpitation, insomnia, dreaminess, heat sensation in the chest and centers of the palms and bottom of the feet, irritability, or even accompanied with mental disorder, scanty menstruation.

Tongue: Red body with little coating.

Pulse: Thready and rapid.

Treatment Principle: Nourish heart and spleen.

Point Prescription & Manipulation:
Primary points:
    BL-15 Xinshu +
    HT-7 Shenmen +
    BL-20 Pishu +

    BL-23 Shenshu +
    SP-6 Sanyinjiao /

Explanation:
- BL-15 Xinshu, the Back-Shu Point of the heart, and HT-7 Shenmen reinforce the heart, tonify blood and calm the mind;
- BL-20 Pishu and SP-6 Sanyinjiao reinforce the spleen and generate blood;
- BL-23 Shenshu and SP-6 Sanyinjiao tonify the kidney and regulate the Chong and Ren Meridians.

Secondary points according to conditions:
1▢ Insomnia — DU-24 Shentin [+], GB-13 Benshen [+] and EX-HN-1 Sishencong [/];
2▢ Palpitation — HT-5 Tongli [/];
3▢ Heat sensation of the chest and centers of the palms and bottom of the feet — PC-8 Laogong [/];
4▢ Mental disorder — DU-26 Shuigou [/] and PC-7 Daling [/].

3. Stagnation of Qi and Phlegm

Manifestations: Obesity, distressed sensation in the chest, spitting of sputum, abdominal distention and fullness, poor appetite, edema, loose stool, scanty and dilute menstruation or profuse menstruation.

Tongue: Sticky coating.

Pulse: Slippery.

Treatment Principle: Promote circulation of qi and dissolve phlegm.

Point Prescription & Manipulation:
Primary points:
    RN-17 Danzhong -
    RN-12 Zhongwan /
    RN-6 Qihai +
    ST-25 Tianshu +
    ST-40 Fenglong -
    SP-6 Sanyinjiao /

Explanation:
- RN-17 Danzhong, the Influential Point of qi, disperses stagnation of qi;
- ST-40 Fenglong, and SP-6 Sanyinjiao reinforce the spleen's function and transform phlegm;
- RN-12 Zhongwan, RN-6 Qihai and ST-25 Tianshu, the Four Door Points, strengthen the spleen and stomach, and remove phlegm and dampness.

Secondary points according to conditions:
1⦆ Distressed feeling in the chest — PC-6 Neiguan [-];
2⦆ Insomnia — EX-HN-16 Anmian [/], ST-8 Touwei [/] and GB-13 Benshen [/].

II. EXPERIENTIAL TREATMENT

Ear Acupuncture

Indication: Menopausal syndrome.

Ear Point Prescription:
Inner Genitalia, Kidney, Liver, Endocrine, Yuanzhong, Subcortex, Shenmen.

Manipulation: See page 255-256

Comment:
Zhenjiu is effective in the treatment of menopausal syndrome. In most cases, it is effective to relieve their symptoms or even cure this disease. Generally, Zhenjiu treatment should be given 7-10 days before menstruation and until the menses comes, and another 1-2 courses of the treatment are needed after the menopausal syndrome disappears in order to consolidate the result. If the patient's menstruation has terminated, namely, she will not have menstruation in the future, the treatment should be given whenever the patient begins her symptoms of menopausal syndrome.

Notes:

64.   Chronic   Pelvic Inflammation

Chronic pelvic inflammation refers to chronic inflammation of the internal genitals, pelvis, peritoneum, and pelvic connective tissues. It always develops from acute pelvic inflammation, and there is often a history of sterility or menstrual disorder. Clinically, it is marked by mild fever, fatigue, pain in the lower abdomen with sinking sensation, lower back pain, and profuse vaginal discharge. According to TCM, chronic pelvic inflammation belongs to categories of Dai Xia (leukorrhea) and Fu Tong (abdominal pain), and it is caused by exogenous or endogenous damp-heat accumulating in the lower-jiao.

Cervicitis, one kind of pelvic inflammation, is seen "65. Cervicitis" because it is frequently seen in clinics and it is necessary to discuss it separately.

I. STANDARD TREATMENT

Chronic pelvic inflammation is usually divided into four types—stagnation and accumulation of damp-heat, damp-cold, blood stasis, deficiency of qi and blood. Points of the Ren and Spleen Meridians are frequently selected in its treatment.

1. Stagnation and Accumulation of Damp-Cold

Manifestations: Dragging sensation and distending pain with coldness in the lower abdomen which are relieved by warmth, and aggravated by cold, profuse and clear leukorrhagia, loose stool.

Tongue: Pale body with white and sticky coating.

Pulse: Wiry and tight.

Treatment Principle: Warm the meridian, dispel cold, remove dampness and arrest leukorrhagia.

Point Prescription & Manipulation:
Primary points:
    GB-26 Daimai -
    SP-6 Sanyinjiao / ^
    RN-4 Guanyuan + ^
    ST-29 Guilai / ^
    BL-54 Zhibian / ^
    SP-8 Diji/ ^
    BL-29 Zhonglushu / ^

Explanation:
*   GB-26 Daimai removes dampness and arrests leukorrhagia;
*   SP-6 Sanyinjiao warms the three Foot-Yin Meridians and removes cold and dampness;
*   RN-4 Guanyuan warms the lower-jiao, dispels cold;
*   ST-29 Guilai and SP-8 Diji reinforce the spleen, remove dampness, regulate menstruation, and arrest leukorrhagia;
*   BL-54 Zhibian warms the lower-jiao and dispels cold and dampness, and arrests leukorrhagia.

Secondary points according to conditions:
1 Loose stools and poor appetite— ST-36 Zusanli [+ ^] and SP-9 Yinlingquan [+ ^].

2. Stagnation and Accumulation of Damp-Heat

Manifestations: Dragging sensation and distending pain in the lower abdomen, profuse, sticky and fetid leukorrhagia that is yellow and white.

Tongue: Red body with yellow and sticky coating.

Pulse: Soft and rapid.

Treatment Principle: Clear heat, promote diuresis, arrest leukorrhagia.

Point Prescription & Manipulation:
Primary points:
    GB-26 Daimai -
    RN-3 Zhongji -
    SP-9 Yinlingquan -
    LR-5 Ligou -
    BL-32 Ciliao -
    BL-30 Baihuanshu -
    ST-28 Shuidao -

Explanation:
*   GB-26 Daimai removes dampness and clears heat in the lower-jiao to arrest leukorrhagia;
*   RN-3 Zhongji and ST-28 Shuidao clear damp-heat from the lower-jiao;
*   SP-9 Yinlingquan reinforces the spleen to remove dampness;
*   LR-5 Ligou clears heat from the Liver Meridian;
*   BL-32 Ciliao and BL-30 Baihuanshu clear dampness from the lower-jiao.

Secondary points according to conditions:
1 Fever — LI-11 Quchi [-] and GB-34 Yanglingquan [-].

3. Blood Stasis

Manifestations: Lower abdominal pain which is stabbing and fixed or accompanied with masses, lower back pain, delayed menstruation with dark blood or clots, yellow and white or even red and white leukorrhagia.

Tongue: Purplish and dark or with ecchymoses on the border.

Pulse: Deep and unsmooth.

Treatment Principle: Activate blood, remove masses.

Point Prescription & Manipulation:
Primary points:
    GB-26 Daimai -
    RN-3 Zhongji -

LR-3 Taichong -
ST-30 Qichong-
BL-32 Ciliao -
LR-6 Zhongdu -
SP-8 Diji -
SP-6 Sanyinjiao /
Ashi Point (the tender point or the region with mass on the lower abdomen) -.

Explanation:
The points may be divided into two groups and they are used alternatively.

- GB-26 Daimai regulates the Dai Meridian and arrests leukorrhea;
- RN-3 Zhongji, BL-32 Ciliao, and Ashi Point (the tender point or the region with mass on the lower abdomen) regulate the lower-jiao, promote qi and blood flow, and remove blood stasis;
- LR-3 Taichong and LR-6 Zhongdu promote flow of qi and blood;
- ST-30 Qichong, the point where the Chong Meridian qi is infused at the body surface, regulates the Chong Meridian, removes blood stasis and resolves accumulation;
- SP-8 Diji and SP-6 Sanyinjiao regulate menstruation and arrest leukorrhagia.

Secondary points according to conditions:
1囗 Severe blood stasis — BL-17 Geshu [-] and SP-10 Xuehai [-].

4. Qi and Blood Deficiency

Manifestations: Dragging and distending sensation in the lower abdomen which is aggravated by exertion or during the menstruation, constant and clear leukorrhagia, dizziness, blurred vision, palpitation, shortness of breath, poor appetite, loose stool, pale complexion without luster.

Tongue: Pale body.

Pulse: Thready and weak.

Treatment Principle: Tonify qi and blood.

Point Prescription & Manipulation:
Primary points:
GB-26 Daimai -
RN-4 Guanyuan + ^
RN-6 Qihai + ^
ST-36 Zusanli + ^
SP-6 Sanyinjiao + ^
DU-20 Baihui ^
SP-8 Diji + ^

Explanation:
The points may be divided into two groups and they are used alternatively.

- GB-26 Daimai regulates the Dai Meridian and arrests leukorrhea;
- RN-4 Guanyuan and RN-6 Qihai tonify primary qi, warm the lower-jiao, and arrest leukorrhagia;
- ST-36 Zusanli, SP-6 Sanyinjiao and SP-8 Diji reinforce the spleen and stomach, tonify qi and blood, regulate menstruation and arrest leukorrhagia;
- DU-20 Baihui raises the sunken qi to arrest leukorrhagia.

Secondary points according to conditions:
1囗 Chronic cases — SP-4 Gongsun [+], BL-18 Ganshu [+ ^] and BL-20 Pishu [+ ^];
2囗 Dizziness, poor memory and palpitation— BL-18 Ganshu [+] and BL-15 Xinshu [+].

II. EXPERIENTIAL TREATMENT

1. Puncturing ST-29 Guilai

Indication: Annexitis, one of the pelvic inflammation conditions.

Point Prescription:
ST-29 Guilai

Manipulation: Insert a 2-cun long needle perpendicularly into the point 1.2-1.5 cun, lift, thrust and rotate the needle with a moderate stimulation. After arrival of qi, retain the needle in the point for 20-40 minutes. The treatment is given once daily, with 10 treatments as a course.

2. Ear Acupuncture

Indication: Chronic pelvic inflammation.

Ear Point Prescription:
Pelvic Cavity, Inner Genitalia, Abdomen, Sanjiao, Spleen, Liver, Endocrine, Shenmen, Apex.

Manipulation: See page 255-256.

Comment:
Zhenjiu is effective in relieving symptoms of pelvic inflammation. When the points on the lower abdomen are punctured, the needling sensation should be induced to radiate to the genitalia region. When acute or tuberculous pelvic inflammation is treated, the patient is prohibited to have sexual life during the treatment period. Chronic pelvic inflammation is obstinate, a comprehensive treatment, including Zhenjiu and herbs in combination, is recommended, and the patient should be advised to decrease frequency of sexual life.

Notes:

65. Cervicitis

Cervicitis, one kind of pelvic inflammation, refers to acute or chronic inflammation of the uterine cervix. Sexually transmitted infections and other infections of the reproductive organs may cause it. Clinically, it is marked by increase of discharge through the vagina. According to TCM, cervicitis belongs to the category of Dai Xia (leukorrhagia), and it is caused by down flowing of damp-heat or deficiency of the spleen or kidney, leading to failure of the Dai Meridian in controlling.

I. STANDARD TREATMENT

Cervicitis is usually divided into four types— down-flow of damp-heat, accumulation of cold and blood stasis, spleen qi deficiency, and kidney yin deficiency. Points of the Spleen, Stomach, and Ren Meridians are frequently selected in its treatment.

1. Down-Flow of Damp-Heat

Manifestations: Profuse, sticky, yellow and fetid leukorrhagia, or blood-tinged leukorrhagia, itching of the external genitalia, yellow and scanty urination, fever, bitter taste in the mouth.

Tongue: Red body with yellow and sticky coating.

Pulse: Smooth and rapid.

Treatment Principle: Clear heat, promote diuresis, arrest leukorrhagia.

Point Prescription & Manipulation:
Primary points:
GB-26 Daimai -
RN-3 Zhongji -
ST-28 Shuidao -
SP-9 Yinlingquan /
LR-2 Xingjian -
BL-30 Baihuanshu -
GB-34 Yanglingquan -

Explanation:
- GB-26 Daimai, RN-3 Zhongji and ST-28 Shuidao clear damp-heat from the lower-jiao;
- SP-9 Yinlingquan removes dampness to arrest leukorrhea;
- LR-2 Xingjian and GB-34 Yanglingquan clear damp-heat from the Liver and Gallbladder Meridians, remove dampness from the lower-jiao;
- BL-30 Baihuanshu regulates the urinary bladder to remove dampness.

Secondary points according to conditions:
1🔲 Fever — LI-11 Quchi [-].

2. Accumulation of Cold and Blood Stasis

Manifestations: Sticky, red and fetid leukorrhagia which is like blood but not blood, or even with clots, lower abdominal distending pain, emotional depression, dark complexion.

Tongue: Pale and purplish body with white coating.

Pulse: Wiry and tight.

Treatment Principle: Warm the meridian, remove blood stasis, arrest leukorrhagia.

Point Prescription & Manipulation:
Primary points:
    GB-26 Daimai / ^
    RN-4 Guanyuan + ^
    LR-3 Taichong -
    SP-6 Sanyinjiao / ^
    ST-30 Qichong + ^
    BL-34 Xialiao + ^
    SP-8 Diji + ^

Explanation:
- RN-4 Guanyuan, GB-26 Daimai and BL-34 Xialiao, the local points, warm and unblock the meridians and collaterals, and dispel cold;

- LR-3 Taichong promotes qi circulation to activate blood;
- SP-6 Sanyinjiao and SP-8 Diji regulate menstruation to arrest leukorrhea;
- ST-30 Qichong, the point where qi of the Chong Meridian is infused, removes blood stasis and resolves accumulation.

Secondary points according to conditions:
1🔲 Chronic cases — SP-10 Xuehai [/ ^];
2🔲 Poor appetite and loose stools — SP-9 Yinlingquan [+ ^] and ST-36 Zusanli[+ ^].

3. Spleen and Stomach Qi Deficiency

Manifestations: Prolonged   profuse leukorrhagia which is white or yellowish, clear and odorless, sallow complexion, poor appetite, abdominal distention, lack of spirit, fatigue.

Tongue: Pale body.

Pulse: Thready and weak.

Treatment Principle: Reinforce the spleen, tonify qi, and arrest leukorrhagia.

Point Prescription & Manipulation:
Primary points:
    RN-4 Guanyuan + ^
    RN-6 Qihai + ^
    GB-26 Daimai + ^
    ST-36 Zusanli + ^
    SP-9 Yinlingquan + ^
    BL-30 Baihuanshu + ^
    SP-6 Sanyinjiao + ^

Explanation:
- RN-6 Qihai warms the Ren Meridian, tonifies qi, and consolidates the kidney;
- GB-26 Daimai warms and consolidates the qi of the Dai Meridian;
- ST-36 Zusanli and SP-9 Yinlingquan reinforce the spleen, tonify qi and raise yang;
- BL-30 Baihuanshu warms the lower-jiao to remove dampness;

- SP-6 Sanyinjiao regulates menstruation to arrest leukorrhea.

Secondary points according to conditions:
1□ Loose stools — ST-25 Tianshu [+ ^].

4. Kidney Yin Deficiency

Manifestations: Red-white or yellow and sticky leukorrhagia, burning sensation of the external genitalia, soreness and weakness of the loins, tinnitus, dizziness, feverish sensation in the chest, palms and soles.

Tongue: Red body with little coating.

Pulse: Thready and rapid.

Treatment Principle: Tonify yin, clear heat, reinforce kidney and arrest leukorrhagia.

Point Prescription & Manipulation:
Primary points:
    BL-23 Shenshu +
    BL-52 Zhishi +
    KI-3 Taixi +
    SP-6 Sanyinjiao +
    KI-12 Dahe +
    GB-26 Daimai +
    KI-6 Zhaohai +

Explanation:
- BL-23 Shenshu, BL-52 Zhishi, KI-3 Taixi, KI-6 Zhaohai and SP-6 Sanyinjiao tonify yin and reinforce the kidney;
- KI-12 Dahe and GB-26 Daimai clear heat from the lower-jiao and consolidate the Dai Meridian to stop leukorrhea.

Secondary points according to conditions:
1□ Chronic cases — RN-4 Guanyuan [+];
2□ Insomnia — EX-HN-16 Anmian [+].

II. EXPERIENTIAL TREATMENT

1. Puncturing EX-LE -23 Zigongjing

Indication: Cervical erosion.

Point Prescription:
    EX-LE-23 Zigongjing, located on the leg, 3 cun above the tip of the internal malleolus, one finger-breadth prior to the Achilles tendon, a little bit posterior to SP-6 Sanyinjiao.

Manipulation: Acupuncture is applied on the bilateral EX-LE-23 Zigongjing. Insert a 2-cun long needle perpendicularly through the skin of the point. Then, horizontally push the needle along the skin upwards 1-1.5 cun. In case meeting resistance or inducing numbness, distention or pain to the patient during pushing the needle, withdraw the needle under the skin, change the direction of insertion a little and push the needle again. Retain the needle for 30 minutes. The treatment is given once daily, with 10 treatments as a course.

2. Puncturing RN-4 Guanyuan, RN-6 Qihai & ST-29 Guilai

Indication: Cervicitis

Point Prescription:
Primary points:
    RN-4 Guanyuan
    RN-6 Qihai
    ST-29 Guilai

Secondary points according to conditions:
1□ Syndrome of liver qi stagnation — BL-18 Ganshu and SP-10 Xuehai;
2□ Syndrome of kidney deficiency — BL-23 Shenshu and DU-4 Minmen;
3□ Syndrome of spleen deficiency — SP-6 Sanyinjiao, SP-9 Yinlingquan and BL-23 Shenshu.

Manipulation: Acupuncture is applied with reinforcing manipulation. The treatment is given once daily, with 10 treatments as a course.

3. Ear Acupuncture

Indication: Cervicitis.

Ear Point Prescription:
Uterus, Bladder, Liver, Spleen, Kidney, Endocrine, Shenmen, Sanjiao.

Manipulation: See page 255-256.

Comment:
Zhenjiu is effective in relieving symptoms of cervicitis. At the early stage, cervicitis is mainly related to damp-heat or cold-dampness, belonging to excess syndrome, and dispelling pathogens should be taken as the main in its treatment, reducing manipulation or uniform reinforcing and reducing manipulation is often performed in acupuncture treatment; while at the late stage, cervicitis is characterized by deficiency of spleen and kidney, thus strengthening the body resistance and reinforce zang fu organs should be main, and reinforcing manipulation is frequently applied in acupuncture treatment. Chronic cervicitis is obstinate, and a comprehensive treatment, including Zhenjiu and herbs in combination, is recommended, and the patient should be advised to decrease frequency of sexual life.

Notes:

66. Prolapse of the Uterus

Prolapse of the uterus refers to descent of the uterus from the normal position, with the cervix dropping to below the level of the ischial spine. In extreme cases, the entire uterus may extrude out of the vaginal opening. Prolapse of the uterus is usually accompanied by prolapse of both the anterior and posterior vaginal walls. In the initial stage, the prolapsed uterus may spontaneously return to normal when a horizontal position is assumed. But with development of the condition, the prolapsed uterus remains exposed outside of the vaginal opening, with accompanying difficulty in defecation, urinary retention or incontinence, or urinary tract infection. According to TCM, prolapse of the uterus, called Yin Ting in Chinese, is caused by frequent deliveries or general asthenia, leading to deficiency and subsequent sinking of qi in the middle-jiao or deficiency of the kidneys.

I. STANDARD TREATMENT

It is usually divided into two types — sinking of spleen qi and failure of kidney in consolidation. Points of the Spleen, Stomach, and Kidney Meridians are frequently selected in its treatment.

1. Sinking of Spleen Qi

Manifestations: Decent of the uterus from the normal position which is aggravated by exertion, dragging sensation in the lower abdomen, weakness of the limbs, shortness of breath, pale complexion.

Tongue: Pale body.

Pulse: Thready and weak.

Treatment Principle: Tonify spleen and stomach, enhance the sinking.

Point Prescription & Manipulation:
Primary points:

DU-20 Baihui   ^
RN-6 Qihai + ^
GB-28 Weidao + ^
ST-36 Zusanli + ^
SP-6 Sanyinjiao + ^
BL-20 Pishu + ^
BL-21 Weishu + ^
EX-CA-1 Zigong + ^

Explanation:
- DU-20 Baihui raises yang and lifts the sunken;
- RN-6 Qihai, a point of the Ren Meridian connecting with the uterus and near the uterus, and GB-28 Weidao, the Crossing Point of the Foot-Shaoyang and Dai Meridians, regulate the Chong and Ren Meridians, consolidate the Dai Meridian, and strengthen the uterus;
- EX-CA-1 Zigong, an experiential point for treating prolapse of the uterus;
- ST-36 Zusanli, SP-6 Sanyinjiao, BL-20 Pishu and BL-21 Weishu reinforce the middle-jiao, tonify qi, and elevate the uterus.

Secondary points according to conditions:
1꜀ Chronic cases — RN-4 Guanyuan [+ ^];
2꜀ Loose stools — ST-25 Tianshu [+ ^] and SP-9 Yinlingquan [+ ^].

2. Failure of Kidney in Consolidation

Manifestations: Decent of the uterus from the normal position, soreness and weakness of the loins and knees, dragging sensation of the lower abdomen, frequent urination which is worse in the night, dizziness, tinnitus.

Tongue: Pale body.

Pulse: Deep, thready and weak.

Treatment Principle: Tonify kidney and restore the uterus in the normal position.

Point Prescription & Manipulation:
Primary points:

RN-4 Guanyuan + ^
EX-CA-1 Zigong + ^
KI-12 Dahe + ^
KI-6 Zhaohai + ^
BL-23 Shenshu + ^
BL-52 Zhishi + ^
DU-3 Yaoyangguan + ^
ST-36 Zusanli + ^

Explanation:
- RN-4 Guanyuan and KI-12 Dahe regulate and reinforce the Chong and Ren Meridians;
- EX-CA-1 Zigong, an experiential point for treating prolapse of the uterus;
- KI-6 Zhaohai, BL-23 Shenshu, BL-52 Zhishi and DU-3 Yaoyangguan reinforce and consolidate the kidney qi;
- ST-36 Zusanli reinforces the middle-jiao and tonifies qi to nourish the kidney.

Secondary points according to conditions:
1꜀ Chronic cases — DU-20 Baihui [+ ^];
2꜀ Edema — KI-3 Taixi [+ ^] and SP-9 Yinlingquan [+ ^].

II. EXPERIENTIAL TREATMENT

1. Puncturing EX-LE-14 Huanshang with the Long Needle

Indication: Prolapse of the uterus.

Point Prescription:
EX-LE-14 Huanshang, located at the point 0.5 cun superior and lateral to EX-LE-13 Huanzhong which is at the midpoint of the line connecting the prominutesence of the great trochanter and the hiatus of the sacrum.

Manipulation: Ask the patient to lie on the side with the leg upper on the position extending and the lower on the position bending. Insert a 6-cun long needle into the point 4-6 cun, with the needle tip towards the uterus, lift and thrust needle and perform bird-pecking manipulation 3-5 times to induce electric shock sensation, which radiates to the perineum and lower abdomen, and enhancing sensation of the uterus to the patient. Then, remove the needle. The treatment is given once daily and on one side, and another side selected in turn. 10 treatments are taken as a course, and next course begins after 3-5 days of interval. Usually 2-4 courses are needed.

2. Acupuncture & Moxibustion on EX-CA-5 Tigong

Indication: Prolapse of the uterus.

Point Prescription:
EX-CA-5 Tigong, located at the point 2-finger breadth directly below the midpoint of the anterior border of the pubic arch.

Manipulation: Ask the patient to lie on the back, insert a 2-cun long needle into the point 1-1.5 cun, lift, thrust and rotate the needle to induce soreness and numbness radiating upwards to the lumber region. Then retain the needle in the point for 15-30 minutes. After removing the needle, apply warming moxibustion with moxa stick on the point for 7-10 minutes. The treatment is given once daily, with 10 treatments as a course. Next course can be given after an interval of 5-10 days.

3. Ear Acupuncture

Indication: Prolapse of the uterus.

Ear Point Prescription:
Internal Genitalia, Pelvic Cavity, Abdomen, Kidney, Spleen, Liver.

Manipulation: See Page 255-256.

Comment:
Zhenjiu is effective in the treatment of prolapse of the uterus. In many cases, Zhenjiu can act to cure the disease. During treatment, the patient should be advised to have longer rest on the bed, and to avoid doing heaving physical exertion.

Notes:

67.   Hysteromyoma   and Oophoritic Cyst

Hysteromyoma, also known as fibroids or myomas, refers to benign growths of muscle cells in the uterus. It is most common among women between the age of thirty and menopause. Its cause is uncertain, although a diet rich in processed and fast foods, the birth control pill and high stress level are closely related to its etiology. Oophoritic cyst refers to cyst in the ovary. It is caused by hormonal imbalances often related to diet, including too much meat, saturated fats and products made from white flour which lacks fiber. Hysteromyoma and oophoritic cyst may not have any symptoms, known only through examination such as routine pelvic examination and ultrasound examination. But some cases may have symptoms including uterine bleeding, abdominal bloating and menstrual cramps. According to TCM, Hysteromyoma and oophoritic cyst often share the same etiology and pathogenesis, thus they are discussed together. They are classified into categories of Zheng Jia (abdominal mass), and they are caused by emotional depression and stagnation of liver qi leading to blood stasis or internal production of phlegm.

I. STANDARD TREATMENT

Hysteromyoma and oophoric cyst is usually divided into three types — stagnation of qi, blood stasis, and damp-phlegm. Points of the Ren, Spleen and Liver Meridians are frequently selected in their treatment.

1. Stagnation of Qi

Manifestations: Hysteromyoma or oophoric cyst is showed under ultrasonic diagnosis. Emotional depression, hypochondriac distending pain, irregular menstruation, lower abdominal distending pain or dysmenorrhea.

Tongue: Purplish body with thin coating.

Pulse: Wiry.

Treatment Principle: Soothe the liver, regulate qi, and resolve mass.

Point Prescription & Manipulation:
Primary points:
> LR-3 Taichong -
> EX-CA-1 Zigong -
> RN-2 Qugu -
> RN-3 Zhongji -
> SP-6 Sanyinjiao /
> PC-6 Neiguan -
> RN-17 Danzhong -
> ST-29 Guilai -

Explanation:
- LR-3 Taichong, PC-6 Neiguan and RN-17 Danzhong soothe the liver and promote qi circulation;
- EX-CA-1 Zigong, an experiential point for treating uterus disorders, RN-2 Qugu and RN-3 Zhongji, points of the Ren Meridian, all of these three points located at region near the uterus, regulate the Chong and Ren Meridians, resolve qi stagnation of the uterus, and eliminate the mass;
- SP-6 Sanyinjiao and ST-29 Guilai regulate the menstruation and resolve the mass.

Secondary points according to conditions:
1□ Bitter taste in the mouth — GB-34 Yanglingquan [-];
2□ Insomnia — EX-HN-16 Anmian [-].

2. Blood Stasis

Manifestations: Hysteromyoma or oophoric cyst is showed under ultrasonic diagnosis. Irregular menstruation, lower abdominal pain which is fixed or stabbing, abdominal mass.

Tongue: Purplish tongue with ecchymoses.

Pulse: Wiry and unsmooth.

Treatment Principle: Promote qi circulation, activate blood circulation, remove blood stasis and resolve mass.

Point Prescription & Manipulation:
Primary points:
> RN-3 Zhongji -
> ST-29 Guilai -
> EX-CA-1 Zigong -
> SP-6 Sanyinjiao /
> LR-3 Taichong -
> LI-4 Hegu -
> PC-6 Neiguan -
> SP-10 Xuehai -
> BL-17 Geshu -
> BL-18 Ganshu /

Explanation:
The points may be divided into two groups and they are used alternatively.

- RN-3 Zhongji, a point of the Ren Meridian, ST-29 Guilai, one of the key points for gynecological disorders, and EX-CA-1 Zigong, an experiential point for treating uterus disorders, all of these three points located at region near the uterus, regulate the Chong and Ren Meridians, resolve blood stagnation of the uterus, and eliminate the mass;
- SP-6 Sanyinjiao regulates the menstruation to activate blood circulation;
- LR-3 Taichong and LI-4 Hegu, the Four Gate Points, regulate qi and blood;
- PC-6 Neiguan soothes the liver to promote blood circulation;
- SP-10 Xuehai, BL-17 Geshu, and BL-18 Ganshu activate blood circulation and remove blood stasis.

Secondary points according to conditions:
1□ Severe blood stasis — SP-21 Dabao and BL-17 Geshu are pricked to bleed.

3. Retention of Damp-Phlegm

Manifestations: Hysteromyoma or oophoric cyst is showed under ultrasonic diagnosis.

Irregular menstruation, abdominal pain, distressed feeling in the chest, poor appetite, and loose stool.

Tongue: Pale and slippery body.

Pulse: Wiry and slippery.

Treatment Principle: Remove dampness and phlegm, resolve mass.

Point Prescription & Manipulation:
Primary points:
    ST-29 Guilai - ^
    RN-6 Qihai + ^
    EX-CA-1 Zigong -
    SP-6 Sanyinjiao / ^
    ST-36 Zusanli + ^
    GB-26 Daimai - ^
    BL-30 Baihuanshu - ^
    ST-40 Fenglong -

Explanation:
The points may be divided into two groups and they are used alternatively.

- RN-6 Qihai, a point of the Ren Meridian, and ST-29 Guilai, one of the key points for gynecological disorders, both of these two points located at region near the uterus, regulate the Chong and Ren Meridians, resolve phlegm of the uterus, and eliminate the mass;
- EX-CA-1 Zigong, an experiential point for treating uterus disorders;
- SP-6 Sanyinjiao, ST-36 Zusanli and ST-40 Fenglong reinforce the spleen, and transform phlegm;
- GB-26 Daimai regulates the Dai Meridian;
- BL-30 Baihuanshu regulates the uterus and dispels dampness.

Secondary points according to conditions:
1☐ Chronic cases — LR-5 Ligou [-];
2☐ Loose stools — ST-25 Tianshu [-];
3☐ Nausea and epigastric distention — RN-12 Zhongwan [- ^].

II. EXPERIENTIAL TREATMENT

Puncturing Points of the Body and Ear

Indications: Hysteromyoma, oophoric Cyst.

Point Prescription:
Points of the body:
    EX-CA-1 Zigong, RN-2 Qugu, KI-11 Henggu, SP-6 Sanyinjiao.

Point of the ear:
    Subcortex.

Manipulation: Acupuncture is applied. After insertion of needles into EX-CA-1 Zigong, KI-11 Henggu, SP-6 Sanyinjiao and RN-2 Qugu, lift, thrust and rotate the needles with uniform reinforcing-reducing manipulation to induce a needling sensation radiating to the perineum or the upper portion of the thigh. Then, retain the needles in the points for 20-40 minutes, and manipulate the needles every 10 minutes. During the retention of the needles, insert a needle into Subcortex 0.1-0.2 cun, perform moderate stimulation and retain the needles in the point for 20 minutes. If there is a tender point around Subcortex, take the tender point to replace Subcortex as the puncturing point, the result will be better. The treatment is given once daily, with 10 treatments as a course. After an interval of 5-7 days, the next course can be done. Usually, before starting the second or the third course, ultrasonic diagnosis is suggested to the patient in order to know the treatment result.

Comment:
Zhenjiu is effective in the treatment of hysteromyoma and oophoric cyst. In many cases, Zhenjiu is effective to cure these diseases. If herb treatment is accompanied, the result will be better.

Notes:

68. Malposition of Fetus

Malposition of fetus refers to abnormal lying of the fetus in the uterus which is found thirty weeks after conception, usually known by prenatal examination and causing no symptoms. According to TCM, malposition of fetus, called Tai Wei Bu Zheng in Chinese, is caused by deficiency of qi and blood or stagnation of qi and blood.

I. STANDARD TREATMENT

Malposition of fetus is usually treated by applying moxibustion on BL-67 Zhiyin.

Manipulation: Ask the patient to have urination firstly, then, loose the girdle and lie on the back. Apply moxibustion with moxa stick on the point bilaterally, fix the lighted end of the moxa stick 2-3 cm away from the point for 15-20 minutes to induce a local congestion. The treatment is given once daily until the position of fetus becomes right. Generally, 7-15 treatments are needed.

II. EXPERIENTIAL TREATMENT

1. Moxibustion on SP-6 Sanyinjiao

Indication: Malposition of fetus.

Point Prescription:
SP-6 Sanyinjiao

Manipulation: Apply moxibustion with moxa stick on the point bilaterally, fix the ignited end of the moxa stick 2-3 cm away from the point for 15-20 minutes, until the local skin becomes flushed. The treatment is given once daily, and usually, within 5 treatments the position will be right. If the result is not satisfactory, moxibustion may be applied on GB-41 Zulinqi and PC-6 Neiguan additionally.

2. Ear Acupuncture

Indication: Malposition of fetus.

Ear Point Prescription:
Uterus, Xiajiaoduan, Liver, Brain, Spleen, Abdomen.

Manipulation: See page 255-256.

Comment:
Zhenjiu is very effective in correcting malposition of the fetus, and causes no side effect to the patient. But to patients with habitual abortion or toxemia of pregnancy, acupuncture, including ear acupuncture, is not suitable. During the treatment period, the patient is advised to loose her belt and lie on the side during sleep.

Notes:

69. Pernicious Vomiting

Pernicious vomiting refers to nausea, vomiting, dizziness, anorexia or prompt vomiting after eating which appear during pregnancy. Generally, it occurs in the early stage of the pregnancy. According to TCM, pernicious vomiting belongs to E Zu (pernicious obstruction), and it is due to deficiency of stomach, attack of stomach by liver heat or obstruction of stomach by phlegm-dampness, leading to failure of the stomach qi in normal descending.

I. STANDARD TREATMENT

Pernicious vomiting is usually divided into three types— spleen and stomach deficiency, attack of stomach by liver heat, damp-phlegm, and deficiency of qi and yin. Points of the Stomach, Spleen and Ren Meridians are frequently selected.

1. Spleen and Stomach Deficiency

Manifestations: Nausea, vomiting, anorexia after conception, tastelessness or vomiting of saliva, lack of spirit, drowsiness.

Tongue: Pale tongue with white and sticky coating.

Pulse: Slippery and weak.

Treatment Principle: Strengthen the spleen, regulate the stomach, and lower the adverse flow of qi to arrest vomiting.

Point Prescription & Manipulation:
Primary points:
    ST-36 Zusanli +
    RN-13 Shangwan /
    RN-12 Zhongwan /
    SP-4 Gongsun /

Explanation:

- ST-36 Zusanli, RN-12 Zhongwan and SP-4 Gongsun reinforce the stomach and regulate qi;
- RN-13 Shangwan regulates qi and checks down adverse flow of qi.

Secondary points according to conditions:
1️⃣ Severe vomiting — PC-6 Neiguan [/];
2️⃣ Abdominal distention and fullness — RN-10 Xiawan [/].

2. Attack of Stomach by Heat of Liver

Manifestations: Vomiting of sour or bitter fluid after conception, distention and pain in the chest and hypochondrium, eructation and sigh, distention of the head, dizziness, excessive thirst and bitter taste.

Tongue: Red body with yellowish coating.

Pulse: Wiry and slippery.

Treatment Principle: Check hyperfunction of the liver, regulate the stomach, and lower the adverse flow of qi to arrest vomiting.

Point Prescription & Manipulation:
Primary points:
    PC-6 Neiguan -
    LR-3 Taichong -
    RN-12 Zhongwan /
    ST-36 Zusanli +
    GB-34 Yanglingquan -

Explanation:
- PC-6 Neiguan, GB-34 Yanglingquan and LR-3 Taichong soothe the liver and lower the adverse flow of qi;
- RN-12 Zhongwan and ST-36 Zusanli strengthen the stomach and regulate the middle-jiao.

Secondary points according to conditions:
1️⃣ Distressed sensation in the chest —RN-17 Danzhong [-];

2) Headache — GB-20 Fengchi [-] and LU-7 Lieque [-].

3. Obstruction of Stomach by Damp-Phlegm

Manifestations: Vomiting of saliva which is worse in the morning after conception, fullness and distress of the chest and upper abdomen, fatigue, drowsiness.

Tongue: White and sticky coating.

Pulse: Soft and slippery.

Treatment Principle: Resolve phlegm, regulate stomach, and lower the adverse flow of qi to arrest vomiting.

Point Prescription & Manipulation:
Primary points:
　SP-9 Yinlingquan /
　ST-40 Fenglong -
　ST-36 Zusanli +
　KI-21 Youmen /
　RN-12 Zhongwan /
　RN-17 Danzhong /

Explanation:
* SP-9 Yinlingquan, ST-40 Fenglong and ST-36 Zusanli reinforce the middle-jiao, tonify qi, remove dampness and transform phlegm;
* KI-21 Youmen, RN-12 Zhongwan and RN-17 Danzhong regulate qi and check down the adverse.

Secondary points according to conditions:
1) Distressed feeling in the chest and nausea-- PC-6 Neiguan [-].

4. Deficiency of Qi and Yin

Manifestations: Repeated vomiting lasting for a long time, vomiting with blood in severe cases, listlessness, fatigue, lusterless complexion, scanty urine.

Tongue: Red body with little coating and no moisture.

Pulse: Thready, slippery and weak.

Treatment Principle: Reinforce and regulate stomach, nourish yin and tonify qi, arrest vomiting.

Point Prescription & Manipulation:
Primary points:
　PC-6 Neiguan /
　ST-36 Zusanli +
　KI-6 Zhaohai +
　RN-12 Zhongwan +

Explanation:
* ST-36 Zusanli reinforces the middle-jiao, tonifies qi, nourishes yin;
* RN-12 Zhongwan and PC-6 Neiguan regulate qi and check down the adverse
* KI-6 Zhaohai nourishes yin.

Secondary points according to conditions:
1) Severe cases — BL-20 Pishu [+] and BL-21 Weishu [+].

II. EXPERIENTIAL TREATMENT

1. Gentle Puncture

Indication: Pernicious vomiting.

Point Prescription:
Primary points:
　RN-17 Danzhong
　PC-6 Neiguan
　RN-12 Zhongwan
　ST-36 Zusanli

Secondary points
1) Profuse sputum — ST-40 Fenglong;
2) Dizziness — DU-20 Baihui.

Manipulation: Acupuncture is applied with gentle manipulation. When puncturing RN-17 Danzhong, insert the needle obliquely with the needle tip downwards; on RN-12 Zhongwan, insert the needle perpendicularly to induce the needling sensation radiating to the umbilicus; on PC-6 Neiguan, insert the needle obliquely with the needle tip upwards to induce the needling sensation radiating to the elbow; and on ST-36 Zusanli, insert the needle perpendicularly. The manipulation on all of the points should be gentle. Retain the needles in the points for 20-40 minutes. The treatment is given once daily, with 5 treatments as a course. Generally, vomiting will be arrested after 2-3 treatments.

2. Puncturing PC-6 Neiguan & ST-36 Zusanli

Indication: Pernicious vomiting.

Point Prescription:
Primary points:
    PC-6 Neiguan
    ST-36 Zusanli

Secondary points according to conditions:
1〇 Stomach deficiency — RN-12 Zhongwan;
2〇 Heat of the liver — LR-3 Taichong;
3〇 Phlegm — ST-40 Fenglong.

Manipulation: Acupuncture is applied. When puncturing PC-6 Neiguan, insert the needle perpendicularly 0.5-1 cun; on ST-36 Zusanli, insert the needle perpendicularly 1.5-2.5 cun; on RN-12 Zhongwan, insert the needle 1-1.5 cun; on Taichong, insert the needle 0.5-1 cun; and on ST-40 Fenglong, insert the needle perpendicularly 1-3 cun. When manipulating, insert the needles slowly and rotate them gently. Retain the needles for 30-40 minutes, and manipulate them 2-3 times during the retention. The treatment is given twice daily at beginning and once daily when the condition becomes milder.

Comment:
Zhenjiu is very effective in the treatment of pernicious vomiting, and causes no side effect. As this reason, it can be taken as the first choice for the patients. But a strong stimulation should not be applied in acupuncture with the filiform

needle in either the body or the ear, so as to avoid inducing constriction of the uterus.

Notes:

CHAPTER FOUR
CHILDREN'S DISEASES

70. Infantile Diarrhea

Infantile diarrhea refers to increased frequency and volume of defecation. Acute diarrhea may be associated with improper intake, bacterial infection or affection by its toxin, or viral infection. The course of diarrhea of persisting type is usually over one month and it is often caused by uncontrolled intestinal infections or induced by flora imbalance resulting from abused antibiotics. According to TCM, infantile diarrhea belongs to the category of Xiao Er Xie Xie (children diarrhea), and it is due to improper diet or attack by pathogenic cold of heat, leading to impairment of the spleen and stomach.

I. STANDARD TREATMENT

Infantile diarrhea is usually divided into five types — damp-heat, impairment by overeating, insufficiency of spleen, spleen and kidney yang deficiency, and wind-cold. Points of the Spleen and Stomach Meridians are frequently selected in its treatment.

1. Wind-Cold

Manifestations: Increased frequency of defecation, watery stool with undigested food, abdominal pain, stuffy nose with watery sneezing, aversion to cold, lower fever.

Tongue: White and moist coating.

Finger Superficial Venules: Red superficial venule of the index finger.

Treatment Principle: Dispel wind and cold, remove dampness, arrest diarrhea.

Point Prescription & Manipulation:
Primary points:
    ST-25 Tianshu / ^
    DU-20 Baihui ^
    ST-37 Shangjuxu / ^
    SP-6 Sanyinjiao + ^

Explanation:
After insertion of the needle, rotate the needle to induce gentle stimulation for 1 minute, and take out the needle without retention. Then, apply moxibustion with moxa stick on each point for 5-10 minutes. The treatment is given once daily and usually within 2-3 treatments diarrhea will be arrested.

- ST-25 Tianshu, the Front-Mu Point of the large intestine, and ST-37 Shangjuxu, the Lower He-Sea Point of the Large Intestine Meridian, remove dampness from the large intestine and arrest diarrhea;
- DU-20 Baihui dispels wind and cold pathogens and raises yang qi to arrest diarrhea;
- SP-6 Sanyinjiao removes dampness and arrests diarrhea.

Secondary points according to conditions:
1 Fever with chills — DU-14 Dazhui [+^] and LI-4 Hegu [/]
2 Extreme diarrhea — SP-4 Gongsun [^] and SJ-5 Waiguan [/].

2. Damp-Heat

Manifestations: Increased frequency of defecation, watery stool with undigested food and mucous fluid, which is green or yellow, red anus and burning sensation, scanty and dark urine, fever.

Tongue: Yellow and sticky coating.

Finger Superficial Venules: Purplish superficial venule of the index finger.

Treatment Principle: Clear heat, remove dampness, arrest diarrhea.

Point Prescription & Manipulation:
Primary points:
　　ST-25 Tianshu -
　　ST-36 Zusanli -
　　ST-44 Neiting -
　　SP-9 Yinlingquan -

Explanation:
After insertion of the needles, gently rotate them for 1 minute. Then, take out the needles without retention. The treatment is given once daily and usually within 2-4 treatments diarrhea will be arrested.

- ST-25 Tianshu, the Front-Mu Point of the large intestine, clears damp-heat from the large intestine and arrests diarrhea;
- ST-36 Zusanli reinforces the middle-jiao;
- ST-44 Neiting clears heat from the Yangming Meridian;
- SP-9 Yinlingquan removes dampness.

Secondary points according to conditions:
1 High fever — LI-4 Hegu [-] and DU-14 Dazhui [-].

3. Impairment due to Overeating

Manifestations: History of overeating, abdominal distention and pain which are relieved after diarrhea, crying and restlessness before diarrhea, diarrhea with an odor as sour as that of putrid eggs, anorexia, vomiting.

Tongue: Thick and sticky coating.

Finger Superficial Venules: Deep and stagnated superficial venule of the index finger.

Treatment Principle: Promote digestion, remove stagnated food, and regulate stomach, arrest diarrhea.

Point Prescription & Manipulation:
Primary points:
　　RN-12 Zhongwan -
　　ST-25 Tianshu -
　　EX-UE-10 Sifeng -
　　ST-36 Zusanli +
　　ST-44 Neiting -

Explanation:
- When puncturing EX-UE-10 Sifeng, prick the point with a thick needle or a three

edged needle, and squeeze the point to let out a little of fluid;

- RN-12 Zhongwan, the Front-Mu Point of the stomach, and ST-36 Zusanli, the He-Sea Point of the Stomach Meridian, regulate the middle-jiao and improve digestion;
- ST-25 Tianshu the Front-Mu Point of the large intestine, clears accumulated food from the large intestine and arrests diarrhea;
- EX-UE-10 Sifeng, an experiential point to remove accumulated food and improve digestion;
- ST-44 Neiting clears heat, which is transformed from accumulated food.

Secondary points according to conditions:

1□ Vomiting — PC-6 Neiguan [-] and RN-13 Shangwan [-];

2□ Abdominal distention and pain — RN-10 Xiawan [-] and LI-4 Hegu [-].

4. Spleen Deficiency

Manifestations: Intermittent or lingering diarrhea, loose stools, or undigested food in the stool with white milky mass or food residues, diarrhea right after food intake, sallow complexion, sleeping with eyes open.

Tongue: Pale body with thin and white coating.

Finger Superficial Venules: Pale and superficial venule of the index finger.

Treatment Principle: Strengthen spleen, arrest diarrhea.

Point Prescription & Manipulation:
Primary points:
RN-12 Zhongwan + ^
ST-36 Zusanli + ^
BL-20 Pishu + ^
BL-26 Guanyuanshu + ^
DU-20 Baihui +
ST-37 Shangjuxu + ^

Explanation:

- RN-12 Zhongwan, the Front-Mu Point of the stomach, ST-36 Zusanli, the He-Sea Point of the Stomach Meridian, and BL-20 Pishu, the Back-Shu Point of the spleen, reinforce the middle-jiao and improve digestion;
- BL-26 Guanyuanshu warms and reinforces the kidney to strengthen the spleen, i.e., tonifies fire to generate earth;
- DU-20 Baihui reinforces qi, raises yang and arrests diarrhea;
- ST-37 Shangjuxu, the Lower He-Sea Point of the Large Intestine Meridian, consolidates the large intestine and arrests diarrhea.

Secondary points according to conditions:

1□ Prolonged course or chronic cases—RN-4 Guanyuan [+ ^] and SP-9 Yinlingquan [+];

2□ Extreme diarrhea — ST-37 Shangjushu [+ ^] and ST-25 Tianshu [+ ^].

5. Spleen and Kidney Yang Deficiency

Manifestations: Intermittent or lingering diarrhea, loose stools, or undigested food in the stool with white milky mass or food residues, diarrhea right after food intake, or prolapse of the rectum, cold limbs, frequent and profuse clear urine, low spirit.

Tongue: Pale body with thin and white coating.

Finger Superficial Venules: Pale and superficial venule of the index finger.

Treatment Principle: Strengthen spleen, arrest diarrhea.

Point Prescription & Manipulation:
Primary points:
RN-8 Shenque ^
ST-37 Shangjushu + ^
BL-20 Pishu + ^
BL-23 Shenshu + ^
DU-4 Mingmen +

Explanation:

- RN-8 Shenque, an experiential point to warm spleen and kidney yang, and BL-20 Pishu, the Back-Shu Point of the spleen, warm yang, reinforce the spleen and kidney;
- BL-23 Shenshu warms and reinforces the kidney to strengthen the spleen, i.e., tonifies fire to generate earth;
- DU-4 Mingmen warms the fire of the life gate to strengthen spleen and kidney yang;
- ST-37 Shangjuxu, the Lower He-Sea Point of the Large Intestine Meridian, consolidates the large intestine and arrests diarrhea.

Secondary points according to conditions:
1 □ Profuse and clear urine — RN-4 Guanyuan [+ ^] and DU-20 Baihui [+];
2 □ Prolapse of rectum — DU-20 Baihui [+ ^] and DU-1 Changqiang [+ ^].

II. EXPERIENTIAL TREATMENT

1. Puncturing DU-1Changqiang and ST-36 Zusanli

Indication: Infantile diarrhea.

Point Prescription:
   DU-1 Changqiang
   ST-36 Zusanli

Manipulation: Acupuncture is applied. When puncturing DU-1 Changqiang, insert the needle horizontally upwards and push the needle under the coccyx-sacral bones 0.5-0.8 cun. Then rotate the needle 4 times, scratch the needle handle with the nail of the thumb 4 times and take out the needle. When puncturing bilateral ST-36 Zusanli, insert the needle 1 cun, manipulate the needle with the same method mentioned above. The treatment is given once daily, usually, within five treatments, diarrhea will be arrested.

2. Puncturing EX-AC-3 Jueyuan

Indication: Acute infantile diarrhea.

Point Prescription:
   EX-AC-3 Jueyuan, located on the upper border of RN-8 Shenque.

Manipulation: Acupuncture is applied. Insert a 1-cun long needle into the point perpendicularly 0.5-0.8 cun, rotate the needle for 15-20 minutes and take out the needle. The treatment is given once daily, usually, only 1-2 treatments are needed to arrest diarrhea.

3. Moxibustion on DU-1 Changqiang

Indication: Infantile chronic diarrhea.

Point Prescription:
   DU-1 Changqiang

Manipulation: Moxibustion is applied. Ignite a matchstick, keep the ignited end of the stick to face to the point, quickly press and touch the point with the end and lift the stick immediately. Usually, only one treatment is needed to arrest diarrhea. In case diarrhea is not arrested by one treatment, the second treatment can be given after an interval of 3-5 days.

4. Pressing with the Finger

Indication: Infantile diarrhea.

Point Prescription:
   DU-1 Changqiang

Manipulation: Ask the patient to lie on the stomach with DU-1 Changqiang exposed fully. Press DU-1 Changqiang with the tip of the thumb, and knead and press the point with right rotating movement 200-300 times. The treatment is given once daily, and usually within 3-5 treatments diarrhea will be arrested.

Comment:
Zhenjiu is very effective in the treatment of infantile diarrhea. In most cases, diarrhea can be arrested by Zhenjiu treatment.

Notes:

71. Children's Enuresis

Children's enuresis refers to unconscious urination during sleep when the children are above the age of three. Its cause may be related to heredity, fright, over physical stress, over excitement, and change of environment. Clinically, it is marked by involuntary emptying of the bladder during sleep once several nights in mild cases and several times in one night in severe cases, and not waking up after enuresis. According to TCM, enuresis, called Yi Niao in Chinese, is mainly caused by deficiency of the bladder leading to failure in controlling urination.

I. STANDARD TREATMENT

Enuresis is usually divided into three types — kidney yang deficiency, qi deficiency of spleen and lung, and damp-heat in the Liver Meridian. Points of the Ren, Spleen and Liver Meridians are frequently selected in its treatment.

1. Kidney Yang Deficiency

Manifestations: Frequent enuresis during sleeping, difficulty in being awakened from sound sleep, frequent light-colored urine, pallor, cold limbs, aversion to cold, weakness of the lower limbs, lassitude of the loins and legs, mental retardation.

Tongue: Pale body with thin and white coating.

Treatment Principle: Warm and tonify the kidney yang, arrest enuresis.

Point Prescription & Manipulation:
Primary points:
    RN-4 Guanyuan + ^
    RN-3 Zhongji + ^
    SP-6 Sanyinjiao + ^
    BL-23 Shenshu + ^
    BL-20 Pishu + ^
    ST-36 Zusanli + ^

Explanation:
- RN-3 Zhongji and RN-4 Guanyuan warm and reinforce the urinary bladder, tonify kidney qi, and arrest enuresis;
- SP-6 Sanyinjiao reinforces and warms the three Foot-Yin Meridians;
- BL-23 Shenshu, the Back-Shu Point of the kidney, warms and tonifies the kidney yang;
- BL-20 Pishu and ST-36 Zusanli reinforce the middle-jiao and consolidate the body constitution.

Secondary point:
1□ Severe cases — DU-20 Baihui [^] and DU-4 Mingmen [+ ^].

2. Qi Deficiency of Spleen and Lung

Manifestations: Enuresis during sleeping, frequent and scanty urination, shortness of breath, disinclination to speak, lassitude and weakness, sallow complexion, poor appetite, loose stool, frequent spontaneous perspiration or night sweat.

Tongue: Pale and tender body with thin and white coating.

Treatment Principle: Tonify spleen and lung, reinforce qi, arrest enuresis.

Point Prescription & Manipulation:
Primary points:
    RN-3 Zhongji + ^
    RN-4 Guanyuan + ^
    ST-36 Zusanli + ^
    SP-9 Yinlingquan + ^
    BL-20 Pishu + ^
    BL-21 Weishu + ^
    BL-13 Feishu + ^

Explanation:
- RN-3 Zhongji and RN-4 Guanyuan warm and reinforce the urinary bladder, tonify qi, and arrest enuresis;
- ST-36 Zusanli and SP-9 Yinlingquan, the He-Sea Points of the Stomach and Spleen

Meridians, and BL-20 Pishu and BL-21 Weishu, the Back-Shu Points of the spleen and stomach, reinforce the middle-jiao and tonify qi;

- BL-13 Feishu reinforces the lung, tonifies qi and controls the upper resource of water to arrest enuresis.

Secondary points according to conditions:
1️⃣ Bad sleeping —HT-7 Shenmen [+] and SP-6 Sanyinjiao [+].

3. Damp-Heat in the Liver Meridian

Manifestations: Enuresis during sleeping, scanty urine with fish-stink odor and yellow color, irascible temperament or feverish sensation in the palms and soles, nocturnal muttering and teeth grinding, flushed face and lips.

Tongue: Yellowish coating.

Treatment Principle: Clear heat and remove dampness from the Liver Meridian.

Point Prescription & Manipulation:
Primary points:
BL-33 Zhongliao -
RN-3 Zhongji -
SP-6 Sanyinjiao -
LR-3 Taichong -
GB-34 Yanglingquan -

Explanation:
- BL-33 Zhongliao and RN-3 Zhongji clear damp-heat from the urinary bladder;
- SP-6 Sanyinjiao, GB-34 Yanglingquan and LR-3 Taichong clear damp-heat from the Liver Meridian.

Secondary points according to conditions:
1️⃣ Chronic cases — LI-4 Hegu [-] and BL-32 Ciliao [-];
2️⃣ Constipation — ST-25 Tianshu [-] and SJ-6 Zhigou [-].

II. EXPERIENTIAL TREATMENT

1. Puncturing EX-LE-19 Yiniao

Indication: Enuresis.

Point Prescription:
EX-LE-19 Yiniao, located on the bottom of the foot, at the midpoint of the interphalangeal transverse crease.

Manipulation: Insert a 0.5-cun long needle perpendicularly into the point, push it to reach the surface of the bone. Rotate the needle with strong stimulation until the patient feels violent pain or lower abdominal distention or burning sensation. Then retain the needle for 30 minutes, and manipulate once during the retention. The treatment is given once daily, and usually the disease will be cured within 3-5 treatments.

2. Acupuncture & Moxibustion on RN-1 Huiyin

Indication: Enuresis.

Point Prescription:
RN-1 Huiyin

Manipulation: Ask the patient to lie on the back with the legs bent. Insert a 2-cun long needle perpendicularly into the point 1-1.5 cun, and apply moxibustion with warming needling method for 5 minutes to induce a sensation of flow of warm current in the head. Then, remove the needle, insert another needle into the point, and push it horizontally upward at an angle of 15 degrees 1-1.5 cun. Apply warming needling moxibustion again for 5 minutes to induce a sensation of flow of warm current in the lower abdomen. Then, remove the needle, insert another needle into the point, and push the needle downward again, horizontally at an angle of 15 degrees 1-1.5 cun. Apply warming needling moxibustion again for 5 minutes to induce warming sensation in the back of the body and legs. The treatment is given once daily, and usually, within six treatments the disease will be cured.

3. Puncturing SP-6 Sanyinjiao

Indication: Enuresis.

Point Prescription:
SP-6 Sanyinjiao

Manipulation: Insert a 1.5-cun long needle through the skin of the point, and push the needle upward horizontally under the skin 1.4 cun. Then, retain the needle for 30 minutes. It is necessary not to manipulate the needle with lifting, thrusting or rotating movement, and not to induce any pain, soreness or distention to the patient. The treatment is given once daily, and usually, one treatment is effective to arrest nocturnal enuresis.

4. Puncturing EX-UE-17 Urine-Controlling Point

Indication: Enuresis.

Point Prescription:
EX-UE-17 Urine-Controlling Point, located on the palmar surface of the hand, at the midpoint of the first transverse crease of the small finger.

Manipulation: Insert a 1-cun long needle perpendicularly into the point 0.3-0.5 cun, rotate the needle to induce pain, soreness, numbness and heaviness to the patient, retain the needle for 5-10 minutes, and manipulate once during the retention. The treatment is given once daily, and generally, 2-3 treatments are needed to cure the disease.

5. Wrist-Ankle Puncture

Indication: Enuresis.

Wrist-Ankle Point Prescription:
Lower 1

Manipulation: Insert a 2-cun long needle through the skin at an angle of 30 degrees, push the needle horizontally under the skin 1-1.5 cun without any other manipulation. There should be no soreness, numbness , distention or pain to the patient. Then, retain the needle for 20-30 minutes. The treatment is given once every other day, and usually five treatments are needed.

Comment:
Zhenjiu is very effective in the treatment of children's nocturnal enuresis. In most cases, it can produce a curative result. Before the treatment, the patient should have urination. Usually, in order to consolidate the treatment result, another 3-5 treatments are needed after the patient has not had enuresis.

Notes:

72. Poliomyelitis and Its Sequels

Poliomyelitis, infantile paralysis or Heine-Medin Disease, refers to an epidemic infantile disease caused by poliovirus. Clinically, it is initially marked by fever, sore throat, cough, sweating or accompany with abdominal pain, diarrhea, general muscular pain, and finally by softness and weakness of the muscles of the diseased limb, leading to flaccid paralysis and atrophy of the diseased limb. According to TCM, poliomyelitis belongs to the categories of Shu Wen (summer fever syndrome) and Shi Wen (damp-warm syndrome), and its sequel belongs to the categories of Wei Zheng (flaccid syndrome) and Wei Bi (flaccid lower limb syndrome).

I. STANDARD TREATMENT

Poliomyelitis and its sequels are generally divided into four types — attack of the lung and stomach by the pathogen, attack of the meridian and collateral by the pathogen, obstruction of the meridian and collateral by blood stasis, and deficiency of qi and blood. Points of the Du, Large Intestine, Stomach and Spleen Meridians and points on the diseased meridians are frequently selected in its treatment.

1. Attack of Lung and Stomach by Pathogen

Manifestations: Fever, cough, general discomfort, poor appetite, abdominal pain, diarrhea, and weakness of the leg.

Tongue: Red body with thin and yellow coating.

Pulse: Soft and rapid.

Treatment Principle: Relieve exterior syndrome and clear heat.

Point Prescription & Manipulation:
Primary points:

DU-14 Dazhui -
LI-4 Hegu-
SJ-5 Waiguan -
LU-5 Chize -
LU-5 Lieque -
ST-36 Zusanli +

Explanation:
- DU-14 Dazhui, LI-4 Hegu and SJ-5 Waiguan relieve exterior syndrome and clear heat;
- LU-5 Chize and LU-5 Lieque dispel pathogens from the lung;
- ST-36 Zusanli reinforce the middle-jiao, nourish and strengthen the muscles and tendons.

Secondary points according to the paralyzed portion and accompanied conditions:

1） Paralysis of the upper limb —LI-15 Jianyu [-], LI-10 Shousanli [-], LI-11 Quchi [-], SJ-5 Waiguan [-], SJ-3 Zhongzhu [-].

2） Paralysis of the lower limb — GB-30 Huantiao [-], ST-32 Futu [-], GB-34 Yanglingquan [-], GB-39 Xuanzhong [-], GB-40 Qiuxu [-].

3） Weakness and flaccidity of the neck — GB-20 Fengchi [-], BL-11 Dazhu [-], SJ-15 Jianzhongshu [-], SI-3 Houxi [-], BL-60 Kunlun [-].

4） High fever — LI-1 Shangyang is pricked to bleed.

2. Attack of Meridian & Collaterals

Manifestations: Fever, soreness and pain of the muscles, sensitivity of the skin, irritability, restlessness, thirst, dark urine.

Tongue: Red tongue with yellow and sticky coating.

Pulse: Soft and rapid.

Treatment Principle: Clear heat, remove dampness, dredge the meridians and activate the collaterals.

Point Prescription & Manipulation:
Primary points:
    DU-14 Dazhui -
    LI-11 Quchi -
    LI-4 Hegu -
    GB-34 Yanglingquan -
    SP-9 Yinlingquan -

Explanation:
- DU-14 Dazhui, LI-11 Quchi and LI-4 Hegu clear heat, activate the meridians and collaterals;
- GB-34 Yanglingquan, the He-Sea Point of the Gallbladder Meridian and the Influential Point of tendons, clears heat, dredges the collaterals and strengthens the tendons;
- SP-9 Yinlingquan reinforces the spleen and removes dampness.

Secondary points according to the paralyzed portion and accompanied conditions:
1① Paralysis of the upper limb —LI-15 Jianyu [-], LI-10 Shousanli [-], LI-11 Quchi [-], SJ-5 Waiguan [-], SJ-3 Zhongzhu [-].

2① Paralysis of the lower limb — GB-30 Huantiao [-], ST-32 Futu [-], GB-34 Yanglingquan [-], GB-39 Xuanzhong [-], GB-40 Qiuxu [-].

3① Weakness and flaccidity of the neck — GB-20 Fengchi [-], BL-11 Dazhu [-], SJ-15 Jianzhongshu [-], SI-3 Houxi [-], BL-60 Kunlun [-].

4① Constipation — ST-Tianshu [-] and SJ-6 Zhigou [-].

3. Obstruction of Meridians & Collaterals by Blood Stasis

Manifestations: Weakness and flaccidity of the diseased limb or paralysis.

Tongue: Purplish body.

Pulse: Uneven or wiry.

Treatment Principle: Promote circulation of qi, activate blood and dredge the meridians and collaterals.

Point Prescription & Manipulation:
Primary points:
    ST-36 Zusanli +
    SP-10 Xuehai   -
    LR-3 Taichong   -
    BL-18 Ganshu +
    BL-17 Geshu -

Explanation:
Acupuncture is applied on 5-7 points (including the secondary points) at each treatment. After inserting the needles through the skin of the points, lift, thrust and rotate them to induce arrival of qi, and remove them without retention. The stimulation from needling should be increased gradually.

- ST-36 Zusanli reinforces the middle-jiao, tonifies qi and nourishes the muscles;
- LR-3 Taichong and SP-10 Xuehai promote qi flow and remove blood stasis;
- BL-18 Ganshu and BL-17 Geshu promote qi and blood circulation, and dredge the meridians and collaterals.

Secondary points according to the paralyzed portion and accompanied conditions:
1① Paralysis of the upper limb —LI-15 Jianyu [-], LI-10 Shousanli [-], LI-11 Quchi [-], SJ-5 Waiguan [-], SJ-3 Zhongzhu [-].

2① Paralysis of the lower limb — GB-30 Huantiao [-], ST-32 Futu [-], GB-34 Yanglingquan [-], GB-39 Xuanzhong [-], GB-40 Qiuxu [-].

3□ Weakness and flaccidity of the neck — GB-20 Fengchi [-], BL-11 Dazhu [-], SJ-15 Jianzhongshu [-], SI-3 Houxi [-], BL-60 Kunlun [-].

4□ Difficulty in breath — BL-17 Geshu [-], LR-14 Qimen [-], SP-21 Dabao [-], RN-22 Tiantu [-].

5□ Retention of urine or incontinence of urine — ST-28 Shuidao [-], RN-3 Zhongji [-], RN-4 Guanyuan [+], BL-39 Weiyang [-], BL-33 Zhongliao [-].

6□ Difficulty in voluntary bowel movement — ST-25 Tianshu [-], RN-6 Qihai [+], BL-25 Dachangshu [-], ST-37 Shangjuxu [-], LI-4 Hegu [-].

7□ Swelling—Tiantu RN 22 [-], Futu LI 18 [-], Tianding 17 [-], Hegu LI 4 [-].

8□ Difficulty in breath — BL-13 Feishu [-], RN- 17 Danzhong [-], LU-5 Chize [-], PC-6 Neiguan [-], RN-1 Huiyin [-];

9□ Strephenopodia—BL-60 Kunlun [/] and GB-40 Qiuxu [/];

10□ Strephexopodia —SP-5 Shangqiu [/], KI-3 Taixi [+], KI-7 Fuliu [+] and SP-6 Sanyinjiao [+].

4. Deficiency of Kidney and Liver

Manifestations: Paralysis with obvious muscular atrophy and coldness of the skin of the diseased limb, dislocation and flaccidity or even deformation of the joint of the diseased limb.

Tongue: Thin and pale or red body.

Pulse: Weak.

Treatment Principle: Tonify the liver and kidney, reinforce the tendons and bones.

Point Prescription & Manipulation:

Primary points:
SP-21 Dabao　+ ^
SP-9 Yinlingquan + ^
GB-39 Xuanzhong　+ ^
BL-11 Dashu　+ ^
SP-6 Sanyinjiao　+ ^
BL-18 Ganshu　+ ^
BL-23 Shenshu　+ ^

Explanation:
• SP-21 Dabao, the Luo-Connecting Point of the general collateral of the spleen, and BL-11 Dashu and GB-39 Xuanzhong, the Influential Points of the bone and marrow, dredge the collaterals, strengthen the bones and reinforce the marrow;

• SP-6 Sanyinjiao and SP-9 Yinlingquan reinforce the middle-jiao and nourish the muscles;

• BL-18 Ganshu and BL-23 Shenshu, the Back-Shu Points of the liver and kidney, tonify the liver and kidney and nourish the tendons and bones.

Secondary points according to the diseased regions:
To paralysis, refer to "3.Obstruction of the Meridians and Collaterals by Blood Stasis" (Page 477).

To dislocation or deformation of the joints, select the following points according to the joints involved:
1□ Dislocation of the shoulder joint — LI-15 Jianyu, SJ-14 Jianliao and LI-16 Jugu;

2□ Hip joint dislocation—GB-30 Huantiao, GB-29 Juliao and ST-31 Biguan;

3□ Strephexopodia — SP-5 Shangqiu, KI-3 Taixi, KI-7 Fuliu and SP-6 Sanyinjiao;

4□ Foot drop — BL-60 Kunlun, GB-40 Qiuxu and BL-59 Fuyang;

5□ Hand drop — SJ-5 Waiguan, SJ-4 Yangchi, LI-5 Yangxi, SI-5 Yanggu.

Acupuncture with reinforcing manipulation and moxibustion are applied.

II. EXPERIENTIAL TREATMENT

Acupuncture and Moxibustion

Indication: Paralysis due to poliomyelitis.

Point Prescription:
According to the diseased region and patients' general condition:

1□ Paralysis of the upper limb — BL-11 Dazhu, SJ-15 Jianzhongshu, SI-11 Quyuan, LI-15 Jianyu, LI-11 Quchi, SJ-5 Waiguan, SJ-3 Zhongzhu, LI-4 Hegu;

2□ Paralysis of the lower limb — BL-23 Shenshu, BL-33 Zhongliao, GB-30 Huantiao, GB-31 Fengshi, ST-32 Futu, GB-34 Yanglingquan, ST-33 Yinshi, ST-36 Zusanli, RN-2 Qugu, GB-39 Xuanzhong, GB-40 Qiuxu, SP-6 Sanyinjiao, LR-2 Xingjian, ST-44 Neiting;

3□ Weakness and facility of the neck and lumber — GB-20 Fengchi, BL-10 Tianzhu, BL-11 Dazhu, BL-23 Shenshu, BL-40 Weizhong, GB-39 Xuanzhong;

4□ Weak constitute — BL-18 Ganshu, BL-20 Pishu, RN-6 Qihai, RN-4 Guanyuan, ST-36 Zusanli, SP-6 Sanyinjiao.

Manipulation: Acupuncture and moxibustion are applied on 5-7 points each treatment. Generally, apply treatment on the points of the diseased side firstly. If there is no result after many treatments, apply the treatment on the points of the healthy side firstly and diseased side secondly or even only on the healthy side. Apply shallow and gentle puncture, insert the needle into the point slowly while rotating it until the needle tip reaches a designed depth, constantly and gently rotate the needle to induce arrival of qi, and remove the needle. Then, apply bird-pecking moxibustion on the punctured points until the local skin becomes flushed. To patients who are in cooperation with the treatment, retain the needles in the points and apply warming needling moxibustion to replace the bird-peck moxibustion during the retention of the needles. The treatment is given once daily with 10 treatments as a course, and next course begins after an interval of 5-7 days. Generally, within three treatment courses, the patient's condition should be improved greatly. If not, the prognosis is bad.

Comment:
Zhenjiu is effective in the treatment of paralysis due to poliomyelitis. In some cases, paralysis due to poliomyelitis can be cured by Zhenjiu treatment. However, generally, Zhenjiu treatment should be carried out with massage in conjunction. If so, the treatment result will be much better. Additionally, the patient should be advised to do physical exercise of the diseased limbs.

Notes:

73. Childhood Anorexia

Childhood anorexia is a digestive disorder. It may be due to improper diet or exposure to cold and dampness, and parasitosis. Clinically, it is marked by long-standing poor appetite or even loss of appetite, and is usually accompanied by pale complexion, emaciation and retardation of growth and development. According to TCM, childhood anorexia belongs to the categories of Shang Shi (injury by over-eating), and Gan Ji (malnutrition due to abdominal retention of food). It is due to weakness of the spleen and stomach or injury due to improper diet, leading to accumulation of undigested food.

I. STANDARD TREATMENT

Point Prescription:
Primary points:
    EX-UE-10 Sifeng   -
    RN-12 Zhongwan +
    BL-20 Pishu   +
    BL-21 Weishu +

Explanation:
Prick EX-UE-10 Sifeng with the three-edged needle, squeeze the local region to let out some yellow mucous out of the punctured hole. Generally, one treatment is effective to cure this disease. If not, the treatment can be repeated once 7 days later.

- EX-UE-10 Sifeng, an experiential point to treat childhood anorexia;
- RN-12 Zhongwan, the Front-Mu Point of the stomach, and BL-20 Pishu and BL-21 Weishu, the Back-Shu Points of the spleen and stomach, strengthen the spleen and stomach, and promote digestion.

Secondary points according to conditions:
1〕 Stools with undigested food — ST-36 Zusanli [+] and SP-3 Taibai [+];

2〕 Diarrhea — RN-11 Jianli [+ ^], ST-25 Tianshu [+ ^] and RN-6 Qihai [+ ^].

II. EXPERIENTIAL TREATMENT

1. Cutting

Indication: Malnutrition due to intractable anorexia.

Point Prescription:
    LU-10 Yuji

Manipulation: Apply local sterilization and anesthesia on the point of both sides, cut the point 0.4 cm. long and 0.2 cm. deep with a surgical knife and squeeze the local region to let out some liquid tissues. Cover the wound with sterilized cotton, band it and press the point with the thumb tightly for 5 minutes in order to prevent bleeding. 5 days later remove the bandage. Usually, only one treatment is needed to improve appetite greatly.

2. Ear Acupuncture

Indication: Malnutrition due to anorexia.

Ear Point Prescription:
    Spleen, Stomach, Small Intestine, Liver, Abdomen, Endocrine, Subcortex.

Manipulation: See page 255-256.

Comment:
Zhenjiu is very effective in the treatment of anorexia. In most cases, it can act to cure this disease. Method of pricking EX-UE-10 Sifeng has been used for treatment of childhood anorexia since ancient times.

Notes:

CHAPTER FIVE
DISEASES OF EYE, EAR, NOSE & THROAT

74. Myopia

Myopia is a visual disorder caused by dysfunction of the optic-dioptric system. Since the visual focus is formed in the front of the retina when parallel light passes through the optic-dioptric system, dysfunction of this system affects the ability to focus normally. Clinically, myopia is marked by poor distance vision and normal near-range vision. The more extreme the condition is, the shorter the range of vision will be. A common cause of myopia is overuse or improper use of the eyes, although severe myopia is usually related to heredity. According to TCM, myopia, called Jin Shi in Chinese, is mainly due to deficiency of the liver and kidney leading to loss of normal nourishment of the eye. In addition, it may also be caused by improper usage of the eyes, which impairs the eyesight.

I. STANDARD TREATMENT

It is usually divided into two types — qi deficiency with impairment of mind and deficiency of kidney and liver. Points of the local region and the Liver and Kidney Meridians are frequently selected in its treatment.

1. Qi Deficiency with Impairment of Mind

Manifestations: Near-sightedness, liability of the eye to become tired, dreaminess, poor memory, fatigue and weakness.

Tongue: Pale body.

Pulse: Weak.

Treatment Principle: Tonify the heart qi, calm the mind and improve eyesight.

Point Prescription & Manipulation:
Primary points:
    BL-1 Jingming /
    ST-1 Chengqi /
    BL-2 Cuanzhu /
    BL-15 Xinshu + ^
    HT-7 Shenmen +

Explanation:
When puncturing points on the eye region such as BL-1 Jingming and ST-1 Chengqi, insert the needle to the correct depth without any lifting, thrusting or rotating manipulation. Take out the needle after 20-40 minutes retention and immediately press the needling holes to prevent bleeding. When puncturing BL-2 Cuanzhu, apply point-to-point method with the needle tip facing BL-1 Jingming and push the needle 0.5-1 cun, or with the needle facing EX-HN-4 Yuyao and push the needle 1-1.5 cun, and perform uniform reinforcing-reducing manipulation. When puncturing the other points, regular reinforcing manipulations are performed, and the needles are retained for 20-40 minutes as well.

- BL-1 Jingming, ST-1 Chengqi and BL-2 Cuanzhu, located around the eye, improve circulation of qi and blood in the local region and improve the eyesight;
- BL-15 Xinshu and HT-7 Shenmen nourish the heart and calm the mind.

Secondary points according to conditions:
1〕 Poor appetite and loose stool — ST-36 Zusanli [+ ^] and BL-20 Pishu [+ ^];
2〕 Dizziness and blurred vision — DU-20 Baihui [^].

2. Deficiency of Kidney and Liver

Manifestations: Near-sightedness, soreness and weakness of the loins and knees, dizziness, blurred vision, nocturnal emission.

Tongue: Thin and red body with little coating.

Pulse: Deep, thready and weak pulse.

Treatment Principle: Tonify the liver and kidney, improve eyesight.

Point Prescription & Manipulation:
Primary points:
   BL-1 Jingming +
   ST-1 Chengqi +
   BL-2 Cuanzhu +

   GB-20 Fengchi /
   GB-37 Guangming +
   BL-23 Shenshu +
   BL-18 Ganshu +

Explanation:
Manipulation of needles in BL-1 Jingming and BL-2 Chuanzhu is the same as above. When puncturing GB-20 Fengchi, push the needle towards the opposite eyeball 1-1.5 cun, and perform uniform reinforcing and reducing manipulation to induce the needling sensation radiating to the eye region.

- BL-1 Jingming, ST-1 Chengqi and BL-2 Cuanzhu, located around the eye, improve circulation of qi and blood in the local region and improve the eyesight;
- GB-20 Fengchi soothes the liver, dredges the collaterals and improves the eyesight;
- GB-37 Guangming, an experiential point for improving the eyesight;
- BL-23 Shenshu and BL-18 Ganshu, the Back-Shu Points of the kidney and liver, tonify the liver and kidney and nourish the eyes.

Secondary points according to conditions:
1〕 Poor appetite and poor sleeping — ST-36 Zusanli [+], SP-6 Sanyinjiao [+] and HT-7 Shenmen [+];
2〕 Night sweating and low grade fever — SP-9 Sanyinjiao [+] and LI-4 Quchi [-].

II. EXPERIENTIAL TREATMENT

1. Puncturing ST-1 Chengqi, EX-HN-14 Yiming, and GB-20 Fengchi

Indication: Juvenile myopia.

Point Prescription:
   ST-1 Chengqi
   EX-HN-14 Yiming
   GB-20 Fengchi

Manipulation: Acupuncture is applied. When applying acupuncture on ST-1 Chengqi, insert a 1.5-cun long needle through the skin of the point, push the needle obliquely about 1 cun and at an angle of 30 degrees with the tip toward BL-1 Jingming. Induce soreness, numbness, dissension and lacrimation to the patient, and retain the needle for 10 minutes. The manipulation should be gentle, with large amplitude of rotation. Lifting and thrusting the needle should be avoided, and the needling hole should be pressed with a cotton ball immediately after removing the needle to prevent bleeding. When puncturing EX-EN-14 Yiming and GB-20 Fengchi, insert a 1-cun needle 0.8 cun deep, perform a rotating, lifting and thrusting manipulation to induce needling sensation, and retain the needle for 10 minutes. The treatment is given once daily, with 10 treatments as a course. Generally, 2-4 treatment courses are needed.

2. Puncturing EX-HN-7 Qiuhou

Indication: Juvenile myopia.

Point Prescription:
    EX-HN-7 Qiuhou

Manipulation: Acupuncture is applied. Ask the patient to lie on his/her back and look upward. Insert a 1.5-cun long needle through the skin of the point, push the needle gently with the needle tip towards the optic foramen until the patient feels local dissension and electric shock sensation. Lifting, thrusting or rotating manipulation is prohibited. If the patient is highly sensitive to acupuncture, retention of the needle is not suggested. For the patient who is moderately sensitive, the needle is retained for 30 minutes, and to the patient who is not sensitive, the needle is retained for 40-50 minutes and the needle handle is scraped several times during the retention. Finally, remove the needle slowly and press the needling hole immediately with cotton ball for 1 minute to prevent bleeding. The treatment is given once daily, with 10 treatments as a course. Generally, two courses are needed.

3. Ear Acupuncture

Indication: Juvenile myopia.

Ear Point Prescription:
    Eye, Eye 1, Eye 2, Liver, Kidney, Heart.

Manipulation: See page 255-256.

Comment:
Zhenjiu is effective in the treatment of juvenile myopia. Most patients who have suffered from myopia not more than 2 years and whose age is less than 18 can improve their eyesight obviously after Zhenjiu treatment. When puncturing the points around the eyes and GB-20 Fengchi, manipulation should be gentle, and the needling sensation should be induced to radiate to the eyeball. The patient should be suggested to pay attention to correct reading habit, and do some massage on the eye region.

Notes:

75.   Epidemic   Acute Conjunctivitis

Epidemic acute conjunctivitis is an acute infectious ophthalmopathy due to bacterial or viral infection. Clinically, it is marked by obvious conjunctival congestion and is of a pandemic nature. According to TCM, epidemic acute conjunctivitis belongs to the categories of Tian Xing Chi Yan (epidemic red eyes) and Huo Yan (fire eyes). It is due to invasion of epidemic pathogens, and accumulation of heat in the lung and stomach, the combination of which attacks the eyes, leading to qi stagnation and blood stasis.

I. STANDARD TREATMENT

Epidemic acute conjunctivitis is divided into two types — wind-heat and over activity of internal heat-toxin. Points of the eye region and of the Shaoyang Meridians are frequently selected in its treatment.

1. Wind-Heat

Manifestations: Redness, itching and sensation of foreign body in the diseased eye, photophobia with lacrimation, headache, fever, sore throat.

Tongue: Thin and yellow coating.

Pulse: Floating and rapid.

Treatment Principle: Dispel wind and clear heat.

Point Prescription & Manipulation:
Primary points:
 EX-HN-5 Taiyang -
 LU-11 Shaoshang -
 BL-1 Jingming -
 GB-20 Fengchi -
 LI-4 Hegu -

Explanation:
First, bleed EX-HN-5 Taiyang and LU-11 Shaoshang with three-edged needle to let out several drops of blood. Then puncture the other points with the filiform needles with reducing manipulation, and retain the needles for 20-40 minutes after arrival of qi.

- EX-HN-5 Taiyang and LU-11 Shaoshang clear heat;
- BL-1 Jingming, located at the eye region, clears heat from the eyes;
- GB-20 Fengchi and LI-4 Hegu dispel wind, clear heat and relieve exterior syndrome.

Secondary points according to conditions:
1○ High fever — LI-11 Quchi [-];
2○ Constipation — SJ-6 Zhigou [-].

2. Fire Toxin

Manifestations: Burning sensation, pain, redness and swelling of the diseased eye, sticky gum, photophobia with lacrimation, scanty and dark urine, and constipation.

Tongue: Red body with yellow coating.

Pulse: Rapid.

Treatment Principle: Cool blood and detoxify poison

Point Prescription & Manipulation:
Primary points:
 EX-HN-5 Taiyang -
 DU-23 Shangxing -
 LU-11 Shaoshang -
 BL-1 Jingming -
 BL-2 Cuanzhu -
 SJ-23 Sizhukong -

Explanation:
First, puncture EX-HN-5 Taiyang, DU-23 Shangxing and LU-11 Shaoshang with a three-edged needle to let out several drops of blood. Then, puncture the other points with filiform needles and use a reducing manipulation and retain them for 20-40 minutes after arrival of qi.

- EX-HN-5 Taiyang, DU-23 Shangxing and LU-11 Shaoshang clear heat, cool blood and detoxify poison;

- BL-1 Jingming, BL-2 Cuanzhu and SJ-23 Sizhukong, located at the eye region, clear heat from the eyes.

Secondary points according to conditions:

1️⃣ Extreme congested eyes — BL-40 Weizhong is pricked to bleed, LI-4 Hegu [-] and LR-2 Xingjian [-];

2️⃣ High fever — LI-11 Quchi [-];

3️⃣ Constipation— SJ-6 Zhigou [-].

II. EXPERIENTIAL TREATMENT

1. Breaking the Reaction Spot

Indication: Any type of acute conjunctivitis.

Point Prescription:
The reaction spot, a small gray-white, red, or dark-brown spot on the scapular region of the healthy side, which is as big as a half grain of rice, is lustrous, and does not extinguish its color after pressure.

Manipulation: Seen page 220.

Generally, only one treatment is needed to cure this disease. If not, apply the same treatment next day.

2. Pricking PC-9 Zhongchong

Indication: Any type of acute conjunctivitis.

Point Prescription:
PC-9 Zhongchong of the diseased side.

Manipulation: Prick the point with a three-edged needle and squeeze the region around the point to bleed 2-4 drops of blood. The treatment is given once daily and generally, the disease will be cured within three treatments.

3. Through Puncturing

Indication: Any type of acute conjunctivitis.

Point Prescription:
ST-43 Xiangu

Manipulation: Insert a 3-cun needle into the point of both sides, slowly rotate and push the needle deeply until its tip arrives under the skin of KI-1 Yongquan. Rotate the needle with reducing manipulation to induce arrival of qi, retain the needle for 20-40 minutes and manipulate it every 10 minutes. Generally, only one treatment is needed to cure this disease. If not, the treatment may be repeated next day.

4. Ear Acupuncture

Indication: Any type of acute conjunctivitis.

Point Prescription:
The apex of the ear on the diseased side.

Manipulation: Prick the point with the three-edged needle 0.1 cun deep, and squeeze the apex to let out 3-5 drops of blood. The treatment may be repeated next day. Generally, only one or two treatments are needed to cure this disease.

Comment:
Acupuncture is very effective in the treatment of acute conjunctivitis, and if properly applied, it can function to cure this disease.

Notes:

76. Central Choroido-Retinitis

Central choroido-retinitis refers to inflammation of the choroid and retina in the macula. Its cause is uncertain. Clinically, it is marked by gradual diminution of vision, appearance of a fixed central shadow in the visual field, metamorphopsia, presence of edema and exudate in the macula. According to TCM, central choroido-retinitis belongs to the categories of Shi Zhan Hun Miao (blurring of vision) and Shi Huo (metamorphopsia). It is due to deficiency of kidney and liver leading to poor nourishment of the eyes, or stagnation of liver qi leading to obstruction of the vessels and collaterals.

I. STANDARD TREATMENT

Central choroido-retinitis is usually divided into three types — kidney-yang deficiency, yin deficiency with over-activity of yang, and depression of liver and qi stagnation. Points on the eye region and the Liver and Kidney Meridians are frequently selected in its treatment.

1. Stagnation of Liver Qi

Manifestations: Blurred vision or diminution of vision, pigment disturbance or pigmentation, dim reflected light of the central fovea in the macula, accompanied by mental depression, chest oppression, hypochondriac dissension.

Tongue: Red body with thin, yellow coating.

Pulse: Wiry.

Treatment Principle: Relieve depressed liver qi and improve eyesight.

Point Prescription & Manipulation:
Primary points:
   BL-1 Jingming -
   EX-HN-7 Qiuhou -
   EX-HN-5 Taiyang -
   BL-2 Cuanzhu -

   LR-3 Taichong -
   BL-18 Ganshu -

Explanation:
When puncturing BL-1 Jingming and EX-HN-7 Qiuhou, insert the needle through the skin and push the needle deeply but gently without lifting, thrusting or rotating manipulation. After removing the needle, press the needle hole immediately to prevent bleeding. When puncturing BL-2 Cuanzhu, apply point-to-point method with the needle tip facing BL-1 Jingming and push the needle 0.5-1 cun, or with the needle facing EX-HN-4 Yuyao and push the needle 1-1.5 cun, and perform uniform reinforcing-reducing manipulation. When puncturing the other points, perform lifting, thrusting and rotating manipulation to induce reducing effect. All needles in the points are retained for 20-40 minutes.

- EX-HN-7 Qiuhou, an experiential point for eye disorders which improves the eyesight;
- BL-1 Jingming, EX-HN-5 Taiyang and BL-2 Cuanzhu, located around the eye region, promote qi and blood circulation and improve the eyesight;
- LR-3 Taichong and BL-18 Ganshu soothe the liver, relieve depressed liver qi and improve the eyesight.

Secondary points according to conditions:
1️⃣ Chronic cases — EX-HN-4 Yuyao [-] and GB-34 Yanglingquan [-];
2️⃣ Stressed feeling in the chest — PC-6 Neiguan [-];
3️⃣ Insomnia — EX-HN-16 Anmian [/].

2. Hyperactivity of Fire due to Yin Deficiency

Manifestations: Blurred vision, slight dissension of the eye causing discomfort, dizziness and tinnitus, retinal edema in the macula accompanied by petachial exudate, disappearance of reflected light of the central fovea.

Tongue: Red body with thin coating.

Pulse: Wiry, thready and rapid.

Treatment Principle: Tonify yin and reduce fire.

Point Prescription:
Primary points:
> BL-1 Jingming +
> EX-HN-7 Qiuhou +
> EX-HN-5 Taiyang +
> BL-2 Cuanzhu +
> KI-3 Taixi +
> BL-18 Ganshu +
> BL-23 Shenshu +

Explanation:
Manipulation on the local points around the eye is the same as above.

- EX-HN-7 Qiuhou, an experiential point for eye disorders;
- BL-1 Jingming, EX-HN-5 Taiyang and BL-2 Cuanzhu, located around the eye region, promote qi and blood circulation, and improve the eyesight;
- KI-3 Taixi, BL-18 Ganshu and BL-23 Shenshu tonify the liver and kidney, nourish yin to reduce deficient fire and improve the eyesight.

Secondary points according to conditions:
1□ Chronic cases — KI-2 Rangu [+] and SI-6 Yanglao [+];
2□ Insomnia — EX-HN-16 Anmian [/];
3□ Headache — GB-20 Fengchi [-].

3. Kidney Yang Deficiency

Manifestations: Blurred vision, black shadow in the visual field, retinal edema in the macula, disappearance of reflected light in the central fovea, soreness and weakness of the lions and knees, light-colored and profuse urination.

Tongue: Pale body with white coating.

Pulse: Deep and weak.

Treatment Principle: Warm yang, tonify kidney and improve eyesight.

Point Prescription & Manipulation:
Primary points:
> BL-1 Jingming +
> EX-HN-7 Qiuhou +
> BL-2 Cuanzhu +
> EX-HN-4 Yuyao +
> RN-4 Guanyuan + ^
> DU-3 Yaoyangguan + ^
> BL-18 Ganshu + ^
> BL-23 Shenshu + ^

Explanation:
To BL-1 Jingming, EX-HN-7 Qiuhou and BL-2 Cuanzhu, apply acupuncture only and perform the same manipulation as above. To the other points, apply both acupuncture and moxibustion with reinforcing manipulation.

- EX-HN-7 Qiuhou, an experiential point for eye disorders;
- BL-1 Jingming, BL-2 Cuanzhu and EX-HN-4 Yuyao, located around the eye region, promote qi and blood circulation, and improve the eyesight;
- RN-4 Guanyuan, DU-3 Yaoyangguan and BL-23 Shenshu tonify the kidney and strengthen yang;
- BL-18 Ganshu reinforces the liver and improves the eyesight.

Secondary points according to conditions:
1□ Edema — SP-6 Sanyinjiao [+ ^] and KI-3 Taixi [+ ^].

II. EXPERIENTIAL TREATMENT

Scalp Acupuncture

Indication: Central choroido-retinitis.

Scalp Line Prescription:
Primary lines:
> Middle Line of Forehead, the posterior 1/3 of the Forehead-Vertex Line, lower 1/3 of the Vertex-Occiput Line.

Secondary lines:
    Line 2 Lateral to Forehead of the left side over-activity of liver fire.

Manipulation: Acupuncture is applied. When puncturing Middle Line of Forehead and Line 2 Lateral to Forehead, insert the needle from the upper downwards; and on puncturing Vertex-Occiput Line, insert 2 needles parallel to each other from the upper downwards. Retain the needles for 60 minutes, lift and thrust the needles using small amplitude for 3-5 minutes, and repeat this manipulation after every interval of 15 minutes during the retention. When manipulating the needles, ask the patient to keep relaxed and calm, press and knead the eyes with hands for 2-3 minutes, loosen the hands, close the eyes gently, and open the eyes. Ask the patient repeat this action during the manipulation and retention of the needles. The treatment is given once daily, with 10 treatments as a course.

Comment:
Zhenjiu is effective in the treatment of central choroido-retinitis. However, since central choroido-retinitis is an obstinate disease, a comprehensive treatment including other therapeutic methods is generally needed.

Notes:

77. Optic Atrophy

Optic atrophy refers to fibroid retrograde degeneration of the optic nerve, caused by optic neuritis or other factors. Clinically, it is marked by gradual diminution of vision, light-colored or pale optic disc and contraction of visual field. According to TCM, optic atrophy belongs to Qing Mang (green blindness) and Shi Wu Hun Miao (blurring of vision). It is due to deficiency of liver and kidney, insufficiency of qi and blood, or depressed emotion, leading to failure of the eyes in nourishment.

I. STANDARD TREATMENT

Optic atrophy may be divided into three types: yin deficiency of kidney and liver, yang deficiency of spleen and kidney, and stagnation of qi and blood. Points of the local regions and the Liver, Kidney and Bladder Meridians are frequently selected in its treatment.

1. Yin Deficiency of Liver and Kidney

Manifestations: Gradual diminution or even loss of vision, soreness and weakness of the lower back and knees, fatigue, listlessness, insomnia, dreaminess.

Tongue: Thin and red body with little coating.

Pulse: Thready and rapid.

Treatment Principle: Tonify the liver and kidney, and improve eyesight.

Point Prescription & Manipulation:
Primary points:
    EX-HN-7 Qiuhou +
    BL-1 Jingming +
    BL-2 Cuanzhu +
    BL-18 Ganshu +
    BL-23 Shenshu +
    GB-37 Guangming +
    ST-36 Zusanli +

Explanation:
On BL-1 Jingming and EX-HN-7 Qiuhou, insert a needle slowly, rotate it at a small amplitude but do not lift or thrust it. Press the needle hole immediately after removing the needle. On the other points, rotate, lift and thrust needles with reinforcing manipulation. Retain the needles for 20-40 minutes.

- EX-HN-7 Qiuhou and GB-37 Guangming, experiential points for eye disorders, improve the eyesight;
- BL-1 Jingming and BL-2 Cuanzhu, located around the eye region, promote qi and blood circulation of the local region and improve nourishment of the eyes;
- BL-18 Ganshu and BL-23 Shenshu, the Back-Shu Points of the liver and kidney, tonify the liver and kidney and improve the eyesight;
- ST-36 Zusanli reinforces the middle-jiao and promotes production of qi and blood.

Secondary points according to conditions:
1꘡ Fullness and distension of the chest and hypochondriac region or emotional depression —LR-3 Taichong [-], GB-20 Fengchi [-] and RN-17 Danzhong [-];
2꘡ Insomnia, palpitation and poor memory— BL-15 Xinshu [+] and HT-7 Shenmen [+].

2. Yang Deficiency of Spleen and Kidney

Manifestations: Gradual diminution or even loss of vision, aversion to cold and cold limbs, shortness of breath, lassitude, frequent night urination, poor appetite, loose stools.

Tongue: Pale body with white coating.

Pulse: Deep, thready and weak.

Treatment Principle: Warm and tonify the spleen and kidney and improve the eyesight.

Point Prescription & Manipulation:
Primary points:
EX-HN-7 Qiuhou +
BL-1 Jingming +
BL-2 Cuanzhu +
BL-23 Shenshu + ^
BL-20 Pishu + ^
ST-36 Zusanli + ^

Explanation:
On BL-1 Jingming, BL-2 Cuanzhu and EX-HN-7 Qiuhou, manipulation is the same as above. On the other points, rotate, lift and thrust the needles with reinforcing manipulation. Retain the needles for 20-40 minutes.

- EX-HN-7 Qiuhou and GB-37 Guangming, experiential points for eye disorders, improve the eyesight;
- BL-1 Jingming and BL-2 Cuanzhu, located around the eye region, promote qi and blood circulation of the local region and improve nourishment of the eye;
- BL-20 Pishu and BL-23 Shenshu, the Back-Shu Points of the Spleen and Kidney Meridians, reinforce the spleen and kidney yang;
- ST-36 Zusanli reinforces the middle-jiao and promotes production of qi and blood.

Secondary points according to conditions:
1꘡ Blood stasis manifested by purple tongue and uneven pulse — BL-17 Geshu [-] and BL-18 Ganshu [-];
2꘡ Impotence and cold sensation in the lower abdomen — RN-4 Guanyuan [+ ^].

3. Stagnation of Qi and Blood

Manifestations: Gradual or sudden diminution or even loss of vision, usually having a head or eye traumatic injury history, headache and poor memory.

Tongue: Purple or dark body.

Pulse: Unsmooth.

Treatment Principle: Promote flow of qi and blood, activate the collaterals and improve the eyesight.

Point Prescription & Manipulation:

Primary points:
> EX-HN-7 Qiuhou /
> BL-1 Jingming /
> BL-2 Cuanzhu -
> BL-17 Geshu -
> RN-6 Qihai +
> GB-37 Guangming   -
> EX-HN-5 Taiyang   -

Explanation:
On BL-1 Jingming, BL-2 Cuanzhu and EX-HN-7 Qiuhou, manipulation is the same as above.

- EX-HN-7 Qiuhou and GB-37 Guangming, experiential points for eye disorders, improve the eyesight;
- BL-1 Jingming and BL-2 Cuanzhu, located around the eye region, promote qi and blood circulation of the local region and improve nourishment of the eye;
- BL-27 Geshu and EX-HN-5 Taiyang activate the collaterals and remove blood stasis;
- RN-6 Qihai reinforces qi to promote its flow.

Secondary points according to conditions:
1〕 Hypochondriac distention—LI-4 Hegu [-] and LR-5 Ligou [-];
2〕 Headache — GB-20 Fengchi [-].

II. EXPERIENTIAL TREATMENT

1. Puncturing EX-HN-23 Xinming 1 and EX-HN-24 Xinming 2

Indication: Optic atrophy.

Point Prescription:
> EX-HN-23 Xinming 1, located on the joint of the ear lobe and check, 0.5 cun anterior and superior to SJ-17 Yifeng;
> EX-HN-24 Xinming 2, located on the forehead, 1 cun above and 0.5 cun lateral to the lateral end of the eyebrow.

Manipulation: When puncturing EX-HN-23 Xinming 1, pull the ear lobe forward and upward, insert the needle obliquely at an angle of 45 degrees quickly and deeply into the point at the posterior-lateral border of the mandibular condyloid process about 1-1.5 cun. Manipulate a needle to induce a needling sensation. Then, rotate the needle with combination of slow lifting and quick thrusting manipulations to induce sensation of warmth, distention and electric shock that radiates to the eyeball. When puncturing EX-HN-24 Xinming 2, insert a needle about 0.5-0.8 cun, manipulate the needle to induce local soreness, distention and heaviness sensation. Then, perform quick rotating manipulation in combination with lifting and thrusting manipulations to induce a heat and distention sensation that radiates to the eyeball. Retain the needles for 20-40 minutes, and manipulate them every 10 minutes. The treatment is given once daily with 10 times as one course.

2. Puncturing EX-HN-7 Qiuhou

Indication: Optic atrophy.

Point Prescription:
> EX-HN-7 Qiuhou of the diseased side.

Manipulation: Insert a needle into the point along the lower border of the orbit, push the needle somewhat obliquely upward 1.5-2 cun to induce soreness and distention in the eye region, or sensation of the eye extruding. Retain the needle for 5 minutes, remove the needle and then press the needle hole immediately with cotton ball for about 30 seconds. When the needle tip meets some resistance, lift the needle a little, change the inserting direction slightly, and push the needle deeply again. When puncturing this point, always use gentle manipulation, in order to avoid injuring the eyeball or inducing bleeding. The treatment is given once daily with 10 treatments as one course.

3. Puncturing Two Groups of Points

Indication: Optic atrophy.

Point Prescription:
> *Group 1*: BL-1 Jingming, EX-HN-23 Xinming 1, BL-18 Ganshu, GB-20 Fengchi, SI-6 Yanglao,   SP-6 Sanyinjiao;

Group 2: EX-HN-7 Qiuhou, EX-HN-24 Xinming 2, BL-23 Shenshu, GB-12 Wangu, LI-4 Hegu.

Manipulation: When puncturing BL-1 Jingming, gently fix the eyeball in a lateral direction with the left hand. Then, insert the needle slowly along the interior border of the orbit about 1-1.5 cun deep. If the needle meets resistance, lift the needle a little, change the insertion direction slightly and push it deep again. Then, rotate the needle slowly and gently to induce a needling sensation which radiates to the eyeball, remove the needle and press the needle hole immediately for over 30 seconds to avoid bleeding. When puncturing EX-HN-7 Qiuhou, EX-HN-23 Xinming 1 and EX-HN-24 Xinming 2, manipulate the needles as the same as in puncturing EX-HN-24 Xinming 2 and puncturing EX-HN-7 Qiuhou mentioned above. When puncturing the other points, perform uniform reinforcing and reducing manipulation, retain the needle for 20-40 minutes and manipulate every 10 minutes. The treatment is given once every day with 10 times as one course.

4. Scalp Puncture

Indication: Optic atrophy.

Scalp Line Prescription:
   The posterior 1/3 of the Line of the Forehead-Vertex
   The lower 1/3 of the Line of the Vertex-Occiput

Manipulation: On the posterior 1/3 of the Line of the Forehead-Vertex, insert two needles into the posterior end of the line. Push the needles horizontally forward along the posterior 1/3 of the line and lift and thrust the needles with reinforcing manipulation. On the lower 1/3 of the Line of the Vertex-Occiput, insert two needles into the upper end of the lower 1/3 of the line. Push the needles horizontally along the line downwards, and lift and thrust the needles with reducing manipulation. Ask the patient to press the eyes with their hands gently for about ten seconds, open the eyes to look forward at a

distance, close the eyes gently, and repeat this course several times during the manipulation of the needle. Retain the needles for 1 hour; manipulate the needles 3-5 minutes every 20 minutes during the retention. The treatment is given once daily with 10 treatments as one course.

Comment:
Optic atrophy is an obstinate disease. Zhenjiu has some effective results in its treatment.

Notes:

78. Color Blindness

Color blindness refers to dyschromatopsia. It is caused by hereditary defect. Clinically, it is marked by disability of the eyes to distinguish color. It is divided into two types, the congenital and the acquired. The former is due to latent genetic variation; and the latter, due to optic atrophy, toxins from smoking or alcohol, or some diseases of the optic fundus. According to TCM, color blindness, called Se Mang in Chinese, is due to congenital deficiency or poor nutrition after birth. This leads to deficiency of the liver and kidney, resulting in failure of the eyes to be nourished. It may also be due to obstruction of the vessels and collaterals leading to failure of essence in being distributed over the eyes.

I. STANDARD TREATMENT

Color blindness is usually divided into three types — deficiency of the liver and kidney, deficiency of the spleen and kidney, and obstruction of the vessels and collaterals. Points of the eye region, the Urinary Bladder, Liver and Kidney Meridians are frequently selected in its treatment.

1. Deficiency of Liver and Kidney

Manifestations: Color blindness, dryness and discomfort of the eyes, dizziness, tinnitus, soreness and weakness of the loins and knees.

Tongue: Pale body.

Pulse: Deep and thready.

Treatment Principle: Nourish the liver, reinforce the kidney and improve the eyesight.

Point Prescription & Manipulation:
Primary points:
   BL-1 Jingming /
   EX-HN-7 Qiuhou /
   BL-2 Cuanzhu /
   EX-HN-14 Yiming +

   BL-18 Ganshu + ^
   BL-23 Shenshu + ^

Explanation:
No lifting, thrusting or rotating manipulation is performed on EX-HN-7 Qiuhou, and the needle hole should be immediately pressed to prevent bleeding after removing the needle.

* EX-HN-7 Qiuhou and EX-HN-14 Yiming, experiential points for eye disorders, improve the eyesight;
* BL-1 Jingming and BL-2 Cuanzhu, located around the eye region, promote qi and blood circulation of the local region and improve the eyesight;
* BL-18 Ganshu and BL-23 Shenshu, the Back-Shu Points of the liver and kidney, reinforce the liver and kidney.

Secondary points according to conditions:
1□ Severe cases — LI-3 Sanjian [/], LR-3 Taichong [/] and KI-3 Taixi [+];
2□ Headache and dizziness — GB-20 Fengchi [+];
3□ Poor appetite — ST-36 Zusanli [+].

2. Deficiency of Spleen and Kidney

Manifestations: Color blindness, Blurred vision, soreness and weakness of the loins and knees, short breath, poor appetite, loose stool.

Tongue: Pale body.

Pulse: Deep and weak.

Treatment Principle: Tonify spleen, reinforce kidney, and improve eyesight.

Point Prescription & Manipulation:
Primary points:
   BL-1 Jingming +
   EX-HN-7 Qiuhou +
   BL-2 Cuanzhu +
   ST-36 Zusanli + ^
   BL-20 Pishu + ^
   BL-23 Shenshu + ^
   RN-4 Guanyuan + ^

Explanation:
Manipulation on EX-HN-7 Qiuhou is the same as above.

- EX-HN-7 Qiuhou, an experiential point for eye disorders;
- BL-1 Jingming and BL-2 Cuanzhu, located around the eye region, promote qi and blood circulation of the local region and improve the eyesight;
- ST-36 Zusanli and BL-20 Pishu tonify the middle-jiao;
- BL-23 Shenshu and RN-4 Guanyuan warm the kidney yang.

Secondary points according to conditions:
1❑ Chronic cases — SP-6 Sanyinjiao [+], KI-6 Zhaohai [+] and LI-3 Sanjian [+];
2❑ Dizziness and insomnia— DU-20 Baihui [+] and EX-HN-16 Anmian [+].

3. Obstruction of the Vessels and Collaterals

Manifestations: Color blindness, distending pain of eyes.

Tongue: Purplish body with ecchymoses.

Pulse: Uneven.

Treatment Principle: Activate collaterals and improve eyesight.

Point Prescription & Manipulation:
Primary points:
  BL-1 Jingming +
  EX-HN-7 Qiuhou -
  ST-1 Chengqi ^
  GB-37 Guangming /
  BL-17 Geshu /
  PC-6 Neiguan /

Explanation:
Manipulation on EX-HN-7 Qiuhou is the same as above.

- EX-HN-7 Qiuhou and GB-37 Guangming, experiential points for eye disorders, improve the eyesight;

- BL-1 Jingming and ST-1 Chengqi, located around the eye region, promote qi and blood circulation and activate the collaterals of the local region;
- BL-17 Geshu and PC-6 Neiguan activate blood circulation and remove blood stasis.

Secondary points according to conditions:
1❑ Dizziness and tinnitus —KI-6 Zhaohai [+];
2❑ Hypochondriac dissension and irritability — LR-3 Taichong [-] and GB-34 Yanglingquan [-].

II. EXPERIENTIAL TREATMENT

1. Puncturing the Points of the Three Groups

Indication: Color blindness.

Point Prescription:
1❑ GB-20 Fengchi, BL-2 Cuanzhu, EX-HN-5 Taiyang, ST-36 Zusanli;

2❑ ST-2 Sibai, LI-4 Hegu, GB-37 Guangming, SJ-23 Sizhukong;

1❑ EX-HN-4 Yuyao, ST-1 Chengqi, KI-3 Taixi, SP-6 Sanyinjiao.

Manipulation: Acupuncture is applied, even reinforcing and reducing manipulation is performed, and the three groups are selected alternatively.

2. Scalp Puncture

Indication: Color blindness.

Scalp Line Prescription:
  Upper-Lateral Line of Occiput, the lower 2/5 of the Posterior Oblique Line of Vertex-Temporal;
  Middle Line of Forehead;
  Line 1 lateral to Forehead.

Manipulation: Acupuncture is applied.

3. Ear Acupuncture

Indication: Color blindness.

Ear Point Prescription:
Eye, Brian Spot, Kidney, Eye, Subcortex, Adrenal Gland.

Manipulation: See page 255-256.

Comment:
Zhenjiu can provide some effective results in the treatment of color blindness.

Notes:

79. Acute Optic Neuritis

Acute optic neuritis includes two types—palilitis of optic nerve and retrobulbar neuritis. Its cause is mainly related to viral infections. Clinically, it is marked by abrupt onset, severe diminution of vision, or even total blindness within 1-2 days, pain of eyes which is aggravated by turning the eyeballs, and tenderness of eyeballs. According to TCM, acute neuritis belongs to the category of Bao Mang (sudden blindness), and it is mainly due to emotional depression and stagnant qi, turning into fire and wind which flames upward to injure the eyes.

I. STANDARD TREATMENT

It is manifested as the syndrome of over-activity of liver fire, and treated by selecting the local points as the main.

Over-Activity of Liver Fire

Manifestations: Sudden diminution of vision, pain of eye and headache, photophobia.

Tongue: Red body with yellow coating.

Pulse: Wiry and rapid.

Treatment Principle: Clear liver fire.

Point Prescription & Manipulation:
Primary points:
EX-HN-7 Qiuhou -
BL-1 Jingming -
BL-2 Cuanzhu -
EX-HN-5 Taiyang -
GB-1 Tongziliao -
SJ-23 Sizhukong -
BL-23 Shenshu +
BL-18 Ganshu /
LR-2 Xingjian -

Explanation:
Acupuncture is applied on EX-HN-7 Qiuhou and other 3-5 points at each time, which are selected alternatively. On EX-HN-7 Qiuhou and

BL-1 Jingming, insert and push the needles gently without lifting, thrusting or rotating manipulation, and press the needle holes immediately after removing the needles.

- EX-HN-7 Qiuhou, an experiential point for eye disorders;
- BL-1 Jingming, BL-2 Cuanzhu, EX-HN-5 Taiyang, GB-1 Tongziliao and SJ-23 Sizhukong, located around the eye region, clear fire from the eye and improve the eyesight;
- BL-23 Shenshu and BL-18 Ganshu, the Back-Shu Points of the kidney and liver, reinforce the liver and kidney to nourish the eyes for protection of the eyesight;
- LR-2 Xingjian clears fire from the Liver Meridian.

Secondary points according to conditions:
1） Red eyes — GB-43 Xiaxi [-];
2） Constipation — SJ-6 Zhizheng [-] and GB-34 Yanglingquan [-];
3） Emotional depression with insomnia— PC-6 Neiguan [-] and HT-7 Shenmen [/].

II. EXPERIENTIAL TREATMENT

1. Puncturing GB-37 Guangming

Indication: Acute optic neuritis.

Point Prescription:
    GB-37 Guangming

Manipulation: Insert a 2-cun needle into the point, lift, thrust and rotate the needle with reducing manipulation to induce arrival of qi, and retain the needle for 15 minutes. Generally, only one treatment is necessary to cure the disease. In severe cases, 2-3 treatments may be needed.

2. Scalp Puncture

Indication: Acute optic neuritis.

Scalp Line Prescription:
    Middle Line of the Forehead

Lateral Line 2 of the Forehead of the left side
The lower 1/3 of the Line of Vertex-Occiput
The posterior 1/3 of the Line of Forehead-Occiput.

Manipulation: On Middle Line of Forehead and the Lateral Line 2 of Forehead, insert needles from the upper downward; on the lower 1/3 of the Vertex-Occiput, insert two needles from the upper downward. Lift and thrust the needles at small amplitude on the above three lines. On the posterior 1/3 of the Line Forehead-Vertex, insert a needle from the posterior towards the anterior, and lift and thrust the needle at small amplitude. During manipulation, ask the patient to breathe in and hold their breath, press his/her eyes with his/her hands for two seconds followed by relaxation, and repeat this action several times. Retain the needles for 1-2 hours, manipulate them every 15 minutes and for 5 minutes each time. The treatment is given once daily, with 10 treatments as a course.

Comment:
Acupuncture is very effective in the treatment of acute optic neuritis, and in most cases, the disease can be cured through proper acupuncture treatment.

Notes:

80. Pigmentary Degeneration of the Retina

Pigmentary degeneration of the retina refers to primary degeneration of the retina epithelium. Its cause is uncertain, but in most cases, it is closely related to a hereditary factor. Clinically, it is marked by binocular onset, night blindness, and contraction of visual field, leading to blindness at the late stage. It is closely related to heredity. According to TCM, it belongs to the category of Gao Feng Que Mu Nei Zhang (pigmentary degeneration of retina with the pupil golden in color), and it is mainly due to deficiency of the kidney, liver and spleen.

I. STANDARD TREATMENT

Pigmentary degeneration of the retina is usually divided into four types — kidney yang deficiency, yin deficiency of liver and kidney, spleen qi deficiency and stagnation of qi and blood. Local points of the eye region, Back Shu Points, points of the Kidney, Liver and Spleen Meridians are frequently selected in its treatment.

1. Kidney Yang Deficiency

Manifestations: Night blindness, contraction of visual field, soreness and weakness of the loins and knees, cold limbs, aversion to cold, profuse and clear urination, impotence.

Tongue: Pale and slippery body with white coating.

Pulse: Deep and weak.

Treatment Principle: Tonify kidney, warm yang, and improve eyesight.

Point Prescription & Manipulation:
Primary points:
 EX-HN-5 Taiyang -
 BL-1 Jingming /
 EX-HN-7 Qiuhou +
 DU-4 Mingmen + ^

 DU-9 Zhiyang + ^
 BL-23 Shenshu + ^
 ST-36 Zusanli + ^

Explanation:
On BL-1 Jingming and EX-HN-7 Qiuhou, insert needles perpendicularly 1-1.5 cun with no lifting, thrusting or rotating manipulation. On EX-HN-5 Taiyang, insert a needle perpendicularly 1.2 cun deep and perform reducing manipulation by rotating the needle.

* EX-HN-7 Qiuhou, an experiential point for eye disorders, improves the eyesight;
* EX-HN-5 Taiyang and BL-1 Jingming, located around the eye region, promote qi and blood circulation and improve the eyesight;
* DU-4 Mingmen, DU-9 Zhiyang and BL-23 Shenshu warm yang and tonify the kidney;
* ST-36 Zusanli reinforces qi to warm yang.

Secondary points according to conditions:
1❑ Impotence — RN-4 Guanyuan [+ ^] and RN-3 Zhongji [+ ^].

2. Yin Deficiency of Liver and Kidney

Manifestations: Night blindness, contraction of visual field, diminution of central vision, dryness and discomfort of the eyes, dizziness tinnitus, soreness and weakness of the loins and knees, insomnia and dreaminess, nocturnal emission.

Tongue: Red body with little coating.

Pulse: Thready and rapid.

Treatment Principle: Tonify liver and kidney, and improve eyesight.

Point Prescription & Manipulation:
Primary points:
 EX-HN-5 Taiyang +
 BL-1 Jingming +
 EX-HN-7 Qiuhou +
 BL-18 Ganshu +
 BL-23 Shenshu +

KI-10 Yingu +
KI-6 Zhaohai +
GB-37 Guangming /

Explanation:
The points on the eye region are punctured with the same manipulation as above.

- EX-HN-7 Qiuhou and GB-37 Guangming, experiential points for eye disorders, improve the eyesight;
- EX-HN-5 Taiyang and BL-1 Jingming, located around the eye region, promote qi and blood circulation of the local region and improve the eyesight;
- BL-18 Ganshu, BL-23 Shenshu, KI-10 Yingu and KI-6 Zhaohai nourish yin and reinforce the liver and kidney.

Secondary points according to conditions:
1□ Insomnia — EX-HN-16 Anmian [+];
2□ Nocturnal emission — RN-3 Zhongji [+];
3□ Dizziness or tinnitus—GB-20 Fengchi [-] and LR-3 Taichong [-] which is punctured towards KI-1 Yongquan with the point-to-point method.

3. Spleen Qi Deficiency

Manifestations: Night blindness, constriction of vision or even blindness, fatigue, shortness of breath, poor appetite, loose stools, pale complexion.

Tongue: Pale body with thin coating.

Pulse: Slow and weak.

Treatment Principle: Tonify spleen, reinforce qi and improve eyesight.

Point Prescription & Manipulation:
Primary points:
EX-HN-5 Taiyang +
BL-1 Jingming +
EX-HN-7 Qiuhou +
BL-20 Pishu + ^
BL-21 Weishu + ^
ST-36 Zusanli + ^

DU-20 Baihui +

Explanation:
The manipulation is the same as that in "Kidney Yang Deficiency".(Page 496)

- EX-HN-7 Qiuhou, an experiential point for eye disorders, improves the eyesight;
- EX-HN-5 Taiyang and BL-1 Jingming, located around the eye region, promote qi and blood circulation of the local region and improve the eyesight;
- BL-20 Pishu and BL-21 Weishu, the Back-Shu Points of the spleen and stomach, reinforce the middle-jiao to promote production of qi and blood;
- ST-36 Zusanli and DU-20 Baihui tonify qi, raise yang and nourish the eye.

Secondary points according to conditions:
1□ Loose stools or diarrhea — SP-9 Yinlingquan [+ ^], RN-6 Qihai [+ ^] and ST-25 Tianshu [+ ^];
2□ Dizziness — EX-HN-1 Sishencong [+];
3□ Insomnia—SP-6 Sanyinjiao [+] and HT-7 Shenmen [+].

4. Stagnation of Qi and Blood

Manifestations: Night blindness, constriction of vision or even blindness, distending pain of the eye.

Tongue: Purplish body.

Pulse: Unsmooth.

Treatment Principle: Promote circulation of qi, activate blood and improve eyesight.

Point Prescription & Manipulation:
Primary points:
EX-HN-7 Taiyang -
BL-1 Jingming /
EX-HN-7 Qiuhou /
BL-17 Geshu -
BL-18 Ganshu /
GB-37 Guangming -
LR-3 Taichong -

Explanation:
On EX-HN-5 Taiyang, BL-1 Jingming, EX-HN-7 Qiuhou, the same manipulation mentioned above is performed. LR-3 Taichong is punctured towards KI-1 Yongquan with the point-to-point method.

- EX-HN-7 Qiuhou and GB-37 Guangming, experiential points for eye disorders, improve the eyesight;
- EX-HN-5 Taiyang and BL-1 Jingming, located around the eye region, promote qi and blood circulation of the local region and improve the eyesight;
- BL-17 Geshu, the Influential Point of blood, promotes blood circulation and removes blood stasis;
- BL-18 Ganshu and LR-3 Taichong soothe the liver, promote qi circulation and improve the eyesight.

Secondary points according to conditions:
1口 Distressed feeling in the chest — PC-6 Neiguan [-];
2口 Insomnia — EX-HN-16 Anmian [/].

II. EXPERIENTIAL TREATMENT

1. Ear Acupuncture

Indication: Pigmentary degeneration of retina.

Ear Point Prescription:
Eye 1, Eye 2, Eye, Liver, Kidney, Spleen and Heart.

Manipulation: See page 255-256.

2. Scalp Puncture

Indication: Pigmentary degeneration of retina.

Scalp Line Prescription:
Visual region.

Manipulation: After inserting a needle through the scalp of the upper end of the line, push the needle 1-2 cun downwards along the scalp, rotate the needle at frequency of 80-120 times per minute for 1-3 minutes. Then, retain the needle for 30 minutes. The treatment is given once every other day, with 10 treatments as a course.

Comment:
Pigmentary degeneration of retina is a very obstinate disease. Zhenjiu has some effective result in relieving its symptoms and signs.

Notes:

81. Ptosis of Upper Eye Lid

Ptosis of upper eyelid refers to a disorder causing failure of the upper eyelid in rising or rising wholly. It is caused by dysfunction or loss of function of the elevator muscle of the upper lid, resulting from trauma or immune disorders. Clinically, it is marked by ptosis of the upper lid and failure of the eye in opening. According to TCM, ptosis of upper lid belongs to the category of Shang Bao Xia Chui (ptosis of the upper lid), and it is due to congenital deficiency, deficiency of spleen and kidney, or obstruction of the collaterals by wind-phlegm which all lead to malnourishment of the upper eyelid.

I. STANDARD TREATMENT

Ptosis of upper lid is generally divided into two types — deficiency of spleen and kidney and spleen deficiency with wind-phlegm. Points of the Stomach, Bladder and Spleen Meridians are frequently selected in its treatment.

1. Deficiency of Spleen and Kidney

Manifestations: Ptosis of the bilateral upper lids, soreness and weakness of the lower back and knees, poor appetite, loose stools.

Tongue: Pale body with white coating.

Pulse: Deep and weak.

Treatment Principle: Reinforce the spleen and warm the kidney.

Point Prescription & Manipulation:
Primary points:
GB-14 Yangbai +
BL-2 Cuanzhu +
EX-HN-5 Taiyang +
EX-HN-4 Yuyao +
PL-20 Pishu + ^
BL-23 Shenshu + ^
ST-36 Zusanli + ^
SP-6 Sanyinjiao + ^
DU-20 Baihui +

Explanation:
- PL-20 Pishu and SP-6 Sanyinjiao reinforce the spleen and tonify qi;
- BL-23 Shenshu warms the kidney yang;
- ST-36 Zusanli and DU-20 Baihui reinforce qi, raise yang and lift the sunken;
- GB-14 Yangbai, BL-2 Cuanzhu, EX-HN-5 Taiyang and EX-HN-4 Yuyao, located at the diseased region, promote nourishment of the upper lid and strengthen the local muscles.

Secondary points according to conditions:
1☐ Impotence — RN-4 Guanyuan [+ ^];
2☐ Loose stools or morning diarrhea — RN-6 Qihai [+ ^] and ST-25 Tianshu [+ ^].

2. Spleen Deficiency with Wind-Phlegm

Manifestations: Ptosis, swelling and numbness of the upper lid, difficulty in moving eyeball, numbness of the limbs, fatigue, poor appetite.

Tongue: Pale body with white and sticky coating.

Pulse: Soft and thready.

Treatment Principle: Reinforce spleen and resolve phlegm.

Point Prescription & Manipulation:
Primary points:
GB-14 Yangbai /
BL-2 Cuanzhu /
EX-HN-4 Yuyao /
ST-36 Zusanli + ^
SP-9 Yinlingquan + ^
ST-40 Fenglong - ^
SP-3 Taibai + ^
GB-20 Fengchi /

Explanation:
- ST-36 Zusanli reinforces stomach qi;
- SP-9 Yinlingquan and SP-3 Taibai reinforce the spleen and remove dampness;
- ST-40 Fenglong transforms phlegm;
- GB-20 Fengchi dispels wind;

- GB-14 Yangbai, located at the diseased region, promotes nourishment of the upper lid and strengthens the local muscles.

Secondary points according to conditions:
1☐ Difficulty in moving eyeball — LR-3 Taichong [/] and LI-4 Hegu [/];
2☐ Oppressive feeling in the chest — PC-6 Neiguan [-];
3☐ Nausea and poor appetite — RN-12 Zhongwan [+ ^].

II. EXPERIENTIAL TREATMENT

1. Puncturing GB-14 Yangbai

Indication: Congenital ptosis of upper lid.

Point Prescription:
GB-14 Yangbai

Manipulation: Insert a 2-cun needle through the skin of the point, push the needle horizontally in three directions: First, laterally to the outer canthus. Second, directly downward to the upper border of the upper lid and. Third, laterally to the inner canthus. In each direction of insertion, manipulate the needle gently to induce a needling sensation, and retain the needle. The treatment is given once every other day, with 10 treatments as one course.

2. Puncturing Some Points

Indication: Ptosis of upper lid due to myasthenia gravis.

Point Prescription:
Primary points:
BL-2 Cuanzhu
GB-14 Yangbai
EX-HN-4 Yuyao

Secondary points according to conditions:
1☐ Double vision — ST-36 Zusanli [^], SP-6 Sanyinjiao [^], EX-HN-5 Taiyang, ST-2 Sibai, BL-1 Jingming and GB-20 Fengchi.

Manipulation: Acupuncture is applied on 3-5 points with all of the primary points and secondary points selected alternatively each treatment. Perform gentle manipulation to induce arrival of qi, and retain the needles for 20-40 minutes. The treatment is given once daily, with 10 treatments as one course. The next course may begin after an interval of 3-5 days.

3. Puncturing Three Points

Indication: Congenital ptosis of upper lid.

Point Prescription:
EX-HN-4 Yuyao
BL-2 Cuanzhu
SJ-23 Sizhukong

Manipulation: Ask the patient to lie in a supine position. Extend the skin of the upper lid with the thumb and index finger of the one hand, and massage the skin gently with the other thumb for about 2 minutes. Then, insert a 1-cun needle into EX-HN-4 Yuyao horizontally at an angle of 10-15 degrees downward. Insert needles into the other two points horizontally with the needle tips towards EX-HN-4 Yuyao, and push the needles 0.3-0.5 cun. Manipulate the needles gently to induce arrival of qi, retain them for 30 minutes, and manipulate them every 5 minutes. The treatment is given once every other day, with 10 treatments as one course.

Comment:
Ptosis of upper lid is an obstinate disorder. Zhenjiu is effective in its treatment in many cases, and in some cases it is even effective to cure this disorder.

Notes:

82. Rhinitis

Rhinitis refers to an inflammatory change of the nasal mucosa. Its cause is mainly related to bacterial or viral infections, certain allergens and environmental irritants. It includes acute rhinitis, chronic rhinitis, atrophic rhinitis and allergic rhinitis. Clinically, it is marked by nasal obstruction, frequent nasal discharge and poor sense of smell. According to TCM, rhinitis belongs to the categories of Bi Yuan (nasal pond) and Bi Zhi (nasal obstruction). It is caused by attack of exogenous pathogenic wind, cold or heat, or by accumulation of phlegm, resulting in disorder of the nasal function.

I. STANDARD TREATMENT

Rhinitis is generally divided into five types — deficiency of lung qi with attack of cold, deficiency of lung qi with retained pathogen, stagnation of qi and blood with retained pathogen, deficiency of lung fluid and spleen deficiency. Points of the Lung, Large Intestine, Bladder, Stomach and Spleen Meridians are frequently selected in its treatment.

1. Deficiency of Lung Qi with Attack of Cold

Manifestations: Sudden onset of itching of the nose, distention of the nose, paroxysmal sneezing, profuse dilute nasal discharge and intermittent or persistent nasal obstruction, accompanied by fatigue, shortness of breath, pale complexion, sweating.

Tongue: Pale body with thin and white coating.

Pulse: Weak.

Treatment Principle: Warm lung, replenish qi and disperse cold.

Point Prescription & Manipulation:

Primary points:
    EX-HN-3 Yintang   -
    GB-20 Fengchi -

    LI-20 Yingxiang -
    BL-13 Feishu + ^
    LU-9 Taiyuan +
    ST-36 Zusanli + ^
    LI-4 Hegu   -

Explanation:
When puncturing LI-20 Yingxiang, after insertion of a needle, push the needle towards EX-HN-8 Bitong along the nasolabial groove 0.5-0.8 cun, and manipulate it until the patient has local distending pain and lacrimation, making the needling sensation radiate to the nose; when puncturing EX-HN-3 Yintang, insert the needle obliquely downwards and push it to reach the root of the nose, making the needling sensation radiate to the nose tip.

- LI-4 Hegu, GB-20 Fengchi and LI-20 Yingxiang dispel pathogenic cold, and remove obstruction from the nose;
- EX-HN-3 Yintang promotes flow of qi and blood of the local region to remove obstruction from the nose;
- BL-13 Feishu and LU-9 Taiyuan warm and reinforce the lung qi;
- ST-36 Zusanli reinforces the middle-jiao and transforms phlegm.

Secondary points according to conditions:
1️⃣ Chills with fever — LI-4 Hegu [-] and DU-14 Dazhui [+ ^];
2️⃣ Profuse nasal discharge — EX-HN-8 Bitong [-], which is punctured subcutaneously towards the nose root 0.5-0.8 cun;
3️⃣ Fatigue — BL-20 Pishu [+ ^] and SP-6 Sanyinjiao [+ ^].

2. Deficiency of Lung Qi with Retained Pathogen

Manifestations: Nasal obstruction and running nose, which are aggravated by cold, cough with thin sputum, shortness of breath, pale complexion.

Tongue: Pale body with thin and white coating.

Pulse: Slow and floating or floating and weak.

Treatment Principle: Reinforce lung, replenish qi, disperse pathogen and remove obstruction.

Point Prescription & Manipulation:
Primary points:
  EX-HN-3 Yintang -
  BL-13 Feishu + ^
  DU-20 Baihui + ^
  LI-20 Yingxiang -
  LU-9 Taiyuan +
  ST-36 Zusanli + ^
  LI-4 Hegu +

Explanation:
When puncturing LI-20 Yingxiang and EX-HN-3 Yintang, the same manipulation as above is performed.

• BL-13 Feishu and LU-9 Taiyuan warm and reinforce the lung qi;
• DU-20 Baihui raises yang qi to help the lung function of dispersing;
• ST-36 Zusanli reinforces the middle-jiao and transforms phlegm;
• LI-20 Yingxiang and EX-HN-3 Yintang promote circulation of qi and blood of the nose region, and remove obstruction from the nose;
• LI-4 Hegu dispels the pathogen.

Secondary points according to conditions:
1️⃣ Severe running nose and cough with phlegm — ST-40 Fenglong [-] and BL-12 Feishu [+ ^];
2️⃣ Liability to catch cold— DU-14 Dazhui [+ ^];
3️⃣ Tight sensation in the chest — PC-6 Neiguan [-];
4️⃣ Shortness of breath — RN-17 Danzhong [-] and RN-6 Qihai [+ ^].

3. Stagnation of Qi and Blood with Retained Pathogen

Manifestations: Swelling of the nose, persistent obstruction of the nose, profuse white or yellow sticky nasal discharge, poor sense of smell, cough with profuse sputum.

Tongue: Red body with purple spots.

Pulse: Wiry and thready.

Treatment Principle: Promote circulation of qi and blood, transform phlegm, and remove obstruction from the nose.

Point Prescription & Manipulation:
Primary points:
  EX-HN-3 Yintang   -
  EX-HN-8 Bitong   -
  LI-20 Yingxiang -
  DU-23 Shangxing -
  LI-4 Hegu -
  ST-40 Fenglong -
  RN-17 Danzhong -
  BL-12 Feishu -
  BL-17 Geshu -

Explanation:
When puncturing LI-20 Yingxiang, EX-HN-8 Bitong and EX-HN-3 Yintang, the same manipulation as above is performed.

• EX-HN-3 Yintang, EX-HN-8 Bitong, LI-20 Yingxiang and DU-23 Shangxing promote circulation of qi and blood of the nose region, and remove obstruction from the nose;
• LI-4 Hegu and BL-12 Feishu regulate the lung and dispel pathogen;
• ST-40 Fenglong transforms phlegm;
• RN-17 Danzhong and BL-17 Geshu promote qi and blood circulation and remove blood stasis.

Secondary points according to conditions:
1️⃣ Obstinate cases—BL-13 Feishu [+] and BL-23 Shenshu [+];
2️⃣ Pain in the forehead—RN-12 Zhongwan [-].

4. Fluid Deficiency of Lung

Manifestations: Atrophy of the nasal mucosa, dry nose, turbid and thick nasal discharge, dryness or itching of the throat and fatigue.

Tongue: Red body with little coating.

Pulse: Thread and rapid.

Treatment Principle: Replenish yin and moisten dryness.

Point Prescription & Manipulation:
Primary points:
    EX-HN-3 Yintang -
    EX-HN-8 Bitong -
    LI-20 Yingxiang /
    LI-4 Hegu /
    KI-3 Taixi +
    LU-9 Taiyuan +
    SP-3 Taibai +

Explanation:
When puncturing LI-20 Yingxiang, EX-HN-8 Bitong and EX-HN-3 Yintang, the same manipulation as above is performed.

- EX-HN-3 Yintang, EX-HN-8 Bitong and LI-20 Yingxiang improve circulation of qi and blood of the nose region and help nourishment of the nose;
- LI-4 Hegu, an experiential point for nose disorders, removes obstruction from the nose;
- LU-9 Taiyuan and SP-3 Taibai, the Shu-Stream Points of the Lung and Spleen Meridians which belong to earth in the five element theory and nourish the metal (the lung), nourish the lung yin.

Secondary points according to conditions:
1▢ Dryness or itching of the throat — KI-6 Zhaohai [+] and LU-7 Lieque [-];
2▢ Constipation — KI-6 Zhaohai, ST-25 Tianshu [-] and SJ-6 Zhigou [-];
3▢ Fatigue — ST-36 Zusanli [+] and SP-6 Sanyinjiao [+].

5. Spleen Deficiency

Manifestations: Atrophy of the nasal mucosa, turbid and sticky nasal discharge, poor appetite, loose stools, fatigue, shortness of breath, pale lips and complexion.

Tongue: Pale body with thin and white coating.

Pulse: Slow and weak.

Treatment Principle: Replenish spleen for nourishing lung.

Point Prescription & Manipulation:
Primary points:
    EX-HN-3 Yintang -
    EX-HN-8 Bitong -
    LI-20 Yingxiang /
    BL-20 Pishu + ^
    BL-13 Feishu + ^
    ST-36 Zusanli + ^
    SP-3 Taibai + ^
    LI-4 Hegu -

Explanation:
- BL-20 Pishu, ST-36 Zusanli and SP-3 Taibai reinforce the spleen (earth) and nourish the lung (metal);
- BL-13 Feishu reinforces the lung;
- EX-HN-3 Yintang, EX-HN-8 Bitong and LI-20 Yingxiang improve circulation of qi and blood of the nose region and help nourishment of the nose;
- LI-4 Hegu, an experiential point for nose disorders, removes obstruction from the nose.

Secondary points according to conditions:
1▢ Loose stools—SP-9 Yinlingquan [+ ^] and ST-25 Tianshu [+ ^]
2▢ Chronic cases—RN-12 Zhongwan [+ ^] and BL-21 Weishu [+ ^].

6. Damp-Heat Accompanied with Spleen Deficiency

Manifestations: Profuse turbid and sticky nasal discharge, long term obstruction of the nasal orifice, declining of smelling ability, dizziness, headache, distention and fullness sensation of the abdomen, poor appetite, loose stools, fatigue, shortness of breath, pale lips and complexion.

Tongue: Red body with yellow sticky coating.

Pulse: Soft.

Treatment Principle: Remove damp-heat, strengthen spleen, and unobstruct the nose.

Point Prescription & Manipulation:
Primary points:
    EX-HN-3 Yintang -
    EX-HN-8 Bitong -
    LI-20 Yingxiang /
    LI-4 Hegu -
    BL-20 Pishu + ^
    ST-36 Zusanli + ^
    SP-3 Taibai -
     ST-40 Fenglong -

Explanation:
When puncturing LI-20 Yingxiang, EX-HN-8 Bitong and EX-HN-3 Yintang, the same manipulation as above is performed.

* BL-20 Pishu, ST-36 Zusanli and SP-3 Taibai reinforce the spleen (earth) and remove dampness;
* EX-HN-3 Yintang, EX-HN-8 Bitong and LI-20 Yingxiang improve circulation of qi and blood of the nose region and help nourishment of the nose;
* LI-4 Hegu an experiential point for nose disorders, and ST-40 Fenglong, an experiential point to resolve phlegm, clear heat, resolve phlegm and remove obstruction from the nose.

Secondary points according to conditions:
1️⃣ Loose stools—SP-9 Yinlingquan [+ ^] and ST-25 Tianshu [+ ^];
2️⃣ Chronic cases—RN-12 Zhongwan [+ ^] and BL-21 Weishu [+ ^].

II. EXPERIENTIAL TREATMENT

1. Puncture EX-HN-3 Yintang

Indication: Rhinitis.

Point Prescription:
    EX-HN-3 Yintang

Manipulation: Puncture horizontally with the needle tip towards the nose tip and insert the needle about 1 cun. Perform rotating, thrusting and lifting manipulation to induce a needling sensation that radiates to the nose. Retain the needle for 20 minutes and manipulate it every 5 minutes. The treatment is given once daily, with 10 treatments as a course, only one or two courses are given.

2. Puncture LI-20 Yingxiang

Indication: Chronic nasal sinusitis.

Point Prescription:
    LI-20 Yingxiang

Manipulation: First, insert a needle into the point 0.2-0.5 cun. Then, push the needle obliquely at an angle of 35-40 degrees until the needle tip reaches the anterior upper tip of the inferior nasal concha, and retain the needle for 40 minutes. The treatment is given once daily, with 3-5 treatments as a course. Usually, within 12 treatments the disease will be cured.

3. Moxibustion on BL-13 Feishu

Indication: Rhinitis.

Point Prescription:
    BL-13 Feishu

Manipulation: Apply moxibustion with moxa stick on the point until the local skin becomes flushed and the patient can not stand the heat, usually for about 30 minutes. The treatment is given twice daily, with 3-5 days of treatment as a course. Usually, only one treatment course is needed.

4. Ear Acupuncture

Indication: Allergic Rhinitis.

Ear Point Prescription:
    Internal Nose, External Nose, Lung, Spleen, Kidney, Endocrine, Adrenal Gland and Apex of Ear.

Manipulation: See page 255-256.

Comment:
Rhinitis is an obstinate disease. Zhenjiu is effective to relieve its symptoms, and in many cases, proper Zhenjiu treatment can lead to curative results.

Notes:

83. Acute Tonsillitis

Acute tonsillitis is an acute nonspecific inflammation of the tonsils. Clinically, it is marked by sore throat aggravated by swallowing, reddened and swollen palatal tonsils, fever and headache. According to TCM, acute tonsillitis belongs to the categories of Feng Re Ru E (swollen tonsil due to wind-heat) and E Feng (swollen tonsil due to wind). It is due to attack of the throat by pathogenic wind-heat or accumulation of fire from the lung and stomach at the throat.

I. STANDARD TREATMENT

Acute tonsillitis is usually divided into three types — wind-heat, fire in the lung and stomach, and upward flaming of deficient fire. Points of the Lung and Large Intestine Meridians are frequently selected.

1. Wind-Heat

Manifestations: Sore throat aggravated by swallow, redness and swelling of the palatal tonsils, fever, aversion to cold, headache.

Tongue: Red body with thin and yellow coating.

Pulse: Floating and rapid.

Treatment Principle: Disperse wind, clear away heat, and relieve throat.

Point Prescription & Manipulation:
Primary points:
    LI-4 Hegu -
    SJ-5 Waiguan -
    LI-18 Futu -
    SI-17 Tianrong -
    LU-11 Shaoshang -

Explanation:
On LI-18 Futu, pay attention to avoid the common carotid artery, insert the needle 1 cun, and rotate the needle at a great amplitude. On

LU-11 Shaoshang, prick with a thick needle or three-edged needle to make bleeding 2-3 drops.

- LI-4 Hegu and SJ-5 Waiguan dispel and clear external pathogenic wind-heat;
- LI-18 Futu and SI-17 Tianrong, near the diseased region; resolve swelling of the tonsil to stop pain;
- LU-11 Shaoshang clears heat from the Lung Meridian, and relieves soreness of the throat.

Secondary points according to conditions:
1〕 High fever—LI-11 Quchi [-];
2〕 Headache—GB-20 Fengchi [-].

2. Fire in the Stomach and Lung

Manifestations: Extreme sore throat, dysphasia, redness and swelling in the palatal tonsils, high fever, thirst, ozostomia, constipation, dark-red urine.

Tongue: Red body with yellow coating.

Pulse: Full and rapid.

Treatment Principle: Clear away heat and toxin, and relieve sore throat.

Point Prescription & Manipulation:
Primary points:
    LU-11 Shaoshang -
    LI-1 Shangyang -
    SJ-1 Guanchong -
    DU-14 Dazhui -
    LI-11 Quchi -
    LI-4 Hegu -
    LI-17 Tianding -

Explanation:
On LU-11 Shaoshang, LI-1 Shangyang and SJ-1 Guanchong , prick with a thick needle or three-edged needle to make bleeding 2-3 drops.

- LU-11 Shaoshang, LI-1 Shangyang and SJ-1 Guanchong clear heat from the three yang meridians of the hand, and relieve high fever;

- DU-14 Dazhui, LI-11 Quchi and LI-4 Hegu clear heat and relieve high fever;
- LI-17 Tianding relieves sore throat.

Secondary points according to conditions:
1〕 Constipation—SJ-6 Zhigou [-] and ST-25 Tianshu [-].

3. Upper Flaming of Deficient Fire

Manifestations: Dryness and slight pain of the throat, swelling of the palatal tonsils, fever and flushed cheek in the afternoon.

Tongue: Red body with little coating.

Pulse: Thready and rapid.

Treatment Principle: Nourish yin, subdue fire and relieve sore throat.

Point Prescription & Manipulation:
Primary points:
    LU-10 Yuji -
    KI-6 Zhaohai +
    KI-7 Fuliu +
    RN-23 Lianquan +
    LI-17 Futu -

Explanation:
- LU-10 Yuji clears heat from the lung;
- KI-6 Zhaohai and KI-7 Fuliu reinforce the kidney yin (water) and subdue heat to help nourishment of the lung (metal);
- RN-23 Lianquan, the Crossing Point of the Ren and Yinwei Meridians and near the throat, nourishes yin and relieves sore throat
- LI-17 Futu, near the throat, relieves sore throat.

Secondary points according to conditions:
1〕 Lower fever — DU-14 Dazhui [-] and PC-5 Jianshi [-];
2〕 Chronic cases—BL-23 Shenshu [+] and KI-3 Taixi [+].

II. EXPERIENTIAL TREATMENT

1. Puncturing LU-10 Yuji

Indication: Acute or chronic tonsillitis.

Point Prescription:
    LU-10 Yuji

Manipulation: After insertion of a needle, rotate the needle gently to induce soreness, numbness and distention to the patient. Then, retain the needle for 20-40 minutes and manipulate it every 5 minutes. The treatment is given once daily, or 2-3 treatments a day are given for acute cases.

2. Moxibustion on SJ-20 Jiaosun

Indication: Acute tonsillitis.

Point Prescription:
    SJ-20 Jiaosun

Manipulation: Ignite a matchstick, poke the point with the lighted end of the stick. Usually, one treatment is effective to cure the disease, but a few cases may need another treatment in the next day.

3. Puncturing PC-6 Neiguan

Indication: Acute tonsillitis.

Point Prescription:
    PC-6 Neiguan

Manipulation: Insert a 1-cun needle into the point 0.5-0.8 cun, lift, thrust and rotate the needle with a big amplitude to induce a needling sensation. Then, retain the needle for 30 minutes, and manipulate it every 5 minutes. If the manifestations do not disappear, it is suggested to give the treatment in the next day. Generally, only 1-3 treatments are needed to cure the disease.

4. Bleeding from LU-5 Chize

Indication: Acute tonsillitis.

Point Prescription:
    LU-5 Chize of the healthy side.

Manipulation: Tap the point region with the fingers to induce local congestion of the blood to the patient, and prick the point with a three-edged needle to cause bleeding. If the result is not obviously effective, the treatment can be given again the next day. Generally, within two treatments, the patient's condition will be greatly improved.

5. Bleeding from the Vein on the Back of the Ear

Indication: Acute tonsillitis.

Point Prescription:
    The most obvious vein on the back of the ear.

Manipulation: Knead the vein region several times with the fingers. Then, fix the vein with the thumb and index finger of one hand, prick the vein with a three-edged needle held by the other hand and release several drops of blood. Finally, press the needling hole with a dry sterilized cotton ball to prevent further bleeding. Generally, one treatment is needed to cure the disease.

Comment:
Acupuncture is very effective in the treatment of acute tonsillitis. In most cases, the disease can be cured by several acupuncture treatments. Among Zhenjiu treatment, pricking to bleed is the most effective method, usually only 1-3 treatments are needed to cure this disease.

Notes:

84. Chronic Pharyngitis

Chronic pharyngitis is a chronic and diffuse inflammation of the pharyngeal mucous. It is always from acute pharyngitis caused by infection. Clinically, it is marked by long-term discomfort, the sensation of a foreign body or obstruction in the throat, dry cough, and itching, dryness, and mild soreness of the pharynx. According to TCM, chronic pharyngitis belongs to the category of Hou Bi (obstruction in the pharynx), and it is due to attack of the exogenous pathogens , or deficiency of the lung and kidney leading to upward flaming of the deficiency fire and failure of the throat in nourishment.

I. STANDARD TREATMENT

Chronic pharyngitis is usually divided into two types — dryness of the lung due to yin deficiency and stagnation of qi and phlegm. Points of the Lung and Kidney Meridians are frequently selected in its treatment.

1. Dryness of Lung due to Yin Deficiency

Manifestations: Dryness, itching and slight pain of the throat, cough without sputum or with a little sticky sputum, congestion, diffuse dark redness and dilatation of the pharyngeal mucous membranes and thickening of the lateral pharyngeal bands.

Tongue: Red body with little coating.

Pulse: Thready and rapid.

Treatment Principle: Nourish yin, moisten the lung and relieve sore throat.

Point Prescription & Manipulation:
Primary points:
    EX-HN-27 Liyan /
    LU-9 Taiyuan /
    LU-10 Yuji /
    BL-13 Feishu /
    KI-6 Zhaohai /

Explanation:

- EX-HN-27 Liyan, an experiential point to treat throat disorders, located at the midpoint of the line connecting the lowest point of the ear lobe and the angle of the mandible;
- LU-9 Taiyuan and LU-10 Yuji clear the lung and relieve sore throat;
- BL-13 Feishu tonifies the lung, nourishes yin and clears deficient heat;
- KI-6 Zhaohai, one of the Eight Confluent Points connecting with the Yinqiao Meridian, which runs to the throat, nourishes the kidney yin and clears the throat.

Secondary points according to conditions:
1□ Soreness of the low back and knees—KI-3 Taixi [+];
2□ Tidal fever and night sweating—BL-43 Gaohuang [+] and HT-6 Yinxi [+].

2. Stagnation of Qi and Phlegm

Manifestations: Sensation of obstruction or foreign body in the throat, which may be aggravated by emotional depression, cough with sputum, distressed feeling and distention in the chest and hypochondria.

Tongue: Flabby body with sticky coating.

Pulse: Wiry and thready.

Treatment Principle: Promote circulation of qi, resolve phlegm, and relieve sore throat.

Point Prescription & Manipulation:
Primary points:
    EX-HN-27 Liyan -
    PC-5 Jianshi -
    LI-3 Sanjian -
    SJ-2 Yemen -
    LU-10 Yuji -
    KI-6 Zhaohai /

Explanation:
- EX-HN-27 Liyan, an experiential point to treat throat disorders, located at the midpoint of the line connecting the lowest point of the ear lobe and the angle of the mandible;
- PC-5 Jianshi, the Jing-River Point of the Pericardium Meridian which has the function of promoting qi circulation and activating blood flow, and LI-3 Sanjian, the Shu-Stream Point of the Large Intestine Meridian, effectively relieve sensation of obstruction or foreign body in the throat when they are used together according to Great Compendium of Acupuncture and Moxibustion;
- SJ-2 Yemen, LU-10 Yuji and KI-6 Zhaohai relieve sore throat.

Secondary points according to conditions:
1□ Cough with sputum—ST-40 Fenglong [-];
2□ Distention and fullness in the chest and hypochondriac region—LR-3 Taichong [-], PC-6 Neiguan [-] and RN-17 Danzhong [-].

II. EXPERIENTIAL TREATMENT

1. Tapping RN-22 Tiantu

Indication: Chronic pharyngitis.

Point Prescription:
    RN-22 Tiantu

Manipulation: Prepare a piece of 4 sides plaster which is 3 cm long in each side, and tape the plaster on the point. Keep the plaster on the point 4 days. After an interval of 1 day, tape a new piece of the plaster on the point again. 5 times of the taping are taken as a course.

2. Ear Acupuncture

Indication: Chronic pharyngitis.

Ear Point Prescription:
    Pharynx, Mouth, Lung, Kidney, Sanjiao, Endocrine and Shenmen.

Manipulation: See page 255-256.

Comment:
Chronic pharyngitis is an obstinate disease. Zhenjiu can provide effective results in its treatment, but the treatment course may be long.

Notes:

85. Vocal Cord Paralysis

Vocal cord paralysis refers to dysfunction of the motor never of the laryngeal muscles. Trauma or viral illness may cause it. Clinically, it is marked by hoarseness in mild cases and loss of voice in severe cases. According to TCM, vocal cord paralysis belongs to the category of Yin (disability in pronounce), and it is due to attack of the laryngeal by external pathogens, adverse upward flow of the liver qi, or external injury of the tongue vessels.

I. STANDARD TREATMENT

Vocal cord paralysis is usually divided into 4 types — obstruction of the lung by pathogenic wind, stagnation of the lung due to adverse flow of qi, yin deficiency of lung and kidney, and impairment of the vessels. Local points and points of the Lung, Kidney and Liver Meridians are frequently selected in its treatment.

1. Obstruction of Lung by Pathogenic Wind

Manifestations: Abrupt attack of hoarseness, aversion to cold, fever, headache, cough with sputum, stuffy nose.

Tongue: White coating.

Pulse: Floating.

Treatment Principle: Dispel wind, relieve the exterior syndrome, ventilate the lung, relieve throat condition.

Point Prescription & Manipulation:
Primary points:
    RN-22 Tiantu -
    RN-23 Lianquan   -
    LI-17 Tianding -
    GB-20 Fengchi -
    BL-12 Fengmen -
    LI-4 Hegu -
    LU-7 Lieque -
    LU-5 Chize -

Explanation:
On RN-22 Tiantu and LI-17 Tianding, perform reducing manipulation by lifting, thrusting and rotating the needle to induce middle-degrees stimulation, and remove the needle without retention. On LU-17 Shaoshang, prick with the three-edged needle to bleed. On the other points, apply strong stimulation and perform reducing manipulation by lifting, thrusting and rotating the needles.

- RN-23 Lianquan, RN-22 Tiantu and LI-17 Tianding relieve the throat condition and improve pronunciation;
- LI-4 Hegu, GB-20 Fengchi and BL-12 Fengmen dispel wind and relieve exterior syndrome;
- LU-5 Chize and LU-7 Lieque promote the lung's dispersing function and relieve throat condition.

Secondary points according to conditions:
1▢ High fever, thirst and red tongue — ST-44 Neiting [-] and LU-11 Shaoshang [-];
2▢ Headache — GB-20 Fengchi [-].

2. Obstruction of the Lung due to Adverse Flow of Qi

Manifestations: Hoarseness or even loss of voice induced by emotional depression or anger, distressed feeling in the chest and hypochondria, irritability, restlessness, insomnia.

Tongue: Purplish body with thin coating.

Pulse: Wiry.

Treatment Principle: Soothe the liver to check the adverse, and disperse obstruction to relieve the throat condition.

Point Prescription & Manipulation:
Primary points:
    LR-3 Taichong -
    GB-43 Xiaxi -
    PC-6 Neiguan -
    RN-22 Tiantu -
    RN-23 Lianquan   -

LI-17 Tianding -

Explanation:
- RN-22 Tiantu, RN-23 Lianquan and LI-17 Tianding relieve the throat condition and improve pronunciation;
- LR-3 Taichong and GB-43 Xiaxi soothe the liver and relieve depression of qi;
- PC-6 Neiguan relieves depression of qi in the chest and calms the mind.

Secondary point:
1□ Sore throat — Yuji LU 10 [-];
2□ Irritability with flashed face — LR-2 Xingjian [-] and GB-34 Yanglingquan [-];
3□ Restlessness and insomnia —DU-20 Baihui [-] and EX-HN-1 Sishencong [-];
4□ Sensation of a foreign body obstructing the throat — ST-40 Fenglong [-] and RN-12 Zhongwan [-].

3. Yin Deficiency of Lung and Kidney

Manifestations: Hoarseness, intractable cough, tidal fever, night sweating, heat sensation in the palms and soles, dry mouth.

Tongue: Red body with little coating.

Pulse: Thready and rapid.

Treatment Principle: Tonify lung and kidney, moisten the throat.

Point Prescription & Manipulation:
Primary points:
RN-22 Tiantu +
RN-23 Lianquan -
LI-17 Tianding +
BL-13 Feishu +
BL-23 Shenshu +
BL-43 Gaohuang +
KI-3 Taixi +

Explanation:
- RN-23 Lianquan, RN-22 Tiantu and LI-17 Tianding relieve the throat condition and improve pronunciation;

- BL-13 Feishu, BL-23 Shenshu, BL-43 Gaohuang and KI-3 Taixi reinforce the lung and kidney and nourish yin.

Secondary points according to conditions:
1□ Night sweating — HT-6 Yinxi [+] and KI-7 Fuliu [+];
2□ Poor appetite — ST-36 Zusanli [+].

4. Impairment of the Collaterals

Manifestations: Hoarseness or loss of voice after surgical operation. In severe cases, difficulty in swallowing and dull sensation of the throat may be accompanied.

Treatment Principle: Dredging the meridian, activate the collaterals, and recover the voice.

Point Prescription & Manipulation:
Primary points:
RN-22 Tiantu + ^
RN-23 Lianquan -
LI-17 Tianding + ^
LI-18 Futu + ^
KI-3 Taixi +
LI-4 Hegu +

Explanation:
On RN-22 Tiantu, RN-23 Lianquan, LI-17 Tianding and LI-18 Futu, apply puncture firstly with reinforcing manipulation by lifting, thrusting and rotating the needles to induce strong stimulation, then apply moxibustion on them until the local skin becomes flushed. On KI-3 Taixi and LI-4 Hegu, apply acupuncture with reinforcing manipulation by lifting, thrusting and rotating the needles to induce strong stimulation. On RN-23 Lianquan, apply acupuncture with reducing manipulation by lifting, thrusting and rotating the needle to induce strong stimulation.

- LI-18 Futu, RN-22 Tiantu, RN-23 Lianquan and LI-17 Tianding promote qi and blood circulation of the throat region, and improve pronunciation;
- KI-3 Taixi nourishes the kidney yin and moistens the throat;

- LI-4 Hegu, one of the Four General Points that has strong effect of clearing and activating the collaterals and meridians, improves pronunciation.

Secondary points according to conditions:
1□ Difficulty in swallowing, dull sensation of the throat — RN-23 Lianquan [-];
2□ Severe cases — RN-17 Danzhong [-] and BL-17 Geshu [-].

II. EXPERIENTIAL TREATMENT

1. Puncturing KI-1 Yongquan

Indication: Hysterical aphasia.

Point Prescription:
    KI-1 Yongquan

Manipulation: Insert a thick needle perpendicularly into the point, and lift, thrust and rotate the needle with great amplitude for 1-10 minutes. Usually, during the treatment the patient can speak.

2. Puncturing PC-6 Neiguan

Indication: Vocal cord paralysis.

Point Prescription:
    PC-6 Neiguan

Manipulation: Insert a needle perpendicularly into the point 0.8-1 cun, and lift, thrust and rotate the needle to induce strong stimulation for 1-5 minutes. Usually, acute vocal cord paralysis can be cured by one treatment.

3. Puncturing ST-9 Renyin

Indication: Chronic vocal cord paralysis.

Point Prescription:
    ST-9 Renyin of the diseased side.

Manipulation: Insert a 2-cun needle perpendicularly into the point 1.2-1.5 cun, manipulate the needle until the patient feels that there is a foreign body in the throat, or soreness and numbness. Retain the needle for 30 minutes. If the patient loses voice or has severe hoarseness, RN-23 Lianquan is punctured additionally. The treatment is given once daily, with 10 treatments as a course.

Comment:
Zhenjiu is effective in the treatment of vocal cord paralysis. In many cases, vocal cord paralysis even can be cured by Zhenjiu treatment. In Zhenjiu treatment, selection of RN-22 Tiantu and LI-17 Tianding has been stressed since ancient times, which can be taken as the key points to treat acute aphasia or acute hoarseness.

Notes:

86. Meniere's Disease

Meniere's disease is a type of auditory vertigo caused by hydrops in the labyrinth of the ear. Its cause is uncertain. It is clinical marked by paroxysmal dizziness aggravated by changes of body position, usually accompanied by tinnitus, hearing loss, parallel nystagmus, nausea, and vomiting. Spontaneous cure and repeated recurrence are often seen in many cases. According to TCM, Meniere's disease belongs to the category of Xuan Yun (dizziness), and it is due to rising of hyperactive liver yang, which disturbs the ears, or due to accumulation of turbid phlegm in the middle-jiao, which obstructs the rising of clear-qi to the ear.

I. STANDARD TREATMENT

Meniere's disease is usually divided into two types — rising of hyperactive liver yang and turbid phlegm obstruction in the middle-jiao. Points around the ear and points of the Liver, Spleen and Kidney Meridians are frequently selected in its treatment.

1. Rising of Hyperactivity of Liver Yang

Manifestations: Abrupt onset of vertigo induced and aggravated by emotional stimulation or fatigue, irritability, restlessness, bitter taste in the mouth, nausea, red eyes.

Tongue: Red body with little coating.

Pulse: Wiry and thready.

Treatment Principle: Check the liver, nourish yin, suppress yang and stop endogenous wind.

Point Prescription & Manipulation:
Primary points:
    BL-18 Ganshu -
    BL-23 Shenshu +
    LR-3 Taichong -
    KI-3 Taixi +
    GB-20 Fengchi -
    SP-6 Sanyinjiao +

Explanation:
- BL-18 Ganshu, LR-3 Taichong and GB-20 Fengchi check the liver, suppress yang hyperactivity, and calm endogenous wind;
- BL-23 Shenshu, KI-3 Taixi and SP-6 Sanyinjiao tonify kidney yin (water) to nourish the liver (wood).

Secondary points according to conditions:
1⃞ Distending sensation of the eye and head— GB-43 Xiaxi [-];
2⃞ Nausea and vomiting — PC-6 Neiguan [-] and LI-4 Hegu [-].

2. Turbid Phlegm Obstructing in the Middle-Jiao

Manifestations: Vertigo and shakiness that are aggravated by movements, sensation of heaviness in the head as if it were tightly wrapped, poor appetite, nausea, vomiting, fatigue.

Tongue: White body with white and sticky.

Pulse: Soft or wiry and smooth.

Treatment Principle: Reinforce spleen, regulate stomach and resolve phlegm.

Point Prescription & Manipulation:
Primary points:
    ST-36 Zusanli + ^
    ST-40 Fenglong -
    SP-6 Sanyinjiao +
    BL-20 Pishu + ^
    BL-21 Weishu + ^
    RN-12 Zhongwan - ^

Explanation:
- ST-40 Fenglong and SP-6 Sanyinjiao resolve phlegm and remove dampness;
- BL-20 Pishu and BL-21 Weishu, the Back-Shu Points of the spleen and stomach, reinforce the middle-jiao, and improve spleen's function of transportation and transformation;

- RN-12 Zhongwan and ST-36 Zusanli harmonize the stomach and check down the adverse flow of stomach qi.

Secondary points according to conditions:
1□ Extreme vertigo — GB-20 Fengchi [/];
2□ Vomiting — PC-6 Neiguan [/]and SP-4 Gongsun [+];
3□ Tinnitus SJ-19 — Tinggong [-] and SJ-17 Yifeng [-].

II. EXPERIENTIAL TREATMENT

1. Puncturing EX-HN-3 Yintang, EX-HN-16 Anmian, and PC-6 Neiguan

Indication: Meniere's disease.

Point Prescription:
Primary points:
EX-HN-3 Yintang
EX-HN-16 Anmian
PC-6 Neiguan

Secondary points according to conditions:
1□ Tinnitus and deafness — SJ-19 Tinggong and GB-20 Fengchi.

Manipulation: Acupuncture is applied with even reinforcing and reducing manipulation.

2. Moxibustion on DU-20 Baihui

Indication: Intractable Meniere's disease.

Point Prescription:
DU-20 Baihui
ST-36 Zusanli

Manipulation: Moxibustion is applied on DU-20 Baihui and acupuncture on ST-36 Zusanli. Cut the hair on DU-20 Baihui region 1 square cm, smear a small amount of Vaseline on the point, put a moxa cone as big as a peanut on the point and ignite the cone for moxibustion. When the patient can not stand the burning sensation caused by ignited cone, press the cone to extinguish the fire and remove the ash. Then, replace a new cone and give moxibustion again.

Repeat the course until 50-70 moxa cones have been used. The whole course generally lasts 1 hour. After moxibustion, puncture ST-36 Zusanli with reducing manipulation immediately. Ask the patient not to wash his/her hair within half month. In case there is a scar left on the point, tell the patient to keep clean in that region. It does not need special treatment and will disappear in its own course within a month. Generally, only one treatment is needed to cure the disease.

3. Ear Acupuncture

Indication: Meniere's disease.

Ear Point Prescription:
Primary points:
Internal Ear, External Ear, Sanjiao, Gallbladder, Subcortex, Shenmen and Occiput.

Secondary points according to conditions:
1□ Rising of hyperactivity of liver yang— Liver and Kidney;
2□ Turbid phlegm obstructing in the middle-jiao — Spleen and Stomach.

Manipulation: See page 255-256.

4. Scalp Puncture

Indication: Meniere's disease.

Scalp Line Prescription:
Vertigo and Aural Area.

Manipulation: Insert a needle through the scalp of the anterior end of the line, push the needle backward under the scalp 4 cm, and rotate the needle with moderate stimulation for 5 minutes. Then, retain the needle for 40 minutes and manipulate once every 5 minutes. The treatment is given once daily, with 5-7 treatments as a course.

Comment:
Zhenjiu is effective in the treatment of Meniere's disease. In most cases, the disease can be cured by Zhenjiu treatment.

Notes:

87. Tinnitus and Deafness

Tinnitus refers to feeling of ringing in the head, and deafness refers to dysaudia or hearing disability. Tinnitus may be accompanied by lowering of hearing ability and deafness may develop from tinnitus. Thus, they are discussed together here. Both of them are clinical manifestations that can be seen in many diseases. According to TCM, tinnitus and deafness respectively belong to Er Ming (ringing in the ear) and Er Long (deafness). They are caused by stagnation of liver qi or overactivity of liver yang transforming into fire to interfere with the clear orifice, over accumulation of internal damp-phlegm which upwardly covers the clear orifice or essence deficiency leading to failure of the brain to be nourished.

I. STANDARD TREATMENT

Tinnitus and deafness are generally divided into three types — over activity of liver yang, upward covering by turbid phlegm and deficiency of kidney qi. Points of the local region and Bladder, Liver and Gallbladder Meridians are frequently selected in their treatment.

1. Hyperactivity of Liver Yang

Manifestations: Sudden onset of tinnitus or even deafness, which is aggravated by bad emotional stimulation, headache, dizziness, flushed face, red eyes, bitter taste, dry throat, irritability, liability to lose temper.

Tongue: Red body with yellow coating.

Pulse: Wiry and rapid.

Treatment Principle: Soothe the liver and restrain the overactivity of yang.

Point Prescription & Manipulation:
Primary points:
LR-3 Taichong -
PC-6 Neiguan -
GB-20 Fengchi -
GB-2 Tinghui -
SJ-3 Zhongzhu -
GB-43 Xiaxi -

Explanation:
- LR-3 Taichong, PC-6 Neiguan, SJ-3 Zhongzhu and GB-43 Xiaxi soothe the liver and restrain overactivity of yang;
- GB-20 Fengchi and GB-2 Tinghui clear the Gallbladder Meridian and open the ear.

Secondary points according to conditions:
1〕 Chronic cases — SJ-17 Yifeng [-] and DU-20 Baihui [-];
2〕 Constipation—SJ-6 Zhigou [-] and ST-25 Tianshu [-];
3〕 Red eyes, bitter taste in the mouth and hypochondriac pain—LR-2 Xingjian [-] and GB-34 Yanglingquan [-].

2. Upward Covering by Turbid Phlegm

Manifestations: Ringing sound in the head, lowering of hearing ability with sensation of stuffiness in the ear tract, distressed sensation in the chest and epigastrium, loose stools.

Tongue: Flabby body with sticky coating.

Pulse: Soft or smooth.

Treatment Principle: Remove dampness and phlegm, and open the orifice.

Point Prescription & Manipulation:
Primary points:
SJ-21 Ermen -
SJ-17 Yifeng -
SJ-5 Waiguan -
ST-40 Fenglong - ^
RN-12 Zhongwan - ^
SP-9 Yinlingquan + ^

Explanation:
- SJ-21 Ermen and SJ-17 Yifeng open the ear and clears the orifice;
- SJ-5 Waiguan dredges the Shaoyang Meridian to benefit the hearing;

- ST-40 Fenglong, RN-12 Zhongwan and SP-9 Yinlingquan resolve phlegm and remove dampness.

Secondary points according to conditions:
1 Poor appetite and distressed feeling in the chest — ST-36 Zusanli [+] and PC-6 Neiguan [-];
2 Chronic cases — RN-6 Qihai [+ ^] and ST-25 Tianshu [+];
3 Dizziness and heaviness sensation in the head — GB-20 Fengchi [-] and BL-20 Baihui [/].

3. Deficiency of Kidney Qi

Manifestations: Prolonged but mild ringing in the head which may be alleviated by pressure, chronic lowering of hearing ability, dizziness, blurred vision, soreness and weakness of the lower back and knees, nocturnal emission, impotence.

Tongue: Red or pale body.

Pulse: Thready and rapid or thready and weak.

Treatment Principle: Nourish the kidney qi.

Point Prescription & Manipulation:
Primary points:
SI-19 Tinggong +
BL-18 Ganshu + ^
BL-23 Shenshu + ^
KI-3 Taixi +
RN-4 Guanyuan + ^
ST-36 Zusanli + ^

Explanation:
- SI-19 Tinggong promotes circulation of qi and blood of the ear region, and improves hearing ability;
- BL-18 Ganshu, BL-23 Shenshu and KI-3 Taixi tonify the liver and kidney to improve hearing ability;
- RN-4 Guanyuan and ST-36 Zusanli reinforce the middle-jiao and tonify qi.

Secondary points according to conditions:

1 Impotence—DU-4 Mingmen [+ ^] and RN-2 Qugu [+ ^];
2 Dizziness—ST-40 Fenglong [+ ^] and BL-20 Baihui [+ ^].

II. EXPERIENTIAL TREATMENT

1. Puncturing EX-UE-14 Xiadu

Indication: Tinnitus.

Point Prescription:
EX-UE-14 Xiadu, on the dorsum of the hand, 0.5 cun proximal to the margin of the web between the 4th and 5th fingers.

Manipulation: Insert a 1.5-cun needle into the point, push it upward along the space between the 4th and 5th metacarpal bones 0.5-1 cun, rotate it 10 times or more until arrival of qi. Generally, puncture the point at the diseased side firstly, and 10 minutes later ringing sensation will be decreased obviously or disappear. If not, puncture the opposite point additionally with the same manipulation. Retain the needle for 40 minutes and manipulate it every 10 minutes. The treatment is given once daily, with 5 times as one course.

2. Puncturing GB-31 Fengshi

Indication: Nervous deafness.

Point Prescription:
GB-31 Fengshi of the diseased side.

Manipulation: Insert a 3-cun needle into the point, slowly lift and thrust the needle to induce arrival of qi, and rotate the needle constantly and slowly for 5-10 minutes to make the needling sensation radiate upward. The treatment is given once daily, with five treatments as one course.

3. Puncturing SI-19 Tinggong

Indication: Nervous deafness.

Point Prescription:
SI-19 Tinggong of the diseased side.

Manipulation: Ask the patient to sit down. Insert a 1-cun needle perpendicularly 0.8 cun, and ask the patient to hold the nose with the fingers tightly until the patient feels that there is sound from the dump of the ears. Then, rotate the needle at small amplitude to make the needling sensation radiate to the interior of the ear, retain the needle for 30 minutes and repeat this course once during the retention. The treatment is given once daily, with 10 treatments as one course.

4. Deep Perpendicularly Thrusting and Lifting of the Needle

Indication: Deafness.

Point Prescription:
SI-19 Tinggong
SJ-17 Yifeng
SJ 21 Ermen
GB-2 Tinghui
SJ-18 Chimai
DU-20 Baihui

Manipulation: Acupuncture is applied. On DU-20 Baihui, insert a 1-cun needle obliquely 0.3-0.5 cun, and perform a reinforcing manipulation. On the other points, insert needles perpendicularly 0.8-1 cun, retain the needles for 30 minutes to induce arrival of qi, and remove the needles slowly. The treatment is given 3 times a week, with 10 treatments as one course.

5. Ear Acupuncture by Needling

Indication: Nervous deafness due to drug poison.

Ear Point Prescription:
External Ear, Kidney, Liver of the right side and Adrenal Gland.

Manipulation: Look for reaction spots around the point regions with the probing needle, insert two needles into the spots around External Ear and Kidney each, push one needle perpendicularly and the other obliquely. Insert a needle into the spot around Liver perpendicularly, and insert a needle into Adrenal

Gland obliquely toward EX-HN-5 Taiyang direction. Rotate the needles to induce strong stimulation, and retain them for over one hour. The treatment is given once daily, with 10 treatments as one course. For nervous deafness, if the treatment is given to cases at the early stage of the disease, the result will be better.

6. Ear Acupuncture by Pasting

Indication: Deafness.

Ear Point Prescription:
Inner Ear, Brain Stem, Kidney, Subcortex and Endocrine.

Manipulation: Look for the sensitive spots around the point regions and paste vaccaria seeds on the spots. Ask the patient to keep the seeds on the ear for 3-5 days and press the points 3-5 times daily. After an interval of 5-7 days, repeat this course.

7. Scalp Puncture

Indication: Sudden deafness, tinnitus or deafness at its early stage.

Scalp Line Prescription:
Primary line:
The lower 1/3 of the Posterior Oblique Line on the Vertex of the diseased side.

Secondary line:
Lateral Line 2 of the Forehead of the left side excessive syndrome;
The posterior 1/3 of the Middle Line of the Vertex.

Manipulation: On the lower 1/3 of the Posterior Oblique Line of the Vertex and Lateral Line 2 of the Forehead, insert needles from the top downwards. Then, on the posterior 1/3 of the Middle Line of the Vertex, insert a needle from the front backwards. Manipulate the needles by thrusting and lifting at small amplitude for 2-3 minutes, and perform the manipulation again every 10 minutes during one hour of the retention of the needles. Ask the patient to breathe in, hold his/her breath, hold his/her nose with the fingers, and do an action of making air in the mouth be sent to the ears several times during the manipulation of needles. The treatment is given once daily, with 10 treatments as a course.

Comment:

Zhenjiu is effective in relieving tinnitus, and has shown to be effective in treating deafness in some cases. According to our experience, self-pressing ears is a good way to treat obstinate tinnitus. In the manipulation, press bilateral ears towards each other with palms simultaneously for 10 seconds, and release the palms. Then repeat this course for 10-30 times. The treatment is given 2-3 times daily, for 30-60 days. Usually, tinnitus will be milder greatly. After an interval of 1-2 weeks, the next course can begin. The treatment can last until no tinnitus.

Notes:

88. Dysfunction of the Tempromandibular Joint

Dysfunction of the tempromandibular joint is a commonly seen oral disease, marked by pain in the tempromandibular joint when opening or closing the mouth, usually aggravated by chewing, or yawning. Articular dyskinesia may be present, with snapping or popping of the joint occurring when opening or closing the mouth. It occurs mainly in young people and adults, and its cause has not been clearly determined. According to TCM, dysfunction of the tempromandibular joint is classified into He Tong (mandible pain), Jia Tong (cheek pain) or Kou Jin Bu Kai (lockjaw) .

I. STANDARD TREATMENT

Dysfunction of the tempromandibular joint is generally divided into four types — attack by pathogenic wind-cold, adverse upward flow of liver qi, external injury of muscles and tendons and kidney deficiency. Points of the Yangming Meridians are frequently selected in its treatment.

1. Attack by Pathogenic Wind-Cold

Manifestations: Pain in the tempromandibular joint which is aggravated by chewing, stiffness and snapping or popping of the joint, difficulty in opening the mouth, headache, general ache.

Tongue: Thin and white coating.

Pulse: Floating and wiry.

Treatment Principle: Expel wind and cold, relieve rigidity of muscles and activate collaterals.

Point Prescription & Manipulation:
Primary points:
    EX-HN-25 Jiaozhong -
    ST-6 Jiache - ^
    SI-19 Tinggong - ^
    ST-7 Xiaguan - ^

LI-4 Hegu -

Explanation:
To local points, Zhenjiu is only given to the diseased side.

- EX-HN-25 Jiaozhong, an experiential point to treat temperomandibular joint disorders, ST-6 Jiache, belonging to the Foot-Yangming Meridian, SI-19 Tinggong, the Crossing Point of the Hand-Taiyang and Hand-Shaoyang Meridians, and ST-7 Xiaguan, the Crossing Point of the Foot-Shaoyang and Foot-Yangming Meridians, all located at the diseased part, regulate and dredge the three facial yang meridians, activate the collaterals and relieve rigidity of the local muscles;
- LI-4 Hegu, the Primary-Source Point of the Hand-Yangming Meridian, activates the collaterals, relieves rigidity of the muscles, alleviates pain and dispels wind and cold.

Secondary points according to conditions:
1▢ Headache—GB-20 Fengchi [-] or EX-HN-5 Taiyang [-].

2. Adversely Upward Flowing of Liver qi

Manifestations: Pain in the tempromandibular joint which is aggravated by chewing, stiffness and snapping or popping of the joint, difficulty in opening the mouth, dizziness, insomnia, irritability, tinnitus.

Tongue: Thin and white coating.

Pulse: Thready and wiry.

Treatment Principle: Soothe the liver and regulate circulation of qi, relieve rigidity of muscles and activate collaterals.

Point Prescription & Manipulation:
Primary points:
  EX-HN-25 Jiaozhong /
  SI-19 Tinggong /
  ST-7 Xiaguan /
  ST-6 Jiache /

  LR-3 Taichong -
  GB-34 Yanglingquan -
  LI-4 Hegu -

Explanation:
To local points, Zhenjiu is only given to the diseased side.

- EX-HN-25 Jiaozhong, an experiential point to treat temperomandibular joint disorders, ST-6 Jiache, belonging to the Foot-Yangming Meridian, SI-19 Tinggong, the Crossing Point of the Hand-Taiyang and Hand-Shaoyang Meridians, and ST-7 Xiaguan, the Crossing Point of the Foot-Shaoyang and Foot-Yangming Meridians, all located at the diseased part, regulate and dredge the three facial yang meridians, activate the collaterals and relieve rigidity of the local muscles;
- LR-3 Taichong and GB-34 Yanglingquan soothe the liver and regulate qi flow;
- LI-4 Hegu, the Primary-Source Point of the Hand-Yangming Meridian, activates the collaterals, relieves rigidity of the muscles and alleviates pain.

Secondary points according to conditions:
1▢ Insomnia—EX-HN-16 Anmian [/];
2▢ Dizziness—GB-20 Fengchi [/].

3. Impairment of the Muscle and Tendon by External Injury

Manifestations: Pain in the tempromandibular joint that is aggravated by chewing, stiffness and snapping or popping of the joint, difficulty in opening the mouth, history of external injury to the cheek, or sprain of the tempromandibular joint by opening the mouth too wide.

Tongue: Purplish body.

Pulse: Wiry.

Treatment Principle: Dredge the meridian, circulate the collaterals and activate blood circulation.

Point Prescription & Manipulation:
Primary points:
  EX-HN-25 Jiaozhong   - ^
  SI-19 Tinggong - ^
  ST-7 Xiaguan - ^
  ST-6 Jiache - ^
  SJ-5 Waiguan -
  LI-4 Hegu -
  Tender point or hard nodule point -

Explanation:
To local points, Zhenjiu is only given to the diseased side.

- EX-HN-25 Jiaozhong, an experiential point to treat temperomandibular joint disorders, ST-6 Jiache, belonging to the Foot-Yangming Meridian, SI-19 Tinggong, the Crossing Point of the Hand-Taiyang and Hand-Shaoyang Meridians, and ST-7 Xiaguan, the Crossing Point of the Foot-Shaoyang and Foot-Yangming Meridians, all located at the diseased part, regulate and dredge the three facial yang meridians, activate the collaterals and relieve rigidity of the local muscles;
- SJ-5 Waiguan, the Luo-Connecting Point and the Crossing Point of the Hand-Shaoyang and Yangwei Meridians, activates the collaterals and dredges the yang meridians of the body;
- LI-4 Hegu, the Primary-Source Point of the Hand-Yangming Meridian, activates the collaterals, relieves rigidity of the muscles and alleviates pain;
- Tender point or hard nodule point activates the collaterals and relieves pain.

Secondary points according to conditions:
1〇 Semiluxation of the tempromandibular joint-- SI-18 Quanliao [-].

4. Kidney Deficiency

Manifestations: Pain in the tempromandibular joint which is aggravated by chewing, stiffness and snapping or popping of the joint, difficulty in opening the mouth, maldevelopment of joints,

loose teeth, fatigue, dizziness, insomnia, tinnitus.

Tongue: Thin and white coating.

Pulse: Thready and weak.

Treatment Principle: Reinforce kidney qi and strengthen tendons and bones.

Point Prescription & Manipulation:
Primary points:
  EX-HN-25 Jiaozhong   + ^
  SI-19 Tinggong + ^
  ST-7 Xiaguan + ^
  ST-6 Jiache + ^
  BL-23 Shenshu +
  ST-36 Zusanli +

Explanation:
To local points, Zhenjiu is only given to the diseased side.

- EX-HN-25 Jiaozhong, an experiential point to treat temperomandibular joint disorders, ST-6 Jiache, belonging to the Foot-Yangming Meridian, SI-19 Tinggong, the Crossing Point of the Hand-Taiyang and Hand-Shaoyang Meridians, and ST-7 Xiaguan, the Crossing Point of the Foot-Shaoyang and Foot-Yangming Meridians, all located at the diseased part, regulate and dredge the three facial yang meridians, activate the collaterals and relieve rigidity of the local muscles;
- BL-23 Shenshu reinforces the kidney qi and strengthens the bones and tendons;
- ST-36 Zusanli reinforces the spleen and stomach to nourish the kidney.

Secondary points according to conditions:
1〇 Dizziness GB-20 Fengchi [/];
2〇 Tinnitus SJ-17 Yifeng [+].

II. EXPERIENTIAL TREATMENT

1. Puncturing A Group of Points

Indication: Various types of tempromandibular joint syndrome.

Point Prescription:
Primary points:
    SI-19 Tinggong
    ST-7 Xiaguan
    ST-6 Jiache

Secondary points according to conditions:
1) Facial paralysis—LI-4 Hegu [-];
2) Dislocation of the joints — GB-34 Yanglingquan [-];
3) Long-term course—BL-23 Shenshu [+];
4) Emotional depression—LR-3 Taichong [-].

Manipulation: Each treatment, the chief points and 1-3 assistant points are punctured. After regular sterilization, SI-19 Tinggong is punctured firstly. With the mouth opened, a 2 cun needle is inserted 1.5 cun (25-40 mm) to make the needling sensation radiating to the cheek. Then, ask the patient to close the mouth and insert a 1.5 cun needle into ST-7 Xiaguan 1-1.2 cun (25-35 mm), with the needle tip directing backwards a little to make the needling sensation radiate to the whole tempromandibular joint. Then, insert a 1.5-cun needle into ST-6 Jiache with its tip upwards a little, to make the needling sensation radiate to the whole cheek. Twisting, thrusting, and lifting manipulations are applied on all of these three points with middle-degree force, and the needles are retained for 20-30 minutes. If the patient has headache and general ache, LI-4 Hegu is punctured additionally with uniform reinforcing-reducing manipulation; LR-3 Taichong and GB-34 Yanglingquan are punctured with reducing manipulation for irritability, insomnia and tinnitus; and BL-23 Shenshu is punctured with reinforcing manipulation for deficiency syndrome. The treatment is given once a day or every other day, 5-7 treatments are needed in one treatment course. If there is no satisfactory effect after the first course, the second course begins after an interval of 3-5 days.

2. Acupuncture and Moxibustion on A Group of Points

Indication: Various types of tempromandibular joint syndrome.

Point Prescription:
Primary points:
    SI-19 Tinggong
    GB-2 Tinghui
    ST-7 Xiaguan

Secondary points according to conditions:
1) Poor appetite—ST-36 Zusanli [+];
2) Facial numbness—BL-18 Ganshu [+];
3) Long-term course—BL-23 Shenshu [+].

Manipulation: The three primary points are used alternatively. After regular sterilization, insert a 1.5 cun filiform needle into the point, rotate, lift and thrust the needle with middle-degrees stimulation to induce arrival of qi. Then, retain the needle, and put a segment of moxa stick 1.5-2.0 cm long on the handle of the needle for moxibustion. After burning out the moxa segment, remove the needle. The assistant points are punctured with reinforcing manipulation. The treatment is given once a day or every other day, with 10 treatments as a course. After an interval of 4-5 days, the second course can be given if the problem does not disappear.

3. Puncturing A Group of Points

Indication: Chronic tempromandibular joint syndrome.

Point Prescription:
    ST-7 Xiaguan
    EX-HN-25 Jiaozhong (located at the midpoint of the line connecting ST-7 Xiaguan and ST-6 Jiache)
    ST-6 Jiache

Manipulation: Insert a 1.5-cun needle perpendicularly into ST-7 Xiaguan 1.0-1.5 cun (25-40 mm), and insert 1 cun needles into Jiaozhong EX-HN-25 and ST-6 Jiache 0.6-0.8 cun (13-20 mm). Rotate, lift and thrust the needles with middle-degrees stimulation, and retain the needles for 30-60 minutes with manipulation of the needles 1-2 times. After removing the needles, press the needle holes with fingers, apply massage along the lower border of the zygomatic arch for 3 minutes, and gently push the cheek upward and downward along the masseter 12 times. The treatment is given once every day, with 10 treatments as one course.

4. Puncturing Two Points

Indication: Tempromandibular joint syndrome with difficulty in opening the mouth.

Point Prescription:
    ST-7 Xiaguan
    ST-6 Jiache

Manipulation: Insert 1.5-cun needles perpendicularly into the points, rotate , lift and thrust the needles to make arrival of qi. Then, connect the needles with electric-acupuncture instrument and give electric stimulation with constant low wave of frequency of 150-200 cycles/minute, at a level the patient can stand, for 20-30 minutes. The treatment is given 2-3 times a week and six treatments are taken as one course.

Comment:
Acupuncture is effective in the treatment of tempromandibular joint syndrome. In acupuncture clinic, needling therapy is usually the first selection, with dredging the meridian and activating the collaterals as the basic treatment principle, and by puncturing the local points as the main in the treatment.

Notes:

89. Toothache

Toothache is a common symptom of various oral problems, including caries, pulpitis, apical periodontal inflammation, pericoronitis, and periodentitis. According to TCM, toothache, called Ya Tong in Chinese, is due to attack of external wind-heat or accumulation of heat in the stomach, leading to obstruction of the vessels and collaterals, or due to upward flaming of deficient fire caused by kidney yin deficiency, resulting in impairment of the vessels and collaterals.

I. STANDARD TREATMENT

Toothache is usually divided into three types — wind-fire, stomach fire and deficient fire. Points of the Yangming Meridians are frequently selected in its treatment.

1. Wind-Fire

Manifestations: Abrupt attack of severe toothache, which is aggravated by heat and relieved by cold, redness and swelling of the gums.

Tongue: Red body with thin and yellow coating.

Pulse: Floating and rapid.

Treatment Principle: Dispel wind, clear heat, relieve swelling and stop pain.

Point Prescription & Manipulation:
Primary points:
    GB-20 Fengchi -
    LI-4 Hegu -

Explanation:
On GB-20 Fengchi and LI-4 Hegu, perform reducing manipulation by lifting, thrusting and rotating the needles for 1-3 minutes, and retain the needles for 30 minutes. If the pain is not relieved obviously by manipulating the needle on the above points, additionally puncture ST-7 Xiaguan for upper toothache and ST-6 Jiache

for lower toothache with manipulation of rotating, lifting and thrusting the needles. During manipulating the needles on ST-6 Jiache or ST-7 Xiaguan, the patient is advised to clench the teeth until the pain is relieved. Then, retain the needles for 20-30 minutes. On DU-14 Dazhui, apply reducing manipulation by lifting, thrusting, and rotating the needle, and retain the needle for 20-30 minutes.

- GB-20 Fengchi, an essential point for dispelling wind, dispels and clears wind and fire;
- LI-4 Hegu, an essential point for relieving toothache, dredges the collaterals, dispels wind-heat and alleviates pain of the tooth.

Secondary points according to conditions:
1️⃣ Pain of the upper tooth—ST-7 Xiaguan [-];
2️⃣ Pain of the lower tooth— ST-6 Jiache [-];
3️⃣ High fever—DU-14 Dazhui [-]

2. Stomach Fire

Manifestations: Severe toothache with red and swelling gums, which is relieved by cold and aggravated by heat, thirst, bad smell from the mouth, constipation, dark urination.

Tongue: Red body with yellow coating.

Pulse: Rapid.

Treatment Principle: Clear fire from the stomach, subdue swelling and relieve pain.

Point Prescription & Manipulation:
Primary points:
    LI-4 Hegu -
    ST-44 Neiting -
    ST-7 Jiache -
    ST-6 Xiaguan -

Explanation:
- LI-4 Hegu, a key point for relieving toothache which belongs to the Large Intestine Meridian, clears heat from the Yangming Meridian, regulates the large

intestine qi, dredges the collaterals, and alleviates pain of the tooth.
- ST-44 Neiting clears heat from the stomach;
- ST-7 Jiache and ST-6 Xiaguan, near the diseased region and belonging to the Yangming Meridian, dredge the Yangming Meridian qi, activate the collaterals, and alleviate pain of the tooth.

Secondary points according to conditions:
1️⃣ Constipation—SJ-6 Zhigou [-] and BL-57 Chengshan [-].

3. Upward Flaming of Deficient Fire

Manifestations: Protractible intermittent and dull pain of the tooth, atrophy of the gums, loose teeth, soreness and weakness of the loins and knees.

Tongue: Red body with little coating.

Pulse: Thready and rapid.

Treatment Principle: Tonify yin, nourish the kidney, check down fire and relieve pain.

Point Prescription & Manipulation:
Primary points:
    LI-4 Hegu -
    ST-6 Jiache -
    KI-3 Taixi +
    KI-2 Rangu +

Explanation:
- LI-4 Hegu, key point for relieving toothache, dredges the collaterals, dispels wind-heat, and alleviates pain of the tooth.
- ST-6 Jiache, near the diseased region, activates the collaterals of the local region and alleviates pain;
- KI-3 Taixi, the Yuan-Source Point of the Kidney Meridian, tonifies the kidney and nourishes yin;
- KI-2 Rangu, the Ying-Spring Point of the Kidney Meridian, tonifies the kidney and clears deficient fire.

Secondary points according to conditions:
1️⃣ Soreness and weakness of the loins and knees — BL-23 Shenshu [+] and BL-52 Zhishi [+]
2️⃣ Tinnitus and dizziness — BL-23 Shenshu [+] and DU-20 Baihui [+].

II. EXPERIENTIAL TREATMENT

1. Puncturing SJ-2 Yemen

Indication: Various types of toothache.

Point Prescription:
SJ-2 Yemen of the diseased side.

Manipulation: Insert a 1.5-cun needle into the point obliquely upward along the space of the carpal bones 0.5-1 cun. Then, rotate the needle to induce a needling sensation until the patient feels local soreness, numbness and distention which radiate to the arm, elbow or tip of the finger, and retain the needle for 20-60 minutes. If the pain is not relieved greatly after retention of the needle for 15 minutes, puncture the opposite SJ-2 Yemen additionally with the same manipulation. Usually, the pain will be stopped only by one treatment.

2. Puncturing EX-UE-22 Yatong (Toothache)

Indication: Various types of toothache.

Point Prescription:
EX-UE-22 Yatong of the diseased side, located on the hand, at the center of the first metacarpophalangeal joint on the dorsum aspect.

Manipulation: Insert a 1-cun needle through the skin of the point and push the needle horizontally upward under the skin 0.5 cun. Then, rotate the needle with a large amplitude to induce a needling sensation which radiates upward to the gums, and retain the needle for 30 minutes. Generally, the pain will be relieved during the puncture and one treatment can be effective to stop pain.

3. Puncturing EX-UE-17 Yatongling

Indication: Various types of toothache.

Point Prescription:
EX-UE-17 Yatongling of the diseased side, located on the palmar aspect of the hand, between the third and fourth metacarpophalangeal joints.

Manipulation: Puncture perpendicularly 0.3-0.5 cun, manipulate the needle to induce arrival of qi, and perform reducing manipulation by rotating the needle. Retain the needle until the pain disappears. Usually, only one or two treatments are needed.

4. Ear Acupuncture on the Earlobe

Indication: Various types of toothache.

Ear Point Prescription:
The base of the ear lobe on the diseased side.

Manipulation: Insert a 1-cun needle perpendicularly into the base of the ear lobe 0.5-0.7 cun. If the patient has upper toothache, puncture with the needle tip directing upward a little; if the patient has lower toothache, with the tip directing downward a little. Lift, thrust and rotate the needle with big amplitude to induce strong stimulation, and retain the needle for 10-30 minutes. Generally, the pain will be relieved during the puncture and one treatment may be effective to stop pain.

5. Ear Acupuncture on A Group Points

Indication: Various types of toothache.

Ear Point Prescription:
Primary points:
Shenmen, Cheek, Apex of Antitragus, Yatongding.
Secondary points according to conditions:
1️⃣ Stomach fire — Stomach, Large Intestine;
2️⃣ Wind-fire — Inner ear, Ear Apex;
3️⃣ Deficiency fire — Kidney

Manipulation: See page 255-256.

Comment:

Toothache is a symptom seen in many diseases. Acupuncture is effective to relieve toothache. However, the diseases causing the toothache should be treated as well.

Notes:

90. Recurrent Ulcer of the Mouth

Recurrent ulcer of the mouth, also known as recurrent canker sore, is the most commonly seen ulcerative condition of the mucous membrane of the mouth. Its cause is uncertain, although it is probably linked to an abnormal immune system response that has been triggered by a deficiency, injury or another problem. Clinically, it is marked by frequently recurring, painful, small, circular or oval ulcers of the mucous membrane of the mouth. The pain is aggravated by exposure of the ulcers to heat, cold, acid, or salt, and may be so severe that it could affect diet and sleep. It may become more severe or recur more frequently in the presence of insomnia, poor diet, or overstrain. According to TCM, recurrent ulcer of the mouth belongs to the categories of Kou Mi (erosion of the mouth) and Kou She Sheng Chuang (ulcer of the mouth and tongue). It is due to over intake of greasy, sweet, and pungent food, or internal injury due to emotional stimulation that leads to generation of excessive fire which flames upward. It may also be due to prolonged illness, overstrain or overindulgence in sexual life which all lead to impairment of yin fluids of the body and generation of deficient fire, which flames upward.

I. STANDARD TREATMENT

Recurrent ulcer of the mouth is divided into two types — excess fire and deficiency fire. Points of the Heart, Kidney, Small Intestine and Yangming Meridians are frequently selected in its treatment.

1. Excess Fire

Manifestation: Recurrent attack of sore of the mouth or tongue with burning sensation, dry throat, strong smell from the mouth, constipation, dark and scanty urine.

Tongue: Red body with yellow coating.

Pulse: Rapid and forceful.

Treatment Principle: Clear heat and reduce fire.

Point Prescription & Manipulation:
Primary points:
> ST-4 Dicang -
> LI-4 Hegu -
> LI-11 Quchi -
> ST-44 Neiting -
> PC-6 Neiguan -
> LR-3 Taichong -
> HT-9 Shaochong -

Explanation:
- ST-4 Dicang , LI-4 Hegu, LI-11 Quchi and ST-44 Neiting clear fire from the Yangming Meridians;
- PC-6 Neiguan and HT-9 Shaochong reduce fire of the heart;
- LR-3 Taichong clears heat from the Liver Meridian.

Secondary points according to conditions:
1〕 Constipation—SJ-6 Zhigou [-] and ST-25 Tianshu [-];
2〕 Irritability and hypochondriac pain—LR-2 Xingjian [-] and GB-34 Yanglingquan [-].

2. Deficiency Fire

Manifestation: Recurrent sore of the mouth and tongue with little pain, dry mouth, sensation of heat of the palms and soles, soreness and weakness of the knees and waist.

Tongue: Red body with little coating.

Pulse: Thready and rapid.

Treatment Principle: Nourish yin and check down fire.

Point Prescription & Manipulation:
Primary points:
> RN-23 Lianquan +
> BL-15 Xinshu +
> KI-1 Yongquan +

> SI-1 Shaoze +
> HT-9 Shaochong +
> KI-3 Taixi +
> KI-6 Zhaohai +

Explanation:
- RN-23 Lianquan nourishes yin to moisten the tongue and mouth;
- BL-15 Xinshu nourishes the heart yin and clears the mind;
- KI-1 Yongquan, SI-1 Shaoze and HT-9 Shaochong tonify the kidney, generate water, and reduce deficient fire from the Heart Meridian;
- KI-3 Taixi and KI-6 Zhaohai nourish the kidney (water) to extinguish the heart fire.

Secondary points according to conditions:
1〕 Insomnia—EX-HN-16 Anmian [+] and HT-7 Shenmen [+];
2〕 Nocturnal emission —BL-23 Shenshu [+].

II. EXPERIENTIAL TREATMENT

1. Puncturing KI-1 Yongquan

Indication: Recurrent ulcer of mouth with deficiency as its syndrome.

Point Prescription:
> KI-1 Yongquan

Manipulation: Select the point on the two sides alternatively. Puncture perpendicularly about 1 cun, thrust and lift the needle gently to induce soreness, numbness and distention to the patient, retain the needle for 20 minutes, and manipulate once during the retention. The treatment is given once daily, and generally, within 5-7 treatments the disease will be cured.

2. Moxibustion on RN-8 Shenque

Indication: Recurrent ulcer of mouth.

Point Prescription:
> RN-8 Shenque

Manipulation: Ignite one end of the moxa stick, and fix the end 2 cm. away from the point for 5-

15 minutes until the local skin become flushed. The treatment is given once daily, and generally three treatments are needed to cure this disease. To some cases, 10 treatments may be needed. Usually, the treatment result will be better if the patient doesn't feel a burning sensation during moxibustion.

3. Ear Acupuncture

Indication: Various types of recurrent ulcer of mouth.

Ear Point Prescription:
Shenmen, Mouth, Tongue, Heart, Synthetic, Spleen

Manipulation: See page 255-256.

Comment:
Acupuncture is effective in the treatment of recurrent ulcer of the mouth. In many cases, their disorder can be cured by acupuncture treatment.

Notes:

CHAPTER SIX
SKIN DISEASES

91. Urticaria

Urticaria is an allergic skin disease with skin wheals as the main manifestation. It is essentially anaphylaxis limited to the skin and subcutaneous tissues and can be due to drug allergy, insect stings or bites, desensitization injections, or ingestion of certain foods (particularly eggs, shellfish. nuts, or fruits). Clinically, it is marked by the appearance of wheals over the skin with abrupt onset and rapid disappearance, severe itching and burning sensation on the diseased region, repeated attack with long course and leaves no trace after recovery. According to TCM, urticaria belongs to Yin Zhen (hidden eruption), Pei Lei (urticaria), Feng Zhen Kuai (wind eruption), or You Feng (wandering wind disorder), and it is due to deficiency of the body resistance, attack of external pathogens, improper food or accumulation of internal heat.

I. STANDARD TREATMENT

Urticaria is usually divided into three types — wind-cold, wind-heat, and spleen and stomach deficiency. Points of the Stomach, Spleen and Urinary Bladder Meridians are frequently selected.

1. Wind-Cold

Manifestations: Abrupt onset of pale or light-colored wheals and severe itching of the diseased region, which are both aggravated by cold or wind, aversion to cold.

Tongue: White coating.

Pulse: Floating.

Treatment Principle: Dispel wind and disperse cold.

Point Prescription & Manipulation:
Primary points:
  GB-20 Fengchi -
  LI-11 Quchi -

BL-12 Fengmen - ^
BL-13 Feishu- ^
SP-10 Xuehai -

Explanation:
- GB-20 Fengchi, the Crossing Point of the Gallbladder Meridian and Yangwei Meridian, controls the exterior of the body, dispels wind and cold and relieves exterior syndrome;
- BL-12 Fengmen, the Crossing Point of the Foot-Taiyang and Du Meridians, and BL-13 Feishu, the Back-Shu Point of the Lung Meridian, improve the exterior yang, regulate the lung and dispel wind and cold;
- LI-11 Quchi and SP-10 Xuehai promote qi flow and activate blood circulation.

Secondary points according to conditions:
1⃞ Repeated attack of intractable cases—ST-36 Zusanli [+ ^], BL-21 Weishu [+ ^] and BL-20 Pishu [+ ^].

2. Wind-Heat

Manifestations: Red wheals, burning sensation and severe itching on the affected region, which become aggravated by heat and milder by cold, thirst, fever, aversion to wind.

Tongue: Thin and yellow coating.

Pulse: Floating and rapid.

Treatment Principle: Expel wind and clear heat.

Point Prescription & Manipulation:
Primary points:
   DU-14 Dazhui -
   LI-11 Quchi -
   SP-10 Xuehai -
   GB-20 Fengchi -

Explanation:
- DU-14 Dazhui, the Crossing Point of the Du and Hand and Foot Yang Meridians, clears heat and dispels wind;

- GB-20 Fengchi, the Crossing Point of the Gallbladder Meridian and Yangwei Meridian which controls the exterior of the body, dispels wind and heat and relieves exterior syndrome;
- LI-11 Quchi and SP-10 Xuehai promote qi flow and activate blood circulation;
- HT-7 Shenmen calms the mind and relieves itching.

Secondary points according to conditions:
1⃞ Insomnia—HT-7 Shenmen [-];
2⃞ Vomiting and diarrhea—PC-6 Neiguan [-] and ST-36 Zusanli [+];
3⃞ Sore throat—LU-10 Yuji [-] and LU-11 Shaoshang [-].

3. Deficiency of Spleen and Stomach

Manifestations: Attack of wheals induced by intake of certain food, cold limbs, aversion to cold, abdominal pain, loose stools, distressed sensation of the epigastrium, poor appetite.

Tongue: Pale body with white coating.

Pulse: Thready and slow.

Treatment Principle: Warm the middle-jiao, reinforce the spleen and regulate yin and wei.

Point Prescription & Manipulation:
Primary points:
   ST-36 Zusanli + ^
   SP-6 Sanyinjiao + ^
   RN-12 Zhongwan + ^
   PC-4 Ximen +
   SP-10 Xuehai + ^

Explanation:
- ST-36 Zusanli and SP-6 Sanyinjiao reinforce the spleen and stomach;
- RN-12 Zhongwan reinforces the middle-jiao and promotes transportation and transformation to nourish qi and blood;
- PC-4 Ximen calms the mind and relieves itching;
- SP-10 Xuehai promotes qi and blood circulation.

Secondary points according to conditions:
1🗌 Palpitation and insomnia—HT-7 Shenmen [+].

II. EXPERIENTIAL TREATMENT

1. Cupping on RN-8 Shenque

Indication: Various types of urticaria.

Point Prescription:
RN-8 Shenque

Manipulation: Ask the patient to lie down on the back. Make cupping on the point for 3-5 minutes, remove the cup, and repeat this course three times. The treatment is given once daily, with three treatments as a course. Usually, within one course of the treatment the disease will be cured. To intractable urticaria, 2-3 courses may be needed.

2. Puncturing SI-3 Houxi

Indication: Various types of urticaria.

Point Prescription:
SI-3 Houxi

Manipulation: Insert a 1-cun long needle perpendicularly into the point 0.8 cun deep. Lift, thrust and rotate the needle for 3-5 minutes and retain the needle for 20-40 minutes. The treatment is given once daily, and usually, within 10 treatments the disease will be cured.

3. Pricking and Cupping on BL-40 Weizhong

Indication: Obstinate urticaria.

Point Prescription:
BL-40 Weizhong of one side.

Manipulation: Prick BL-40 Weizhong and make cupping on the point for 5 minutes to make about 10 ml of bleeding. The treatment is given once daily, and usually the disease will be cured by 2-3 treatments. In case the treatment result is not effective, the opposite BL-40 Weizhong can be treated the same way.

4. Ear Acupuncture

Indication: Various types of urticaria.

Ear Point Prescription:
The most painful point, Lung, Adrenal Gland, Shenmen, Endocrine, Anti-Sensitive Point and the Point corresponding to the Diseased region.

Manipulation: See page 255-256.

Comment:
Zhenjiu is effective in treatment of urticaria. In most cases, their disease can be cured by Zhenjiu treatment.

Notes:

92. Eczema

Eczema is a commonly seen allergic inflammatory dermatosis. Its cause is closely related to heredity, improper diet and emotional stress. Clinically, it is marked by itching on the affected part, polymorphic skin lesion, orrhorrhea and frequent recurrences. According to TCM, eczema belongs to different categories according to its location and the patient's age. It Includes Nai Xiang (tinea due to milk appearing in infants), Chan Er Chuang (boils appearing on the external ear), Shen Lang Feng (wind in the kidney sac appearing on the scrotum), Si Wan Feng (wind in the four turning regions appearing on the elbows and knees), and Shi Du Chuang (carbuncle due to noxious dampness appearing on the local region but with a severe condition). It is due to attack of the skin and muscles by exogenous pathogenic damp, heat, and noxious factors, or blood deficiency leading to poor nourishment of the skin.

I. STANDARD TREATMENT

It is usually divided into two types—damp-heat and blood deficiency. Points of the Taiyang, Yangming and Taiyin Meridians are frequently selected in its treatment.

1. Damp-Heat

Manifestations: Diffuse redness, clusters of red papulae, blisters, erosion, exudations with burning sensation of the skin, severe itching.

Tongue: Red body with yellow and sticky coating.

Pulse: Soft and rapid.

Treatment Principle: Clear heat and dampness.

Point Prescription & Manipulation:
Primary points:
    LI-4 Hegu -
    SP-9 Yinlingquan -
    LI-11 Quchi -
    SP-10 Xuehai -
    SP-6 Sanyinjiao -

Explanation:
- LI-4 Hegu and LI-11 Quchi clear heat;
- SP-9 Yinlingquan and SP-6 Sanyinjiao remove dampness;
- SP-10 Xuehai clears heat from the blood and promotes blood flow.

Secondary points according to conditions:
1〕 High fever — DU-14 Dazhui [-];
2〕 Extreme itching — HT-7 Shenmen [-];
3〕 Itching and rashes in the anterior yin region (the region around the external genitalia)— LR-5 Ligou [-];
4〕 Obstinate cases —ST-40 Fenglong [-].

2. Blood Deficiency

Manifestations: Thick and rough skin with skin desquamation, pigmentation and sensation of severe itching that is aggravated in the night.

Tongue: White coating.

Pulse: Thready and weak.

Treatment Principle: Nourish the blood, moisten the dryness.

Point Prescription & Manipulation:
Primary points:
    LI-11 Quchi -
    SP-10 Xuehai +
    SP-6 Sanyinjiao +
    BL-17 Geshu +
    ST-36 Zusanli +

Explanation:
- LI-11 Quchi clears heat from the blood for relieving itching;
- SP-10 Xuehai and BL-17 Geshu nourish blood and activate blood flow;
- SP-6 Sanyinjiao and ST-36 Zusanli reinforce the spleen and stomach and promote production of blood.

Secondary points according to conditions:
1⊡ Palpitation and poor memory — HT-7 Shenmen.

II. EXPERIENTIAL TREATMENT

1. Ear Acupuncture

Indication: Various types of acute or chronic eczema.

Ear Point Prescription:
The point corresponding to the diseased portion, Lung, Spleen, Sanjiao, Large Intestine, Endocrine, Heart, Shenmen, Erzhong, Adrenal Gland.

Manipulation: See page 255-256.

2. Hydro-Puncture

Indication: Intractable chronic eczema.

Point Prescription:
ST-36 Zusanli
LI-11 Quchi

Manipulation: Inject 0.1 mg of vitamin B12 to each point. The treatment is given once daily with 10 treatments as a course. The next course can be given after an interval of 5-7 days. Generally, the disease can be cured within one therapeutic course.

Comment:
Zhenjiu is effective in treatment of eczema. In many cases, eczema can be cured by Zhenjiu treatment. However, for most cases of chronic eczema, a long term of treatment is needed. It is important to advise the patient not to take hot taste food, not to eat chicken and fish, and not to drink alcohol during treatment period. Also it is important to persuade the patient avoiding to scratch the itching skin or to have hot shower for a long period.

Notes:

93. Herpes Zoster

Herpes zoster is a kind of acute herpetic skin infection caused by the herpes zoster virus. Clinically, it is marked by abrupt onset of groups of crowded blisters arranged in zonary fashion along one side of the nerve distribution, accompanied with nervous pain in the diseased region. According to TCM, herpes zoster belongs to the categories of Chan Yao Dan (erysipelas along the waist), Huo Dai Chuang (fire-strip boil) and She Chuang (boil with snake shape). It is caused by attack of pathogenic heat or damp-heat, or depressed liver qi turning into fire.

I. STANDARD TREATMENT

Herpes zoster is generally divided into three types — wind-fire of the liver and gallbladder, damp-heat, and stagnation of qi and blood. Points of the Liver and Gallbladder Meridians and local points are frequently selected in its treatment.

1. Wind-Fire of Liver and Gallbladder

Manifestations: Abrupt onset of groups of papular eruptions at the affected part with pain and heat sensation and accompanied by restlessness, thirst, bitter taste in the mouth.

Tongue: Red body with yellow coating.

Pulse: Wiry and rapid.

Treatment Principle: Clear heat from the liver and gallbladder, cool blood, and stop pain.

Point Prescription & Manipulation:
Primary points:
GB-34 Yanglingquan -
LR-8 Ququan -
GB43 Xiaxi -
LR-2 Xingjian -
SP-10 Xuehai -
3-4 points surrounding the diseased region

Explanation:
- GB-34 Yanglingquan, GB-43 Xiaxi, LR-8 Ququan and LR-2 Xingjian, the He-Sea Points and Ying-Spring Points of the Gallbladder and Liver Meridians, clear heat from the gallbladder and liver;
- SP-10 Xuehai cools blood and removes blood stasis;
- 3-4 points surrounding the diseased region promote qi and blood flow in the local region, remove heat and toxin, and relieve pain.

Secondary points according to conditions:
1☐ Constipation — SJ-6 Zhigou [-];
2☐ Skin lesion appearing on the face and neck —GB-20 Fengchi [-], LI-4 Hegu [-] and SJ-5 Waiguan [-].

2. Damp-Heat

Manifestations: Erythema, pain, burning sensation, clusters of blisters or exudation at the affected part, restlessness, poor appetite, loose stools.

Tongue: Red body with yellow and sticky coating.

Pulse: Soft and rapid.

Treatment Principle: Clear heat and dampness, stop pain.

Point Prescription & Manipulation:
Primary points:
    SP-10 Xuehai -
    SP-9 Yinlingquan -
    SP-6 Sanyinjiao -
    LR-3 Taichong -
    GB-34 Yanglingquan -
    ST-44 Neiting -
    3-4 points surrounding the diseased region -

Explanation:
- SP-10 Xuehai cools blood, improves blood flow and relieves itching;
- SP-9 Yinlingquan and SP-6 Sanyinjiao remove dampness;

- LR-3 Taichong and GB-34 Yanglingquan clear heat from the liver and gallbladder;
- ST-44 Neiting clears heat;
- 3-4 points surrounding the diseased region promote qi and blood flow in the local region, remove heat, dampness and toxin, and relieve pain.

Secondary points according to conditions:
1☐ Skin lesion appearing on the face and neck—GB-20 Fengchi [-], LI-4 Hegu [-] and SJ-5 Waiguan [-].

3. Stagnation of Qi and Blood

Manifestations: Crust formation of the blisters with some red, brown spots and pigmentation on the diseased region, persistent stabbing local pain.

Tongue: Dark-red tongue with purple spots.

Pulse: Wiry and thready.

Treatment Principle: Soothe liver, promote blood circulation, activate collaterals and stop pain.

Point Prescription & Manipulation:
Primary points:
    SP-10 Xuehai -
    LR-3 Taichong -
    PC-6 Neiguan -
    LI-4 Hegu -
    BL-17 Geshu -
    GB-34 Yanglingquan -
    BL-18 Ganshu -
    3-4 points surrounding the diseased region -

Explanation:
- LR-3 Taichong, PC-6 Neiguan and LI-4 Hegu promote qi flow;
- SP-10 Xuehai, BL-17 Geshu and BL-18 Ganshu activate blood and remove blood stasis;
- GB-34 Yanglingquan dredges the Shaoyang Meridian and promotes qi flow;
- 3-4 points surrounding the diseased region promote qi and blood flow in the local

region, remove hardness and toxin, and relieve pain.

Secondary points according to conditions:
1□ Skin lesion appearing on the face and neck —GB-20 Fengchi [-], and SJ-5 Waiguan [-].

II. EXPERIENTIAL TREATMENT

1. Moxibustion with Cotton

Indication: Herpes zoster at early or middle stage.

Point Prescription:
The diseased region.

Manipulation: Cover the diseased region with a thin layer of the cotton, ignite the cotton and let it burn on its own course. Usually, only one treatment is effective to cure this disease. If not, repeat the treatment next day.

2. Moxibustion on EX-B-10 Herpes Zoster Point

Indication: Herpes zoster.

Point Prescription:
EX-B-10 Herpes Zoster Point, locating on the midline of the back, at the point where the ends of a thread, which is as long as the patient's head circumference, reach when the line circles the neck with its ends at the midline of the back.

Manipulation: Place a piece of garlic on the point, and a moxa cone on the garlic, ignite the cone for moxibustion. Usually, only one treatment is effective to cure this disease. If not, repeat the treatment next day.

Comment:
Zhenjiu is very effective in treatment of herpes zoster. In most case, the disorder can be cured by Zhenjiu treatment in a short period.

Notes:

94. Contact Dermatitis

Contact dermatitis refers to an acute inflammatory reaction on the skin or mucous membrane through contact of certain substances. Clinically, it is marked by the skin lesion being limited to the contacted parts. According to TCM, contact dermatitis belongs to Qi Chuan (dermatitis rhus), Hua Fen Chuang (pollen sore), Gao Yao Feng (adhesive plaster dermatitis) and Ma Tong Xiang (contact dermatitis of buttocks). It is caused by attack of toxic pathogen and deficiency of body resistance.

I. STANDARD TREATMENT

Contact dermatitis is generally divided into three types — toxic heat, damp-heat, and blood dryness. Points of the Liver and Gallbladder Meridians and local points are frequently selected in its treatment.

1. Toxic Heat

Manifestations: Red maculae and red populous with burning sensation or pricking pain in the affected region, fever, thirst, scanty and dark urine, constipation.

Tongue: Red body with yellow coating.

Pulse: Wiry and rapid.

Treatment Principle: Clear heat, remove toxin and cool the blood.

Point Prescription & Manipulation:
Primary points:
LR-3 Taichong -
ST-44 Neiting -
GB-34 Yanglingquan -
LI-11 Quchi -
SP-10 Xuehai -
GB-31 Fengshi -

Explanation:
* GB-31 Fengshi, LR-3 Taichong and GB-34 Yanglingquan soothe the liver and clear heat;
* ST-44 Neiting and LI-11 Quchi clear heat and remove toxin;
* SP-10 Xuehai cools blood and relieves itching.

Secondary points according to conditions:
1□ High fever — DU-14 Dazhui [-];
2□ Constipation — SJ-6 Zhigou [-].

2. Damp-Heat

Manifestations: Erythemata, blisters, erosion, exudation and limited edema on the affected region, accompanied by itching, heat sensation and pain, poor appetite, abdominal distention, distressed sensation in the epigastric region.

Tongue: Red body with yellow and sticky coating.

Pulse: Soft and rapid.

Treatment Principle: Clear dampness and heat.

Point Prescription & Manipulation:
Primary points:
    GB-34 Yanglingquan -
    SP-9 Yinlingquan -
    SP-10 Xuehai -
    SP-6 Sanyinjiao -
    LI-11 Quchi -

Explanation:
* GB-34 Yanglingquan and LI-11 Quchi clear heat;
* SP-9 Yinlingquan and SP-6 Sanyinjiao remove dampness;
* SP-10 Xuehai cools blood and relieves itching.

Secondary points according to conditions:
1□ Severe itching — GB-35 Fengshi [-].

3. Blood Dryness

Manifestations: Chronic and inflammatory infiltration with brown spots, cracked and lichenoid change on the affected region, local itching.

Tongue: Red body with yellow coating.

Pulse: Wiry.

Treatment Principle: Nourish blood, activate blood circulation, moisten dryness and disperse wind.

Point Prescription & Manipulation:
Primary points:
    SP-10 Xuehai +
    SP-6 Sanyinjiao +
    ST-36 Zusanli +
    LI -4 Quchi -
    LR-3 Taichong -
    KI-3 Taixi +

Explanation:
* SP-10 Xuehai and SP-6 Sanyinjiao tonify yin and nourish blood;
* ST-36 Zusanli promotes production of qi and blood;
* LI-4 Quchi clears heat from the blood and relieves itching;
* LR- 3 Taichong clears heat from the liver;
* KI -3 Taixi generates water and moistens dryness.

Secondary points according to conditions:
1□ Insomnia and palpitation — HT-7 Shenmen[+].

II. EXPERIENTIAL TREATMENT

1. Cupping on RN-8 Shenque

Indication: Contact dermatitis.

Point Prescription:
    RN-8 Shenque

Manipulation: Apply cupping with a glass cup until the umbilicus becomes purplish, usually after 5-10 minutes. The treatment may be given once every other day, with four treatments as a course.

Precaution:
The cupping should be used cautiously on children to avoid protrusion of the umbilicus.

2. Acupuncture and Moxibustion on DU-14 Dazhui

Indication: Contact dermatitis.

Point Prescription:
DU-14 Dazhui

Manipulation: Puncture DU-14 Dazhui and manipulate the needle to induce arrival of qi, retain the needle for 30 minutes and apply cupping on the point during the retention of the needle. The treatment is given once daily with five treatments as a course.

Comment:
Zhenjiu is effective in treatment of contact dermatitis. However, in some severe cases, Zhenjiu usually is not the first choice.

Notes:

95. Neurodermatitis

Neurodermatitis refers to a chronic skin disease with pruritic inflammation, which is usually induced by mental injury or localized physical irritation. Its cause is uncertain. Clinically, it is marked by lichenoid skin lesions accompanied by paroxysmal itching. In the initial stage, there is localized itching, with dense groups of falciform pimples occurring as the result of extensive scratching, As the condition develops, deep dermatoglyph, dermal ridging, and brown pachyderma appear. According to TCM, neurodermatitis, called Niu Pi Xiang in Chinese, is caused by attack of exogenous pathogens such as wind, dampness and heat, leading to obstruction of flow of qi and blood in the skin, or by deficiency of blood, leading to internal generation of wind and insufficient nourishment of the skin.

I. STANDARD TREATMENT

Neurodermatitis is generally divided into two types — wind-heat and blood dryness. Points of the Large Intestine, Spleen and Liver Meridians are frequently selected in its treatment.

1. Wind-Heat

Manifestations: Paroxysmal itching, reddish crowds of papulae on the skin.

Tongue: Red body with thin, yellow coating.

Pulse: Wiry and rapid.

Treatment Principle: Clear heat, disperse wind, cool blood and stop itching.

Point Prescription & Manipulation:
Primary points:
LI-4 Hegu -
LI-11 Quchi -
GB-20 Fengchi -
SP-10 Xuehai -
GB-31 Fengshi -

Explanation:
- LI-4 Hegu and GB-20 Fengchi dispel wind;
- LI-11 Quchi and GB-31 Fengshi clear heat and relieve itching;
- SP-10 Xuehai cools blood and relieves itching.

Secondary points according to conditions:
1⬚ High fever — DU-14 [-].

2. Blood Dryness

Manifestations: Paroxysmal itching, thick, rough and dry skin with fine and broken scurf, irritability, and insomnia.

Tongue: Red body with little coating.

Pulse: Thready.

Treatment Principle: Replenish blood, moisten dryness, calm wind and stop itching.

Point Prescription & Manipulation:
Primary points:
SP-10 Xuehai +
SP-6 Sanyinjiao +
ST-36 Zusanli +
LI-4 Hegu /
LR-3 Taichong /
PC-6 Neiguan /

Explanation:
- SP-10 Xuehai and SP-6 Sanyinjiao tonify yin, nourish blood and moisten dryness;
- ST-36 Zusanli promotes production of qi and blood;
- LI-4 Hegu and LR-3 Taichong calm wind due to blood deficiency to relieve itching;
- PC-6 Neiguan calms the mind.

Secondary points according to conditions:
1⬚ Poor memory and palpitation — HT-7 Shenmen [+], EX-HN-1 Sishencong [+];
2⬚ Severe itching — GB-31 Fengshi [-].

II. EXPERIENTIAL TREATMENT

1. Puncturing ST-36 Zusanli , etc.

Indication: Neurodermatitis.

Point Prescription:
ST-36 Zusanli
The courses of the Bladder Meridian on the upper back
Affected region

Manipulation: Firstly, puncture ST-36 Zusanli with middle-degree stimulation, manipulate the needles to induce arrival of qi, and retain the needles for 20 minutes. Then, during the retention, tap the courses of the Bladder Meridian on the upper back and the affected region with a seven star needle until there is slight bleeding. The treatment is given once daily, 10-15 treatments are needed in curing this disease.

2. Acupuncture and Moxibustion on HT-5 Tongli

Indication: Prolonged or intractable neurodermatitis.

Point Prescription:
HT-5 Tongli
Affected region

Manipulation: Firstly, puncture HT-5 Tongli 1-1.5 cun deep, with the needle tip towards the midline of the forearm, perform the needles with reducing manipulation, and remove the needles without retention. Secondly, tap the affected skin from its border gradually to center, making slight bleeding. Lastly, apply moxibustion with moxa stick on the affected skin from its border to center gradually until the patient can not stand, usually for 20-50 minutes. The treatment is given twice per week. Usually, 5-20 treatments are needed for cure this disease.

3. Ear Acupuncture

Indication: Neurodermatitis.

Ear Point Prescription:
Lung, Liver, Endocrine, Adrenal Gland, Wind Stream, Heart, Shenmen, Occiput, Subcortex and Apex of Ear.

Manipulation: See page 255-256.

Comment:
Acupuncture is effective to relieve itching and other symptoms of the neurodermatitis. In some cases, their neurodermatitis can be cured by acupuncture treatment. But neurodermatitis is an obstinate disease. Usually, recent result may be good, but late result may be not satisfactory because it is easy to reoccur. Therefore, a long-term treatment course is often needed in its treatment. Mental factors affect this disease strongly. Usually, such poor mental conditions as emotional depression, grief, or irritability aggravates the patient's symptoms and signs. Thus, a doctor should let the patient know it and try to avoid or overcome poor emotional state.

Notes:

96. Cutaneous Pruritis

Cutaneous pruritis refers to a kind of dermatosis which has a sensation of self-conscious itching on the affected part, which may occur secondary to various diseases such as endocrine dysfunction, parasitosis, diabetes mellitus, hepatic illness, nephritic disorders, or tumors. According to TCM, cutaneous pruritis belongs to Yang Feng (itching due to wind), and it is caused by dryness due to blood deficiency leading to failure of the skin in nourishment, attack by exogenous wind pathogen, or stagnation of heat in the blood leading to internal production of wind.

I. STANDARD TREATMENT

Cutaneous pruritis is usually divided into three types — wind-dryness due to blood deficiency, wind-dryness due to heat in the blood, and accumulation of damp-heat. Points of the Spleen, Stomach and Large Intestine Meridians are frequently selected.

1. Wind-Dryness due to Blood Deficiency

Manifestations: Paroxysmal itching on the affected part of the skin which becomes worse in the night, dry skin, atrophic, thick and lichenoid skin lesion.

Tongue: Pale body.

Pulse: Thready.

Treatment Principle: Nourish blood, moisten the dryness, dispel wind and arrest itching.

Point Prescription & Manipulation:
Primary points:
SP-10 Xuehai +
SP-6 Sanyinjiao +
GB-20 Fengchi +
SP-9 Yinlingquan +
ST-36 Zusanli +

Explanation:
- SP-10 Xuehai nourishes blood and promotes blood flow;
- SP-6 Sanyinjiao and SP-9 Yinlingquan reinforce the spleen , nourish blood and moisten dryness;
- GB-20 Fengchi dispels wind and relieves itching;
- ST-36 Zusanli reinforces the middle-jiao to promote production of qi and blood.

Secondary points according to conditions:
1️⃣ Extreme itching — HT-7 Shenmen [+];
2️⃣ Poor memory and palpitation — DU-20 Baihui [+] and HT-7 Shenmen [+].

2. Wind-Dryness due to Heat in Blood

Manifestations: Severe itching and burning sensation of the affected skin which are aggravated by heat, thirst, dark urination.

Tongue: Red body with yellow coating.

Pulse: Rapid.

Treatment Principle: Clear heat, cool the blood, dispel wind and arrest itching.

Point Prescription & Manipulation:
Primary points:
   GB-20 Fengchi -
   SP-10 Xuehai -
   LI-11 Quchi -
   DU-14 Dazhui -
   SP-6 Sanyinjiao -
   LI-4 Hegu -

Explanation:
- LI-4 Hegu and GB-20 Fengchi dispel wind and relieve itching;
- SP-10 Xuehai, LI-11 Quchi and DU-14 Dazhui clear heat from the blood;
- SP-6 Sanyinjiao nourishes yin and moistens dryness.

Secondary points according to conditions:
1️⃣ Severe itching — HT-7 Shenmen [-] and PC-6 Neiguan [-].

3. Accumulation of Damp-Heat

Manifestations: Itching, swelling, redness and exudation in the external pudendum, bitter taste in the mouth.

Tongue: Red body with yellow and sticky coating.

Pulse: Slippery.

Treatment Principle: Clear heat, promote diuresis and arrest itching.

Point Prescription & Manipulation:
Primary points:
   SP-9 Yinlingquan -
   SP-6 Sanyinjiao -
   LR-5 Ligou -
   LI-11 Quchi -
   ST-40 Fenglong -
   LR-2 Xingjian -
   RN-10 Xiawan -

Explanation:
- SP-9 Yinlingquan and SP-6 Sanyinjiao remove dampness;
- LR-2 Xingjian, LR-5 Ligou and LI-11 Quchi clear heat;
- ST-40 Fenglong transforms phlegm and relieves itching;
- RN-10 Xiawan regulates the middle-jiao and removes dampness.

Secondary points according to conditions:
1️⃣ Constipation — SJ-5 Zhigou [-].

II. EXPERIENTIAL TREATMENT

1. Puncturing SP-10 Xuehai

Indication: General cutaneous pruritis.

Point Prescription:
   SP-10 Xuehai

Manipulation: Insert a needle into the point until the operator feels a tight, heavy and difficult sensation in the area around the needle tip. Perform reinforcing manipulation by slow-rapid insertion and lifting to patients belonging in deficiency category, and use reducing manipulation by slow-rapid insertion and lifting to the cases with excessive syndrome. Retain the needle for 20-40 minutes. The treatment is given once daily, with 10 treatments as a course.

2. Puncturing EX-UE-14 Xiadu

Indication: General cutaneous pruritis.

Point Prescription:
EX-UE-14 Xiadu of the diseased side, on the dorsum of the hand, between the 4th and 5th metacarpal bones, and proximal to the joint of the metacarpophalangeal joint.

Manipulation: Insert a needle into the point along the space of the carpal bones 0.5-1 cun deep, rotate the needle to induce arrival of qi, retain the needle for 20-40 minutes, and manipulate it every 10 minutes. If the patient still feels itching during the retention of the needle, puncture the opposite Xiadu EX-UE-14 with the same manipulation additionally. The treatment is given once daily, with 10 treatments as a course.

3. Ear Acupuncture

Indication: General cutaneous pruritis.

Ear Point Prescription:
The point corresponding to the diseased region, Lung, Spleen, Liver, Heart, Shenmen, Subcortex, Middle Ear and Apex.

Manipulation: See page 255-256.

Comment:
Acupuncture is effective to relieve itching and other symptoms of cutaneous pruritis. In some cases, it can be cured by acupuncture treatment.

Notes:

97. Acne Vulgaris

Acne vulgaris is a chronic inflammation of hair follicle and sebaceous glands which is a common problem of adolescence. It is mainly caused by hormonal disturbances, improper diet and chronic constipation. Clinically, it is marked by papulae, nodules and acne on the face. According to TCM, acne vulgaris belongs to the categories of Fei Feng Fen Ci (acne due to attack of the lung by wind), or Fen Ci (acne). It is caused by exogenous wind-heat invading the lung or by indulgence in spicy or greasy food, resulting in accumulation of heat in the stomach and intestines.

I. STANDARD TREATMENT

Acne vulgaris is generally divided into three types—heat in blood, accumulation of phlegm, and toxic heat. Points of the Large Intestine, Lung and Stomach Meridians are frequently selected in its treatment.

1. Heat in Blood

Manifestations: Red papules, tubercles, acne and inflammatory infiltration around them on the face.

Tongue: Red body with thin and yellow coating.

Pulse: Smooth and rapid.

Treatment Principle: Clear heat and cool blood.

Point Prescription & Manipulation:
Primary points:
SP-10 Xuehai -
SP-6 Sanyinjiao
LI-4 Hegu -
ST-44 Neiting -
LI-11 Quchi -
LR-3 Taichong -

Explanation:
- SP-10 Xuehai and SP-6 Sanyinjiao nourish yin and cool blood;
- LI-4 Hegu, ST-44 Neiting and LI-11 Quchi clear heat from the Yangming Meridians which distribute on the face;
- LR-3 Taichong clears heat from the liver and cools blood.

Secondary points according to conditions:
1□ Severe or chronic cases — BL-40 Weizhong and DU-10 Lintai are punctured with reducing manipulation and the area around the needle holes are squeezed to let out several drops of blood immediately after removing the needles;
2□ Bitter taste in the mouth — GB-34 Yanglingquan [-].

2. Accumulation of Phlegm

Manifestations: Acne, indurative acne or cystic acne on the face.

Tongue: White and sticky coating.

Pulse: Smooth.

Treatment Principle: Transform phlegm, resolve masses.

Point Prescription & Manipulation:
Primary points:
    LI-4 Hegu -
    ST-40 Fenglong -
    SP-6 Sanyinjiao /
    RN-12 Zhongwan /
    ST-36 Zusanli +

Explanation:
- LI-4 Hegu promotes circulation of qi of the Yangming Meridian and resolves masses on the face;
- ST-40 Fenglong transforms phlegm and resolves nodules;
- SP-6 Sanyinjiao, RN-12 Zhongwan and ST-36 Zusanli reinforce the spleen, regulate stomach, and transform phlegm.

Secondary points according to conditions:
1□ Obesity—SP-9 Yinlingquan [-] and ST-25 Tianshu [-];
2□ Constipation—SJ-5 Zhigou [-].

3. Toxic Heat

Manifestations: Facial malar flush, scattered inflammatory nodules, acne, abscesses and furuncles on the face, thirst, bitter taste in the mouth, scanty urine, constipation.

Tongue: Red body with yellow coating.

Pulse: Smooth and rapid.

Treatment Principle: Clear heat, cool blood, detoxify poison and resolve nodules.

Point Prescription & Manipulation:
Primary points:
    SP-10 Xuehai -
    ST-44 Neiting -
    LI-4 Hegu -
    GB-34 Yanglingquan -
    LR-2 Xingjian -
    ST-40 Fenglong -

Explanation:
- SP-10 Xuehai cools blood and resolves blood stasis;
- ST-44 Neiting reduces fire and detoxifies poison;
- LI-4 Hegu clears heat from the Yangming Meridian, which distributes on the face;
- GB-34 Yanglingquan and LR-2 Xingjian clear heat from the liver and gallbladder and detoxify poison;
- ST-40 Fenglong transforms phlegm and resolves nodules.

Secondary points according to conditions:
1□ Severe or chronic cases—BL-40 Weizhong and DU-10 Lintai are punctured with reducing manipulation and the area around the needle holes are squeezed to let out several drops of blood immediately after removing the needles;
2□ Constipation—SJ-5 Zhigou [-].

II. EXPERIENTIAL TREATMENT

1. Breaking the Reaction Points

Indication: Acne vulgaris.

Point Prescription:
The reaction points on the back. Like rushes, they are 2-4 mm in diameter, usually with dark-yellow, green-dark-yellow, reddish, or white color. Their distribution lies over the region from 0.5 cun lateral to the spinal column to 3 cun lateral to the spinal column and from the first to the 12th thoracic vertebra.

Manipulation: Ask the patient to sit down in a chair and to expose his/her back as much as possible. Rub the bilateral sides of the spinal column with the palm several times and look for the reaction spots. Then, fix the skin around the spot with the thumb and index finger of one hand, hold the three-edged needle with the other hand, quickly prick and break the skin of the spot at an angle of 15-30 degrees that is formed between the needle and skin. Continuing, insert the needle deeply into the subcutaneous tissue, make the needle shaft tilt and then gently move it upward to break some of fibrous tissues. Squeeze the local skin to make a little bleeding. Finally, cover the operated region with sterilized cotton and fix the cotton on the skin. Each time 1-2 reaction spots can be broken and the next operation may be done 5-7 days later. Usually 3-8 treatments are needed for curing this disorder.

2. Puncture and Cupping on DU-14 Dazhui

Indication: Acne vulgaris.

Point Prescription:
DU-14 Dazhui

Manipulation: Ask the patient to sit down on a chair to expose his/her DU-14 Dazhui region fully. Puncture DU-14 Dazhui with the needle tip obliquely downward, manipulate it to induce needling sensation, and retain the needle for 40 minutes Then, apply cupping on the point during the retention for 20-30 minutes. The treatment is given once daily, with 10 treatments as a course. Usually 1-3 courses are needed.

3. Ear Acupuncture

Indication: Acne vulgaris.

Ear Point Prescription:
Lung, Stomach, Large Intestine, Endocrine, Midpoint of Rim, Adrenal Gland and Apex of Ear.

Manipulation: See page 255-256.

Comment:
Acupuncture is effective in treatment of acne vulgaris and in some cases can cure it. During treatment, the patient should be advised to keep the bowel movement regular to prevent constipation.

Note:

CHAPTER SEVEN
OTHER DISEASES OR
CONDITIONS

98. Tobacco Addiction

Cigarette addiction is a big medical and social problem. It seriously affects health of the human being. There are almost 100 kinds of various poisoning materials produced by smoking, which can induce or cause hypertension, heart diseases, chronic bronchitis, congenital diseases, cancers, etc., shorten the life span, cause fatal malformation. However, the underlying causes of alcoholism are not fully understood. To persons who hope to give up smoking, the following methods can be applied.

1. Puncturing EX-UE-21 Tianweixue

Indication: Addiction to tobacco but hope to give up smoking.

Point Prescription:
EX-UE-21 Tianweixue, located on the hand, at the midpoint of the line connecting LU-7 Lieque and LI-5 Yangxi.

Manipulation: Insert a 1-cun needle perpendicularly into the point 3-4 mm deep while asking the patient to breathe in. Then, manipulate the needle to induce a sensation of numbness and distention in the wrist or even arm, or a feeling of drowsiness or happiness, or the sensation of having a metallic or some other taste in the mouth, and retain the needle for 15 minutes. The treatment is given once daily, and usually 1-2 treatments are effective to help the patient to give up smoking.

2. Ear Acupuncture

Indication: Addiction to tobacco but hope to give up smoking.

Ear Point Prescription:
Mouth, Tongue, Lung, Liver, Chest, Subcortex, Shenmen, Occiput, Trachea.

Manipulation: See page 255-256.

Comment:
Long-term smokers often experience withdrawal

symptoms such as restlessness, anxiety, irritability, insomnia, feelings of emptiness, and weight gain when they suddenly stop smoking. Acupuncture therapy has been shown to be very effective for relieving these symptoms. Additionally, acupuncture therapy can act to change the person's taste to the tobacco, making the person feel that the tobacco taste becomes tasteless and dislike smoking.

Notes:

99. Alcoholism

Alcoholism is a big medical and social problem. The long-term effects of alcohol on the body are serious for heavy or chronic users of alcohol. Alcohol affects the brain and nervous system, which control behavior and body functions, as well as the pancreas and liver. No body system is left untouched by the effects of chronic alcohol use. Irregular heartbeats, polyneuropathy causing tingling and numbness, and stomach pain from inflammation of the stomach lining are not uncommon. Impotence is typical. Alcohol also affects the immune system and hinders resistance to disease. The underlying causes of alcoholism are not fully understood. It is well known that an inability to deal with an emotional problem is often a trigger, since alcoholism is more likely to begin at emotionally difficult periods of life.

To persons who want to give up drinking, the following methods can be selected.

1. Puncturing Some Points

Indication: Addiction to drinking but hope to give up drinking.

Point Prescription:
   SP-6 Sanyinjiao
   ST-40 Fenglong
   ST-44 Neiting
   LR-3 Taichong
   PC-6 Neiguan
   SP-9 Yinlingquan
   RN-12 Zhongwan
   HT-7 Shenmen

Manipulation: Acupuncture is applied with reducing manipulation. The treatment is given once daily, with 10 treatments as a course. Usually, three courses are needed.

2. Puncturing DU-25 Suliao

Indication: Drunk.

Point Prescription:
 DU-25 Suliao

Manipulation: Insert a 0.5-cun long needle into the point 0.2 cun deep, lift, thrust and rotate the needle gently for 3-10 minutes.

3. Ear Acupuncture

Indication: Addiction to drinking but hope to give up drinking.

Ear Point Prescription:
 Mouth, Stomach, Sanjiao, Endocrine, Shenmen, Occiput, Subcortex, Apex.

Manipulation: See page 255-256.

Comment:
Long-term drinkers often experience withdrawal symptoms such as restlessness, irritability, anxiety, feelings of emptiness, or even paroxysmal attack of trembling, sweating, illusion, or convulsion when they suddenly stop drinking. Acupuncture therapy has been shown to be effective for relieving these symptoms. Therefore, it has action to help drinkers to give up drinking.

Notes:

100. Drug Addiction

Drug addiction is a big medical and social problem. To patients who want to give up drug, the following methods are helpful.

1. Puncture A Group of Points

Indication: Addiction to drug.

Point Prescription & Manipulation:
 HT-7 Shenmen /
 PC-6 Neiguan /
 LR-3 Taichong -
 ST-40 Fenglong -
 LI-4 Hegu /
 ST-36 Zusanli /
 SP-6 Sanyinjiao /

2. Puncturing EX-UE-21 Tianweixue

Indication: Addiction to drug.

Point Prescription:
 EX-UE-21 Tianweixue, locating on the hand, at the midpoint of the line connecting LU-7 Lieque and LI-5 Yangxi.

Manipulation: Insert a 1-cun needle perpendicularly into the point 3-4 mm deep while asking the patient to breathe in. Then, manipulate the needle to induce a sensation of numbness and distention in the wrist or even arm, or a feeling of drowsiness or happiness, or the sensation of having a metallic or some other taste in the mouth, and retain the needle for 15 minutes The treatment is given once daily, and usually 1-2 treatments are effective to help the patient to give up using drugs.

3. Ear Acupuncture

Indication: Addiction to drug.

Ear Point Prescription:
 Lung, Large Intestine, Kidney, Stomach, Spleen, Subcortex, Forehead, Liver, Chest, Shenmen, Occiput.

Manipulation: See page 255-256.

Comment:
Drug withdrawal refers to the physiological and psychological process of overcoming addiction to drugs such as heroin or other narcotics, barbiturates, or amphetamines, by complete cessation of use. It has been shown that acupuncture can abolish both the physical symptoms and psychological craving present during the withdrawal process. Through the acupuncture treatment, usually, the patients will fell less drowsy, more interested in their surroundings, and quickly regain interest in conversation and reading. Appetite and bowel function both will be improved. In addition, lacrimation, running nose, wheezing, stomach cramps, and feelings of aching bones and cold will be usually disappeared after 10-15 minutes of auricular stimulation.

Notes:

101. Obesity

Obesity is a commonly seen condition caused by various factors including nervous dysfunction, endocrine disorder, metabolic disturbance, improper diet, drugs, or heredity.

The standard of normal body weight is generally taken as the follows:

- Male: The body weight (Kg) = The body length (cm) -105
- Female: The body weight (kg) = The body length (cm) - 100

If a female person, for example, is 165 cm high, her standard weight is 165-100=65 (kg).

If the body weight is increased by 20% or more to the standard, it is considered obesity. According to TCM, obesity, called Fei Pang in Chinese, is due to dysfunction of the spleen and kidney, leading to accumulation of phlegm and dampness in the body.

I. STANDARD TREATMENT

Obesity is generally divided into three types — heat in the stomach, spleen deficiency and kidney deficiency. Points of the Spleen and Stomach Meridians are frequently selected in its treatment.

1. Heat in Stomach

Manifestations: Overweight, excessive appetite, abdominal distention, constipation, flashed face.

Tongue: Yellow and sticky coating.

Pulse: Slippery and forceful.

Treatment Principle: Clear heat from the stomach

Point Prescription & Manipulation:
Primary points:
   LI-11 Quchi -

LI-4 Hegu -
ST-44 Neiting -
SP-6 Sanyinjiao /
ST-40 Fenglong-

Explanation:
Three to five points are selected for puncture with the filiform needle each time. After insertion of the needle, it is twisted, lift and thrust with strong manipulation to induce reducing effect. After arrival of qi, it is retained for 20-40 minutes, and manipulated once every 5 minutes with strong stimulation, or is connected with electric therapeutic instrument for electric stimulation.

- LI-11 Quchi, LI-4 Hegu and ST-44 Neiting clear heat in the Yangming Meridians, and restrain overactivity of the stomach qi;
- SP-6 Sanyinjiao, the Crossing Point of the Liver, Spleen and Kidney Meridians, soothes the liver, promotes the splenic function of transportation and transformation and removes dampness;
- ST-40 Fenglong transforms phlegm.

Secondary points according to conditions:
1囗 Constipation—ST-25 Tianshu [-];
2囗 Gastric discomfort with acid regurgitation, and liability of hunger—RN-12 Zhongwan [-] and ST-34 Liangqiu [-].

2. Spleen Deficiency

Manifestations: Overweight, pale face, listlessness, fatigue, heaviness of the limbs, poor appetite, abdominal distention, constipation.

Tongue: Pale with white coating.

Pulse: Deep and thready.

Treatment Principle: Tonify qi and reinforce the spleen, resolve phlegm and dampness.

Point Prescription & Manipulation:
Primary points:
    BL-20 Pishu + ^
    BL-21 Weishu + ^

    ST-36 Zusanli + ^
    RN-6 Qihai + ^
    RN-4 Guanyuan + ^
    SP-6 Sanyinjiao + ^

Explanation:
- BL-20 Pishu and BL-21 Weishu, the Back-Shu Points of the spleen and stomach, reinforce the function of the spleen and stomach, and remove dampness;
- ST-36 Zusanli reinforces the spleen and stomach;
- RN-6 Qihai and RN-4 Guanyuan warm yang and transform dampness;
- SP-6 Sanyinjiao reinforces the spleen to remove dampness.

Secondary points according to conditions:
1囗 Abdominal distention and poor appetite— RN-12 Zhongwan [+ ^];
2囗 Scanty urination and edema — SP-9 Yinlingquan [+ ^].

3. Kidney Deficiency

Manifestations: Over weight, fatigue, listlessness, pale complexion, weakness and soreness of the waist and knees, aversion to cold.

Tongue: Pale body with tooth prints on its border

Pulse: Deep and slow.

Treatment Principle: Warm the kidney, strengthen yang, reinforce the spleen, and dispel dampness.

Point Prescription & Manipulation:
Primary points:
    BL-23 Shenshu + ^
    BL-20 Pishu + ^
    DU-4 Mingmen + ^
    SP-6 Sanyinjiao + ^
    KI-3 Taixi + ^
    ST-40 Fenglong - ^

Explanation:
- BL-23 Shenshu, BL-20 Pishu and DU-4 Mingmen warm and tonify the spleen and kidney to treat its root;
- SP-6 Sanyinjiao and KI-3 Taixi reinforce the spleen and kidney, and remove dampness and relieve edema;
- ST-40 Fenglong transforms phlegm.

Secondary points according to conditions:
1☐ Impotence RN-4 Guanyuan [+ ^].

II. EXPERIENTIAL TREATMENT

1. Puncturing the Ear Points

Indication: Obesity.

Ear Point Prescription:
   Sympathetic, Endocrine, Uterus, Adrenal Gland, Heart, Shenmen, Stomach, Spleen and Mouth.

Manipulation: Two to four points are employed each treatment session, medium strength stimulation is applied and the needles are retained at the Otopoints for 20 minutes. The treatment is given once daily with 10 treatments as a course, and the next course begins after an interval of 5 days. Alternatively, the thumbtack needles are embedded into the Otopoints or the vaccaria seeds are stuck on the Otopoints. The needles or the seeds are kept in the Otopoints for 3-5 days, and during the period they are pressed by the patient himself/herself 4-5 times daily. The Otopoints are replaced by some other ones in next session.

2. Puncturing and Embedding on ST-34 Liangqiu and SP-4 Gongsun

Indication: Obesity with excessive appetite.

Point Prescription:
   ST-34 Liangqiu
   SP-4 Gongsun

Manipulation: One point is employed each treatment session, and these two points are employed alternately. Reducing manipulations are applied by twisting, lifting and thrusting the needle until comparatively strong needling sensation is induced to the patient. Then, the needle inserted in the point is connected with a lead from an electropuncture unit, and electric stimulation with a contiguous wave is given for 20 minutes. The intensity of the electric stimulation is adjusted so as to be strong but tolerable to the patient. Following withdrawal of the needle, an wheat-grain-sized intradermal needle is inserted into the point 1 cm deep, and it is fixed in the skin with a piece of adhesive plaster and kept there for 3 days. The patient is asked to press the point 2 or 3 times daily and for 1or 2 minutes each time, and additionally, to press the point forcefully whenever the patient himself/herself feels hungry or 10 minutes before eating, to induce a strong sensation. The treatment is given once every 3 days with 10 times as course.

3. Embedding the Needle into Ear Points:

Indication: Obesity.

Ear Point Prescription:
   Sanjiao, Lung, Endocrine.

Manipulation: After a routine and local sterilization, a thumb-tack needle held by a pair of small-sized homeostatic forceps is embedded into the point and fixed to the skin with adhesive plaster. The needle is kept there for 5-6 days, during which, the patient is asked to press is 3 or 4 times daily. After removing it, another point is employed with the same way. The three Otopoints are employed alternately, and only one otopoint is employed each session. The embedding is performed once per 5 days, with six sessions as a course.

4. Taping Ear Points

Indication: Overweight with disorder of endocrine system.

Ear point Prescription:
   Endocrine, Ovary, Sympathetic, Heart, Shenmen, Adrenal Gland.

Manipulation: See page 255-256.

5. Comprehensive Therapy

Indication: Obesity due to various factors.

Point Prescription:
- *Acupoints of the body*: ST-40 Fenglong, SP-9 Yinlingquan, ST-25 Tianshu, HT-7 Shenmen, PC-6 Neiguan, SP-6 Sanyinjiao, ST-28 Shuidao.
- *Ear points:* Hungry point, Mouth, Sanjiao, Endocrine.

Modification: Some points are added according to the patient's condition.

Manipulation: Three to five acupoints of the body are punctured with the filiform needle each treatment session. After insertion of the needle, it is rotated, lifted and thrust with a large amplitude and strong enough force to induce needling sensation to the patient. After arrival of qi, the needle is retained in the point for 30-50 minutes and manipulated once every 5-10 minutes with strong stimulation. If the patient's condition belongs to yang deficiency, dampness or phlegm with no obvious heat symptoms or signs, moxibustion is applied on the point during the retention period. The acupuncture on the points of the body is given once daily. In cooperation, vaccaria seeds are plastered on the Otopoints of the one side , and kept there 4-6 days. During the period, the patient is asked to press the points 4-5 times daily, before eating and whenever feeling hungry. After the seeds are removed, the Otopoints of the other side are plastered with the same way and the two sides are selected alternately.

Comment:
Generally, obesity is an obstinate disorder, and no very satisfactory therapeutic method in its treatment has been fund by now. Zhenjiu has some effective result to most cases, and in some cases, even their weight can be restore to the normal level through Zhenjiu treatment. During the treatment, the patient should be advised to have a proper diet, including taking food in regular time and with regular amount, avoiding over eating of greasy food and sweet food, especially in dinner, to have more physical exercise.

Notes:

102. Infertility

A woman is deemed infertile if she fails to conceive after three or more years of marriage with a healthy companion, or if she remains a number of years without conceiving again after once or twice pregnant.

I. STANDARD TREATMENT

Infertility is usually divided into four types—Kidney Deficiency, Blood Deficiency, Retention of Cold in the Uterus, and Phlegm and Blood Stagnation, and the points of the Ren, Liver, Kidney and Spleen Meridians are frequently selected for its treatment.

1. Kidney Deficiency

Manifestations: Infertility, irregular or scanty menstruation with dark color, lassitude, soreness of the back, weak legs, dizziness, tinnitus.

Tongue: White coating,

Pulse: Deep and weak pulse.

Treatment Principle: Tonify and replenish kidney qi to regulate the Chong and Ren Meridians.

Point Prescription & Manipulation:
Primary points:
> BL-23 Shenshu +
> KI-13 Qixue +
> KI-2 Rangu +
> SP-6 Sanyinjiao +

Explanation:
- BL-23 Shenshu, the Back-Shu Point of kidney, strengthens kidney;
- KI-13 Qixue and KI-2 Rangu reinforce kidney and regulate Chong and Ren Meridians;
- SP-6 Sanyinjiao strengthens spleen, nourishes yin and regulates menstruation.

Secondary points according to conditions:
1〕 Poor appetite — ST-36 Zusanli [+].

2. Blood Deficiency

Manifestations: Infertility, scanty and pale menstruation, sallow complexion, general physical weakness and mental lassitude, dizziness and tinnitus.

Tongue: White body with thin coating.

Pulse: Deep and thready.

Treatment Principle: Tonify and replenish essence and blood to regulate the Chong and Ren Meridians.

Primary points:
    RN-4 Guanyuan + ^
    ST-13 Qihu + ^
    EX-CA-1 Zigong + ^
    SP-6 Sanyinjiao + ^
    ST-36 Zusanli + ^

Explanation:
- RN-4 Guanyuan, the Crossing Point of the Chong, Ren and three Foot-Yin Meridians, tonifies the essence and blood;
- ST-13 Qihu and EX-CA-1 Zigong are experiential points for infertility;
- SP-6 Sanyinjiao and ST-36 Zusanli nourish and reinforce the source of generation and transformation to tonify blood.

Secondary points according to conditions:
1〕 Palpitation and poor memory — HT-Shenmen [+];
2〕 Dizziness — BL-15 Ganshu [+] and DU-20 Baihui [+].

3. Retention of Cold in the Uterus

Manifestations: Infertility, delayed menstruation with scanty dark menses, cold pain in the lower abdomen, cold body and limbs, sometimes also accompanied with soreness of the back and weakness of the legs, clear abundant urination.

Tongue: Pale body with thin coating.

Pulse: Deep and slow.

Treatment Principle: Warm the uterus to disperse cold.

Primary points:
    RN-7 Yinjiao + ^
    RN-2 Qugu + ^
    DU-4 Mingmen + ^
    RN-6 Qihai + ^

Explanation:
- RN-7 Yinjiao and RN-2 Qugu warm the Chong and Ren Meridians and dispel cold;
- DU-4 Mingmen warms yang and dispels cold;
- RN-6 Qihai warms the uterus and improves reproductive function.

Secondary points according to conditions:
1〕 Late menstruation—ST-25 Tianshu [+] and ST-29 Guilai [+];
2〕 Soreness of back and weakness of legs— BL-23 Shenshu [+] and EX-B-7 Yaoyan [+]

4. Phlegm and Blood Stagnation

Manifestations: Infertility, late periods, obstructed menstrual flow with blood clots, fullness of the chest and hypochondrium, restlessness and irritability, or obesity, dizziness, palpitations, abundant leukorrhea of thick, sticky consistency.

Tongue: Dark or blood-specked body.

Pulse: Slippery or choppy.

Treatment Principle: Resolve phlegm and remove stagnation.

Primary points:
    RN-3 Zhongji - ^
    ST-30 Qichong - ^
    KI-14 Siman - ^
    SP-6 Sanyinjiao /
    ST-40 Fenglong -

Explanation:
- RN-3 Zhongji, KI-14 Siman and ST-30 Qichong remove blood stagnation from the Chong and Ren Meridians, and improve the reproductive function;
- SP-6 Sanyinjiao strengthens spleen, removes dampness, and regulates menstruation;
- ST-40 Fenglong transforms phlegm.

Secondary points according to conditions:
1) Obstructed menstrual flow—SP-8 Diji [-];
2) Fullness in the chest and hypochondrium— LR-3 Taichong [-] and PC-6 Neiguan;
3) A lot of clots in menses—BL-17 Geshu [-] and SP-10 Xuehai[-];
4) Abundant leukorrhea — BL-33 Zhongliao [-].

II. EXPERIENTIAL TREATMENT

Ear Acupuncture

Indication: Infertility.

Ear Point Prescription:
   Endocrine, Kidney, Uterus, Ovary.

Manipulation: See page 255-256.

Comment:
Zhenjiu is effective in treatment of infertility, especially, when Zhenjiu is accompanied with undergoing herbal treatment. It is the recommendations for optimum recovery that patients should avoid emotional upsets and excessive sexual activities, and should lead an orderly life and get appropriate rest, aside from Zhenjiu and herbal treatment.

Notes:

103. Depression

Depression is characterized by a persistent sadness and lethargy, which remove the desire and courage to carry out ideas and activities. The pleasures and interests in life suddenly seem to be missing. Easily changing moods and weeping without cause are outward signs of a mild depression. Low self-esteem causes the person to give up more easily than usual. There are feelings of loneliness, and isolation from family and friends may become evident. Apathy and helplessness cause a cycle of passivity and indecisiveness, which further undermine self-confidence and cause feelings of guilt.

Depression affects individuals very differently. More obvious outward signs are changes in routine, such as sleep and eating habits. Difficulties falling asleep or staying asleep are common problems, though others use sleep as an escape from problems. Eating habits become extreme, triggering either a poor appetite and weight loss, or strong cravings for sweets and junk foods.

Many physical symptoms occur as a result of this emotional problem. Abdominal distention or pain, headache, constipation and low or no sex drive are just a few of the more common symptoms.

As an emotional problem, depression is becoming increasingly common in modern times. This illness may affect individuals of either sex, but is more common in women. Teenagers are susceptible to it too, and even young children can become depressed.

In TCM, depression may belong to category of Yu Zheng, melancholia, and is due to emotional injury resulting in disharmony of the activity of the zang-fu organs.

Depression is usually divided into four types— stagnation of liver qi, transformation of depressed qi into fire, stagnation of phlegm and blood deficiency. Points on the Liver, Spleen, Heart and Bladder Meridians are frequently selected in its treatment.

1. Stagnation of Liver Qi

Manifestations: Mental depression, distress in the chest, hypochondriac distending pain, abdominal distention, belching, poor appetite, abnormal bowel movement, susceptibility to fatigue.

Tongue: Thin or sticky coating.

Pulse: Wiry.

Treatment Principle: Soothe liver, relieve depressed qi and strengthen middle-jiao.

Point Prescription & Manipulation:
Primary points:
   LR-3 Taichong -
   BL-18 Ganshu /
   RN-17 Danzhong -
   ST-36 Zusanli +
   SP-4 Gongsun +

Explanation:
- LR-3 Taichong, Yuan-Source Point of Liver Meridian, BL-18 Ganshu, the Back-Shu Point of liver, and RN-17 Danzhong, the Influential Point of qi, soothe liver, regulate flow of qi and remove depression;
- ST-36 Zusanli, one of the key points to regulate and strengthen stomach, and SP-4 Gongsun, Luo-Connecting Point of the Spleen Meridian, strengthen the middle-jiao.

Secondary points according to conditions:
1□ Irregular menstruation — SP-6 Sanyinjiao [/];
2□ Oppressive feelings in chest — PC-6 Neiguan [-];
3□ Epigastric distention and belching—RN-12 Zhongwan [-];
4□ Constipation or loose stools — ST-25 Tianshu [-].

2. Transformation of Depressed Qi into Fire

Manifestations: Irritability, headache, dryness and bitter taste in the mouth, distress in the chest, hypochondriac distention or pain, constipation, tinnitus, red eyes.

Tongue: Red tongue with yellow coating.

Pulse: Wiry and rapid.

Treatment Principle: Soothe liver, reduce fire and regulate stomach

Point Prescription & Manipulation:
Primary points:
   LR-2 Xingjian -
   GB-43 Xiaxi -
   GB-34 Yanglingquan -
   SJ-6 Zhigou -
   RN-13 Shangwan -

Explanation:
- LR-2 Xingjian and GB-43 Xiaxi, the Ying-Spring Points of the Liver and Gallbladder Meridians, clear fire from the liver and gallbladder;
- GB-34 Yanglingquan and SJ-6 Zhigou relieve distress of the chest, hypochondriac distention, biter taste in the mouth and constipation;
- RN-13 Shangwan harmonizes the stomach and regulates flow of qi.

Secondary points according to conditions:
1□ Irregular menstruation — SP-6 Sanyinjiao [/];
2□ Oppression in chest—PC-6 Neiguan [-];
3□ Headache and tinnitus — GB-20 Fengchi [-].

3. Stagnation of Phlegm and Qi

Manifestations: Mental depression, distress in the chest, heaviness of the body, desire for sleep often, fatigue, poor appetite, loose stools, weight increase.

Tongue: Enlarged tongue body with sticky coating.

Pulse: Wiry or slippery.

Treatment Principle: Soothe liver, regulate middle-jiao and transform phlegm.

Point Prescription & Manipulation:
Primary points:
    LR-3 Taichong -
    PC-6 Neiguan -
    RN-17 Danzhong -
    ST-40 Fenglong -
    RN-12 Zhongwan -

Explanation:
- LR-3 Taichong, PC-6 Neiguan and RN-17 Danzhong soothe liver, promote qi flow and relieve distress in chest and hypochondriac region;
- ST-40 Fenglong, one of the key points to transform phlegm, and RN-12 Zhongwan, the Back-Shu Point of stomach, regulate the middle-jiao and transform phlegm.

Secondary points according to conditions:
1□ Irregular menstruation — SP-6 Sanyinjiao [/];
2□ Poor appetite and increase of weight — ST-36 Zusanli [+] and ST-25 Tianshu [-].

4. Blood Deficiency

Manifestations: Mental depression, grief for no reason, capricious joy or anger, suspicious feelings, easy to get frightened, palpitation, insomnia, dizziness, vertigo, pale complexion, fatigue.

Tongue: Pale tongue with thin coating.

Pulse: Thready and weak.

Treatment Principle: Tonify blood, nourish heart and calm mind.

Point Prescription & Manipulation:
Primary points:
    RN-14 Juque +
    HT-7 Shenmen +
    SP-6 Sanyinjiao +
    LR-3 Taichong +

Explanation:
- LR-3 Taichong soothes the liver and removes depression;
- RN-14 Juque, the Front-Mu Point of heart, and HT-7 Shenmen, the Yuan-Source Point of the Heart Meridian, nourish heart and calm mind;
- SP-6 Sanyinjiao strengthens spleen to generate blood, and nourishes yin and calms mind.

Secondary points according to conditions:
1□ Dizziness, blurred vision and soreness of lumbar region and knees—BL-18 Ganshu [+] and BL-23 [+];
2□ Palpitation and insomnia—BL-15 Xinshu [+];
3□ Poor appetite and fatigue—ST-36 Zusanli [+] and SP-9 Yinlingquan [+].

Comment:
Zhenjiu is effective in treating depression. If some other relaxation techniques, such as massage, are combined with Zhenjiu, the treatment will provide better result. As drugs, caffeine, cigarettes and contraceptives induce depression, and analgesics or any toxic chemicals are also capable of producing symptoms of depression, it is better not to use them.

Notes:

104. AIDS & HIV

AIDS is a new disease, but it has spread very quickly and is widespread. it is now in all five continents with a very high death rate. AIDS has been called "super-cancer" and a "world wide epidemic disease". It damage greatly threatens the health of the human race.

AIDS is an acronym for Acquired Immune Deficiency Syndrome. This is a breakdown in human immunity caused by the human immunodeficiency virus (HIV) resulting in a clinical syndrome of numerous opportunistic infections and cancers. However, HIV is not AIDS, nor does every person with HIV develop AIDS. Each person's immune system will respond differently to the HIV, which may or may not result in a symptomatic disease—AIDS.

HIV is present in four types of body fluids: blood, semen, vaginal fluid and breast milk. HIV can only be transmitted to another person if these fluids get into his/her body. There are three main ways of transmitting HIV. The first is through unprotected anal or vaginal sex. The second method is through blood to blood contact, such as in the sharing of needles among intravenous drug users, and through blood transfusions and infected blood products. The third way is from mother to baby, any time during pregnancy, birth or breast-feeding.

Many research studies have shown that Zhenjiu is able to improve the immunity of the body and inhibit viruses. Based on these well established facts, the treatment and prevention of AIDS with Zhenjiu has drawn increasingly more attention from both Zhenjiu practitioners and AIDS patients or persons with HIV.

Based on AIDS' clinical manifestations, it has three stages — AIDS latent stage, i.e., asymptomatic virus-carrying stage, AIDS-related complex (ARC) stage and full blown AIDS stage.

I. AIDS LATENT STAGE

In the initial stage of AIDS infection, there is usually a transient period of weight loss, fatigue, night sweats, diarrhea, lymphadenopathy, and other infectious symptoms. They may be so mild that the patient does not pay any attention to them. Then the patient recovers and enters the asymptomatic virus-carrying period. In this period, the virus usually has a latency stage of up to 5 years or more without any signs of disease. However, such virus carriers have a high chance of developing clinical AIDS, and also may infect other people with HIV in this latent stage. This stage can only be diagnosed by blood tests for human immune deficiency virus antibodies. Zhenjiu treatment is given according to the blood test diagnosis and clinical manifestations, and in order to remove the virus, improve the body immune system, and prevent the progression to AIDS. Usually there are three types in this stage—deficiency of qi and blood, stagnation of liver qi and hiding of evil qi due to strong body resistance.

1. Deficiency of Qi & Essence

Manifestations: Weakness,   fatigue, susceptibility   to   diseases,   poor   memory, insomnia and pale complexion.

Tongue: Pale body with thin coating.

Pulse: Weak and Thready.

Treatment Principle: Tonify qi and essence, stabilize body surface and calm the spirit.

Point Prescription & Manipulation:
Primary points:
    ST-36 Zusanli + ^
    RN-4 Guanyuan + ^
    BL-23 Shenshu + ^
    DU-14 Dazhui + ^
    HT-7 Shenmen +

Explanation:
- ST-36 Zusanli reinforces the middle-jiao, supplements and boosts the postnatal root and hence strengthens body resistance to diseases;
- RN-4 Guanyuan and BL-23 Shenshu

reinforce kidney yin and yang, and supplement and boost prenatal essence and hence strengthen body resistance to diseases;

- DU-14 Dazhui, the Crossing Point of all seven yang meridians in the fourteen meridians, strengthens yang qi of the entire body and hence strengthens body resistance to diseases;
- HT-7 Shenmen nourishes the heart and calms the spirit.

Secondary points according to conditions:
1〕 Fever with chills—BL-13 Feishu [+] and LI-4 Hegu [-];
2〕 Mental depression—LR-3 Taichong [-] and PC-6 Neiguan [-];
3〕 Insomnia —EX-HN-16 Anmian [+].

2. Stagnation of Liver Qi

Manifestations: Mental depression, easily frightened and feelings of loneliness, chest oppression, sighing, hypochondriac distention and fullness.

Tongue: Purplish body with thin coating.

Pulse: Wiry.

Treatment Principle: Soothe liver, relieve depression, calm spirit and strengthen body constitute.

Point Prescription & Manipulation:
Primary points:
LR-3 Taichong -
PC-4 Neiguan -
ST-36 Zusanli + ^
RN-4 Guanyuan + ^
BL-23 Shenshu + ^
HT-7 Shenmen /

Explanation:
- LR-3 Taichong and PC-4 Neiguan soothe the liver, promote qi flow and relieve depression;
- ST-36 Zusanli reinforces the middle-jiao, supplements and boosts the postnatal root

and hence strengthens body resistance to diseases;

- RN-4 Guanyuan and BL-23 Shenshu reinforce kidney yin and yang, and supplement and boost prenatal essence and hence strengthen body resistance to diseases;
- HT-7 Shenmen tranquilizes the heart and calms the spirit.

Secondary points according to conditions:
1〕 Fever or fever with chills—LI-4 Hegu [-] and DU-14 Dazhui [-];
2〕 Insomnia—EX-HN-16 Anmian [+].

3. Hiding of Evil Qi due to Strong Body Resistance

Manifestations: No symptoms.

Tongue: Normal.

Pulse: Normal.

Treatment Principle: Strengthen body resistance and remove evils.

Point Prescription & Manipulation:
Primary points:
ST-36 Zusanli + ^
RN-4 Guanyuan + ^
DU-14 Dazhui + ^
LI-4 Hegu -
LI-11 Quchi -

Explanation:
- ST-36 Zusanli reinforces the middle-jiao, supplements and boosts the postnatal root and hence strengthens body resistance to diseases;
- RN-4 Guanyuan reinforces kidney yin and yang, and supplements and boost prenatal essence and hence strengthens body resistance to diseases;
- DU-14 Dazhui, the Crossing Point of all seven yang meridians in the fourteen meridians, strengthens yang qi of the entire body and hence strengthens body resistance and removes evils;

- LI-4 Hegu and LI-11 Quchi regulate qi of Yangming Meridian to remove evils.

Secondary points according to conditions:
1☐ Insomnia—EX-HN-16 Anmian [+].

II. THE STAGE OF AIDS-related COMPLEX (ARC)

In patients who progress from asymptomatic, latent viral infection to AIDS-related complex, there may be fever, sweating, aversion to cold, emaciation, poor appetite, prolonged diarrhea, lymphadenopathy and other similar symptoms. There may be seven types in this stage according to TCM differentiation — qi deficiency with fever due to attack by external pathogen, yin deficiency with fever due to attack by external pathogen, deficiency of lung qi, deficiency of spleen qi, liver depression with spleen deficiency, kidney yin deficiency and kidney yang deficiency.

1. Yin Deficiency with Fever due to Attack by External Pathogen

Manifestations: General weakness, hot sensation in palms, soles and heart, soreness of low back and knees, nocturnal emission, premature ejaculation, low fever, cough with little sputum, lymphadenopathy in the back of the neck, underarms, and groin.

Tongue: Red body with little coating.

Pulse: Floating, thread and rapid.

Treatment Principle: Nourish yin and transform phlegm, clear heat and relieve exterior.

Point Prescription & Manipulation:
Primary points:
   LU-7 Lieque -
   SI-7 Zhizheng -
   BL-13 Feishu +
   KI-7 Fuliu +
   SP-6 Sanyinjiao +
Explanation:

- LU-7 Lieque, Luo-Connecting Point of the Lung Meridian, and BL-13 Feishu, Back-Shu Point of the lung, dispel wind and relieve exterior, disperse the lung and transform phlegm;
- SI-7 Zhizheng, the Luo-Connecting Point of the Small Intestine Meridian, dispels superficial pathogen from the Taiyang Meridian, clears heat and relieves exterior;
- KI-7 Fuliu and SP-6 Sanyinjiao nourish yin and generate fluids.

Secondary points according to conditions:
1☐ High fever—LI-4 Hegu [-] and DU-17 Dazhui [-];
2☐ Insomnia—HT-7 Shenmen [+] and EX-HN-16 Anmian [+].

2. Qi Deficiency with Fever due to Attack by External Pathogen

Manifestations: General weakness, lassitude, listlessness, spontaneous sweating, shortness of breath on exertion, fever or slight aversion to wind, cough with scanty sputum, general aches and/or lymphadenopathy.

Tongue: Pale body with thin coating.

Pulse: Weak.

Treatment Principle: Reinforce qi and stabilize exterior, transform phlegm and clear heat.

Point Prescription & Manipulation:
Primary points:
   LU-7 Lieque -
   LI-4 Hegu -
   GB-20 Fengchi -
   LB-13 Feishu +
   LB-20 Pishu +
   ST-36 Zusanli + ^

Explanation:
- LU-7 Lieque, LI-4 Hegu and GB-20 Fengchi dispel wind, clear heat and relieve exterior;
- LB-13 Feishu and LB-20 Pishu, Back-Shu Points of the lung and spleen which

generate and control qi, reinforce qi and resolve phlegm;

- ST-36 Zusanli reinforces the source of generating qi and strengthens the body constitution.

Secondary points according to conditions:

1☐ High fever and constipation — ST-44 Neiting [-], SJ-6 Zhigou [-] and DU-17 Dazhui [-];

2☐ Insomnia—HT-7 Shenmen [+] and EX-HN-16 Anmian [+].

3. Deficiency of Lung Qi

Manifestations: General weakness, faint voice, fear of wind, spontaneous sweating, shortness of breath, liability to catch cold, pale complexion.

Tongue: Pale body with thin coating.

Pulse: Weak.

Point Prescription & Manipulation:
Primary points:
    BL-13 Feishu + ^
    BL-41 Gaohuang + ^
    ST-36 Zusanli + ^
    RN-4 Guanyuan + ^

Explanation:
- BL-13 Feishu and BL-41 Gaohuang reinforce lung qi;
- ST-36 Zusanli reinforces the middle-jiao to tonify qi;
- RN-4 Guanyuan reinforces primary qi to strengthen body constitution.

Secondary points according to conditions:
1☐ Loose stools and poor appetite—BL-20 Pishu [+ ^] and SP-9 Yinlingquan [+ ^];

2☐ Insomnia—HT-7 Shenmen [+] and EX-HN-16 Anmian [+].

4. Deficiency of Spleen Qi

Manifestations: General weakness, listlessness, fatigue, poor appetite, loose stools, sallow complexion, spontaneous sweating.

Tongue: Pale body with thin coating.

Pulse: Weak.

Treatment Principle: Strengthen the middle-jiao and tonify qi.

Point Prescription & Manipulation:
Primary points:
    ST-36 Zusanli + ^
    BL-20 Pishu + ^
    RN-4 Guanyuan + ^
    RN-12 Zhongwan + ^

Explanation:
- ST-36 Zusanli, one of the most important points of reinforcing the middle-jiao and strengthening body resistance, BL-20 Pishu, the Back-Shu Point of spleen, and RN-12 Zhongwan, the Front-Mu Point of stomach, strengthen the middle-jiao and reinforce qi;
- RN-4 Guanyuan reinforces primary qi and strengthens the bodily constitution.

Secondary points according to conditions:
1☐ Insomnia—HT-7 Shenmen [+] and EX-HN-16 Anmian [+];

2☐ Prolonged diarrhea and dizziness—DU-20 Baihui [+ ^];

3☐ Kidney yang deficiency manifested by prolonged diarrhea with shortness breath, soreness of low back and knees, edema or impotence—DU-20 Baihui [+ ^] and BL-23 Shenshu [+ ^];

4☐ Blood deficiency manifested by dizziness, blurred vision and palpitation — SP-6 Sanyinjiao [+], BL-17 Geshu [+] and SP-10 Xuehai [+];

5☐ Heart deficiency manifested by palpitation, insomnia, excessive dreams, anxiety and agitation — BL-15 Xinshu [+], HT-7 Shenmen [+] and PC-6 Neiguan [/];

6☐ Retention of dampness manifested by nausea, vomiting, abdominal distention and fullness, diarrhea and white and sticky tongue coating—SP-9 Yinlingquan [+] and ST-25 Tianshu [-].

5. Liver Depression with Spleen Deficiency

Manifestations: Emotional depression, frequent sighing, restlessness, hypochondriac distention and stuffiness, insomnia, general weakness, poor appetite, diarrhea, sallow complexion.

Tongue: Pale body with white coating.

Pulse: Wiry and thready.

Treatment Principle: Soothe liver, resolve depression and strengthen spleen.

Point Prescription & Manipulation:
Primary points:
    ST-36 Zusanli + ^
    BL-20 Pishu + ^
    LR-3 Taichong -
    PC-6 Neiguan -
    RN-17 Danzhong -

Explanation:
- ST-36 Zusanli and BL-20 Pishu strengthen spleen, harmonize stomach and regulate the middle-jiao;
- LR-3 Taichong and PC-6 Neiguan soothe liver and relieve depression;
- RN-17 Danzhong, the Influential Point of qi, promotes qi flow and regulates qi.

Secondary points according to conditions:
1□ Insomnia and restlessness—HT-7 Shenmen [+] and EX-HN-16 Anmian [+].

6. Kidney Yin Deficiency

Manifestations: Exhausted spirit, weakness, fatigue, tinnitus, insomnia, night sweating, dry mouth and throat, low back and knee soreness, nocturnal emission, and mental depression.

Tongue: Thin and red body with little coating.

Pulse: Thready and rapid.

Treatment Principle: Reinforce kidney and nourish yin.

Point Prescription & Manipulation:
Primary points:

    BL-23 Shenshu +
    SP-6 Sanyinjiao +
    KI-3 Taixi +
    ST-36 Zusanli +
    HT-7 Shenmen +

Explanation:
- BL-23 Shenshu and KI-3 Taixi reinforce kidney;
- SP-6 Sanyinjiao nourishes yin;
- ST-36 Zusanli strengthens the middle-jiao and supplements the postnatal root;
- HT-7 Shenmen nourishes heart and calm spirit.

Secondary points according to conditions:
1□ Severe insomnia—EX-HN-16 Anmian [+];
2□ Loose teeth, falling and dull-colored hair, tinnitus and blurred vision — RN-4 Guanyuan [+] and BL-18 Ganshu [+].

7. Kidney Yang Deficiency

Manifestations: General weakness, aversion to cold, cold limbs, clear and copious urine, impotence, diarrhea in the early morning, soreness of low back and knees, pale complexion.

Tongue: Pale or enlarged body with white coating.

Pulse: Weak, deep and slow.

Treatment Principle: Strengthen kidney and warm yang.

Point Prescription & Manipulation:
Primary points:
    BL-23 Shenshu + ^
    RN-4 Guanyuan + ^
    DU-4 Mingmen + ^
    ST-36 Zusanli + ^
    ST-25 Tianshu + ^

Explanation:
- BL-23 Shenshu, RN-4 Guanyuan and DU-4 Mingmen strengthen kidney and warm primary yang;

- ST-36 Zusanli strengthens the middle-jiao and supplements the postnatal root to reinforce the prenatal root;
- ST-25 Tianshu regulates stomach and arrests diarrhea.

Secondary points according to conditions:
1 Insomnia—HT-7 Shenmen [+] and EX-HN-16 Anmian [+];
2 Edema—SP-9 Yinlingquan [+ ^].

III. THE FULL BLOWN STAGE OF AIDS

The clinical manifestations of patients in the full-blown AIDS stage are extreme weakness, emaciation, various opportunistic infections and various kinds of malignant tumors. There may be four types in this stage liver stagnation with blood stasis, retention of turbid phlegm, internal stirring of liver-wind and deficiency of both yin and yang.

1. Liver Stagnation with Blood Stasis

Manifestations: Distention and pain in hypochondrium and chest, masses in the hypochondrium or abdomen with fixed pain, emotional depression, dark complexion, dark purplish lips and nails, fatigue.

Tongue: Dark-purplish body and/or with ecchymotic spots.

Pulse: Thready and unsmooth.

Treatment Principle: Soothe liver, activate blood and remove blood stasis.

Point Prescription & Manipulation:
Primary points:
> RN-17 Danzhong -
> LI-4 Hegu -
> PC-6 Neiguan -
> LR-13 Zhangmen -
> BL-17 Geshu -
> SP-10 Xuehai -

Explanation:
- RN-17 Danzhong, the Influential Point of qi

and located on the chest, soothes the chest and regulates qi;
- LI-4 Hegu and PC-6 Neiguan promote qi flow and soothe the chest and hypochondrium;
- LR-13 Zhangmen, the Influential Point of zang organs and the Front-Mu Point of spleen, soothes liver and regulates spleen;
- BL-17 Geshu and SP-10 Xuehai promote blood flow and remove blood stasis.

Secondary points according to conditions:
1 Insomnia—HT-7 Shenmen [+] and EX-HN-16 Anmian [+];
2 Poor appetite—ST-36 Zusanli [+] and RN-12 [+].

2. Retention of Turbid Phlegm

Manifestations: Cough with little or copious yellow and sticky phlegm, chest pain and distress, subcutaneous nodules of varying size, and poor appetite.

Tongue: Enlarged body with thick and sticky coating.

Pulse: Wiry or slippery.

Treatment Principle: Transform phlegm and scatter nodules.

Point Prescription & Manipulation:
Primary points:
> ST-36 Zusanli +
> ST-40 Fenglong -
> SP-9 Yinlingquan /
> HT-10 Tianjing -

Explanation:
- ST-36 Zusanli strengthens spleen, harmonizes stomach and transforms phlegm;
- ST-40 Fenglong, the key point of transforming phlegm;
- SP-9 Yinlingquan strengthens spleen, resolves dampness and transforms phlegm;
- HT-10 Tianjing, an empirically proven point for the treatment of scrofula, scatters

nodulation.

Secondary points according to conditions:
1️⃣ Insomnia—HT-7 Shenmen [+] and EX-HN-16 Anmian [+];
2️⃣ Damp-heat syndrome manifested by bitter taste in the mouth, dark urine, diarrhea with loose and foul-smelling stools, red tongue with stick coating, and slippery and rapid pulse—DU-14 Dazhui [-], LI-11 Quchi [-] and GB-34 Yanglingquan [-].

3. Internal Stirring of Liver-Wind

Manifestations: Emotional depression, dizziness and distention feeling in the head, sever vertigo, soreness and weakness of waist and knees, deviated mouth and eyes, unclear speech, spasms and convulsion.

Tongue: Red body with sticky coating.

Pulse: Wiry.

Treatment Principle: Subdue liver and extinguish wind.

Point Prescription & Manipulation:
Primary points:
ST-40 Fenglong -
LR-3 Taichong -
LI-4 Hegu -
DU-20 Baihui /
KI-7 Fuliu +

Explanation:
- ST-40 Fenglong, the key point of transforming phlegm;
- LR-3 Taichong and LI-4 Hegu, the Four Gate Points, move qi, clear heat, soothe liver and extinguish wind;
- DU-20 Baihui subdues adverse upward flow of yang and extinguishes wind;
- KI-7 Fuliu enriches kidney water to nourish liver wood, calming the wind.

Secondary points according to conditions:
1️⃣ Insomnia—HT-7 Shenmen [+] and EX-HN-16 Anmian [+];

2️⃣ Flushed face with red eyes, irritability and constipation—SJ-6 Zhigou [-] and LR-2 Xingjian [-].

4. Deficiency of Both Yin and Yang

Manifestations: Emaciation, withered spirit, heat trunk with cold limbs, palpitation, dizziness, tinnitus.

Tongue: Thin and red or enlarged and pale body, dry coating or no coating.

Pulse: Extremely thready.

Treatment Principle: Reinforce qi and generate blood, and strengthen yang and nourish yin.

Point Prescription & Manipulation:
Primary points:
ST-36 Zusanli + ^
RN-4 Guanyuan + ^
DU-4 Mingmen + ^
SP-6 Sanyinjiao +
BL-18 Ganshu +
BL-23 Shenshu +

Explanation:
- ST-36 Zusanli reinforces qi and nourishes blood;
- RN-4 Guanyuan strengthens primary qi to nourish yin and yang;
- DU-4 Mingmen warms the fire of the Gate of Life to prolong life;
- SP-6 Sanyinjiao nourishes yin;
- BL-18 Ganshu and BL-23 Shenshu tonify liver and kidney, and nourish essence and blood.

Secondary points according to conditions:
1️⃣ Insomnia — HT-7 Shenmen [+] and EX-HN-16 Anmian [+].

Comment:
It has been proved that Zhenjiu treatment can provide positive help to patients with AIDS in relieving their pain, mental depression and other symptoms, improving their immune system functions, prolonging their life, and to

asymptomatic HIV-carriers (those who have been infected by HIV but have no AIDS clinical manifestations,) in preventing it from developing into AIDS. Moreover, Zhenjiu treatment can provide better result if it is combined with proper Chinese herbal therapy.

Notes:

105. Emergency Conditions

I. FAINTING DUE TO PUNCTURING

See "4.Needling Fainting" in "PRECAUTIONS & MANAGEMENT OF POSSIBLE ACCIDENTS IN ZHENJIU TREATMENT" (Page 237).

II. COMA

Coma refers to a state of unconsciousness caused by some severe diseases or conditions, such as severe infectious disease, cerebral diseases, metabolism diseases, toxin due to medicine or chemical products, and prolonged shock, which greatly interfere with the functions of the brain. In TCM, it is usually divided into two types — Bi Zheng (blockage syndrome) and Tuo Zheng (collapse syndrome).

1. Blockage Syndrome

Manifestations: Fits when the patient is prostrated, loss of consciousness, locked jaw, clenched fists, no incontinence, stiffness and spasms of the limbs.

Tongue: Sticky coating.

Pulse: Wiry and smooth.

Treatment Principle: Open the obstruction and restore consciousness.

Points Prescription & Manipulation:
Primary points:
  DU-26 Shuigou -
  DU-20 Baihui -
  KI-1 Yongquan -
  Twelve Jing-Well Points on both hands -

Explanation:
Perform continued manipulation with strong stimulation until the patient recovers his/her consciousness. Prick the Jing-Well Points to bleed.

- DU-26 Shuigou and DU-20 Baihui open the orifice of the mind and effect resuscitation;
- KI-1 Yongquan aids DU-26 Shuigou and DU-20 Baihui in inducing resuscitation;
- Twelve Jing-Well Points regain consciousness.

Secondary points according to conditions:
1️⃣ Clenched jaws — ST-6 Jiache [-] and LI-4 Hegu [-].

2. Collapse Syndrome

Manifestations: Fall in a fit, loss of consciousness, closed eyes, open mouth, feeble breathing, relaxed hands, cold limbs, profuse and incessant sweating, incontinence, flaccid limbs.

Tongue: Hypokinesia.

Pulse: Feeble, thready and fainting.

Treatment Principle: Restore yang, promote resistance.

Points Prescription & Manipulation:
Primary points:
    RN-8 Shenque ^
    RN-6 Qihai ^
    RN-4 Guanyuan ^

Explanation:
Apply heavy moxibustion until the patient recovers his/her consciousness.

- These three points are located on the lower abdomen along the Ren Meridian and are the main points effective for collapse.

Secondary points according to conditions:
1️⃣ Incontinence of urine — DU-20 Baihui [+ ^], RN-3 Zhongji [+ ^] and SP-6 Sanyinjiao [+ ^].

Comment:
Coma is an emergency condition, and the patient's life is usually dependent on whether the first aid is given in time or not. Usually, the

earlier a correct first aid measure to induce resuscitation is given, the bigger and more the opportunity of rescuing the patient's life is. Zhenjiu treatment has been proved to be effective to induce the resuscitation to many patients with coma. Therefore, when a patient has sudden coma in clinic, the practitioner can immediately apply the Zhenjiu methods mentioned above to save the patient's life. However, coma is a very serious condition and other emergency measures should be combined if they are available.

III. SHOCK

Shock is a state in which blood flows to and perfuses peripheral tissues, and inadequate to sustain life because of insufficient cardiac output or maldistribution of peripheral blood flow, usually associated with hypotension and oliguria. It is usually caused by severe dehydration, blood loss, megalgia, toxin and allergic reaction.

Manifestations: Dizziness, fatigue, lethargy, confusion, somnolence, or restlessness, pale complexion, profuse sweating, cold limbs, cyanoses, shallow and quick breathing, falling of blood pressure, or even unconsciousness which may lead to coma.

Treatment Principle: Restore devastated yang.

Points Prescription:
    DU-25 Suliao
    PC-6 Neiguan
    KI-1 Yongquan

Manipulation: Puncture DU-25 Suliao obliquely upwards 0.5 cun, and puncture the other points perpendicularly 1 cun. Constantly manipulate the needles until the systolic blood pressure is elevated to over 90 mm Hg.

Comment:
The patient should be kept warm, with legs raised slightly to improve venous return. The patient's head should be turned to avoid aspiration if emesis occurs.

Not treated in time, shock is usually fatal, because when shock persists, impaired organ function is followed by irreversible cell damage and death. The patient's life is usually dependent on whether the fist aid is given in time or not. Usually, the earlier a correct first aid measure is given, the bigger and more the opportunity of rescuing the patient's life is. Zhenjiu treatment has been proved to be effective to rescue many patients from shock. Therefore, when a patient has sudden shock in clinic, the practitioner can immediately apply the Zhenjiu methods mentioned above to save the patient's life. However, shock is a very serious condition and other emergency measures should be combined if they are available.

IV. SYNCOPE

Syncope is marked by a sudden, brief loss of consciousness due to decreased cerebral blood flow (with resultant cerebral hyperemia). It is usually induced by fright, fatigue, weakness, hunger, emotional stimulation, sudden standing up, etc. The patient can gradually recover consciousness soon after the outbreak, without the sequel of hemiplegia, dysphasia and deviation of the mouth and eyes. However, sever cases may lead to coma and death.

Manifestations: Falling down in a fit, loss of consciousness, pale complexion, cold limbs and sweating.

Pulse: Slow and weak or fast and weak.

Treatment Principle: Open the orifices and restore consciousness.

Immediate Treatment Methods:
a. Arrange the patient in a horizontal posture with the legs elevated. Most patients will be regained from the syncope episode by this posture. If not,

b. Press and pinch PC-9 Zhongchong forcefully to induce strong stimulation. Usually the patients will quickly recover their consciousness by this method. If not,

c. Puncture PC-6 Neiguan, DU-26 Shuigou and SP-6 Sanyinjiao, and lift, thrust and rotate the needles with strong force until the patient recover their consciousness.

Comment:
The immediate treatment methods mentioned above are very effective to syncope. As syncope may lead to coma and death if it is severe and lasts for a long period, the treatment methods should be given as earlier as possible, and other emergent measures should be combined if they are available.

V. SEVERE ATTACK OF EPILEPSY WITH UNCONSCIOUSNESS

See "1. Liver-Wind with Accumulation of Phlegm" and "2. Blockage of Orifice by Phlegm-Fire" of "I. STANDARD TREATMENT" in "29. Epilepsy"(Page 367)

VI. SEVERE SUNSTOKE WITH UNCONSCIOUSNESS

See "2. Collapse of Qi and Yin" of "I. STANDARD TREATMENT" in "38. Sunstroke"(Page 393).

Notes:

INDEXES

INDEX 1: ACUPOINTS IN CHINESE PINYIN

1. THE REGULAR POINTS

2. THE EXTRA POINTS

3. THE EAR POINTS

INDEX 2: SYMPTOMS AND DISEASES KNOWN TO WESTERN MEDICAL SCIENCE

INDEX 3: DISEASES KNOWN TO TCM IN CHINESE PINYIN AND CHARACTERS

图书在版编目（CIP）数据

现代高级中国针灸治疗学：中高级学习实用手册：英文/尹钢林，刘正华编著. — 北京：新世界出版社，2000.1

ISBN 7-80005-558-2

I. 现… II. (1)尹… (2)刘… III. 针灸疗法-英文 IV. R245-0

中国版本图书馆CIP数据核字（1999）第68509号

现代高级中国针灸治疗学
—中高级学习实用手册
　　　　　（英文版）

主　　编：尹钢林，刘正华
责任编辑：李淑娟
封面设计：唐少文
责任印刷：黄厚清
出　　版：新世界出版社
社　　址：北京百万庄大街24号
邮政编码：100037
电　　话：68326644-2569
传　　真：68326679
电子邮件：nwpcn@public.bta.net.cn
印　　刷：北京外文印刷厂
发　　行：中国国际图书贸易总公司
地　　址：北京车公庄西路35号，北京邮政信箱第399号
邮政编码：100044
开　　本：787×1092（毫米）1/16
印　　张：39
插　　图：83
版　　次：2000年1月第一版　2000年第一次印刷
书　　号：ISBN 7-80005-558-2/R·046
定　　价：09600
14E-3354S